Integrative Nursing

Integrative Medicine Library

Published and Forthcoming Volumes

SERIES EDITOR

Andrew Weil, MD

Integrative Nursing

EDITED BY

Mary Jo Kreitzer, PhD, RN, FAAN
Director, Center for Spirituality and Healing
Professor, School of Nursing
University of Minnesota
Minneapolis, Minnesota

Mary Koithan, RN-C, PhD, CNS-BC
Associate Professor, College of Nursing
Associate Dean, Professional and Community Engagement
University of Arizona
Tucson, Arizona

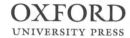

OXFORD
UNIVERSITY PRESS

OXFORD
UNIVERSITY PRESS

Oxford University Press is a department of the University of Oxford.
It furthers the University's objective of excellence in research, scholarship,
and education by publishing worldwide.

Oxford   New York
Auckland   Cape Town   Dar es Salaam   Hong Kong   Karachi
Kuala Lumpur   Madrid   Melbourne   Mexico City   Nairobi
New Delhi   Shanghai   Taipei   Toronto

With offices in
Argentina   Austria   Brazil   Chile   Czech Republic   France   Greece
Guatemala   Hungary   Italy   Japan   Poland   Portugal   Singapore
South Korea   Switzerland   Thailand   Turkey   Ukraine   Vietnam

Oxford is a registered trademark of Oxford University Press
in the UK and certain other countries.

Published in the United States of America by
Oxford University Press
198 Madison Avenue, New York, NY 10016

Library of Congress Cataloging-in-Publication Data
Integrative nursing / edited by Mary Jo Kreitzer, Mary Koithan.
p. ; cm. — (Integrative medicine library)
Includes bibliographical references and index.
ISBN 978-0-19-986073-9 (alk. paper)
I. Kreitzer, Mary Jo, editor of compilation.   II. Koithan, Mary, editor of compilation.
III. Series: Weil integrative medicine library.
[DNLM: 1. Nursing Care.   2. Integrative Medicine—methods.   3. Nursing Process. WY 100]
RT51
610.73—dc23
2013019034

This material is not intended to be, and should not be considered, a substitute for medical or other
professional advice. Treatment for the conditions described in this material is highly dependent on
the individual circumstances. And, while this material is designed to offer accurate information with
respect to the subject matter covered and to be current as of the time it was written, research and
knowledge about medical and health issues is constantly evolving and dose schedules for medications
are being revised continually, with new side effects recognized and accounted for regularly. Readers
must therefore always check the product information and clinical procedures with the most up-to-date
published product information and data sheets provided by the manufacturers and the most recent
codes of conduct and safety regulation. The publisher and the authors make no representations or
warranties to readers, express or implied, as to the accuracy or completeness of this material. Without
limiting the foregoing, the publisher and the authors make no representations or warranties as to the
accuracy or efficacy of the drug dosages mentioned in the material. The authors and the publisher do
not accept, and expressly disclaim, any responsibility for any liability, loss or risk that may be claimed
or incurred as a consequence of the use and/or application of any of the contents of this material.

3 5 7 9 8 6 4

Printed in the United States of America
on acid-free paper

This book is dedicated to Dr. Earl E. Bakken whose inventions, creativity and dreams have made the world a better place. As a mentor and friend, he has inspired me to dream impossible dreams and to advance spirituality and healing around the globe. —MJK

FOREWORD BY SERIES EDITOR
ANDREW WEIL

The term "integrative nursing" is almost redundant. Nurses have long embraced the principles of integrative medicine; often, they have been way ahead of physicians. Because they work more closely with patients, nurses are much more likely to be aware of mind/body interactions; to note correlations of emotional ups and downs with fluctuations in the course of disease. They tend to be more open to natural therapies. They have embraced therapeutic touch and other complementary therapies that physicians rarely consider. They understand the importance of the relationship between practitioner and patient and of "healing presence." They are more comfortable than most physicians with including the spiritual dimension of human life in their professional work.

Unfortunately, nurses have also long been disempowered in modern medical settings, given "orders" by mostly male physicians, and unable to openly advocate for more integrative care of patients. Some colleges of nursing have been reluctant to join integrative medicine initiatives, fearing loss of their own professional identity. As founder and director of the University of Arizona Center for Integrative Medicine, I have always believed that we should first integrate our own health care facilities—creating new collaborative models among doctors, nurses, and pharmacists—before we try to bring in practitioners of Chinese medicine, Ayurveda, and other alternative systems and treatments. That remains an unrealized goal, although I am pleased that a number of nurse practitioners have graduated from our fellowship training.

Publication of this key volume in the Oxford University Press Integrative Medicine Library series represents significant progress. My long-time friend and colleague, Dr. Mary Jo Kreitzer, was an obvious choice as senior editor. She was a founder of the Consortium of Academic Health Centers for Integrative Medicine, and as founder and director of the University of Minnesota's Center for Spirituality and Healing, her career has bridged the medical and nursing professions, infusing both with a robust integrative perspective. Together with Dr. Mary Koithan of the University of Arizona College of Nursing she has assembled a distinguished roster of contributors to this groundbreaking effort to define the principles and practices of integrative nursing.

Health care in the United States is in great disarray. Americans pay more per capita on health than any other people in the world; health care expenditures are creeping toward 20% of our gross domestic product (GDP), which is simply not sustainable. Most of this enterprise is concerned with the management of existing disease, most of it lifestyle related and therefore preventable. Health care of the future must focus on health promotion and disease prevention, and we must break our dependence on costly, high-tech methods of managing the chronic diseases that now absorb so many of our dollars. In other words, health care of the future must be integrative.

Nurses have a critical role to play in transforming health care in this country and others. In order to do that most effectively, their education must stress the principles so clearly stated in this volume. But nursing practice need not wait to make use of the practical advice in these pages to improve patient care and outcomes. Integrative nursing is already a reality here and abroad. It has a solid theoretical base and the wisdom of collective experience. And it has a great deal to offer.

Tucson, Arizona
May, 2013

PREFACE

The expanding role of nursing is an essential element of our changing healthcare system. Embraced for their wisdom and ability to provide outstanding compassionate and patient-centered care, nurses are now optimally positioned to influence and help lead our national and global healthcare systems into the future.

This book offers a practical, point-of-care guide for students, practitioners, and leaders of caregiving in the twenty-first century. Evidence-based integrative nursing interventions and assessment tools are provided for a wide range of conditions. Furthermore, the authors and editors of this book have brought together a national and international panel of nursing leaders to offer readers forward-looking approaches, strategies, and solutions to many of our healthcare system's manifest inadequacies.

As patients, providers, and policy-makers, we are fortunate to live in an exciting and transitional time in healthcare. Integration (stemming from the Latin verb *integrare*, "to complete, make whole") is bringing previously disconnected components together as the desired modus operandum for health delivery. Our approach to healthcare has swung, like a pendulum, back towards addressing, incentivizing, and restoring the humanity in care. It is with great hope that we see a renewed emphasis on reenergizing the core values within the healthcare profession, a renewed vigor that will nourish patient-oriented and holistically minded care into the future.

Along these lines, the Consortium of Academic Health Centers for Integrative Medicine (CAHCIM) advances the principles and practices of integrative healthcare within U.S. academic institutions. They define integrative medicine as "the practice of medicine that reaffirms the importance of the relationship between practitioner and patient, focuses on the whole person, is informed by evidence, and makes use of all appropriate therapeutic approaches, healthcare professionals and disciplines to achieve optimal health and healing."

From the nursing profession's humble beginnings in the early 1900s, these hands-on providers have been guided by the foundational principle of putting the patient in the best possible condition for healing to occur. Although the practice of nursing has grown considerably, the root mission remains the same: to view the patient in his or her entirety, or whole context, providing vertically integrated care on the level of the individual, the family, the community, and the population. At the very cornerstone of this historically modest profession lies the emphasis upon healing—attending to patients with a gentle and genuine presence to evoke a sense of personal wholeness and wellbeing, while coordinating interdisciplinary provider teams and using the best of scientific knowledge to guide practice.

Essential to our quest for new answers in healthcare is the need to reexamine present approaches to disease and illness. Our traditional healing insight today is able to draw upon a globally connected, modern scientific research community, with a systems-based theoretical approach to assess and plan for our increasingly complex and evolving local and global healthcare needs. Current medical systems take us part of the way there. The challenge of the twenty-first century will be to provide personalized and patient-centered care that continually responds and adapts to the growing complexities we will face. As a team, we—the patients, providers, and policy-makers—are working towards solutions that align clinical models with highly diverse financial and institutional incentives.

This book brings together the insights and wisdom of nursing within the global framework of healthcare, spanning the levels of care from individuals to communities and populations. This is the first complete roadmap to integrative nursing, weaving together different authors' knowledge and perspectives to connect with the underlying concepts and skills of the integrative nursing provider. It provides a step-by-step guide to assess and clinically treat conditions and view-optimizing health through a variety of combined methodologies including wellness, lifestyle enhancement, and nutrition. This text puts forth both the skills and theoretical frameworks for multidisciplinary leaders to consider and implement integrative healthcare strategies within institutions, including several case studies involving practical nursing-led initiatives.

Furthermore, this guide significantly builds on the successful and productive years of professional nursing development. Distinguished nursing leaders provide critical commentary on the profession's commitment to training future healthcare pioneers and advancing nursing science. Reflecting upon the years of professional development, it is clear that, as a field, nursing has demonstrated the immense motivation, strength, adaptability, and expertise necessary to lead healthcare change.

As distinguished visionaries in healthcare with accomplished careers in education and research, the authors and editors of this text, Dr. Mary Jo Kreitzer and Dr. Mary Koithan, have dedicated their careers to nursing excellence with passion and innovation.

Dr. Kreitzer is the founder and director of the Center for Spirituality and Healing, and co-director of the Doctorate in Nursing Practice (DNP) program in Integrative Health and Healing, at the University of Minnesota. Her advocacy for the nursing profession and for integrative healthcare in research and policy, fortified by her international profile and visibility, has distinguished the University of Minnesota as a preeminent leader in nursing science and education.

Dr. Koithan is an associate professor and an associate dean for professional and community engagement in the College of Nursing at the University of Arizona. With expertise in research methodologies, theory development, and health response testing, she is known for her accomplishments as a distinguished leader within whole-systems approaches to healing.

Both Dr. Kreitzer and Dr. Koithan exemplify the highest principles and values of nursing and medicine. With grace and eloquence, they have bridged tensions between inspiring ideas and provided valuable insights into what the future may hold.

Nursing history has demonstrated a strong ability to adapt to changing healthcare needs. With more than 3 million nurses in the United States and nearly 20 million nurses worldwide, this group of providers represent healthcare's largest workforce. Nationally and globally, nurses have evolved into a vast multitude of roles in almost every setting conceivable—from direct care, to educating future providers, to participating in health policy and delivery decisions.

From its inception in the Crimean War, the nursing profession has been known for bringing compassionate care to their patients. In recent years, advances in basic nursing science and theory have increased the technical sophistication of nursing in ways that enrich and do not detract from or dilute the core of compassionate care. Curriculum development within our higher education nursing institutions at the undergraduate, graduate, and post-graduate levels are strongly evidence-based. More than 250,000 nurses in the United States are considered "advanced practice nurses," with master's or doctoral-level training. There is increasing evidence to support the multiplication of nurse practitioners as a cost-saving strategy, providing "safe, high-quality primary care" to many millions of Americans who would not otherwise have access. A recent report issued by the National Academy of Sciences' Institute of Medicine and the Robert Wood Johnson Foundation has seen the leading changes within nursing as part of the solution to our primary-care shortage, calling for the creation of residency training programs and recommending that the number of nurses who pursue doctorates be doubled by the year 2020. The nursing profession continues to position itself as the profession that is ready to provide and lead the provision of high-quality, affordable, and accessible care within our national and global healthcare systems.

For those of us who assist from the outer boundaries of nursing, the most exciting aspect of this compendium lies in its demonstration of the progress that nursing has made. The growth of this field has stemmed directly from the foresight of these and other nursing leaders. Someday, we will look back upon this period of nursing's history as a pivotal time, leading to a future of unparalleled progress.

Michele Mittelman RN, MPH
Nursing Advocate
Co-Founder and Editor, *Global Advances in Health and Medicine*

Supplementary references for this title are available online. These can be found by going to http://oxfordmedicine.com/page/288. This title will also be published at oxfordmedicine.com by March 2014, at which time the supplementary references will be available as part of that publication.

ACKNOWLEDGMENTS

I am deeply grateful to my colleagues at the University of Minnesota Center for Spirituality and Healing and the School of Nursing, who have supported my work for decades. In writing this book, I want to highlight the contributions of Layla Nereson, who masterfully coordinated many logistical details, and Andrea Uptmor, who provided invaluable editing assistance. I also want to thank my husband, Joe, who has quietly and patiently supported by career as we strived to balance very full careers and parenthood. For me, family has always riveted me to reality and what is most important in life. I am grateful to my children: David and his wife, Stacey; Kathryn; Rebecca; and Thomas and wife Sara for their support and am proud of them all as they head off in brilliant careers and pursuits of their own. And finally, I am blessed and grateful to have the joy of two grandchildren—Keigan, and the newest addition to our family, Poppy Lou.

—Mary Jo Kreitzer

My heartfelt thanks to my patients, who have quietly taught me and guided my steps; my colleagues and students, who have supported and encouraged me to find my voice; and my family and lifelong friends, who have loved me and taught me to live fully.

—Mary Koithan

CONTENTS

III   Symptom Management and Integrative Nursing

IV   Integrative Nursing Applications

V   Integrative Nursing: Models of Education

VI   Integrative Nursing: Global Perspectives—State of the Practice

VII   Conclusion

CONTRIBUTORS

Ranier Ammende, B.A. (Hons), Diplom-Pflegepädagoge
Academy Munich Municipal Hospital
Munich, Germany

Jane Anderson, DNP, ANP-C, FNP-C, RN
Assistant Clinical Professor, School of Nursing
Assistant Professor, Center for Spirituality and Healing
University of Minnesota
Minneapolis, Minnesota

Judith Aufenthie, RN, PhD, HNB-BC
Integrative Health Specialist, Center for Health and Healing
Mayo Clinic Health System—Franciscan Healthcare
La Crosse, Wisconsin

Deva-Marie Beck, PhD, RN
International Co-Director
Nightingale Initiative for Global Health (NIGH)
Neepawa, Canada

Iris R. Bell, MD, PhD, MD(H)
Professor Emeritus, Family and Community Medicine
Research Professor, College of Nursing
University of Arizona
Tucson, Arizona

Melinda Bors, RN, BSN, MA
University of Minnesota Physicians
Minneapolis, Minnesota

Angela Bradshaw, MA, BA, RN, RM, NDN (Cert)
Associate, Choice Dynamic International
Pontefract, West Yorkshire
England

Kathy Chappell, MSN, RN
Director, Accreditation Program
American Nurses Credentialing Center
Silver Spring, Maryland

Linda L. Chlan, PhD, RN, FAAN
Distinguished Professor of Symptom Management Research, College of Nursing
The Ohio State University
Columbus, Ohio

Corjena Cheung, PhD, RN
Assistant Professor, School of Nursing
University of Minnesota
Minneapolis, Minnesota

Lynette Crane, MA
Certified Life Coach
Creative Life Changes
Minneapolis, Minnesota

Norma G. Cuellar, PhD, RN, FAAN
Professor, Capstone College of Nursing
University of Alabama
Tuscaloosa, Alabama

**Susanne M. Cutshall, DNP, RN,
ACNS-BC, AHN-BC, WHE, HWNC-BC**
Integrative Health Specialist
Assistant Professor of Nursing
College of Medicine
Mayo Clinic
Rochester, Minnesota

Patrick J. Dean, EDD, RN, OSTJ
Clinical Assistant Professor, School of Nursing
University of Minnesota
Rochester, Minnesota

Louise Delagran, MA, MEd
Education Specialist, Center for
Spirituality and Healing
University of Minnesota
Minneapolis, Minnesota

**Connie W. Delaney, PhD, RN,
FAAN, FACMI**
School of Nursing Professor & Dean
Academic Health Center
Director, Biomedical Health
Informatics (BMHI)
Associate Dir. CTSI-BMI
Acting Dir. of the Institute for Health
Informatics (IHI)
University of Minnesota
Minneapolis, Minnesota

**Barbara M. Dossey, PhD, RN, AHN-BC,
FAAN, HWNC-BC**
Co-Director, International Nurse Coach
Association
International Co-Director, Nightingale
Initiative for Global Health
Santa Fe, New Mexico

Diana Drake, DNP RN WHNP
Clinical Assistant Professor
School of Nursing
University of Minnesota
Director of Faculty Practice and
Program Director
Womens Integrative Health, Women's
Health Specialists Clinic, UMMC
Minneapolis, Minnesota

Torkel Falkenberg, PhD, BSc
Associate Professor, Karolinska Institutet
Solna, Sweden

Mary Farrell, MS, PCC
Exercise Physiologist, Certified Health
and Wellness Coach
Penny George Institute for Health and
Healing
Allina Health Systems
Minneapolis, Minnesota

Jayne Felgen, MPA, RN
PresidentCreative Health Care
Management
Minneapolis, Minnesota

**Mary V. Fenton, RN, DrPH,
AHN-BC, FAAN**
Professor, School of Nursing
Texas Tech University Health
Science Center
Lubbock, Texas

Judith Fouladbakhsh, PhD, APRN, BC, AHN-BC, CHTP
Associate Professor, College of Nursing
Wayne State University
Detroit, Michigan

Sebahat Gözüm, PhD, RN
Professor, Faculty of Nursing
Akdeniz University
Antalya, Turkey

Thora Jenny Gunnarsdottir, PhD, RN
Assistant Professor of Nursing, School of Health Sciences
University of Iceland
Reykjavik, Iceland

Linda L. Halcón, PhD, MPH, RN
Associate Professor, School of Nursing
University of Minnesota
Minneapolis, Minnesota

Arlene Horner, DNP, RN, GCNS-BC
Gerontological Clinical Nurse Specialist
Sanford Medical Center
Sioux Falls, South Dakota

Mats Jong, PhD, RN
Senior Lecturer in Nursing Science
Department of Nursing
Mid Sweden University
Sundsvall, Sweden

Miek C. Jong, PhD
Associate Professor in Health Science
Department of Nursing
Mid Sweden University
Sundsvall, Sweden

Merrie J. Kaas, DNSc, RN, PMHCNS
Associate Professor, School of Nursing
University of Minnesota
Minneapolis, Minnesota

Julie Katseres, DNP, RN, CPNP, FNP-BC, CCAP
Nurse Practitioner, Hospice and Palliative Care
Minneapolis VA Health Care System
Minneapolis, Minnesot

Jayson King, BS, RN, HNB-BC
Integrative Health Inpatient Manager
Art of Healing Program Manager
Penny George Institute for Health and Healing
Allina Health System
Minneapolis, Minnesota

Lori Knutson, RN, BSN, HN-BC
Director, Health and Wellness Services
Touchstone Mental Health
Minneapolis, Minnesota

Matthew Koithan, BS, LMT, NCTM, CHFS, CKPT
Physical Therapy Technician
ProActive Physical Therapy
Massage Therapist
Tucson, Arizona

Gisli Kristofersson, PhD, MS, RN, CNS
Clinical Assistant Professor, School of Nursing
University of Minnesota
Minneapolis, Minnesota

Laurie Kubes, DNP, RN, GNP-BC
Nurse Practitioner, Diabetes Care
Minneapolis VA Health Care System
Minneapolis, Minnesota

Cheryl J. Leuning, MS, PhD
Professor and Chair, Department of Nursing
Augsburg College
Minneapolis, Minnesota

Valerie Lincoln, PhD, RN, AHN-BC
Director, Integrative Services
Acute Care Hospitals of the Health
East System Woodwinds Health Campus
Woodbury, Minnesota

Ruth Lindquist, PhD, RN, FAAN
Professor, School of Nursing
University of Minnesota
Minneapolis, Minnesota

Susan Luck, MA, RN, HNB-BC, CCN,
HWNC-BC
Director, Earthrose Institute
Co-Director, International Nurse Coach
Association
Adjunct Faculty, University of Miami
Miami, Florida

Susan Masemer, MS
Exercise Physiologist and Manager,
Penny George Institute for Health and
Healing LiveWell Fitness Center
Allina Health System
Minneapolis, Minnesota

Martin McNamara, EdD, MA, MEd,
MSc, BSc, RNT, RGN, RPN
Dean of Nursing and Head
UCD School of Nursing, Midwifery and
Health Systems
UCD Dublin
Dublin, Ireland

Karen A. Monsen, PhD, RN, FAAN
Assistant Professor, School of Nursing
University of Minnesota
Minneapolis, Minnesota

Marie Napolitano, PhD, ARNP,
FNP-C, FAANP
Director—Doctor of Nursing Practice
Program
School of Nursing, University of
Portland
Portland, Oregon

Kathleen A. Nelson, RN, CNS, ACHPN
Hospice and Palliative Care Consult
Service
Minneapolis VA Health Care System
Minneapolis, Minnesota

Barbara Peterson, PhD, RN,
PMHCNS-BC
Clinical Assistant Professor, School of
Nursing
University of Minnesota
Minneapolis, Minnesota

Nurgün Platin
Emeritus Professor in Nursing,
Ankara, Turkey

Teddie Potter, PhD, RN
Clinical Associate Professor, School of
Nursing
University of Minnesota
Minneapolis, Minnesota

Janet F. Quinn, PhD, RN, FAAN
Director, HaelanWorks
Lyons, Colorado

Debbie Ringdahl, DNP, RN, CNM
Clinical Assistant Professor, School of
Nursing
University of Minnesota
Minneapolis, Minnesota

Patricia A. Roach, MS, RN, NEA-BC
Senior Vice President and Chief Nursing
Officer
Faxton St. Luke's Healthcare
Ilion, New York

Rebecca L. Ross, PhD, PMHNP-BC, RN
Assistant Professor
University of Arizona College of Nursing
Tucson, AZ

Mary M. Rowan, PhD, RN, CNM
Clinical Professor, School of Nursing
Director of Pre-licensure Programs
University of Minnesota
Minneapolis, Minnesota

Cynda H. Rushton, PhD, RN, FAAN
Anne and George Bunting Professor of
Clinical Ethics
Professor of Nursing and Pediatrics
Johns Hopkins University
Baltimore, Maryland

**Laura Sandquist, DNP, ANP-C,
GNP-C, RN**
Nurse Practitioner, Functional Medicine
Newbridge Clinic
Minneapolis, Minnesota

Constance Schein, RN, MSc
National Director of Health Services
The Goodman Group
Chaska, Minnesota

Ellen L. Schellinger, MA
Administrative Director
DeGroot Center: Bioethics, Humanities
and the Healing Arts
Sanford Medical Center
Sioux Falls, South Dakota

**Michael Shannon, PhD, MBA, BSc,
RGN, RPN**
Director of Nursing and Midwifery,
Health Service Executive
Adjunct Associate Professor, UCD
School of Nursing, Midwifery and
Health Systems
UCD Dublin
Dublin, Ireland

**Susan Smith, DBA, MBA, BSc Hons,
RN, RM, RHV**
Owner and Chief Executive Officer
Choice Dynamic International
Pontefract, West Yorkshire
England

Beth Somerville, MHA, BS
Business Development, Center for
Spirituality and Healing
University of Minnesota
Minneapolis, Minnesota

**Janina Sweetenham, MA, DipN
(Lond), DipEd, DipNEd, FETC**
Partner, Sweetenham Bywater
Associates
Summercourt, Cornwall
England

Susan G. Szczesny, MS, RN, BC, NP
Clinical Instructor, College of Nursing
Wayne State University
Detroit, Michigan

Renate Tewes, PhD, RN, RNSc
Professor, Nursing Science
University of Applied Science
Director, CROWN Coaching
International
Dresden, Germany

Susan Thompson, DNP, MBA, RN
Integrative Nurse Consultant
Thompson Integrative Health, Inc.
Eden Prairie, Minnesota

Sue Towey, RN, CNS, MS, LP
Graduate Minor Faculty, Center for
Spirituality and Healing
University of Minnesota
Minneapolis, Minnesota

Andrea Uptmor, MA, MFA
Editor/Writer, Center for Spirituality and
Healing
University of Minnesota
Minneapolis, Minnesota

Lisa M. Van Getson, RN, DNP, FNP-BC,
APHN-BC, MAT, WHE
Directress of Hermitage Farm Center for
Healing Rochester, MN
Family Nurse Practitioner Cardiac
Surgery/Instructor Medical Ethics
College of Medicine
Mayo Clinic
Rochester, Minnesota
Interim Director of Transcultural,
Holistic and Integrative DNP Family
Nurse Practitioner Program
Augsburg College
Minneapolis, MN

Judy L. Wagner, DNP, RN,
NP-C, GNP-BC
Congestive Heart Failure Clinic
Minneapolis VA Healthcare System
Minneapolis, Minnesota

Jean Watson, PhD, RN, AHN-BC, FAAN
Founder/Director Watson Caring
Science Institute
Distinguished Professor Emerita–Dean
Emerita, College of Nursing
University of Colorado—Denver
Denver, Colorado

Elizabeth Fine Weinfurter, MLIS
Liaison and Instruction Librarian
University of Minnesota
Minneapolis, Minnesota

Bonnie L. Westra, PhD, RN,
FAAN, FACMI
Associate Professor, University of
Minnesota, School of Nursing & Institute
for Health Informatics
Director Center for Nursing Informatics

Dawn R. Witt, MPH
Health Promotion Specialist
Minneapolis Heart Institute Foundation
Minneapolis, Minnesota

Terri Zborowsky, PhD, EDAC
Adjunct Instructor
University of Minnesota
Minneapolis, Minnesota

INTRODUCTION

In many ways, the inspiration for this book came from nurses literally around the world who told us stories about their yearning to practice nursing in a different way. While the historical legacy of nursing is deeply rooted in a tradition of caring and healing, and it is that "essence" that attracts millions of men and women to enter this noble profession, the lived reality of many who receive nursing care and who practice nursing is quite different. Many nurses describe hierarchies and bureaucracies that have removed them from the point of care, be that the bedside in a hospital or the home, replacing them with less skilled workers and filling their time with documentation and other administrative tasks.

Patients tell this story from a different point of view. Many experience a long parade of "care providers" who are too busy to actually care, and spend much of their time managing a process, the outcome of which is often quite unsatisfactory from a patient, clinical, and fiscal perspective. This really hit home for me when a friend was hospitalized in a "good" hospital, and I had the opportunity to sit at her bedside for many hours over an extended period of time. One would expect to encounter nurses who vary in their skill, competence, and capacity for caring, and I saw that. I had the honor to witness exquisite nursing care. What astounded me, however, was the extent to which much of the focus of the nurses' attention had shifted from the patient to everything that surrounds the patient. Nurses would enter the room scarcely greeting or even having eye contact with the patient and family and move almost immediately to the machines. There were times that the nurses had more faith in the numbers coming from the monitors than from what the patient was saying or indicating that she needed. These were not bad nurses by any stretch; rather, it felt like they had lost focus on the intended recipient of their care.

A more recent experience hit even closer to home when a family member gave birth. It was a long labor followed by a difficult C-section. There was concern that the mother had an infection that could have been transmitted to the baby, so both were put on antibiotics. Inadequate local anesthesia resulted in general anesthesia, so the mother was not awake when the baby was born. When I arrived at the hospital about ten hours post-birth, I visited the mom first, who was moving around and doing quite well and had not yet seen her baby. Fearing that something might be seriously wrong, I went to the nursery. While on antibiotics, the baby was doing fine, albeit quite hungry. Told that the baby could not leave the nursery, I asked if the mother could come in. Of course, they said, any time! What no one seemed to have noticed was that this mother, ten hours after the birth, had not even seen her baby yet. Mother and baby individually seemed to be getting fine care, but no one had connected the dots to see the bigger picture. This occurred in an urban hospital in 2013.

"Integrative nursing" was born out of the desire to honor the legacy and contemporary practice of nurses who are committed to caring for people, families, and communities in a different way. In our research, we found countless examples of nurses who were creatively—and sometimes in the face of great obstacles—practicing integrative nursing, while not calling it by any name. They were providing whole person/whole system care that was relationship-based, person-centered, and that focused on improving health and wellbeing. Many used what are now often called *integrative therapies*, formerly called *complementary* or *alternative therapies*, but saw them as yet an additional intervention that could be offered to increase people's functional capacity and expand their potential. It was about the people, and not the therapies.

From the lived experience and practice of nurses, we identified what we believe are the core principles and concepts of integrative nursing. Our intention in writing the book was to bring those ideas to life in a way that could strengthen and invigorate the profession while demonstrating that integrative nursing is applicable in all settings. Our hope is to reach both practicing professionals as well as students who are enrolled in undergraduate or graduate nursing programs. We have strived to balance academic rigor with very practical and relevant content that can be readily implemented in practice.

We live in global society, so it matters a great deal how nursing is practiced in other parts of the world. We have much to learn from each other, and were very grateful to have colleagues from many European countries contribute to the first edition of *Integrative Nursing*. In future editions, we hope to add voices from other continents on the globe. I have been blessed to be part of an international learning community of nurses for close to a decade now and continue to be fascinated at how much I learn about nursing even in my own country through their eyes.

The vision and scope of this book required an extraordinary group of collaborators. I was both grateful and relieved when Dr. Mary Koithan agreed to serve as co-editor. Mary brought a wealth of nursing experience and above all, critical thinking. She did a wonderful job both challenging and supporting the team throughout the process. Together, we created a "wisdom circle," including Dr. Janet Quinn, Dr. Debbie Ringdahl, Dr. Linda Halcon, and Lori Knutson, that helped us set an intention and conceptualize the book, and from which we sought advice on numerous occasions.

We were fortunate to hold writing retreats at Charleson Meadows, a site that offered inspiration and nurturing.

Our hope was to lift up many voices within the nursing community, and we were delighted to have as contributors nurses who are very senior in the field as well as relatively new graduates, colleagues from academic and clinical institutions, and writers from across the United States and Europe. Rather than creating a unified voice, we aspired to create a chorus. We were enormously grateful that two of nursing's most prominent wisdom voices—Dr. Barbara Dossey and Dr. Jean Watson—readily agreed to lend their vision and perspective and support.

The world needs nursing. We hope that the book inspires you individually and collectively to advance health and wellbeing in the world through your nursing lens, practice, and leadership.

Mary Jo Kreitzer
Shoreview, Minnesota
March 26, 2013

Integrative Nursing

I
_____

Foundations of Integrative Nursing

1

Concepts and Principles of Integrative Nursing

MARY KOITHAN

From its very beginnings, nursing has been an integrative healing discipline. Florence Nightingale recognized the integral nature of the person–environment system, urging nurses to assist in the reparative processes of nature by "putting the patient in the best condition for nature to act upon him" (Nightingale, 1859/1946, p. 75). Throughout time, nursing theorists have embraced the complex, holistic nature of the human being, stating that the focus nursing is on the totality of the human response to potential or actual health problems (American Nurses Association (ANA), 2010). Daily, nurses across the globe engage in whole-person health promotion and healing, harnessing principles from the health sciences, basic sciences, environmental sciences, arts, and literature to help individuals, families, and communities find comfort and meaning in their lives and to alleviate physical, psychological, social, and spiritual suffering. Integration is the cornerstone of nursing as a discipline and a practice: it guides our thinking, our actions, and our relationships.

In English, the word *integrate* means to "put things together to form something new" (Merriam-Webster, 2012). Entities that are integrated are not characterized by their distinct pieces and parts; rather, they are viewed as new wholes that resemble "living organisms in organization and development" (Merriam-Webster). At each level of organization, integrated wholes uniquely come together as information is shared and relationships among parts are developed. Thus, a person is not a biological, psychological, social, and spiritual being, but a bio-psycho-social-spiritual being. Likewise, communities are not composed of individuals living and working in separate spaces, but are functional wholes with unique properties and characteristics. You cannot know a community by examining each of its members, just as you cannot understand an individual being by examining their mind or the body systems.

Etymologically, the word *integrate* is derived from the Latin *integrare*, which means "to form into one whole, to complete or to begin anew" (http://www.etymonline.com, last accessed 6/1/12). Of particular interest, we note the action inherent in the language of integration. Integrating wholes *work* at the process of integration, a process that involves sharing and exchanging information, creating new relationships based on this information, and formulating new structures. As such, integration is active, creative, ever-beginning, and ever-changing. We are not simply "whole"; we are continually becoming whole and beginning anew.

Integrative nurses form relationships with individuals, families, groups, and communities to promote health and healing and to improve wellbeing. Together, they assess the condition of the system to identify priorities, integrate possible therapies from different disciplines and traditions (e.g., the arts, spiritual traditions, pharmacology, biological and physiological sciences, architecture) to create and implement interventions. Integrative nurses structure unique treatment options, using evidence from a variety of knowledge sources.

Nurses also work to integrate diverse disciplines and perspectives within the healthcare system to create a coordinated healthcare experience for our patients. Nurses integrate the biomedical perspective of physicians, surgeons, and pharmacists with the social needs of individuals and families. Nurses utilize social services when they realize that a family cannot pay for the recommended treatments and medications. They seek out spiritual leaders or provide counseling when those treatments are not consistent with the health beliefs or culture of the person. In a caring relationship, nurses integrate the often-disparate recommendations of providers within our healthcare systems, creating a person-centered plan of care that honors, supports, and heals the whole unique being. Therefore, *integrative nursing is a way of being-knowing-doing that advances the health and wellbeing of persons, families, and communities through caring/healing relationships. Integrative nurses use evidence to inform traditional and emerging interventions that support whole person/whole systems healing.*

Integrative Nursing's Meta-theoretical Perspective

Integrative nursing is closely aligned with complex systems science (CSS), or a complexity meta-theoretical perspective. Nursing leaders, particularly those in administrative and educational leadership positions, have identified this perspective as a "thinking approach" that honors the old, provides for new ways of being-doing, and illuminates what nurses have known for years about the human health experience, our healthcare systems, and the best ways to care for people (Zimmerman, Lindberg, & Plesk, 2008, pp. iii–iv). Complexity encourages interprofessional practice, offers multiple voices and approaches, and encourages us to be innovative, contemplative, and interpretive.

Complex systems science explores "how the parts of a system give rise to the collective behaviors of the system and how the system interacts with its environment" (Bar-Yam, 2004; http://necsi.org/guide/study.html; last accessed Oct 31, 2011). Complex adaptive systems (CAS) are open systems that exchange information with the environments within which they exist. These systems are interdependent and self-organizing, with emergent properties that are different from and greater than those of the attendant parts (Kauffman, 1993). Moreover, a CAS exhibits nonlinear patterns of evolution and change. A small change in one aspect of the system delivered at the right moment may produce disproportionately large effects in both local and global arenas of experience (Bar-Yam, 1997; Guastello, Koopmans, & Pincus, 2009). Because change in a CAS involves complex information exchange, timing plays a very prominent role when conceptualizing when to deliver an intervention (or change stimulus) and predicting the manner and magnitude of system response (Bar-Yam, 2004; Erdi, 2008; Guastello, Koopmans & Pincus, 2009; Miller & Page, 2007).

Koithan et al. (2012) identified six basic tenets of CSS that are directly applicable to the discipline of nursing. They proposed that complex adaptive systems are: (1) *whole systems* that (2) *change over time*. They are characterized by (3) *emergence, connectivity,* and *mutual causation,* which creates a global or holistic "order" that is (4) *not predictable by the properties of the parts but is a function of the whole system.* Emergence is often nonlinear; therefore change can be exponential and potentially synergistic, driven by (5) *self-organization.* Change feeds back into the system across all levels of organization, allowing the system to self-tune for adaptive purposes, giving rise to a sense of edge-of-chaos existence wherein (6) *stability and flexibility are critically paired* to create an continuously shifting or *integrating system* across all levels of existence (individual and collective).

Because of its focus on emergent outcomes, complex systems science helps explain why outcomes to nursing interventions, however well-researched, are often unpredictable in practice. CSS suggests that when planning care, integrative nurses must consider (a) the intervention timing, (b) the readiness for the intervention by the system, and (c) how that system receives/processes information provided by the intervention in its own inherent healing trajectory. This meta-theoretical perspective provides a plausible explanation for the age-old adage that interventions must be considered within the context of the whole of the situation; what works in one case is not guaranteed success in another. Thus, CSS provides a scientific basis that validates nursing's individualized, person-centered approach to care that supports the innate healing potential of the individual, family, or community. Furthermore, the concepts and principles of CSS and the emerging research methodologies aligned with this science provide a meta-theoretical basis for the science, practice, and art of the discipline of nursing.

Integrative Nursing and Contemporary Healthcare Systems

While nursing has historically valued integrative or holistic approaches to healthcare, the larger healthcare system has only recently begun to explore and acknowledge the possibilities of a whole person/whole systems approach to care. Imagine a healthcare system that considers the person within the context of his or her social, cultural, and spiritual environments (whole person) and designs care that meets the needs not only of individuals but of populations, communities, and nations (whole-system). Nursing appears to be almost perfectly situated at this time in our global healthcare crisis to lead the way in integrative healthcare. Nursing's theoretical and scientific traditions have long held the keys to our preferred healthcare future.

The voices calling for change in healthcare are increasingly diverse, and they are rooted in changing technology, increasing access to information and transforming dysfunction across healthcare systems. Evidence clearly indicates that multiple determinants affect health outcomes, including the complex interaction of a person's social, economic, psychological, and physical environments as well as his or her underlying biology and sensitivity to both illness susceptibilities and treatments (Centers for Disease Control, 2013; World Health Organization, 2012). Technological advances at the point of care facilitate marshalling our burgeoning complexity of health information to formulate coherent, whole person/whole systems assessments and engage in patient-provider shared decision-making and interprofessional team care. At the same time, systems biology and advances in genomics provide an opportunity to personalize and target medical treatments; rather than a one-size-fits-all approach, our new biology almost begs for the individualized care that supports each person's innate and very unique healing (Abu-Asab et al., 2012; Bruggeman & Weserthoff, 2006; Cortese, 2007; Jonas, 2005).

Thus, the current healthcare-reform dialogue points to a global readiness to adopt the values of integrative medicine. These values (e.g., patient-provider partnering, use of appropriate therapies to support innate healing processes, consideration of whole person/whole system influences on health and wellbeing, patient and provider self-care/self-healing) (Schultz, Chao & McGinnis, 2009; Maizes & Caspi, 1999; Weil, 2012) are consistent with the historical values of nursing. Therefore, integrative nursing would agree with Boon et al.'s (2004b) suggestion that the term *integrative medicine* be broadened to *integrative healthcare*, recognizing that medicine is but one part of the healthcare system. "Integrative healthcare" describes our vision of system that is focused on whole person/whole systems care that is grounded in relationships and prevention and is delivered by interprofessional teams that include conventional (allopathic) as well as complementary/alternative therapies. This book will describe integrative nursing's contributions to integrative healthcare and our vision forward.

The Principles of Integrative Nursing

Six principles provide a foundation for integrative nursing practice. These principles are based on meta-theoretical perspectives consistent with historical nursing values, beliefs and theoretical perspectives, complex systems science, and the values, beliefs, and practices of integrative healthcare (Boon et al., 2004a, 2004b; Kligler et al., 2004; Maizes et al., 2002; Weil, 2012).

1. HUMAN BEINGS ARE WHOLE SYSTEMS, INSEPARABLE FROM THEIR ENVIRONMENTS

Historically, nursing theorists have consistently claimed that human beings must be understood within the context of their environments. Today, nurses share a belief that caring requires a consideration of the person's needs within the whole of their situation (ANA, 2010). Martha Rogers first proposed that human and environmental energy fields are inseparable and multidimensional in 1970. She hypothesized that human beings are "irreducible wholes that evolve…through dynamic, nonlinear process[es] characterized by increasing diversity and complexity" (Rogers, 1989, p. 184). Naming this process "homeodynamics," she identified three principles (resonancy, helicy, and integrality) that characterize how human/environmental fields change and grow over time and how others can recognize pattern manifestations. Her Science of Unitary Human Beings describes these complex, evolving wholes as the very substance and focus of nursing as a discipline.

Many nurse theorists have built upon Rogers' premises, offering ways to structure care, improve the wellbeing of patients, and promote the health of communities and populations (Barrett, 1990; Newman, 2008; Parse, 1999). Newman (1999) posited that health is an unfolding emergence of consciousness (defined as "information networks") with fluctuating patterns of order/disorder. Parse's theory of Human Becoming (1999, p. 68) claims that human–environmental fields do not simply coexist, but actively co-create the future (identified as "becoming") through "living, valuing and choosing freely". As such, the human–environmental system is a complex network of continuous possibilities and options with human beings who continually "become" something new, unique, and increasingly diverse as information resulting from choices is enfolded into their being. Thus, human beings are dynamic systems that continuously change as a result of an enfolding/unfolding process of transforming possibilities (Parse, 1999).

Principle 1 advances nursing's historical understanding of the human–environmental field transaction by applying the principles of complex systems science to nursing's holistic ontology. Complex adaptive systems (CAS) are self-sustaining entities that comprise nested networks of relationships organized hierarchically across levels of scale (Figure 1.1). Each level of scale is composed of entities from the level below. The essential nature of each level takes shape because of the information from the relationships created at the previous level. For example, the cardiovascular system cannot be understood by studying the heart muscle, the cardiac circulation, the valves, or the condition of the systemic circulation (the organs and tissues that comprise it). The condition of the cardiovascular system can only be known by assessing how it is organized and functions as a whole. Similarly, integrative nurses can certainly assess various systems of the person (body, mind, and spirit), but in order to under the person as a whole, they must stand back and ask—"how is this 'bodymindspirit' doing as a whole?"

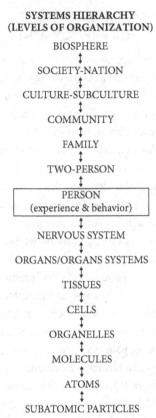

SYSTEMS HIERARCHY
(LEVELS OF ORGANIZATION)

BIOSPHERE
↕
SOCIETY-NATION
↕
CULTURE-SUBCULTURE
↕
COMMUNITY
↕
FAMILY
↕
TWO-PERSON
↕

> PERSON
> (experience & behavior)

↕
NERVOUS SYSTEM
↕
ORGANS/ORGANS SYSTEMS
↕
TISSUES
↕
CELLS
↕
ORGANELLES
↕
MOLECULES
↕
ATOMS
↕
SUBATOMIC PARTICLES

FIGURE 1.1 This figure illustrates a hierarchical biopsychosocial model of human-environmental systems. Changes at any level of a system lead to changes at other levels above & below the level that changed. (Adapted from Engel, G. L. The need for a new medical model: A challenge for biomedicine. *Science* (1977), *196*(4286), 129–136.).

Typically, integrative nurses focus their healing interventions on the personal, family, and community/national levels of scale (Figure 1.1). This has often been referred to as a *whole person/whole systems* approach to care (Kreitzer, 2009; Quinn et al., 2003; Ritenbaugh et al., 2003; Verhoef et al., 2005). Whole-person healing is defined as a focus on overarching, patient-centered outcomes such as wellbeing, energy, happiness, clarity, and purpose, rather than a focus on physiological biomarkers or specific symptoms (Koithan et al., 2007; Mulkins & Verhoef, 2004; Ritenbaugh et al., 2011). Whole systems healing is described as an approach to healing that takes into account the interconnectedness of all living systems. In a whole systems healing approach, integrative nurses are aware that the health of individuals depends on the health of the ecosystem as well as the communities and social systems within which people live and work (Zabrowsky & Kreitzer, 2009). Therefore, the integrative community health nurse may focus well beyond the individual to be concerned about the integrity of our environments, the hopefulness of our communities, and the safety of our population.

Thus, integrative nursing embraces the complexities of the human–environmental system and focuses on the emerging whole. Integrative nurses assess the whole person/whole system, remembering to tend to the whole bodymindspirit as an unfolding living organism. We recognize that human systems are dynamic, individualistic, and complex; they cannot be reduced to diagnoses, symptoms, and deviations from the norm.

2. HUMAN BEINGS HAVE THE INNATE CAPACITY FOR HEALTH AND WELLBEING

Health and wellbeing is an emergent property of the whole person/whole system. Health is not additive; rather, health naturally evolves as the whole person/whole system lives in the world. This principle is based on a primary tenet of complex systems science, which states that change is an inherent quality of the CAS and is characterized as nonlinear and unpredictable (Guastello & Liebovitch, 2009; Koithan et al., 2012). A CAS, responding to new information provided through its set of increasingly varied relationships, shifts and moves in a manner similar to an undulating wave to create a system that is efficient and resilient (Pincus, 2009). This process, born out of self-preservation, entails creating or finding the right (or best-fit) relationships for the system, which are just at the edge of the chaos/order continuum and provide the momentum to sustain system growth and prosperity.

The CAS concept of continual systems change and emergence is consistent with nursing's definition of health as a continual process of "being or becoming whole" (Quinn, 1989). It is also consistent with Parse's (1999) description of health as enfolding/unfolding human becoming, wherein the human–environmental system actively becomes more organizationally coherent through a process of valuing and freely choosing from multiple possibilities. Thus, health is an innate property of the system; all persons have an innate capacity for whole person/whole systems wellbeing across all dimensions of experience (bodymindspirit).

This is not a new idea for nursing; its roots can be found in Nightingale's writings, which encourage nurses to "assist the reparative process which Nature has instituted" (1859/1946, p. 6). This principle is also consistent with Parse's perspective of health as human becoming. "Becoming (health) is a process of human unfolding, an intersubjective process of transcending with the possibilities which is co-constituted with human-universe interrelationships" (Parse, 1999). A similar perspective is Watson's (2011) contention that health is bodymindspirit harmony that occurs as the person seeks greater connectedness between self and universal consciousness, transforming from what is to what is not yet. Kreitzer (Chapter 10) conceptualizes health as wellbeing defined as an alignment of bodymindspirit that supports and maximizes whole person/whole system capacity and potential.

No matter the particulars, the perspective is the same. Complex systems (human and social) intrinsically seek the path that maximizes resources (efficiency, parsimony) and supports the growth and flourishing of the system (resilience) (Guastello & Liebovitch, 2009). Thus, health is an emergent property of the whole; human beings as CAS have the innate capacity for health and wellbeing. The role of the integrative nurse is to support this unfolding process, to facilitate the system's search for balance and right relationship in all dimensions of existence, thereby advancing health and wellbeing. Integrative nursing interventions across level of scale (person- to community-focused) support the natural whole person/whole systems healing processes.

3. NATURE HAS HEALING AND RESTORATIVE PROPERTIES THAT CONTRIBUTE TO HEALTH AND WELLBEING

Recent literature points to the negative consequences of our society's increasing alienation from nature (Buzzell & Chaltquist, 2009). Because human beings are complex adaptive systems that are inseparable from their environments, they are "hard-wired" to interact with the natural environment—water, plants, air, and animals. Our growing cities with islands of concrete, steel, and glass continuously change our natural environment, isolating us from substances that have historically created who we are, within which "we were embedded" (Buzzell, 2009). While some may argue that our increasing technology enhances our ability to connect to others, others claim that this technology is yet another way that we are becoming even more isolated from the natural environment. As a result, we long for "home."

Ulrich (2004) claimed that people have a "biologically prepared disposition to respond favorably to nature because we evolved in nature. Nature was good to us, and we tend to respond positively to environments that were favorable to us." Studies consistently report that when people are stressed or depressed, they seek natural settings or the outdoors (Huelat, 2003; Kahn et al., 2009). Recent systematic literature reviews also support the evidence that being in nature is tied to reduction in blood pressure as well as reduced heart rate and respiratory distress/shortness of breath, with preliminary evidence pointing to changes in biological markers associated with the stress response and changes in neurological activity and brain activation (Devlin & Arneill, 2003; Drahota, 2012; Ulrich, 2008).

Human beings find meaning in nature. It reminds us of the enormousness of the universe, the place of human beings within creation, and our interdependence with the larger whole. Nature supports our spiritual growth and self-knowing, providing "space within which we can connect" (Kreitzer, 2012). In short, nature inspires (Kellert & Wilson, 1993).

Integrative nurses are not surprised by these findings and have long advocated the "biophilia hypothesis," which proposes an instinctive bond between human beings and other living systems (Kellert & Wilson, 1993; Wilson, 1984). Jean Watson (2011) states that the goal of nursing practice is to help people gain a sense of purpose, a meaning for their existence through self-knowledge, self-reverence, self-healing, and self-care. Nature is essential to self-healing and self-care; there are "things that human beings cannot do without, at least not without deep suffering and the diminishing of one's nature.... One of these is...nature and the feeling of our place within it" (Watson, 1999, p. 41). She claims that, without nature, we become machines.

According to Watson (1989), transpersonal, human, caring relationships, the foundation of nursing practice, incorporate ten "carative" factors that support and nurture the person's ability to grow, to transcend what is to what is not yet, and to heal. "Transpersonal caring is the full actualization of the carative factors in a human-to-human transaction.... Such a transaction helps to promote self-knowledge and meaning" (p. 232). Nurses are encouraged by Watson to include art, nature, and beauty in their creation of caring transactions. She notes that "probably no profession more than nursing is aware that some human problems are insoluble" (p. 215). When this occurs, it is incumbent upon the nurse to help the patient look into the mysteries of human life and to find meaning. Often this occurs through the power of arts and nature. "Beauty heals; by showering each other with beauty, we bring out the beauty of one another" (Watson, 1999, p. 193). Art and nature transform; each "moves us into a space where we can create visions of others ways of being-doing"; they integrate the soul (Watson, 1999, pp. 195–96).

Watson (2005) also notes that it is impossible to enter into altruistic caring-healing relationships without cultivating personal sensitivity and self-understanding. The arts (painting, poetry, sculpture) help us access our feelings and our humanness. The aesthetics of the natural beauty around us awaken our senses and infuse our beings so that we can authentically hear the voice of "the other" in relationship. The aesthetics of the arts and nature sensitize us and create within the nurse the ability to heal.

4. INTEGRATIVE NURSING IS PERSON-CENTERED AND RELATIONSHIP-BASED

Integrative nurses co-create caring/healing relationships with individuals, families and communities to support the emergence of health and wellbeing. Nursing has always focused on the unique patient–provider relationship that forms the basis of caring transactions. The ANA Social Policy Statement (2003) states that "true partnership," relationships that extend to both patients and other healthcare professionals, is a core value of the profession. ANA defines partnership as a "relationship in which power is valued by both and shared, with recognition of the strengths, limitations, and contributions of both parties" (p. 33).

Nightingale (1859/1946) specifies the nature of this patient–nurse relationship as assistive, aiding the person to "perform unaided if he had the necessary strength, will or knowledge...and to do so in such a way as to help him gain independence" (p. 8).

Nurses are guided in this relationship by an ethos of self-determination and choice tempered by values of respect, equality, and social justice. The integrative nurse provides options that support the person's growth and healing, recognizing that every caring moment is a complex whole that both parties enter into freely. Person-centered nursing occurs when the unique nature of the individual, family, or community is known in its entirety with all of its attendant strengths, resources, and potentials.

Rosemarie Parse (1992) offers the most theoretically complete perspective on the nature of person-centered, relationship-based care. Her practice methodology proposes that the nurse–patient dyad co-authors health experiences (1992, p. 39). She proposes that practice occurs within three dimensions (illuminating meaning, synchronizing rhythms, and mobilizing transcendence) that are powered by three distinct processes (explicating, dwelling with, and moving beyond). She envisions relationship-based nursing as a true presence with attentive listening that encourages co-creation of new ways of being-knowing-doing in both nurse and patient. "The nurse in true presence moves with the flow, not as a guide or a beacon but rather as an attentive presence that calls the other to illuminate meaning" (Parse, 1992, p. 40).

Relationship-based care and partnership is not confined to the way the integrative nurse attends to patients. It extends to nature of collaborative relationships that nurses have with others in the healthcare team. Nurses approach their professional relationships from a perspective of shared power, recognizing that authentic power is formed within the immediate, person-centered relationship (as opposed to a discipline-centered, hierarchically structured relationship) that is focused on the healing outcome for a person, family, or community. Integrative nurses co-create healing teams in order to creatively move the whole system forward. Team leadership is shared, and it rotates based on system needs and opportunities, always with the recipient of care or their representative firmly in control.

5. INTEGRATIVE NURSING PRACTICE IS INFORMED BY EVIDENCE AND USES THE FULL RANGE OF THERAPEUTIC MODALITIES TO SUPPORT/AUGMENT THE HEALING PROCESS, MOVING FROM LEAST INTENSIVE/INVASIVE TO MORE, DEPENDING ON NEED AND CONTEXT

The goal of nursing practice is to support the innate healing capacity and growth of the individual, family, or community. Interventions are focused on the whole person/ whole system, recognizing that change in a complex adaptive system occurs both locally and globally, dependent on the condition of the system (i.e., readiness and sensitivity) at the time of the intervention (Bell & Koithan, 2006; Koithan et al., 2012). Therefore, the integrative nurse engages in interventions expecting that the recipient of care will respond in unique and perhaps unexpected ways. A massage, while intended to bring about relief and physical wellbeing, might also release pent-up emotions.

Cleansing a wound may facilitate healing the skin but may also communicate regard and respect, which contribute to self-understanding and acceptance of a changed body. The integrative nurse bears witness to this healing process, supportive of whole-person outcomes (intended as well as unintended) that occur in response to the intent to heal.

Integrative nurses make use of the full complement of therapies when constructing a plan of care for their patients. Traditional healing practices (meditation, herbal remedies and tinctures, aromatherapies, healing foods, massage) are melded with the newer interventions suggested by Western science (medications, respiratory support, surgical therapies) dependent upon the needs, context, and readiness and desires of the patient. Integrative nurses also consider the evidence when making decisions about a particular therapy, making their selection based on outcomes evidence and the proposed mechanism of action.

Nursing practice is informed by multiple sources of evidence—empirical, aesthetic, ethical, personal, political, and unknowing (Carper, 1978; Meleis, 2012; Watson, 2005; White, 1995). Nurses have long been informed by the wisdom of the ages, which teaches us how to use herbal remedies, essential oils, human touch, and intention to facilitate healing. Our knowledge is not limited to evidence-created empirical sciences; we value equally the types of information gained through personal experiences, the existential knowing of the lived-body/lived-world of those who suffer, and the clinical knowing-doing found every day in patient care. Nurses recognize that healthcare needs to be informed by all kinds of knowledge, each valuable in its own right, each contributing to the whole that informs our practice (Jonas, 2001). The wise nurse acknowledges the usefulness of multiple forms of evidence when selecting an intervention for a patient.

Because interventions are supportive in nature and are used by the innate intelligence of the human–environmental system, integrative nurses proceed from least invasive to more invasive with the intent to support healing in the most natural and least disruptive way possible. Interventions are structured to begin with relatively non-invasive treatments, such as those with the fewest side effects or greatest potential to alter the bodymindspirit of the recipient of care. Interventions move systematically to more invasive treatments when there is a lack of system response or an inability of the system to use the information conveyed by the therapy to find that balance necessary for system growth and wellbeing.

6. INTEGRATIVE NURSING FOCUSES ON THE HEALTH AND WELLBEING OF CAREGIVERS AS WELL AS THOSE THEY SERVE

Quinn (1984) proposes that the caregiver's use of self is the most powerful instrument for healing. Yet, in order to be engaged in healing, the caregiver must also be fully engaged in his or her own journey of self-discovery and unfolding. Therefore, integrative nursing recognizes the critical nature of the wellbeing of our healthcare workforce and their need to be nurtured and cared for in the same manner that they care for patients. To support the other, the caregiver must likewise be supported.

Watson (1999; 2005) notes that in order to engage in a transpersonal caring-healing, person-centered relationship, nurses must consciously awaken to their own humanity and the sacred nature of their own lives. In addition to cultivating knowledge and skills, nurses must be engaged in cultivating self. Quinn (2009) identifies the nurse as the healing environment, the space within which caring and healing occurs. As such, integrative nurses need to attend to their own wellbeing, consider their own limitations, and seek out activities that feed their bodymindspirit so that they might flourish.

Educators in the health professions have long maintained that empathy is developed by students who examine their own moral convictions and conflicts, feelings and emotional responses to human struggles and dilemmas, and their own mortality and the fragility of life itself (Kozier & Erb, 2011; Potter & Perry, 2012). Additionally, health professionals have encouraged using self-reflection as a method to gain access to feelings, responses, and experiences of caring for others. Reflection helps the healer identify his or her own vulnerabilities and negativities (the "shadow side" of our relationships and lives) as well as appreciate the blessings found within the work, the positive aspects of being in caring-healing relationships (Schon, 1984). Yet, the kind of self-care and self-knowing that is requisite for the integrative healer goes beyond these classical approaches (Quinn, 2009; Watson, 2005).

Watson (2005) calls the healer to engage in a journey of loving remembrance that is both personal and professional. By remembering, we cultivate a true state of "Belonging-Being-Becoming." We learn to honor and love life with all of its negatives and positives, struggles and blessings; we learn about our relationship with living (pp. 70–75). By facing our own humanity, we understand how our "face mirrors the human experience" (Watson, 2005, p. 78). Thus, the nurse becomes the "environment" within which human encounters occur, that space where healing takes place as we authentically listen and consider ways to support the recipients of our care so that they flourish.

Summary

Integrative nursing is active. In order to engage in being-knowing-doing that advances the health and wellbeing of persons, families, and communities through caring/healing relationships, the integrative nurse continuously translates these six principles into a practice that supports the innate healing capacity of the human–environmental system within the current healthcare environment. The integrative nurse selects interventions based on evidence from multiple sources, typically using the most natural, effective, and least-invasive therapy that can be identified.

Therefore, while the definition of *nursing* states that "nursing protects, promotes and optimizes health and abilities, prevents illness and injury, [and] alleviates suffering through the diagnosis and treatment of human responses," integrative nurses implement this social covenant in unique ways (ANA, 2003, p. 6). The integrative nurse attends to suffering and human responses by assessing the bodymindspirit of the recipient of care, recognizing that simply assessing system components (mind, body, and spirit) does not adequately address the complexity of the whole person/whole system. Neither does the integrative nurse assess the "wholeness" of the person without understanding the intricate relationships and continual processing of information that composes the ever-evolving nature of this complex system. Figure 1.2 represents how the integrative nurse assesses the recipient of care and the overall approach to care. Rather than the more simplistic approaches offered by historical biomedical and holistic traditions, integrative nursing recognizes that that there are multidirectional interactions of parts and wholes that generate emergent outcomes, including health and wellbeing.

Integrative nurses use assessment findings to identify interventions that support the natural healing processes, distinguishing healing and health from curing and absence of disease. We use the human being's natural affinity for nature and other living systems to strengthen connectedness and meaning, which in turn fosters purpose, self-understanding, and growth. Nursing care is informed by evidence, uses a full range of therapeutic modalities, and is delivered within a caring-healing relationship by someone who is actively engaged in his or her own healing journey.

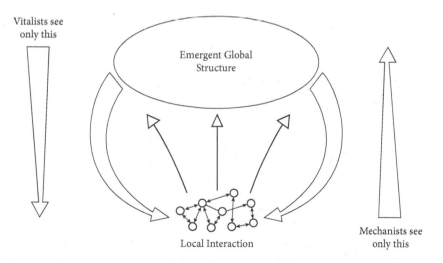

FIGURE 1.2 This figure depicts the ontological perspective of integrative nursing (based on complex systems science) offering an alternative to traditional mechanistic and holistic approaches to patient care. (Koithan et al., 2012, reprinted with permission.)

SELECTED REFERENCES

Boon, H., Verhoef, M., O'Hara, D., Findlay, B., & Majid, N. (2004b). Integrative health-care: Arriving at a working definition. *Alternative Therapies, 10*(5), 48–56.

Kligler, B., Maizes, V., Schachter, S., Park, C., Gaudent, T., Benn, R., et al. (2004). Core competencies in integrative medicine for medical school curricula: A proposal. *Academic Medicine, 79*(6), 521–531.

Koithan, M., Bell, I. R., Niemeyer, K., & Pincus, D. (2012). A complex systems science perspective for whole systems of CAM research. *Forschende Komplementarmedizin und Klassische Naturheilkunde, 19*(Supplement 1), 7–14.

Maizes, V., & Caspi, O. (1999). The principles and challenges of integrative medicine. *Western Journal of Medicine, 171*, 148–149.

Pincus, D. (2009). Coherence, complexity, and information flow: Self-organizing processes in psychotherapy. In Guastello, S. J., Koopmans, M., Pincus, D. (Eds.), *Chaos and Complexity in Psychology. The Theory of Nonlinear Dynamical Systems* (pp. 335–369). Cambridge, UK: Cambridge University Press.

Quinn, J. F., Smith, M., Ritenbaugh, C., Swanson, K., Watson, M. J., (2003). Research guidelines for assessing the impact of the healing relationship in clinical nursing. Quoted in Jonas, W. B., & Chez, R. A. (eds.), Definitions and standards in healing research, *Alternative Therapies in Health and Medicine*, Special Supplement, 9(3): A65–A79.

Rogers, M. (1989). Nursing: A science of unitary human beings. In J. P. Riehl-Sisca(Ed.), *Conceptual models for nursing practice* (3rd ed., pp. 181–188). Norwalk, CT: Appleton & Lange.

Wilson, E. (1984). *Biophilia.* Cambridge, MA: Harvard University Press.

Zabrowsky, T., & Kreitzer, M. J. (2009). People, places and process: The role of place in creating optimal healing environments. *Creative Nursing, 15*(4), 186–190.

Zimmerman, B., Lindberg, C., & Plesk, P. (2008). *Edgeware: Lessons from Complexity Science for Healthcare Leaders.* Washington, DC: Plexus Institute.

2

The Integrated Nurse: Wholeness, Self-Discovery, and Self-Care

JANET F. QUINN

Integrative nursing focuses on the health and wellbeing of caregivers as well as those they serve.

—*(Integrative Nursing Principle 6)*

The Case for Nurse Self-Care

There is no shortage of information available about how to promote and maintain health. For example, one can find a multitude of online health assessments, informational websites, self-help videos, and health tracking programs, many of them run by outstanding universities, hospital systems, and insurers. One excellent example is the website hosted by the Center for Spirituality and Healing at the University of Minnesota (http://www.csh.umn.edu/). If nurses are not taking care of themselves—and research suggests many are not (Letvak, Ruhm, & Gupta, 2012; Aronsson, 2000)—it can be assumed that it is not for lack of adequate information.

The purpose of this chapter is to increase commitment to nurse self-care by increasing awareness of its critical role in integrative nursing and to assist integrative nurses in cultivating deeper self-knowledge and new *bodymindspirit* (Quinn, 2000) skills to fulfill that commitment. We will approach the topic of nurse wholeness and self-care, not as an issue of information-deficit, but rather as an experiential opportunity to increase capacity in self-awareness and self-knowledge as the foundation, not only for self-care, but also for truly integrative nursing. From that expanded awareness, integrative nurses can make choices in their lives and in their work that are in greater alignment with optimal health and wellbeing.

Integrative Nursing Requires Integrated Nurses

One of the most fundamental perspectives undergirding integrative nursing is that human beings are irreducibly whole and inseparable from their environment.

Unpacking that language a bit, we often refer to the whole person as *bodymindspirit* inseparable from the environment. This is a kind of shorthand pointing to the immensely complex system that is the multidimensional human being in relationship with all that is. Figure 2.1 illustrates this model, demonstrating that, no matter where one enters into contact with the person—through the body, the mind, or the spirit—one always connects with and impacts the whole bodymindspirit. From this point of view, there are not *more* or *less* holistic treatments. All treatments impact the totality of bodymindspirit. There are more or less natural treatments, or more or less invasive treatments, but no treatments have a more holistic impact than the others, because there is no way *not* to impact the whole. There *may* be more or less awareness of the intrinsic wholeness of being, and so more or less holistic/integrative perspectives, approaches, assessments, and plans of care. This is what integrative nursing is about.

Integrative nurses facilitate healing of whole persons as the emergence of right relationship at or between the multidimensional levels of the human experience (Quinn, 1984, 1989, 2013). As specified in the definition and the fourth principle of integrative nursing, the work of facilitating healing is accomplished through person-centered, caring/healing relationships. "Practitioners' relationships with their patients, their patients' communities, and other practitioners are central to health care and are the

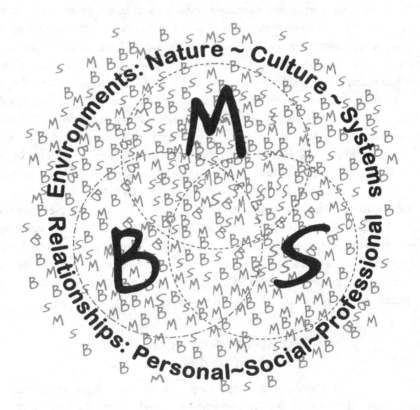

FIGURE 2.1 Bodymindspirit

vehicle for putting into action a paradigm of health that integrates caring, healing, and community" (Pew Fetzer Task Force, 1994, p. 24).

The caring/healing relationship is a particular way of being-doing-knowing that is characterized by (at least) empathy, caring, love, warmth, trust, confidence, credibility, honesty, courtesy, respect, and authentic communication (Dossey, 2003; Quinn et al., 2003). These relationships depend on the health and wholeness of the integrative nurse, without which the nurse's relationship with the patient (or family, community, or system) may devolve into functional, depersonalized transactions that simply convey competent technical procedures addressing the signs and symptoms of disease. Such transactions do not have the capacity to tend whole persons or to facilitate their multidimensional healing. The simple addition of complementary and alternative forms of care into a treatment model that continues to focus only on a cure and is delivered by a healthcare professional who is not truly present, alive, and whole does not make care integrative. Renowned American philosopher Ken Wilber explains it clearly:

> The crucial ingredient in any integral [healing] practice is not the integral medical bag itself—with all the conventional pills, and the orthodox surgery, and the subtle energy medicine, and the acupuncture needles—but the holder of that bag...the doctors and nurses and therapists [who] have opened themselves to an entire spectrum of consciousness—matter to body to mind to soul to spirit—and who have thereby acknowledged what seems to be happening in any event. Body and mind and spirit are operating in self and culture and nature, and thus health and healing, sickness and wholeness, are all bound up in a multidimensional tapestry that cannot be cut into without loss. It is the health professional who is healed and wholed [sic] first, not merely by learning new and complementary techniques, but by inhabiting a new consciousness that makes room for new techniques; and how that integrity then expresses itself...might vary considerably. (Wilber, 2005)

Enhancing Nurse Wholeness: Increased Self-Awareness and Self-Knowledge

One's own self is well hidden from one's own self: Of all mines of treasure, one's own is the last to be dug up.

—*Friedrich Nietzsche*

Self-awareness is at the center of "emotional intelligence," defined by Daniel Goleman as "the capacity for recognizing our own feelings and those of others, for motivating ourselves, and for managing emotions well in ourselves and in our relationships" (Goleman, 1998). In discussing the need for emotional intelligence for nurse leaders, Schaffner and Ludwig-Beymer write that "emotional intelligence (EI) is the differentiator between a good nurse leader and a great nurse leader" (2003).

Self-awareness and self-reflection are prerequisites for skillful, integrative care. In holistic and integrative nursing, we are called to create caring/healing relationships that require authentic presence and the holding of sacred space for healing (Quinn, 1992; Halldorsdottir, 1991; Watson, 2005). These requirements are far more about who we are than what we do or say. Thus, to practice integrative nursing requires ongoing inquiry into and cultivation of the true self, along with a careful tending of that self, which is the instrument for healing.

Self-awareness is at the heart of reflexive practice—noticing our own inner experience as we engage in our work—and without it, care can become automatic and symptom/disease-focused, rather than person-centered and relationship-based. For example, lack of self-awareness may prevent nurses from seeing their biases against certain classes of patients, such as the very obese, the very thin, the homeless, the smoker, the atheist, the fundamentalist, and so on. Unconscious biases can lead to biostatic relationships characterized by subtle neglect, or worse, to "biocidic" relationships that are actually outright abusive (Halldorsdottir, 1991).

Self-Care Requires Self-Awareness

In the context of self-care, lack of self-awareness may prevent a nurse from even knowing that self-care is necessary until full-blown burnout manifests as illness or chronic depression. The Pew Fetzer Task Force on Relationship-Centered Care (1994) suggests that, for healthcare practitioners to work effectively within multiple levels of relationship, they must develop knowledge and skills in several key areas, the first of which includes self-awareness, self-knowledge, continuing self-growth, and self-care: "Self-care is essential: over the course of a lifetime of service, the practitioner is a resource for an enormous number of people. It is only reasonable that practitioners should treat themselves with the same respect and care given to any important resource."

Thus, self-awareness and self-knowledge are at once ends in themselves, but also the means of providing truly integrative nursing care that includes nurse self-care. Next, we will address these essential components of integrative nursing by using a gentle self-inquiry process.

First Things First: What/Who Is the "Self"?

Knowing yourself is the beginning of all wisdom.

—Aristotle

This question "What or who is the self?" is the fundamental existential question of life. It rests at the heart of numerous fields of academic inquiry, study, and research, and it is central to the spiritual journey across the world's traditions. Clearly, the full

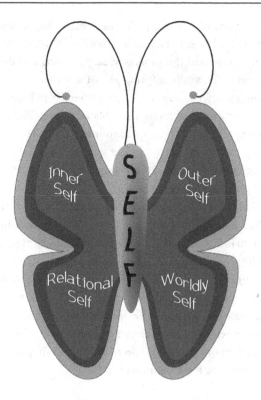

FIGURE 2.2 Four Dimensions of the Self

exploration of this question is beyond the scope of this chapter. Yet the question invites reflection and provides a perfect opportunity to practice a process of inquiry for increased self-awareness.

Figure 2.2 shows a butterfly with four wings as a metaphor for the self. All of the wings emerged as an integrated wholeness out of what was once a caterpillar, and none is more the real butterfly than any other. While the wholeness of bodymindspirit cannot be reduced to the sum of its parts, we can, for this self-inquiry, consider four broad dimensions of the self as we experience them—an outer self (physical and energy bodies), an inner self (mind and spirit), a self in relationships, and a self in the world. The "wings" (dimensions) are loosely based on the quadrants that compose one aspect of the integral framework developed by Ken Wilber (1995) and applied in nursing by several authors (Quinn et al., 2003; Fiandt, 2003; Newman, 2003; Baye, 2005; Clark, 2006, 2012; Jarrin, 2006, 2007, 2012; Dossey, 2007; Watson, 2005, pp. 108–111).

Next, you are invited to expand your self-awareness in each dimension through a gentle inquiry process. This process is a powerful one that can be used to explore any question we are sitting with, as well as a tool that we can use to help others in their healing.

Begin with a deep inhalation and a full exhalation. Bring your awareness to the breath itself. Notice just breathing—the rising and falling of your chest, the movement of air just outside your nostrils, the gentle shift as in-breathing becomes out-breathing. What is the quality of the breath? Is it easy and flowing, or tight and tense? Rhythmic or irregular? Just notice. Repeat this process of easy inhaling and deep exhaling a few times until you begin to feel yourself letting go just a bit, moving attention into your center, however you experience that. Experience yourself as being present here and now, just noticing your breath, allowing thoughts to drift by like clouds on a breezy day. Take your time here before moving on to your inquiry in each specific dimension. When you are ready, please proceed to the next section.

Table 2.1 offers guiding questions for self-inquiry in each of the four dimensions. From this place of centering in the present moment, gently allow yourself to choose one of the dimensions as the starting place for your inquiry. Then begin with the first question on the list, noticing whatever arises in your awareness in response. Allow whatever comes up to just be. There is no right or wrong answer; remain open and curious. You are just interested in learning more about yourself by noticing what arises all by itself. Take your time with this question. You might want to journal your responses for review later. Use this same process with any of the remaining questions in each of the dimensions. Choose to explore another question now, or return to this exercise as an ongoing practice in self-inquiry for greater self-awareness. If you wish to complete this inquiry practice for now, take several deep breaths and simply sit in awareness and appreciation for yourself for these moments of self-care.

Enhancing Nurse Health/Wholeness Through Self-Care

The only way to ensure the best quality for our patients is to have an expert staff of qualified nurses who are healthy enough to offer that kind of care. We can't ignore nurses' health anymore.

—Susan Letvak et al.

Integrative nurse self-care is multidimensional, addressing vulnerabilities, needs, and areas of sub-optimal health, as well as impulses toward creative unfolding that are trying to emerge in each of the dimensions of the self that we have just explored. During the guided inquiry, you may have noticed particular areas that called out for attention, either because they need support or healing, or because they are new impulses toward greater self-expression and wholeness. Take a moment now to complete another brief inquiry, checking in with each of the dimensions of yourself for a few seconds to a minute. Allow the deep wisdom of your integrated self to answer, without censoring or judging the response, the following question: *What is most important for me to attend to in this dimension of myself for my greater wholeness and wellbeing?* Take a few moments with this, and then journal your responses.

Table 2.1: Integrative Self-Awareness

Guiding questions to explore the Inner Self—the mind and spirit dimensions of bodymindspirit	*Guiding questions to explore the Outer Self—the body dimension of bodymindspirit*
Who am I as a thinking, feeling, spiritual being?	Who am I as an embodied, material being?
What is my overall sense/experience of my inner self right now, and usually?	What is my overall sense/experience of my outer self now, and usually?
What is the quality of my mind now, and usually?	Am I satisfied with this experience?
What is the quality of my feelings/emotions right now, and usually?	How does my body feel now, and usually?
What is my sense of my spiritual self right now, and usually?	If it had a voice, what would my body say right now?
What is my sense of the sacred, divine, higher power, or whatever I name the ultimate mystery?	Who am I as an energy being?
What matters most to me?	Am I aware of my subtle energy body?
What are my core beliefs and values?	What is the quality of my energy now, and usually?
Is there healing work I need for/with my outer self?	Who am I as a doing/accomplishing being?
What wants to emerge in/as/through my inner self?	What makes my body feel strong, vital, and happy?
Are there ways of being-knowing-doing in my other dimensions that are helpful or hurtful to me here?	What makes my body feel less than well?
	Is there healing work I need for/with my outer self?
	What wants to emerge in/as/through my outer self?
	Are there ways of being-knowing-doing in my other dimensions that are helpful or hurtful to me here?

Guiding questions to explore the Relational Self	*Guiding questions to explore the Worldly Self*
Who am I in the many relationships and cultures of which I am a part?	Who am I as a being in the outer world?
What is my overall sense/experience of my relational self in this moment and usually?	What is my overall sense/experience of my worldly self in this moment, and usually?
What worldview, values and beliefs do I share in my relationships?	Who am I in the context of the person–environment relationship?
What are my most satisfying relationships and what makes them satisfying?	Who am I in the context of nature?
What are my most challenging relationships and what makes them challenging?	Who am I in the context of my various communities, including my work community?
Is there healing work that I need to do within any of my relationships?	Who am I in the context of my professional groups and the healthcare system?
What is my experience of intersubjectivity (shared energy, consciousness, connection) in my relationships?	What is the usual quality of my experience in my workplace?
What wants to emerge in/as/through my relational self?	What is my sense of my role in my profession?
Are there ways of being-knowing-doing in my other dimensions that are helpful or hurtful to me here?	Is there healing work that I need to do that will benefit my worldly self and/or my communities?
	What wants to emerge in/as/through myworldly self?
	Are there ways of being-knowing-doing in my other dimensions that are helpful or hurtful to me here?

Self-Care, One Degree at a Time

I learned a powerful lesson about change from a camel in middle of the Australian outback, eight hours in any direction from anywhere. This camel was running for his life out in front of our minibus as we bounced down the narrow, red washboard road behind him. The other camels in his herd had already slowly peeled off the road one by one, disappearing into the vast expanses of bush on either side of the path. Making a one-degree change of course in any direction would have relieved this remaining camel from his stress and brought him into the same freedom and ease being enjoyed by his friends. Instead, he just kept going the way he always went, just faster and with more duress. Poor camel! It did not escape me then, nor does it now, that I often do the same thing. I keep running, faster and harder and with increasing duress, on habitual paths that are not getting me what I want, when just a one-degree change in direction is all I need to gain limitless choice and spaciousness.

The process of making changes in our ways of being-knowing-doing can be challenging even when we know our self-care requires it. One way of approaching this challenge is to think in terms of very small, one-degree changes that are actually doable and that over time will lead to greater freedom of choice and improved wellbeing in our whole bodymindspirit. To continue with the process of self-discovery as a foundation for self-care, you are now invited to reexamine the responses you received in the last inquiry. Again returning to the image of the butterfly, turn toward each dimension of yourself and consider the following question: *Is there a one-degree change that I can make in this dimension of myself that would bring me into more wholeness/healing/right relationship?* Once again, gently allow whatever comes in response. Try to be open and willing to be surprised by your inner wisdom and guidance.

It might be useful to use Table 2.2 as you consider the question. It organizes various approaches to self-care by the dimension in which they originate, with the effects impacting the whole self. Some of the strategies have been used clinically for improving healthcare-professional wellbeing. For example, in a review of sixty-four studies on stress-management interventions offered in the workplace, Bormann and her colleagues report that the most common techniques used are progressive muscle-relaxation, mindfulness meditation, transcendental meditation, biofeedback, and cognitive-behavioral skills (2006). In the same paper, the authors report that the use of a *mantram* (silent repetition of a sacred word) at work helped improve the emotional and spiritual wellbeing of healthcare workers. Yong and colleagues found that a spiritual training program that included instruction in mantra meditation, slowing down, and one-pointed attention was effective in improving the psychosocial and spiritual wellbeing of middle managers (2011).

See if there are any strategies on the list that jump out at you, and trust your intuition. If they seem too big for a one-degree change, imagine what the very first, smallest step toward the strategy would be. Journal about your responses, and consider whether or not you need to prioritize the one-degree change(s) you want to make so that you

Table 2.2: Integrative Self Care for Bodymindspirit

Inner Self (Mind and Spirit) Self-Care *Listen to your bodymindspirit and follow guidance for Inner Self self-care, which might include:*	**Outer (Body and Energy) Self-Care** *Listen to your bodymindspirit and follow guidance for Outer Self self-care, which might include:*
Inquiry practice Reading and studying Prayer and/or meditation Journaling Centering prayer Affirmations and positive thinking Mindfulness practice Self-reflection on beliefs, values, etc. Mental training practices Cultivating trust of inner guidance Coming to know your false self Participation in meaningful spiritual practices/rituals/groups Cultivate and honor intuition Creating space daily for stillness Retreat	Using online wellness assessments and plans Healthy nutrition Weight management Aerobic exercise Strength training Being in nature Adequate rest/sleep Recreational sports Movement/dancing/singing Yoga Tai Chi Qigong Other subtle energy practices Eye Movement Desensitization and Reprocessing (EMDR) Emotional freedom technique Being with pets and other animals
Relational Self Self-Care *Listen to your bodymindspirit and follow guidance for Relational Self self-care, which might include:*	**Worldly/Work Self Self-Care** *Listen to your bodymindspirit and follow guidance for Worldly/Work Self self-care, which might include:*
Working to increase social/interpersonal intelligence through: Self-reflection, reading, and studying Reflecting on the health of current relationships and making changes as needed Using typologies and other tools to discover your preferred relational styles and needs Emotional intelligence training Attending workshops, retreats, conferences Seeking professional help to heal old emotional wounds that are impacting current relationships Forgiveness Joining support groups and/or caring circles	Adequate physiology breaks Repetition of silent mantras or prayers Mindfulness applied to workplace Ceaseless centering Practicing kindness and generosity toward self and others Initiating or participating in organizational initiatives to promote staff wellbeing Working to create optimal healing environments/ habitats for healing Creating staff serenity spaces Practicing kindness and generosity Cultivating biogenic relationships with self/others Applying emotional, intrapersonal, and social intelligence to arising work situations

don't get overwhelmed. Remember that the guidance you are seeking may come hours from now, or days, as the question continues to live in you. Inspiration can arrive quite suddenly from almost anywhere—from words you overhear, or something you see on a nature walk, or even in a dream. Stay open.

Once you are clear about the one-degree change you wish to make, consider formalizing a statement of commitment or a vow to yourself or to share with a trusted guide or friend. Or write affirmations that you can post or carry with you as reminders of your self-caring choices, your conscious participation in the unfolding mystery of your life.

Integrative Nursing: Both the End and a Means of Self-Care at Work

The increased self-awareness and self-knowledge that is at the heart of integrative nursing practice is also the most important resource we have for self-care. Self-awareness and a capacity for reflexive practice may become the means by which we can remain vital and energized, rather than being drained, in our work.

The same gentle turning toward the self outlined in the previous exercises, noticing what is present in the bodymindspirit and making choices about how to respond, may be applied in clinical practice to help us respond to the demands of nursing practice in ways that support our wholeness and wellbeing. "Wellbeing is created at the subtle level," write Chopra and Tanzi.

> As raw data stream into your brain through the five senses, what turns them into something nourishing or something toxic depends on the quality, flavor and emotional mood that you add...what is primary is the person who is interpreting every experience as it is happening....Learn to rely on the most holistic power you have, which is feeling. Feeling comprises the underpinning of everything. *(Chopra & Tanzi, 2012)*

The following is a model, summarized in Figure 2.3, for accomplishing this that has been developed over many years of working with nurses to support their wellbeing in the workplace. Many other models propose strategies directed at stress-management or preventing burnout that are practiced away from the work setting, such as meditation, relaxation exercises, support groups, and so on. However, in this model, we use the moment-to-moment awareness of our own bodymindspirit to alert us to the need for a course correction, and then to make a shift so that we are energized and not depleted in that moment.

Ways of Responding to the Demands for Energy (Time, Caring, Skill, Relationship)

I have observed that there are two primary modes of responding that most nurses use in an attempt to protect their energy and prevent being drained by the incessant needs and demands that surround them. These two modes may be thought of as the *defensive mode* and the *sympathetic mode*. Both of these ways of responding tend to be unconscious, and neither of them is very effective in accomplishing the task at hand; namely, to protect the nurse from being drained in her or his work. I am using the term *the one-demanding* to represent any persons who have needs to be met and are making demands.

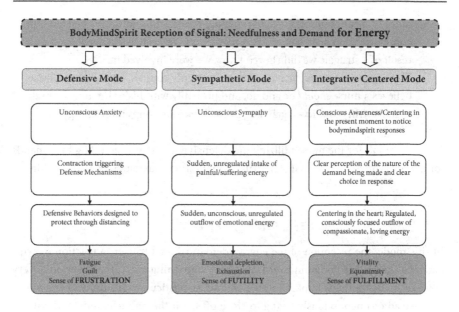

FIGURE 2.3 Adapted from: Quinn, J. F., Client care and nurse involvement in a holistic framework; in Krieger, D., *Foundations for Holistic Nursing*. Philadelphia, PA: J.B. Lippincott, 1981. ©Janet F. Quinn, All Rights Reserved.

THE DEFENSIVE MODE

When the demand for energy (time, caring, skill, relationship, and so on) is registered within the bodymindspirit of the nurse, anxiety is aroused, but, in my experience, typically not noticed. It is as if the demand triggers an unconscious fear of being hooked and drained. This anxiety produces a quality of defensiveness. In experiential exercises, nurses describe the feeling as "tight," "constricting," "closed," and "tense." This manifests in a variety of defensive behaviors, which may include emotional distancing and withdrawal, avoidance of the one-demanding, labeling of or judging the patient or other and thus justifying withdrawal, inappropriate levity and jocularity, false reassurance, or becoming angry with the one-demanding. The possible behaviors that may be utilized as defense mechanisms are as varied as the nurses who use them.

Experience suggests that none of these behaviors helps keep the nurse from being drained, for several reasons:

1. The nurse can never be closed off to the environment. As open systems, whether we are aware of it or not, we are continually exchanging energy with those around us, even when we are deliberately trying not to.
2. Resisting engagement or relationship actually costs us energy. It is a lot of work to maintain defense mechanisms, and a lot of energy is spent in attempting to do so.

3. Since this entire process is to varying degrees unconscious, it is beyond our conscious awareness, control, and regulation. We may end up suffering as a result of a struggle we didn't even know we were involved in.

4. This approach toward clients will most certainly conflict with what the nurse believes a nurse *should* be and do, and probably with his or her image of self as nurse. This conflict—again largely unconscious—saps more energy.

Thus, the result for the nurse utilizing the defensive mode of responding to demands for energy is often fatigue, guilt, and frustration, rather than vitality and flourishing.

THE SYMPATHETIC MODE

In this mode, the reception of the energy-demand signal triggers a reaction of sympathy in the nurse's bodymindspirit. It is as if something about the situation is very close to home, perhaps hooking into a wound or particular sensitivity of the nurse. So, instead of unconsciously trying to close off from the one-demanding, the nurse responds (still unconsciously) with sympathy. "Sympathy" may be defined as the quality of being affected by the state of another with feelings correspondent in kind.

In feeling sympathy, the nurse is literally allowing himself or herself to feel *as* the client does. The client's fears, pain, anxiety, and depression soon become the nurse's. The transfer of these feelings occurs as the energy fields of the client and nurse interact and interpenetrate each other, which they do continually. But in a sympathetic state, it is as if the nurse were taking in the emotionally charged energy of the client and retaining it, rather than dispersing or grounding it. Another way to express this, consistent with some nursing theories, is to say that the nurse's energy field has taken on the pattern of the disturbances in the patient's energy field (Rogers, 1990; Cowling, Smith, & Watson, 2008).

In addition to taking on the pattern of the energies of the client, the sympathetic response includes an outpouring of the nurse's emotional energies in the deep, often unconscious, longing to relieve the suffering being witnessed. The combination of these two factors leaves the sympathetic nurse emotionally drained, exhausted, and often feeling futile, for in reality, sympathy is of little use, even to the patient/one-demanding.

THE INTEGRATIVE CENTERED MODE

When a nurse is practicing from a centered stance, he or she is interacting from a highly conscious and aware perspective. One cannot be more perceptive of the environment without also being more perceptive of oneself; conversely, one does not develop greater self-awareness without also becoming more sensitive to others in the process. It is this very phenomenon that serves to protect the nurse from being drained when interacting with the one-demanding in the integrative centered mode.

As the demand for energy registers in the nurse's bodymindspirit, rather than remaining unconscious, it is recognized at a conscious level because the nurse is in an open, receptive/perceptive state of awareness. This awareness of one's own response can provide a warning signal that there is potential for becoming drained at that moment. The nurse can take a few moments to regroup, or to re-center in the present moment if necessary, before proceeding any further with the one-demanding.

In the centered state, the nurse's sensitivity to self and others is enhanced. The vague awareness of the demand may become more defined. Thus centering serves a dual purpose: (1) to more deeply attune to the state of the other's bodymindspirit and energy, and (2) to give the nurse conscious control of his or her response to the felt demand.

From here, as a further step that will enhance both self-care and optimum response to the one-demanding, the nurse can consciously choose to center in the heart of unconditional love and compassion and make the intention to be an instrument for healing for self and others. The nurse can intentionally generate these feelings of unconditional love and compassion by remembering persons, places, or things that bring one into such a state of being.

Having shifted the state of her or his own bodymindspirit, the nurse may now choose to become an instrument for healing by allowing these energies of love and compassion to simply overflow, as if carried on the out-breath, toward the other. This is the first step in many healing interventions, such as Therapeutic Touch (Quinn, 1994). The centered nurse is able to consciously open to and draw upon the vital energies in the environment and in the subtle realms that surround us, so that as he or she gives energy to the client, he or she is simultaneously replenished. It is like turning on the faucet of the bathtub at the same time that the plug has been pulled. There is neither a tub of stagnating water (the defensive mode) nor a rapidly draining tub (the sympathetic mode). In the integrative centered mode, the outflow of the nurse's energies becomes a conscious, focused, and regulated process, in contrast with the automatic, unconscious, and unregulated reactions that characterize the defensive mode and the sympathetic mode.

Responding to needs and demands in the integrative centered mode usually results in feelings of vitality, equanimity, and fulfillment, making it a powerful tool for self-care.

Using the "Modes of Responding" Model for Self-Discovery and Self-Care

Practice noticing the felt sense of your body at random times. Notice your body when you are feeling happy, energized, sad, angry, peaceful, and so on. If you do this often, you will become very skillful in hearing what your body is saying about your bodymindspirit response to any situation you are in. Your body can thus become a great ally by letting you know when you are about to be drained by mostly unconscious responses to needs of those around you. You can become even more familiar with those responses through the following exercise, which invites you to experience three different scenarios, one for each mode of responding. It will take about five minutes.

Begin by taking several deep breaths, letting go of thoughts and feelings until you come to a centered state in bodymindspirit that can serve as your baseline for this exercise. When you feel you are ready, move on to the first scenario.

1. Imagine someone trying to take something that belongs to you. It doesn't matter what it is. Just let yourself have a vivid sense of a situation in which someone is trying to take something that you don't want to give. Notice your response to this. Where in your body do you notice a response, and what does it feel like? For example, do you notice sensations in your belly, or your jaw, or head, or chest? Do you feel open or closed, expansive or contracted? Is this feeling familiar? Do you like it? Does it seem like a state of being that would help you remain happy and well? Do this for a minute or two to become aware of how your body signals that you are going into the defensive mode of responding. Take a breath and release this experience, coming back to your baseline.

2. Next, imagine being with someone you really feel sorry for; someone (or something—animals, groups of people, the earth itself) in a situation that really hooks you. Repeat the exercise of noticing your body's response to this as you did in the previous scenario. Continue with this inquiry for a few minutes to become aware of how your body signals that you are in the sympathetic mode of responding. Take a breath and release this experience, coming back to your baseline.

3. Last, imagine a person, place, pet, God or higher power, or other being that evokes feelings of unconditional love. Let yourself feel that exchange of love without any expectations. Repeat the exercise of noticing your body's response to this as you did in the previous scenario. Continue with this inquiry for a few minutes to become aware of how your body signals that you are in a centered and loving mode of responding. If you choose, allow this feeling to stay with you as you continue.

This brief exercise demonstrates several things that can be extremely useful to nurse self-care. First, by the end of this exercise, one will have experienced three distinct states of bodymindspirit, all generated, not by what is happening in the environment, but by one's own thoughts and imagination. Thus we witness the fact that our entire being responds to what we are *thinking*, which provides a powerful tool for self-care. Second, one will have experienced the tremendous power for wellbeing that is available to anyone, at any time, simply by allowing the self to center in a state of unconditional love and compassion. With practice, such a state can be generated with just a few breaths and an intention, making it an extremely useful self-care strategy that goes with us wherever we are and whatever the nature of the stressors in our environment.

To apply this exercise in the course of your day:

1. Notice when your body is signaling a defensive and/or a sympathetic response in a situation.
2. Use your breath to center yourself in the present moment.
3. If you choose, center in unconditional love and compassion and become an instrument for healing.

Summary

Nursing within an integrative framework offers a unique opportunity and an exciting challenge. The opportunity is to engage with other human beings at the deepest levels of their existence. It calls us to utilize our whole selves, bodymindspirit, with all of our being-knowing-doing, in assisting people to grow toward increased health and wellbeing. In using ourselves as instruments for healing toward this end, we cannot help but flourish ourselves.

The deepest challenge of integrative nursing may ultimately be one of expanding our self-awareness, self-knowledge, and self-caring. Involvement with people at the level that we have been discussing involves commitment: a commitment to exploring our motivation for such involvement; a commitment to learning about our own limitations and frailties as human beings; a commitment to being honest with ourselves and to accepting ourselves for who we really are without illusion; a commitment to exploring our own depths so that we will not project our fears, uncertainties, judgments, and biases onto our clients; and finally, a commitment to practicing regular and unrelenting self-care both in our personal lives and in our practice, so that we keep ourselves—the instruments for healing—vital, whole, and flourishing.

The process of knowing one's self takes a lifetime. We are never the same person for very long; we are always growing and changing, often more than we expect to (Quoidbach, Gilbert, & Wilson, 2013). But the more deeply we come to know ourselves, the more deeply we can come to know, understand, and care for others. The beauty of nursing within an integrative framework is the realization that we are not ever separate from those we serve, that there is a mutuality in all of our interactions through which we stand to gain every bit as much as those we serve.

SELECTED REFERENCES

Clark, C. (2006). An integral nursing education: Exploration of the Wilber Quadrant Model. *International Journal of Human Caring, 10*(3), 23–29.

Cowling, R., Smith, M., Watson, J. (2008). The power of wholeness, consciousness and caring: A dialogue on nursing science, art and healing. *Advances in Nursing Science*, 31(1), E41–E51.

Goleman, D. (1998). *Working with Emotional Intelligence*. New York: Bantam Books.

Jarrin, O. F. (2012). The integrality of situated caring in nursing and the environment. *Advances in Nursing Science*, 35(1), 14–24.

Letvak, S. A., Ruhm, C. J., Gupta, S. N. (2012). Nurses' presenteeism and its effect on self-reported quality of care and costs. *Am J Nurs*, 112(2), 30–38.

Newman, M. A. (2003). A world of no boundaries. *Advances in Nursing Science*, 26(4), 240–245.

Quinn, J. F. (1994). Caring for the caregiver. In Watson, J. (ed.), *Applying the Art and Science of Human Caring*. New York: National League for Nursing Press, Pub. No. 42–2647.

Quinn, J. F. (1992). Holding sacred space: The nurse as healing environment. *Holistic Nursing Practice*, 6(4):26–36.

Tresolini, C. P. and the Pew-Fetzer Task Force. (1994). *Health Professions Education and Relationship-centered Care*. San Francisco, CA: Pew Health Professions Commission.

Watson, M. J. (2005). *Caring Science as Sacred Science*. Philadelphia, PA: FA Davis.

Wilber, K. (2005). The integral vision of healing. In Schlitz, M., Amorak, T., Micozzi, M. *Consciousness and Healing: Integral Approaches to Mind-Body Medicine*, xv–xxxv. Philadelphia, PA: Elsevier.

3

The Integrated Nurse: Way of the Healer

JANET F. QUINN

*It is the use of self, in a loving and compassionate way, which provides us
with our most powerful instrument for healing.*

—*Quinn, 1984*

A focus on healing whole persons, bodymindspirit, through creating and maintaining caring/healing relationships is a hallmark of nursing. The nurse and the healer are one and the same in the integrated, holistic nurse. Yet many of us have forgotten our heritage as healers as we have become immersed in the sick–cure paradigm that continues to dominate healthcare. We find ourselves increasingly removed from authentic, caring relationships with our patients, and so from the very source of what has meaning and purpose in our work (Quinn, 2000).

There is a profound opportunity for nurses embedded in the movement toward a more integrative healthcare system focused on health promotion and the healing of whole persons through relationship-centered care and the full range of conventional and integrative modalities. The invitation is to reclaim our roots as healers in the lineage of Florence Nightingale, including an unapologetic acknowledgment that what we do is sacred, that who we are is sacred, that the ground we walk on in this work is sacred. We can embrace this knowledge within our own unique and deeply personal understandings of and language for the sacred.

With what is now an interdisciplinary movement, we have a renewed opportunity to recover the *self-as-healer*, an identity embracing the power of our own being, bodymindspirit, as an instrument for healing. Across all the models for an integrative approach to healthcare, we find the practitioner as the starting point. Whole-person healthcare, attending to the full, integral human being, cannot be delivered by practitioners who remain focused on only one dimension of the whole, or who are cut off from their patients' and their own full humanity. To manifest a true healing healthcare system, true healers are necessary.

Healing

WHAT IS HEALING?

Definitions of holistic and integrative medicine and nursing all include healing as a primary focus. The word "heal" comes from the Anglo-Saxon *hælan*, meaning "to be or to become whole," and most nursing literature acknowledges that this is fundamentally what healing is about. Operationalizing this conceptualization, healing has been defined as "the emergence of right relationship at one or more levels of the human experience" (Quinn, 1989, 1992, 1997, 2000, 2013), where the "levels" are the dimensions of being "better represented linguistically as bodymindspirit" (Quinn, 2000) to convey the integral, unitary nature of the whole human being. As the second principle of integrative nursing affirms, healing is an emergent property or process of the whole system. No matter at which level the "right relationship" has emerged, healing will include an increase in the wholeness, order, coherence, and creativity of the whole system (Quinn, 1997, 2013; Dossey, 2003; Siegel, 2012).

Siegel (2012) writes that integration is the fundamental mechanism of health and wellbeing and that the movement of an integrated system, in comparison to one that is disintegrating toward chaos, is in harmony with a sense of coherence. He shares that "An acronym to embrace one interpretation of coherence...is the word itself, COHERENCE: Connected, Open, Harmonious, Engaged, Receptive, Emergent, Noetic, Compassionate, and Empathic" (pp. 16–5).

HEALING VERSUS CURING

Healing may be distinguished from *curing* in several important ways. Perhaps the most important difference is that healing may occur without curing. Healing is the larger construct (Figure 3.1) and may occur without any change, or even a worsening, of the signs and symptoms of disease, as with the chronically ill, the disabled, or the dying. This difference, while widely acknowledged in holistic and integrative nursing and medical literature, continues to provide a challenge for integrative practitioners, because while it seems obvious from a conceptual point of view, there is very little translation of the concept into actual clinical practice.

Tools for assessing healing, as an emergent property or process of whole systems that may or may not have any observable or measureable correlates, have yet to emerge (Quinn et al., 2003, p. A71), and there is no easy way to record such observations on an electronic medical record. Yet on its website the American Nurses Association specifies in its definition of *nursing* that the "provision of a caring relationship that facilitates health and healing" is the first essential feature of professional nursing.

Integrative nurses have this disciplinary mandate as one justification to claim time and attention for whole-person/whole-system healing, despite the challenges of

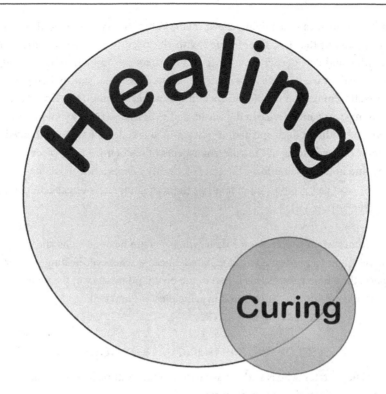

FIGURE 3.1 Healing and Curing

measuring its achievement. In addition, integrative nurses could form meaningful research questions related to healing from their clinical practice, an approach to research recommended by the Institute of Medicine (Olsen, Aisner, & McGinnis, 2007). My colleagues and I have proposed using the integral framework for this purpose (Quinn et al., 2003).

The second difference between healing and curing is that healing is always possible, whereas curing may or may not be possible. Because a right relationship (any shift within the system that manifests the qualities of healing identified earlier) can emerge within, between, and among any dimension(s) of the system, there is no limit to when, where, or how healing manifests, up to and including the moment of death; some would say that death itself is a healing. Sometimes the acceptance that curing is an unlikely outcome opens the door for a person to begin what becomes a true healing journey to new levels of wholeness previously unimagined. Such was the case for physician Deb Zucker, who shares her integral healing experience:

> This healing journey, which is ongoing, has been one of awakening to what it is to be embodied, although by no means did I have that perspective when my journey began. At first the focus was simply on my physicality, the symptoms,

and the remedies that might relieve them. When the symptoms did not resolve, I found that I was confronted with the need to broaden my focus of attention and dive deeper. Thus I began a conscious examination of my "self," and how the various parts were contributing to my current state of being. I explored the contexts of my life, my meaning making, my emotions, my relationships, my work and service in the world, and over time arrived at holding these elements within a deep spiritual inquiry and surrender. I have experienced a complex interweaving of the different aspects of my being. I have come to understand how they all inform the state of vitality I experience, and how a shift in one facet can profoundly influence others in completely unexpected ways. (Zucker, 2011, p. 131)

Sometimes when people pursue their whole-person healing, signs and symptoms of disease are in fact mitigated or eliminated, because whenever healing is emerging, it impacts the whole system. This is part of the profound mystery of the innate healing response affirmed by integrative nursing principles one and two.

WHO OR WHAT IS THE SOURCE OF HEALING?

Echoing Hippocrates, who is said to have written that "Natural forces within us are the true healers of disease," Nightingale instructed thusly:

It is often thought that medicine is the curative process. It is no such thing; medicine is the surgery of functions as surgery is that of limbs and organs. Neither can do anything but remove obstructions; neither can cure. Medicine, so far as we know, assists nature to remove the obstruction but does nothing more. Nature alone cures. (Nightingale, 1859/1969, p. 133)

This understanding is as relevant today as it was when Nightingale, the founder of modern nursing, wrote it. All healing—and curing in the sense that Nightingale is discussing—emerges from/as the unfolding, unitary life process of the whole, complex, adaptive system that is manifesting right relationship. This emergence is sometimes assisted by, but not due to, what healing practitioners bring into the system through any of its dimensions. Medicines and treatments, traditional or complementary and alternative, may be *necessary* causes of healing or curing, but they are not *sufficient* causes. Only the bodymindspirit that is the one-healing can utilize the inputs provided to unfold a healing response, and even that one is not in complete control. "All a good doctor or therapist can do is arrange circumstances to increase the probability of healing" (A. Weil, *The Healer Archetype*, http://www.altjn.com/ideas/healer_archetype.htm (accessed 5/20/2012 2:10:52 PM).

WHAT IS THE ROLE OF THE INTEGRATIVE NURSE
IN HEALING?

Integrative nurses facilitate healing by following Nightingale's directive to "put the patient in the best condition for nature to act upon him" (Nightingale, 1859/1969, p. 133). This is the organizing principle that guides our integrative approach. But what does Nature want to do, and how do we help facilitate that?

Through studying billions of years of evolution, scientists observe that nature wants to move individuals and systems in the direction of increasing complexity and diversity, towards increasing wholeness, integration, and transcendence (Quinn, 2000; Rogers, 1990; Wilber, 1996; Siegel, 2012). This teleological impulse toward wholeness *is* the innate self-healing capacity of every living system, yet it has often been dismissed as "just" the placebo effect, the bane of researchers attempting to find "real" effects through controlled clinical trials of drugs. To offer a counter-position, one that honors rather than dismisses the total, organismic response in the direction of increasing wholeness and integration, I have called this response the Haelan Effect (Quinn, 1989, 2013).

With this understanding, eliciting the Haelan Effect becomes the primary goal toward which all of our care is directed. Once the source of healing is recognized to be the one-healing and not the practitioner or the treatments, then there are no longer "real" and "fake" treatments. As the fifth principle of integrative nursing suggests, there are simply more or less natural, more or less invasive, and more or less effective facilitators of the innate healing response, or Haelan Effect. To view nursing practice in this way would be a paradigm shift of major proportion, empowering nurses and all health-care practitioners to, among other things, actively develop the self-as-healer.

It may be that such a paradigm shift is underway. Recently there has been increasing interest in studying the placebo effect to understand the self-healing capacity of living systems. The front page of the April 2012 issue of the *Harvard Health Letter* carried this headline: "Putting the Placebo Effect to Work—Rather than dismiss it, we should try to understand the placebo and harness it when we can." The lead article reported on research at the Program in Placebo Studies and the Therapeutic Encounter, founded in 2011 by Harvard University Medical School and hosted at Beth Israel Deaconess Medical Center. The program's website explains its purpose:

> For many years, the placebo effect was considered to be no more than a nuisance variable that needed to be controlled in clinical trials. Only recently have researchers redefined it as the key to understanding the healing that arises from medical ritual, the context of treatment, the patient-provider relationship and the power of imagination, trust and hope. Although our biomedical health care system often considers these humanistic dimensions of care as secondary to the administration of pharmaceuticals and procedures, the emerging field of

placebo studies is producing scientific evidence that these more intangible elements of medicine may fundamentally contribute to the improvement of patient outcomes. (http://programinplacebostudies.org; accessed 5-21-12)

It should be noted that, as of this writing, nursing is not represented in the list of disciplines engaged with the Center, and there are no nurse researchers listed in the roster of members, in spite of the fact that most literature on the healing relationship is in nursing. This is an area of system change that integrative nurses could and should engage.

Reviewing the previous ten years of research literature on placebos, authors of a 2010 paper published in *Lancet* concluded that:

Placebo effects are genuine psychobiological events attributable to the overall therapeutic context, and these effects can be robust in both laboratory and clinical settings. There is also evidence that placebo effects can exist in clinical practice, even if no placebo is given. (Finniss et al., 2010, p. 686)

In a 2011 commentary on recent placebo research, Brody and Miller wrote that practitioners have multiple means of helping to activate "powerful inner pathways that assist healing" (p. 2613). Walach and Jonas (2004) noted that many attempts to define the placebo effect all have one thing in common—they all define placebo effects as something negative. The authors call for redefining the placebo effect as the effect that is due to the meaning of a therapeutic intervention for a particular patient and context. They suggest that, instead of viewing the placebo effect as a problem, it "should be seen as a ubiquitous healing response mediated by expectations and conditioning. Thus it can be utilized to enhance or interfere with healing in many clinical settings. By understanding the meaning response, we might understand how optimal healing can be fostered" (p. 103).

The authors provide a table of "ways to enhance *healing responses*" (emphasis added) found in the placebo literature, some of which are shown in Box 3.1. The reader will recognize these strategies as part of regular, expert nursing care since the time of Nightingale.

HOW DO INTEGRATIVE NURSES FACILITATE HEALING?

Putting the patient in the best condition to elicit and support the emergence of the healing response, or the Haelan Effect, is the goal of all nursing. Seen in this way, with the source of healing clearly located within the one-healing, the integrative nurse is called to be a facilitator/instrument of healing (Quinn, 1984, 2000, 2013).

Within the integrative framework, paralleling Dossey's "Era III medicine" (Dossey, 1999) and Newman's "unitary-transformative paradigm" (Newman, 1994, 2008), the

Box 3.1 Ways to Enhance The Healing Response

- Deliver therapies in a warm and caring way.
- Deliver therapies with confidence and in a credible way.
- Determine what treatment your patient believes in or not.
- Deliver a benign but frequent conditioned stimulus along with the effective therapy.
- Inform the patient what they can expect.
- Incorporate reassurance, relaxation, suggestion, and anxiety reduction methods into the delivery.
- Listen and provide empathy and understanding.
- Touch the patient.

(*Source*: Walach and Jonas, 2004)

nurse is not a separate other, but is integral with the healing process via shared consciousness and energy. Through the healing relationship, the nurse can become both "medicine" and a healing environment for whole-person healing, a process through which both nurse and patient are made more whole (Quinn, 1992, Watson, 2005). Recalling principles four and five for integrative nursing, integrative nurses include and transcend the traditional tools of competent care to bring the fullness of their own integral being-knowing-doing into the service of healing. Box 3.2 identifies some of the ways of being-knowing-doing that integrative nurses use to facilitate healing.

EXEMPLAR: HEALING INTO DEATH

An example of healing in the absence of curing comes from my private practice. It involves a woman whom I met first by phone and then in person on the evening before her brain surgery. She had been referred to me because I am both a nurse and a spiritual director. Pat had been diagnosed with a brain tumor that was almost assuredly a glioblastoma, and was having the procedure to confirm and stage the cancer. I was met by this seventy-six-year-old woman at the door of her hospital room. Pat was wearing her own bathrobe, a brightly colored hat from her daughter, and a huge smile. As we sat together in the solarium, with the fish as our silent witnesses, I listened to her story unfold. Among other things, I learned that she had a decades-long practice of "centering prayer" (a contemplative practice out of the Catholic tradition) and also engaged in a wide variety of other meditative processes from across traditions. In addition, she enjoyed reading about consciousness and "awakening" from different spiritual perspectives. After a while, I suggested that we take five minutes in silence together to first quiet ourselves, and then to invite the deep knowing within her being to arise. I asked

> ## Box 3.2 The Integrative Nurse Facilitates Healing Through (at Least) the Following Ways of Being-Knowing-Doing
>
> - Caring
> - Holding sacred space and becoming the environment in which healing may emerge
> - Creating caring/healing relationships with self and others, including patients, families, and colleagues
> - Paying attention and focusing intention for healing and wholeness during ordinary nursing care procedures
> - Using the full range of available therapeutic modalities, moving from least intensive/invasive to more, depending on need and content (Principle 5 of Integrative Nursing)
> - Cultivating and practicing love

Pat to simply be aware of whatever arose, without effort or judgment. After five minutes, I used a gentle gong to bring her awareness back to the solarium.

She opened her eyes, and I will never forget the radiance of being that I was privileged to encounter in that moment, and in fact, in every moment I spent with her until her death a mere seven weeks later. Pat was utterly and completely at peace with the diagnosis and the prognosis. She told me that she was in no way inclined to "fight this." She saw the tumor as an agent of her unfolding journey, bringing a "final adventure" that she was curious about and felt equipped to meet. In her view, the tumor was an uninvited guest that nevertheless was not intrinsically evil but was just being itself, and which had arrived to gently escort her home. I was reminded of a Rumi poem called "The Guest House," and I asked her if she knew it. She laughed, and said it was one of her favorites.

Pat maintained this same friendliness toward the tumor even as it very quickly took away function after function. This was a woman who was dying of a brain tumor, healed. She was flourishing in the fullness of her own being and in her deepening relationship with God, inviting her family and all those around her to the same.

> "The Guest House"
> This being human is a guest house
> Every morning a new arrival.
> A joy, a depression, a meanness,
> some momentary awareness comes
> as an unexpected visitor.
> Welcome and entertain them all!

Even if they are a crowd of sorrows,
who violently sweep your house
empty of its furniture,
still treat each guest honorably.
He may be clearing you out for some new delight.
The dark thought, the shame, the malice,
meet them at the door laughing, and invite them in.
Be grateful for whoever comes,
because each has been sent
as a guide from beyond.

(From: *The Essential Rumi*, by Coleman Barks, [HarperOne, 2004], p. 109, used with permission.)

The Way of the Healer

Not all healthcare professionals are healers, although healthcare practice provides fertile ground for the cultivation of the self-as-healer in one who aspires to it. The healer is a major archetypal pattern or potential, one of many that reside in the collective unconscious described by Carl Jung (1951). In her study of archetypes, Carolyn Myss writes that "the healer archetype manifests as a passion to serve others through repairing of the body, mind and spirit." She adds that the archetype can manifest in people in any occupation, not just through professionals in the healthcare system (Myss, http://www.myss.com/library/contracts/archetypes.asp, accessed 1/14/13). The converse, as one can readily observe in clinical practice, is also true; namely, that being a healthcare professional does not necessarily mean that one is a healer in this full archetypal sense. One can do his or her job every day, more or less effectively, without walking the way of the healer. What makes the difference?

As an archetype, the healer is unconscious potential. I would suggest that *the way of the healer* is a conscious activation of that archetypal pattern of energy and inspiration. The way of the healer is a consciously chosen and actively cultivated path that puts one in service to life, self, others, and creation as an instrument for healing (Quinn, 1984). Box 3.3 identifies some of the characteristics of healers across cultures.

Walking the way of the healer goes beyond expert clinical competence to involve the integrated, whole being who aspires to move through life, not just work, with and as a healing presence. Arrien describes the healer as the one who pays attention to what has heart and meaning (1993). The way of the healer is chosen as the guiding direction for one's life because one feels called and impelled to follow. For such a person, not following the call to be of service as a healer would amount to a profound self-betrayal, because the call is from the deepest dimensions of being, which some would call the soul.

Box 3.3 Characteristics or Commonalities of Healers Across Cultures

1. A sense of calling or vocation—the feeling that this is one's destiny, that one would do this even if one didn't get paid; longing to serve. There is a love of the work itself.
2. A world view that:
    a. embraces mystery and uncertainty—an awe for all that is unknown and a respect for it, rather than seeking certainty and predictability.
    b. is holistic and global versus particularistic and local.
    c. acknowledges non-material reality or spiritual realities.
    d. invites partnership and participation versus control and domination.
    e. places him or her in the role of nature's helper versus nature's master. Non-heroic.
3. Self-awareness and impeccable integrity.
4. Detached commitment—which goes with trusting the process.
5. Curiosity.
6. Genuine love for people; motivated by love and compassion, the genuine and deep enjoyment and appreciation of people as infinitely worthwhile and deserving of joy, love, healing, and wholeness.
7. Non-judgement—allowing people to find their own path in their own time in their own style.
8. ALLOW—*Always, Love Leaves Others Whole.*

Nurses and other healthcare professionals who continue to consciously remain fully present and offer authentic care, in spite of overwhelming challenges, are walking the way of the healer. They don't necessarily use this language or recognize what they do as a way or a path. Yet when it has been named in hundreds of speeches and workshops I've presented, they are often moved to tears in recognition and acknowledgement. This is one reason that the way of the healer is important to name—to support and acknowledge what some nurses are already doing and help them further develop the self-as-healer. Another is to give language and a context that can invite and empower all nurses to claim their work as sacred path and to consciously cultivate it.

RECOGNIZING AND TENDING TO THE HEALER'S VULNERABILITY

There is profound vulnerability associated with our work as healers. Every working day, nurses put their bodies on the line for others; for example, through exposure to toxic pathogens and chemicals; lifting, pushing, and long, back-to-back shifts without adequate time for breaks, proper nutrition, and enough rest. Add to this the physical and emotional stress of working with too few nurses and increasing numbers of really sick patients, a problem created by the healthcare system. Nurses frequently work when they themselves are not well, a practice known as *presenteeism*, which is costly to nurses, and also to patients and systems, while the rate of depression in some groups of nurses is as much as twice the rate in the general population (Letvak et al., 2012). Burnout and compassion fatigue are well-known and significant problems.

If we are truly engaged in the inter-subjective openness that the caring/healing relationship requires, we are emotionally and spiritually vulnerable. In this space, we are witnesses to and participants in the sorrows, trials, pains, and struggles of the people in our care. We are vulnerable, too, to our own suffering arising in response, and to the suffering of our friends and colleagues. Finally, all health professionals carry the burden of knowing that every hour we work holds the possibility of making an error, which is a profound vulnerability.

Sometimes we are made vulnerable in our work, and yet redeemed by patients. I recall such an instance from when I was a very young nurse, working evenings on a general medical surgical unit. I followed the physician's orders to "D/C continuous bladder irrigation" on a patient who had just undergone a transurethral prostatectomy procedure a few hours before, by taking out his Foley catheter. My charge nurse saw me walking down the hallway with the irrigation set up and the Foley and, not quietly, asked me, "What have you done?" I suddenly realized my error, and I almost fainted.

After sitting down and gathering myself, I had to go in and tell this man that not only had I made a mistake, but now he would have to undergo the reinsertion of a catheter. I was utterly humiliated and felt nauseous. I had wanted to be a nurse since I was five years old, and here I was, already a failure, causing more pain to someone who trusted me to care for him. Maybe he would scream at me. Maybe I would be sued. Maybe I would lose my job. I went in to his room and sat down by his bed, trying to find the right words. "What's the matter? you look like you've seen a ghost," he said, with genuine concern. I explained what I had done, and what would have to be done, and I apologized over and over, asking for his forgiveness. He took my hand, looked me right in the eye and said, "Everyone makes mistakes, it's not the end of the world!" I burst in to tears as he absolved me from my overwhelming guilt, lifting me out of my vulnerability. I have never forgotten that kindness, nor the humility it taught me.

Not all stories of nurse vulnerability end with this kind of redemption. So in walking the way of the healer, we must redeem ourselves, and each other; heal ourselves, and each other; be tender to ourselves, and each other; nurture ourselves, and each other; love ourselves, and each other. Using inquiry as a practice to move through the body, mind, and spirit dimensions of our being, we can notice and name the vulnerabilities we feel and take measures to address them.

It is hard work, but it is crucial because it is the naming of our vulnerabilities that allow them to be met with deep appreciation, self-love, and self-compassion.

Unacknowledged vulnerability and unnamed pain makes one defensive, cold, hard, and harsh. It leads to depression, burnout, increased illness, and decreased flourishing. It is our sacred duty to stay in touch with our whole self and to do what we need to do to tend ourselves well as we walk the way of the healer (see Chapter 2, "The Integrated Nurse," for many ways to address nurse self-care). Without this self-care, we cannot continue to be an effective instrument for healing.

The reclamation of our call to be healers can provide a powerful antidote to the burnout and loss of meaning that seems epidemic in our modern healthcare system. As discussed earlier, this is one of the great opportunities of the integrative movement in nursing and medicine for all healthcare professionals. The inner and outer work of growing more integrated manifests in our own increased flourishing as well as in the quality we bring to all of our relationships and communities. It translates directly to our ability to assess, plan, implement, and evaluate nursing care from an integrative perspective.

Since the caregiver and the caring/healing relationship are seen as essential elements of the integrative model, nurses have an opening, actually a mandate, to explore the full meaning and potential of the self-as-healer.

THE WAY OF THE HEALER AS SPIRITUAL PRACTICE: THE ULTIMATE POSSIBILITY OF INTEGRATIVE NURSING

Nursing is a special case of loving.

—Sidney Jourard

The world's spiritual traditions tell us that love is both purpose and path on the spiritual journey. Love is the means by which we can come into closer relationship with the divine, the Holy Mystery, the Nameless that is called by many names across time and cultures. Love, we are also told by many traditions, is the nature of the Divine itself. Thus love is both that which we seek and the path by which we seek it.

Angeles Arrien (1990), an anthropologist who has studied indigenous healers across cultures, writes that "healers in all major traditions recognize that the power of love is the most potent healing force available to all human beings. Effective healers from any culture are those who extend love, and all the arms of love—gratitude, acceptance, recognition, validation, and acknowledgement."

Dean Ornish, the cardiologist who first demonstrated that heart disease can be reversed, concurs with Arrien and summarizes the literature about love and health when he writes: "I am not aware of any other factor in medicine—not diet, not smoking, not exercise, not stress, not genetics, not drugs, not surgery—that has a greater impact on our quality of life, incidence of illness, and premature death from all causes" (1998, p. 3).

The desire that all beings be well and free from suffering is at the very heart of the way of the healer. It is the healer's deepest wish and his or her most compelling motivation, and it is a definition of love. It is the reason that nurse-healers persist in their profoundly challenging work. And this is why the way of the healer is a deep spiritual practice, capable of helping us develop into the fullness of our potential as compassionate, loving human beings. Nightingale was unequivocal about this call of nurses when she wrote: "Strive to awaken the divine spirit of love in yourself, to awaken it in doing your present work, however you may have erred in the past"(Nightingale, 1860/1994, p. 96).

Here is our hope and the full potential of the emerging model of integrative nursing. No matter how far we have drifted from the way of the healer, no matter how burned out we might have felt, we can begin again. Intention by intention, breath by breath, we can strive to develop our capacity for love in service of life and healing. And in the process, we will inevitably be transformed.

We are assured by the wisdom traditions that if we take up spiritual practice, eventually we will notice a new depth of compassion arising. Out of our own fierce and tender struggle comes a deep longing for humanity, for the creatures, and for the earth itself. It is the hope that is so beautifully expressed in the loving-kindness practice that comes to us from the Buddhist tradition: that all beings be happy, well, peaceful, and free from suffering.

This arising compassion can become a source of energy for new or reignited action in the world, action that Andrew Harvey (2009) has called "sacred activism." Through our sacred activism, walking the way of the healer, integrative nurses heal and transform themselves, and in so doing, heal and transform the world.

> Could it be that the human heart and the world's heart are one? We believe that they are. As we grow in love and strength, we become vehicles for the world's growth. We bring new sustenance to our families, new joy to our friends, new light to our places of work. We enhance the physical things around us, and the earth itself.... It becomes more and more evident that our own wellbeing is indissolubly linked to the health of society and our environment. It is possible, now more than ever before, to see that our own growth is rooted in, and furthers, the whole world's advance. (Leonard & Murphy, 1995 p. xi).

SELECTED REFERENCES

Arrien, A. (1993). *The Four-Fold Way: Walking the Paths of the Warrior, Teacher, Healer, and Visionary.* New York: HarperOne.

Brody, H., & Miller, H. G. (2011). Lessons from recent research about the placebo effect—from art to science. *JAMA. 306*(23), 2612–2613.

Letvak, S. A., Ruhm, C. J., & Gupta, S. N. (2012). Nurse presenteeism and its effects on self-reported quality of care and costs. *Am J Nurs, 112*(2): 30–38.

Quinn, J. F. (1992). Holding sacred space: The nurse as healing environment. *Holistic Nursing Practice*, 6(4), 26–36.

Quinn, J. F. (1997). Healing: A model for an integrative health care system. *Advanced Practice Nursing Quarterly*, 3(1), 1–7.

Quinn, J. F. (2013). Transpersonal human caring and healing. In Dossey, B.M., Keegan, L. (eds.). *Holistic Nursing: A Handbook for Practice*, 6th ed. Burlington, MA: Jones & Bartlett Learning.

Rogers, M. E. (1990). Nursing: Science of unitary, irreducible, human beings. In Barrett, E. A. M., ed., *Visions of Rogers' Science-Based Nursing*. pp. 5–11. New York: National League for Nursing.

Siegel, D. J. (2012). *Pocket Guide to Interpersonal Neurobiology*. New York: Norton.

Watson, J. (2005). *Caring Science as Sacred Science*. Philadelphia, PA: FA Davis.

Wilber, K. (1996). *A Brief History of Everything*. Boston: Shambhala.

4

Whole-Systems Healing:
A New Leadership Path

MARY JO KREITZER, WITH EXEMPLAR BY JAYNE FELGEN
AND PATRICIA A. ROACH

Integrative nursing embodies a whole person and whole-systems approach to advancing the health and wellbeing of people, organizations, communities, and the environment. It is a whole-systems healing approach that at the core is based on the simple yet profound understanding that all living systems are interconnected; thus a change in any part of the system creates change in other parts of the system. This chapter focuses on leadership, the changing environments in which we work, and the competencies that leaders need to embody to be effective within organizations and systems that are increasingly complex and turbulent. Understanding how to work effectively within a system is critical to advancing integrative nursing.

The Changing Nature of Work Settings

The days of command and control leadership have evaporated.

—David Gergen,
Director of the Harvard
University Center for Public Leadership

For decades, the hierarchical command and control style of leadership was embraced as the most effective way to tackle problems and lead change. The authority of leaders came from their positional power, and it was seen as the role of the leader to hold the vision, tell subordinates what to do, maintain stability, and fix problems. Whether this approach to leadership ever worked effectively is open to debate. What is now clear is that the nature of our work settings and the problems that we face require a fundamentally different approach.

Many of the issues and challenges we face in workplaces and society as a whole have been described as "wicked problems." Wicked problems are not just complicated and messy; they are complex, driven by forces we often cannot see or control, and they are not resolved by routine and predictable solutions. As noted by Brown et al. (2010), wicked problems are not solved by fixed trajectories of preexisting research pathways. They demand that decision makers explore the full range of investigative avenues. "Tame" problems may be complicated, but they have occurred before, are known or routine and predictable solutions can be readily applied to resolve them.

Healthcare today faces an abundance of wicked problems. There are many external forces that make the healthcare environment particularly uncontrollable, unpredictable, and volatile. The acronym VUCA is being used to describe environments or conditions that reflect volatility, uncertainty, complexity, and ambiguity (Johansen, 2007). Worldwide, healthcare costs are escalating, health disparities are growing, and gaps in systems are widening. There is an epidemic of lifestyle-related diseases and enormous uncertainty as to which models and reimbursement structures will endure. Pouring more money and resources into existing systems is unlikely to produce different results. Increasingly, there is a recognition that we need a fundamentally different approach that embraces new models—such as integrative nursing—that is interdisciplinary, and that has as a goal whole-systems healing.

Whole-Systems Healing

Whole-systems healing (Kreitzer, 2012) is a much bigger and more expansive way to view the world. It is a way of addressing problems and cultivating the health and wellbeing of individuals, organizations, communities, and the environment by living and acting with awareness of the wholeness and the interconnectedness of all living systems. It requires an understanding of several critical key concepts:

- Complexity Science/Chaos Theory: All living systems, from individual humans and communities, to the ecosystem of the planet, are complex systems that are constantly adapting and evolving in response to changing conditions from within and outside.
- Social Networks: Social networks are social structures made up of individuals or organizations that are connected or interrelated. The ties can be social, economic, or organizational.
- Social Change: Social change is a process whereby values, attitudes, or institutions of society become modified.
- Gentle Action: As articulated by David Peat (2005), gentle action is the use of grassroots efforts and collective intelligence to focus many small, coordinated efforts on the best point of leverage within a given system. It is the strategic implementation of highly coordinated, low-intensity actions.

Whole-systems healing is not only a way to address problems or resolve issues, it is an approach, as described in the exemplar highlighted in this chapter, of shifting the culture within an organization. Within many organizations, embracing or adopting integrative nursing or relationship-based care is a culture change that also calls for bold and innovative leadership.

Whole-Systems Leadership

In describing the type of leadership that is now required in organizations, Adam Kahne (2007), author of *Solving Tough Problems: An Open Way of Talking, Listening and Creating New Realities*, notes that leadership must be systemic, participative, and emergent.

- Systemic—not piecemeal or based on a "silo" mentality
- Participative—involving many people's ideas, energy, talent, and expertise
- Emergent—able to move and adapt nimbly in a minefield of uncertainty

Whole-systems leadership embraces this approach and is a departure from conventional leadership, as illustrated in Table 4.1. In the whole-systems framework,

Table 4.1: Conventional and Whole-Systems Leadership

	Conventional View of Leadership	*Whole-Systems Leadership*
Leadership is...	a position or role of authority	an activity or behavior that can arise anywhere in a human system
Leadership flows...	in one direction: from the top down	in all directions
Leadership is exercised...	by individuals with special leadership traits	collectively by groups and/or by individuals informed by the collective
Effective leadership comes from...	accurately anticipating a predictable path to a predetermined outcome	recognizing and influencing patterns that are present in human systems at all levels
Leadership requires...	certainty, clear vision, and the power of persuasion and control	willingness to embrace uncertainty, listen to all voices, and take adaptive action, often in collaboration with others
Leadership creates...	harmony and stability	conditions that are conducive to groups' moving forward—which sometimes means disrupting the habitual patterns of engagement so that groups, communities, or organizations can set the conditions for a preferred future
The purpose of leadership is to...	fix problems and leverage opportunities to achieve goals	enable adaptability, learning, and innovation so that groups make progress on the issues they care about—even in unpredictable and changing conditions
Leadership can make a difference through...	one large strategic intervention designed to fix a problem or achieve a goal	recognizing emerging patterns in human systems and making meaning out of many small changes

Source: Morris, 2011

leadership is viewed as a behavior that can show up any place in the organization. It is not tied to having a role or a position with authority. While a conventional leadership approach focuses on control and stability, a whole-systems approach recognizes that disrupting habitual patterns may be just what is needed to move the organization forward. A conventional leadership approach may direct time and attention to fixing problems and leveraging opportunities to achieve goals. While goal-oriented as well, a whole-systems approach would also be focused on assuring that the organization is building capacity for adaptability, learning, and innovation.

Reflect and Discuss: Do you agree with Adam Kahne that these times demand leadership that is systematic, participative, and emergent? What else do you think would be helpful for leadership in these dynamic and challenging times?

WHOLE-SYSTEMS LEADERSHIP COMPETENCIES

Leaders who embody whole-systems leadership have knowledge, skills, and attitudes that enable them to generate appropriate and effective responses to complex situations. The six core competencies (Morris, 2011) include:

1. *Deep listening:* Conversations have the power to transform our understanding and generate innovative options for action. A key component of successful conversations is "deep listening," which means listening to learn and temporarily suspending judgment.
2. *Awareness of systems:* Whole-systems leadership understands communities, organizations, and groups as adaptive, changing systems. With an awareness of systems, you get a fuller perspective of the situation, which expands and refines your options for action.
3. *Awareness of self:* Developing self-awareness is the necessary beginning to developing skillful ways to respond to situations. If you are not aware of your motivations, feelings, and beliefs, you cannot make effective decisions about how to behave.
4. *Seeking diverse perspectives:* A whole-systems approach thrives on the respectful inclusion of all voices. From this viewpoint, conflicting opinions do not present a problem; rather, they present a potential resource that can sharpen thinking and lead to innovative options for action.
5. *Suspending certainty, embracing uncertainty:* Suspending certainty enables you to see beyond your habitual lenses to get a broader and potentially more

accurate view of what is going on. It also creates room for diverse views so that new or different knowledge can come forth.

6. *Taking adaptive action:* Adaptive action means learning from everything you do. It means taking time to recognize patterns and reflect on their meaning before jumping to a solution. It balances an inclusive, deep listening approach with a bias towards action.

The following exemplar brings these competencies to life in describing a change process in a hospital in Utica, New York, where visionary leaders made a sustained, long-term commitment to build a new organization out of the consolidation of two struggling hospitals. The story highlights how deep grief, disconnection, and a struggling financial bottom line was transformed into an organization-wide commitment to improving relationships, a shared vision around excellence in patient care, and the emergence of leadership from literally every corner of the organization.

A Story of Whole-Systems Leadership: The Soul Has Left the Building
Jayne Felgen and Pat Roach

When Faxton Hospital and St. Luke's Memorial consolidated, staff felt as though they had no choice in the matter. They were two beleaguered hospitals, both struggling financially: one union and the other non-union, former competitors poised to come together whether any of the individuals involved wanted to or not. Shortly after the consolidation, one of the staff physicians remarked, "It feels like the soul has left the building." Painful as they were, the words rang true.

A primary concern in the midst of all the change was patient care. During the most disruptive phases of the physical consolidation, teams felt perilously disconnected. It was only a matter of time before it was anticipated that patient outcomes would reflect a lack of communication and inadequate collaboration. Leaders in the organization recognized that they could not sustain the delivery of quality patient care unless they worked directly on improving the quality of relationships everywhere in the organization.

Leaders had heard of *relationship-based care* (RBC) (Koloroutis, 2004) and believed that it had value, but they were uncertain whether the executive team could be convinced that improving relationships could transform the culture. There was agreement that more than a quick fix was needed, and it seemed that RBC had the potential to create a long-term, sustainable benefit.

In some organizations, RBC had been implemented as a "nurses only" model, but it was always the intention in this institution for it to be interdisciplinary. The initiative started with nursing before opening it up to other disciplines. After the first wave of implementation, however, it was evident to the whole team that every person in the organization, regardless of job description, needed to be engaged in order to sustain the change that was desired. A decision was made that RBC would be multidisciplinary, and the principles underlying this philosophy were introduced in such a way that they were as relevant to a staff person who didn't provide direct patient care as they were to a bedside nurse. The leadership team modeled the change they wanted to see. They were visible, accessible, and willing to be flexible to better serve patient and their families. Staff were invited to co-create the new shared vision.

The magnitude of the culture shift was evident when, in a celebration of RBC six years post-implementation, staff from every corner of the hospital stepped up to talk about what their practice meant to them. In some cases, the "practice" had little to do with direct patient care. A leader emerged from the cleaning service; he built relationships with every patient and family on his floor and had taken the initiative numerous times to take up collections for families in need, once helping to deliver a new bed to a family whose home and belongings were infested with bedbugs. He understood how his role was integral to the corporate vision for patient care—that every person and position matters.

A poignant story was shared at the celebration of how staff in three departments, including risk-management, collaborated to help a young father-to-be who was deployed in Afghanistan participate in the birth of his child via Skype. This story was pivotal in that it reflected "a new soul coming into our building" and a way of working together that demonstrated a transformed culture. In the old organization—one that was rule bound and relationship-hampered—the capacity would not have been there to respond to a patient or family need in this way. It was a fitting story to tell on a day that celebrated how very far the organization had come. It was clear that day that the spirit of the hospital had really changed. There was more love and compassion everywhere and a strong focus on relationships—all relationships. RBC helped the staff in the organization reconnect with the sacredness of their work.

The cost of this endeavor was not trivial. In addition to consultant time, staff from every department were compensated for participating in educational sessions. In addition to patient and staff outcomes, there was also a financial return on investment. Two-thirds of the hospitals in New York State presently operate in the red. This hospital is in the black.

Reflection on Whole-Systems Healing and Leadership

As we look back on what it took to bring about the extraordinary cultural transformation at Faxton St. Luke's, we can see that the framework embraced by whole-systems leadership provides us with a helpful lens. Here's how the six WSL practices played out in the Faxton St. Luke's consolidation and continue to do so to this day.

DEEP LISTENING

Deep listening shows up everywhere in relationship-based care. First, it's about listening to the patient. What is each person's unique story, and what of real value do I have to offer this person today? Each day, we ask patients to tell us about their goals and to name for us their primary concern. During the consolidation (and beyond), it was also extremely important for us to listen to the staff. In the beginning of our consolidation journey, the staff felt that decisions were being made without their input. That turned around pretty quickly, however, when we started asking people about their work. Over time, our most productive question turned out to be, "What is your favorite workaround?" "If you don't have the supplies you need," for example, "what do you do?" If our inquiry revealed that they sometimes went to another floor to get supplies, we knew we had to fix their supply issues. When we ask about people's practice and make visible changes based on their input, they begin to see what an important part they play in helping things run better.

AWARENESS OF SYSTEMS

Every person in an organization is connected to everyone else, and every department is connected to every other department. We have what we call "report outs" by Unit Practice Council (UPC) representatives from every department so that people can see the interconnectedness of the actions on the whole. At one UPC check-in meeting, a representative from laundry services held up a "sharps container." He shook it to show that it was half full of sharps (e.g., scalpels, suture needles), all of which had come down the laundry chute wrapped in sheets and surgical towels. The people in the laundry were being exposed to dirty needles and bloody surgical blades. Everyone could see that they needed to reflect on their practice and make some changes in order to keep the laundry staff safe.

AWARENESS OF SELF

We did a lot of self-reflection as part of the consolidation process. We learned early on to check in with ourselves about our own motives. We would pause and ask, "Who are we really doing this for?" Creative Health Care Management's *Re-Igniting the Spirit of Caring* workshop was key in helping all of us—especially those in leadership positions—remember that we are all here to be healers, even if we aren't working directly in patient care.

SEEKING DIVERSE PERSPECTIVES

At Faxton St. Luke's, every council leader gets a chance to let the entire organization know what's important in his or her world. In 2004, as we started the consolidation, people said they wanted a voice. Now people from every corner of the organization have a voice in the organization. We're always asking, "What assistance do you need from the leadership team?" The executive team takes every issue seriously, and we do everything possible to come to the best conclusion.

SUSPENDING CERTAINTY, EMBRACING UNCERTAINTY

If you're going to be a decision maker in the chaotic world of healthcare, it's important to get comfortable with being uncomfortable. You make decisions that you believe will have the best long-term benefits. Then you stay on top of it and see what the best next steps will be. You can try to make a decision that fixes a problem "once and for all," but in an always-changing organization, there's no such thing.

TAKING ADAPTIVE ACTION

In healthcare (whether you're contending with a consolidation or not) no two days are the same. There is constant variety in our leadership responsibilities, and there is constant variety on the units. We have discovered that when individuals in the organization feel connected, there is a pervasive sense that "we're all in this together." We're in it for the right reasons. We're all focused on doing what's best for patients and families, and we're ready and willing to be as agile as necessary to do that.

The WSL practices are effective because they are all practices that help people be in authentic human relationships with each other. At Faxton St. Luke's, all of these practices came to life through our organization-wide commitment to Relationship-Based Care.

Summary

Skillful leadership is critical to moving integrative nursing forward. To be successful, deeply embedded in the organization, and sustainable, it needs to align with organization-wide vision, values, and priorities. The "whole person" orientation extends not only to patients and their families, but also to staff. As the Faxon St. Luke's exemplar so richly captured, staff need to feel valued and affirmed.

The exemplar also captured the reality that culture change requires systems change. It would not be effective to have Relationship-Based Care end at a particular door or corridor. Likewise, if integrative nursing is to become a reality within a patient care unit, clinic, or program, it doesn't become an "option" for nurses to practice in this way. It becomes embedded in the systems of the organization and is evident in recruitment, orientation, standards of care, clinical practice guidelines, and performance reviews.

Whole-systems leadership focuses on preparing leaders to be agents of healing and transformation that extends to people, organizations, communities, and the environment. It is deeply aligned philosophically and practically with integrative nursing.

SELECTED REFERENCES

Brown, V., Harris, J., & Russell, J. (2010). *Tackling Wicked Problems Through Transdisciplinary Imagination*. London: Earthscan Ltd.

Johansen, B. (2007). *Get There Early: Sensing the Future to Compete in the Present*. San Francisco, CA: Berrett-Koehler Publishers.

Kahne, A. (2007). *Solving Tough Problems: An Open Way of Talking, Listening and Creating New Realities*. San Francisco, CA: Berrett-Koehler Publishers.

Koloroutis, M. (ed.). (2004). *Relationship-Based Care: A Model for Transforming Practice*. Minneapolis, MN: Creative Health Care Management.

Kreitzer, M. J. (2012). *Whole Systems Healing*. Retrieved April 9, 2013, from http://www.csh.umn.edu/wsh/.

Morris, W. (2011). *Whole Systems Leadership*. Retrieved April 9, 2013, from http://www.csh.umn.edu/wsh/Leadership/.

Peat, D. (2005). *Gentle Action: Bringing Creative Change to a Turbulent World*. Pari, Italy: Pari Publishing.

5

Building an Integrative Health Program

MARY JO KREITZER AND BETH SOMERVILLE

In their 1993 book *Through the Patient's Eyes: Understanding and Promoting Patient-Centered Care*, Margaret Gerteis and her colleagues broke new ground in summarizing data obtained from thousands of patients through surveys and focus groups that advanced the perspective that "institutional" does not need to be synonymous with "impersonal." Seven areas were identified as important to improving the patient experience: respecting patients' values and preferences, coordinating care, providing information and education, attending to physical comfort, providing emotional support, involving family and friends in care, and ensuring continuity among providers and treatment settings. As fundamental and basic as these core tenets of patient-centered care are, many healthcare institutions paid little attention to them or to providing holistic, integrative care (Gerteis, 1993).

Over the past decade, consumers have expressed increased dissatisfaction with the cost of care, poor outcomes, and lack of coordination and continuity of care. They have also communicated growing expectations for whole-person care that is inclusive of integrative therapies and healing practices. Access, cost, and quality issues have also been the focus of numerous governmental reports (e.g., *Crossing the Quality Chasm: A New Health System for the 21st Century; National Healthcare Disparities Report 2008;* and *Best Care at Lower Cost: The Path to Continuously Learning Health Care in America*) and have captured the attention of the corporate world that is concerned about the rising cost of healthcare for its employees. Increasingly, there is consensus that the current strategy is no longer sustainable. This has resulted in a changing context that has created incentives and interest in new approaches and models of care that are consistent with integrative health and medicine.

Context for Organizational and System Change

The primary driver behind emerging incentives is focused on what is frequently called the "triple aim." The Triple Aim initiative, a program of the Institute for Healthcare Improvement (IHI), focuses on the simultaneous pursuit of three aims: improving the health of the population, enhancing the patient experience of care (including quality, access, and reliability), and reducing the per capita cost of care. While it started in the United States, the initiative expanded in 2007 when IHI began working with a group of fifteen organizations in America, England, and Sweden, and today it boasts over 100 organizations in Scotland, Australia, New Zealand, and Singapore (Institute for Healthcare Improvement, 2013).

The Triple Aim is consistent with team-based care, focusing not so much on which healthcare professional provides which service, but on whether positive health outcomes are achieved. This might mean offering acupuncture or mindfulness-based stress-reduction to patients with chronic pain. If a patient is struggling with making lifestyle changes, a health coach may help support them in working toward goals.

As the system begins to shift from a fee-for-service model that incentivizes healthcare professionals to provide more services, tests, and procedures, to reimbursement based on cost, quality, and outcomes, new care and reimbursement models and metrics are emerging within the private and public sectors.

VALUE-BASED CONTRACTS

Employers, health plans, and healthcare systems are collaborating to establish value-based contracts. Under value-based contracting, there is shared financial risk that is tied to attaining positive health outcomes. For example, a portion of a provider's total potential payment may be tied to cost efficiency and quality-performance measures. Under some systems, a provider may be paid a fee-for-service for a portion of their payments but still be eligible to receive a bonus or to have payments withheld, depending on whether cost and quality targets have been achieved. In some systems, reimbursement is tied to cost and quality targets and bundles of services, a strategy that encourages team-based care and use of whatever services and providers that will maximize the best outcomes. There are many variations of value-based contracting, which may also be called "pay for performance" (P4P).

Geisinger is a nationally known example of a health system that has been using bundles of services to reduce costs and better serve patients. An integrated health services organization, Geisinger serves more than 2.6 million residents throughout forty-four counties in central and northeastern Pennsylvania. As noted in a report by the *Financial Times*,

> Geisinger physicians are paid a salary with bonuses if their patients don't have to come in for further treatment. Other hospitals operate on a fee-for-service model, giving doctors a financial incentive to do more tests and procedures even if not absolutely necessary. And, rather than charging for each component of

treatment, as is the norm elsewhere, Geisinger offers bundled packages where the cost does not advance, regardless of what is done. This gives the hospital the incentive to be as error-free as possible because it will have to cover any costs beyond the pre-determined package price....This system has helped Geisinger bring down costs. (*Financial Times*, 2010)

ACCOUNTABLE CARE ORGANIZATIONS

In the United States, health reform legislation passed in 2010 that included provisions for establishing what are called accountable care organizations, or ACOs. ACOs are groups of physicians, hospitals, and other healthcare professionals working together to coordinate care and share in certain savings and losses for Medicare beneficiaries assigned to their group, which may be called a medical or healthcare home. As a form of value-based contracting in the public sector, the primary goal of the program is to improve quality and lower costs for patients enrolled with the Centers for Medicare and Medicaid (CMS) in original Medicare Parts A and B programs (fee-for-service). The Medicare Shared Savings Program that went into effect in January of 2012 is part of the Patient Protection and Affordable Care Act ("Obamacare") of 2010. This act also includes provisions focused on reducing preventable hospital readmissions by lowering Medicare payments to hospitals with relatively high preventable readmission rates.

MEANINGFUL USE, METRICS, AND MEASURES

While most healthcare providers in the United States still use medical-record systems based on paper, there are strong and compelling incentives from the government and health plans to switch to electronic health records (EHRs). EHRs enable healthcare providers to have complete and accurate patient information and to share that information among clinics, hospitals, and across health systems with the goal of improved health outcomes and better coordination of care. EHRs also empower patients, a goal consistent with integrative health and medicine, by enabling them to receive copies of their records and share that information securely over the Internet with their families (HealthIT.gov).

At this stage of EHR implementation, there is considerable focus on what is called "meaningful use." Under the provisions of another piece of health reform legislation under the American Recovery and Reinvestment Act of 2009, eligible hospitals participating in Medicare and Medicaid programs may be eligible to receive incentive payments if they demonstrate meaningful use of certified electronic health record technology. Details regarding these programs can be found at the CMS website (CMS. gov, 2013).

The electronic capture and reporting of healthcare data is quickly becoming a way that consumers can access information to help inform their decision making. Health Grades (http://www.healthgrades.com/business/information/) is an example of a tool that enables consumers to access provider information, including the type of practice, whether they are board-certified, patient feedback, types of insurance accepted, and location information.

Another example of publicly reported data is the HCAHPS survey (Hospital Consumer Assessment of Healthcare Providers and Systems). This is the first national, standardized, publicly reported survey of patients' perspectives of hospital care. The survey was designed to allow meaningful and objective comparisons of hospitals that consider factors important to consumers. The survey asked patients about communication with doctors and nurses, the responsiveness of hospital staff, the cleanliness and quietness of the hospital environment, pain management, communication about medications, discharge information, and overall ratings of the hospital. The survey (www.hcahpsonline.org) is available in multiple formats (mail, telephone, active interactive voice recognition) and in five different languages. For each participating hospital, HCAHPS results on ten measures (six summary measures, two individual items, and two global ratings) are publicly reported on the *Hospital Compare* website, found at www.hospitalcompare.hhs.gov.

The landscape for healthcare organizations is rapidly changing, requiring organizations to create new strategies that will enable them to be responsive to increasing demands for transparency and outcomes. More than a tweak to the system, the change required is transformative in nature and inclusive of significant culture change. Emerging models of care are collaborative and team-based, patient-centered and -directed, and inclusive of integrative approaches to health and medicine.

Designing the Care Model, Program, or Service

Designing clinical services and programs or new care models is a creative endeavor that requires engagement by many stakeholders, including the population that will be served. Rather than an abstract and linear process done by experts alone in a boardroom, increasingly the tools and practices of design thinking are being embraced. As described by Brown (2009), *design thinking* is a human-centered planning process that includes three overlapping steps:

- inspiration (the search for solutions)
- ideation (the process of generating developing and testing ideas)
- implementation (the path leading from project room to market)

It is an iterative, nonlinear process that involves continuously testing and re-visiting assumptions and adhering to a philosophy of "fail earlier to succeed sooner."

The foundation of design thinking is planning around three overlapping criteria:

Desirability—What makes sense to people, and what is needed or desired?
Feasibility—What is functionally possible?
Viability—What is likely to be sustainable?

In designing integrative health and medicine programs, understanding the needs of the patient population and the capabilities and constraints of the staff and system will lead to models that are relevant and sustainable.

While there are "best practices" that can be gleaned and models that are replicable, directly engaging both the recipients and providers of care is a critical step toward securing engagement and ultimately support. This results in a variety of different types of integrative health programs, rather than "cookie-cutter" models, while offering greater flexibility and responsiveness to the needs of patients and the demands of the organization.

Within clinical settings, for example, there are several approaches that have been successfully used in developing an integrative health program. First is a model wherein integrative modalities are provided by front-line clinical staff to patients and their families as part of their regular care. In this model, integrative care is embedded in the clinical care model. Second is a model wherein integrative modalities are provided by "experts" (massage therapy, Healing Touch, acupuncture, music therapy) upon referral. Whether or not the services are provided free of charge or for a fee and if they are provided by volunteers or paid staff varies depending on the organization. The breadth and depth of implementation of this model depends on the availability of the expert(s) and the knowledge of staff to make an appropriate referral. A third model often used is a fee-for-service model wherein integrative services are available and referrals are made, but the service is not an integral part of the organization. For instance, a clinic may have a massage therapist or nutritionist who rents office space in the clinic, but the provider makes his or her own appointments and handles all billing.

Ultimately, the goal is to create a program that is strategically aligned with the organization's vision, mission, and goals; has successful outcomes, including identified patient outcomes, staff satisfaction, and financial viability; and is sustainable financially and in terms of organizational acceptance and availability of educated and informed staff.

THEORY U

Otto Scharmer describes in his book *Theory U* (Scharmer, 2007) a process that he describes as "leading from the future as it emerges." Completely resonant with design thinking, the process begins as illustrated in Figure 5.1, with *co-initiating*—building common intent. The second step of the process is *co-sensing*, which is described as

Theory U Process

1. Co-initiating:
uncover common intent
stop and listen to others and to
what life calls you to do

5. Co-evolving:
embody the new in ecosystems
that facilitate acting
from the whole

2. Co-sensing:
observe, observe, observe
connect with people and places
to sense the system from the whole

4. Co-creating:
prototype the new
in living examples to explore
the future by doing

3. Presencing:
connect to the source of inspiration and will
go to the place of silence and allow the inner knowing to emerge

This work is licensed by the Presencing Institute · Otto Scharmer, www.presencing.com/permissions.

 PRESENCING INSTITUTE

FIGURE 5.1 This work is licensed by the Presencing Institute—Otto Scharmer: www. presencing.com/permissions.

observing and deep listening. This requires suspending judgment and assumptions and being open to what needs to emerge. The step of *presencing* is opening up to inner knowing, being mindful of intuition and the source of inspiration. The final steps are *co-creating*, which includes prototyping, and *co-evolving*, or implementing in a system that continues to evolve. Scharmer's work captures a rich and dynamic interplay between personal and organizational transformation.

Assessment

The Theory U model starts with co-initiating and co-sensing, both of which require a deep assessment. What is desirable? What do patients, families, staff, the community, and the organization need and want? While it is tempting to skip over or shorten this step, it is vitally important to the creation of a successful and sustainable clinical care model.

Co-initiating is a process wherein the common intent of key partners is determined. This is the moment when the vision of integrative health is defined and an understanding of how that vision aligns with the organizational mission and priorities arises. This step is not about selecting any particular modality or defining program details; instead, it is about creating overarching goals, such as reduction in patient stress and anxiety, increase in nursing staff retention, or finding non-pharmacological options for symptom management.

Co-sensing is the core of the assessment process and requires the ability to listen deeply to what is said and what is left unsaid. It demands open-hearted engagement with all participants—leaders, staff, and patients—to obtain a sense of the whole system. On a practical level, this observation should lead to an understanding of the capacity of the organization, including current skills and expertise from both leadership and clinical perspectives as well as the financial resources available, whether from philanthropy, fees for services, or administrative funds. Some of the key questions to answer are: "Who are the internal champions?" "What is the level of interest among clinicians?" and "Who are the internal and external strategic partners?"

A useful tool in the assessment process is a *gap analysis*. A gap analysis is a

technique that businesses use to determine what steps need to be taken in order to move from its current state to its desired, future state. It consists of (1) listing of characteristic factors (such as attributes, competencies, performance levels) of the present situation ("what is"), (2) listing factors needed to achieve future objectives ("what should be"), and then (3) highlighting the gaps that exist and need to be filled. (*Business Dictionary*, 2013)

READINESS FOR CHANGE AND DIFFUSION OF INNOVATION

Part of the assessment is to determine where to begin within an organization. Unit-based, service line or program-focused, or system-wide strategies can all be successful. Where to start will depend to a great extent on readiness for change. Organizations are often change-resistant, and long-term employees may be supporters and champions of change or may cling to the status quo. Key supporters may, through their own fears, create barriers to program development and implementation. Other individuals and departments originally not involved may be more flexible and open to innovation. One of the factors to assess is who historically have been early adopters or innovators. Another key factor to consider is if disruptive change is already occurring (i.e., anticipated reductions in third-party reimbursement, staffing changes due to financial constraints, or new regulatory requirements). It is also worthwhile to note the overall pace of change within the organization, differentiating between departments, if that is significant.

At the completion of the assessment phase, the Theory U process rests in "presencing"—a point where the future can emerge. This is a place where something new can be glimpsed and the plan for moving forward is generated.

Program Development

The key to successful program development is a co-creation process that includes all stakeholders. Everyone brings his or her own expertise to the table, whether that is as a nurse, administrator, or patient. Co-creation fosters an environment where support for implementation follows naturally. Since the assessment stage identified how the integrative-care vision is in alignment with the overarching organization's vision, any plan should be clear to senior leadership. A vital success strategy is to create engagement and support—including front-line staff, for example, can assist in creating a program that meets their concerns and provides tools for more effective and efficient patient care and self-care. Patient-centered care demands that the voice of the patients and families be considered when shaping any program. All these factors contribute to the development of a unique solution that matches the culture within which it is embedded.

EDUCATION

Education is a multi-pronged strategy that forms the foundation of successful programs. Educational efforts often include leadership, medical and clinical staff, and the community. The key to long-term sustainability is to build capacity within the system, which requires careful consideration of individuals' educational needs and ability to coordinate education in the long term. Education is never a one-time event. A comprehensive plan includes orientation, basic education, and ongoing continuing education. In many organizations, external resources may be tapped for initial education with the plan to use a "train-the-trainer" model to build internal capacity.

POLICIES AND PROCEDURES

Successful implementation requires the creation of appropriate standards, protocols, and organizational procedures. These are created during the planning process and can require approval committees, leadership teams, or other bodies. At least one person on the planning team should be familiar with organizational standards, protocols, and policies as well as the creation and revision of same to anticipate roadblocks, ensure appropriate formatting, and shepherd the approval process. Such approvals may be required prior to any clinical implementation, but they might be done contiguous with continuing education.

Protocol development can include the creation of educational aids to assist staff implementation. Such aids can show the symptom (e.g., pain, nausea, anxiety), the integrative modality (e.g., acupressure, imagery, aromatherapy), and the specific intervention to be used (e.g., acupressure point L4, use of lavender oil, or quick hand massage). See Table 5.1 for an example of an aromatherapy aid.

DOCUMENTATION

Documentation of integrative care is a necessary part of implementation that is becoming easier through the use of EHRs. Such recordkeeping can be part of demonstrating outcomes and return on investment. Larger and more mature organizations

Table 5.1: Holistic Heart Care Clinical Use of Essential Oils: St. Joseph's Hospital (permission to use granted by Jamie St. Michel, RN, MA, AHN-BC, CCAP, Integrative Services Holistic Nurse Clinician, St. Joseph's Hospital)

Clincal Presentation	Essential Oil	Clinical Effect
Pain Insomnia Difficulty sleeping Anxiety	LAVENDER Blend	Supports rest and relaxation Reduces stress and anxiety Headache reduction Universal oil Antiseptic Antispasmodic—sedative
Excess mucous Nausea Anxiety Digestive problems	GINGER Blend	Mucolytic Universal anti-nausea Antispasmodic Supports respiratory problems
Nausea Insomnia Anxiety Digestive problems	MANDARIN (Citrus Reticulate)	Antiemetic Sedative Relaxant Digestive

with integrative health programs may have developed proprietary data or flow sheets in their EHR. Newer programs that don't have specialized flowsheets may have to use comment fields or other options within their EHR.

Items to be documented include the modality used, what symptom indicated its use, the dose (i.e., which essential oil, length and type of massage, type of imagery used) and, if relevant, any immediate effect. Defining a standard format for documenting this information will permit its more efficient use in program and outcome evaluations.

CREDENTIALING

Many integrative modalities can be provided by nurses to patients and families as part of standard care; no credentialing is required. Some integrative services, like acupuncture or chiropractic care, have licensure guidelines that require the providers to be credentialed by the healthcare organization. This is done to ensure that services are provided by qualified practitioners and eligible to obtain third-party reimbursement where applicable. In these instances, providers must meet certain qualifications, including training and experience, to be eligible for credentialing. Each institution has a unique process that has to be navigated, and sometimes the approval process is extensive. Thus it is imperative to start this process early.

DEPLOYMENT OF SERVICES: DECENTRALIZED, CENTRALIZED, NETWORKED

Just as there are many unique ways to include integrative services, deployment is also unique and will reflect the needs of the system. A decentralized approach permits individual units or departments to create and implement services specifically designed to meet their needs. Such an approach can lead to rapid implementation in those areas where interest is high (such as pain-management and oncology) and permits areas where barriers exist to move at a slower pace. In those instances where integrative modalities are seen as part of standard care, a decentralized approach may be most effective if an "every patient, every shift" model is used.

A centralized approach requires system-wide coordination. It can offer effective deployment of limited resources. This approach is useful in supporting efforts to scale implementation system-wide as successes and barriers can be more easily identified and no unit has to "re-invent the wheel." This approach does not mean that units cannot individualize how integrative care is offered; rather, it supports efforts to provide the most effective care based on the unit's individual requirements.

In a networked system, patients have access to individual programs and services that are funded and managed as discrete units. Ideally, the services are well coordinated. For example, a networked system might include a separate outpatient clinic providing integrative services, a wellness center including physical therapy, and a volunteer program offering Healing Touch and Reiki. Networking permits a healthcare organization to develop numerous options, leverage strengths, and spread the risk across different departments, divisions, or hospitals. This is also a way to institutionalize integrative programs that might have already been in existence or developed in a grassroots fashion.

Implementation

Implementation should be considered an iterative process, one where prototyping, responding flexibly to feedback, and continued improvement are not only welcome but encouraged. Pilot programs provide an opportunity to test implementation strategies and make programmatic changes. Demonstration of successful outcomes provides a foundation for broader implementation. For example, a Minneapolis children's hospital recently began implementation of integrative services on a Pediatric Bone Marrow Transplant unit. The expectation is that what is learned from the successes from that unit will form the basis for a system-wide implementation plan.

Evaluation

Evaluation and assessment are key components of new programming and ongoing sustainability. Funders and administration will want to know that the integrative modalities are making a difference. This is crucial if the initial offering is a pilot program with its broader implementation resting on demonstrated success.

It is important to create methods by which patient outcomes can be measured. The most successful outcome measures are those integrated with the standard documentation and reporting process. This is not always possible with pilot projects or new programming. Since recordkeeping can feel like a burden to front-line staff, finding the most efficient way to record outcome measures is a key step in the evaluation process.

A program evaluation, which covers education, compliance with protocols, and a review of program goals, ensures that aspects of the program are implemented in the most effective and efficient manner. Such an evaluation can also verify if the program is implemented as originally intended, or where and why revisions were made. Furthermore, such an evaluation can provide valuable information on scalability, further barriers to implementation, and areas for improvement.

Securing Partnerships

Implementation of integrative modalities can be facilitated through partnerships with other organizations. Educational institutions for integrative modalities can arrange for students to provide free or reduced-fee services under the supervision of experienced teachers. The benefit to the educational institution includes providing to students an in-the-field practical experience, offering services to the public, and increasing awareness and acceptance within the healthcare organization. The benefit to the healthcare organization includes an institutionally cost-effective method to offer integrative care, often at a significantly reduced fee. It can also serve as a vehicle to increase awareness of the positive outcomes realized through use of the modality.

Integrative programs can also benefit from working with universities that offer a Doctor of Nurse Practitioner (DNP) program. DNP programs require projects based in the community, and a DNP candidate interested in integrative therapies can provide valuable assistance in the organizational assessment, strategic planning, and continuing education as part of his or her degree requirements. For instance, DNP candidates with a concentration in integrative therapies at the University of Minnesota have been placed at several senior care facilities, where they can support the organizations' efforts to implement integrative care, not only by doing an assessment and preparing a proposed action plan, but by providing hands-on, bedside education in integrative modalities. Staff at the participating facilities, initially concerned about the proposed changes in their roles, were able to witness the ease with which such modalities can be used and the benefits received by residents. This increased their interest and acceptance.

Partnering with educational institutions also provides an opportunity for participation in research. For instance, a National Institutes of Health National Center for Complementary and Alternative Medicine funded clinical study on music therapy with ventilated patients allowed multiple sites to offer this modality to patients, who benefitted with a reduction in anxiety (Heidersheidt, Chlan, & Donley, 2011). The clinical study funding was provided to a university that partnered with healthcare organizations in a classic win-win scenario.

While depending on financial support from philanthropy is not a sustainable model, such funds at the beginning of a project can provide the needed "jump-start." Funds can cover consultation services, initial continuing education, supplies, and community programming to generate interest. Philanthropy can also fund the initial expansion of services, ongoing continuing education, and capital development. For instance, funding from the George Family Foundation was the impetus for the creation of the Penny George Institute for Health and Healing at Allina's Abbott Northwestern Hospital. Now a nationally known and outpatient clinic, it serves as the touch point for research and expansion of inpatient services.

Summary

Transformation of clinical care is a current imperative for health systems. Changes in reimbursement are providing opportunities for innovative solutions that provide more cost-effective and patient-centered care. The principles found in *Theory U* can provide a roadmap to creating successful and sustaining programs that meet and are unique to the individual needs of an organization.

SELECTED REFERENCES

Agency for Healthcare Research and Quality. (2008). *National healthcare Disparities Report, 2008*. Rockville, MD: Agency for Healthcare Research and Quality.

Brown, D. (2009). *Change by Design: How Design Thinking Transforms Organizations and Inspires Innovation*. New York: Harper Business.

Centers for Medicare and Medicaid Services (CMS). (2013). EHR incentive programs. Retrieved March 8, 2013, from http://www.cms.gov/Regulations-and-Guidance/Legislation/EHRIncentivePrograms.

Gerteis, M., Edgeman-Levitan, S., Daley, J., et al. (1993). *Through the Patient's Eyes: Understanding and Promoting Patient-Centered Care*. San Francisco: John Wiley & Sons.

Heidersheidt, A., Chlan, L., & Donley, K. (2011). Instituting a music listening intervention for critically ill patients receiving mechanical ventilation: Exemplars from two patient cases. *Music Medicine, 3*(4), 239–246.

Institute for Healthcare Improvement. (2013). The IHI triple aim. Retrieved March 8, 2013, from http://www.ihi.org/offerings/Initiatives/TripleAim/Pages.

Institute of Medicine. (2001). *Crossing the Quality Chasm: A New Health System for the 21st Century*. Washington, DC: The National Academies Press.

Institute of Medicine. (2012). *Best Care at Lower Cost: The Path to Continuously Learning Health Care in America*. Washington, DC: The National Academies Press.

Scharmer, O. C. (2009). *Theory U: Leading from the Future as It Emerges*. San Francisco: Berrett-Koehler Publishers, Inc.

Scharmer, O. C. (n.d.). Tools. Retrieved March 8, 2013, from http://www.ottoscharmer.com/tools.

6

Transforming the Healthcare Environment Through a Hospital-Based Integrative Health Initiative: Sanford Medical Center

ARLENE HORNER AND ELLEN L. SCHELLINGER

Sanford Medical Center

Sanford Medical Center (SMC) is a 547-bed tertiary care hospital in Sioux Falls, South Dakota. SMC serves as the primary teaching institution for the Sanford School of Medicine of the University of South Dakota. A full-service community-owned hospital for over 100 years, Sanford Medical Center employs almost 4,200 staff and provides a full complement of medical and surgical care, both inpatient and outpatient, in all specialties. Centers of Excellence include Heart and Vascular, Orthopedics and Sports Medicine, Women's, Children's, Cancer, and Diabetes. While integrative therapies had been available for many years within various units within the hospital, there was no institution-wide strategic vision or unified effort. An inventory of services showed pockets of activity, such as biofeedback for behavioral management, art and music therapy in pediatrics, massage for oncology inpatients, and centering pregnancy in the labor and delivery department. Within some areas, integrative therapies were available for health promotion as well as chronic disease management. This chapter details the transformational journey we embarked on at Sanford Medical Center as we launched a major institution-wide effort to bring integrative therapies to the bedside.

Building Awareness and Creating a Vision

While staff within the nursing department were fairly familiar with the growing interest in integrative health and medicine across the United States, we felt that it was important to expand awareness and inspire interest in integrative medicine at the medical center and throughout the system. Mary Jo Kreitzer, director of the Center for Spirituality and Healing at the University of Minnesota (UMN), was invited to present an overview of integrative health care in the United States, including current trends and future projections. Over sixty institutional leaders attended, representing the broad scope of the system: vice-presidents, physicians, directors, nurse practitioners, and case managers from all pediatric and adult services in the clinic and hospital settings, as well as representatives from support departments such as pharmacy, rehabilitation therapies, dietary, counseling, and social work.

Shortly after this consultation, a leadership group visited other acute care settings to explore various models. Two very different institutions were visited: a newer, eighty-six-bed community hospital designed to incorporate the principles of a healing environment and staffed with practitioners who use integrative, holistic healing as an integral part of their practice; and a much larger urban hospital with a centralized integrative therapy program that housed massage therapists, nutritionists, and other holistic medicine practitioners.

Following this consultation and the site visits, key stakeholders from the hospital and clinic developed a strategic vision for Sanford Medical Center: to position itself as a care system that offers patients comprehensive, personalized, and holistic care that includes integrative therapies.

Assessment

UNDERSTANDING PATIENTS' AND FAMILIES' NEEDS

Patient attitudes and beliefs regarding the potential use of integrative therapies were studied. A survey was distributed to clinic patients to gauge the needs, expectations and interests of the community. This survey confirmed that there was an expectation that integrative therapies be available that could assist patients in optimizing their own ability to heal, improve their resilience, and provide them with choices in managing their personal health and wellness. The survey exposed gaps between therapies sought, therapies used for coping, and therapies currently available. Patients, in effect, were robbed of their coping mechanisms when they arguably needed them the most. For instance, massage is an intervention frequently utilized on an outpatient basis, yet in-house is only available on a specific hospital unit, supported by limited, donated funds.

BUILDING INTERNAL CAPACITY

In addition to assessing the needs of patients and families, we also evaluated our internal resources to better understand the expertise of the staff. It became clear that while there was considerable interest in integrative therapies, there was limited expertise. Because the hospital is located in a primarily rural Great Plains state, access to integrative medicine practitioners was limited. Therefore, steps were taken to bolster institutional expertise. First, a group of six clinical and administrative leaders attended a week-long immersion course offered by the Center for Spirituality and Healing at UMN. The goal was to better understand the application of integrative health and healing to provide an optimal healing environment in clinical settings. This course provided knowledge of evidence-based research and skills needed to lead the effort of integrating complementary healing modalities into the fabric of care. The team was tasked with weaving integrative practices into the warp and weft of the institution.

Developing the Strategy to Support the Vision

To achieve the vision of offering patients comprehensive, personalized, and holistic care that includes integrative therapies, decisions needed to be made regarding how to deploy resources. Three priorities were identified:

- Develop a cost-effective, self-sustaining model.
- Provide integrative therapies that are evidence-based.
- Offer integrative therapy to every patient.

Unlike other institutional models seen during site visits, Sanford Medical Center's culture supported a non-centralized, integrated approach. The decision was made to focus on the nursing practice and provide on-site education to nurses, as opposed to hiring individual specialized practitioners. The role of integrative therapy within the registered nurse (RN) scope of practice was discussed with the State Board of Nursing.

Program Development

The next step was to develop an action plan to systematically educate and incorporate integrative therapies and theories into the system of care via nurses. This team evolved into the Integrative Therapy Nursing Practice Committee, whose purpose and goals are listed below.

PURPOSE

- Offer comprehensive, personalized, and holistic care that includes integrative therapies.
- Optimize each person's inherent resilience and ability to heal while expanding their choices for managing their health and wellness.

GOALS

Strengthen and expand the Nursing Professional Practice Model of Person-Centered Holistic Care by recognizing that:

- Many integrative therapies fall within the scope of nursing practice. Identify therapies and practices that will be consistently and systematically offered to patients across the continuum of care.

- Embed integrative therapies in the care delivery system so they are a continuous part of assessment, diagnosis, treatment, and evaluation founded in the concepts of the healing relationship.
- Have clear expectations of appropriate certifications and cross-training of practitioners.

ENHANCE STAFF DEVELOPMENT

- Expand the knowledge and skills of direct caregivers across the system with particular emphasis on areas where integrative therapies are being offered within comprehensive clinical programs.
- Develop in-depth expertise of a cadre of staff, including advanced-practice nurses and other providers who can become internal resources and experts.
- Encourage employee self-care efforts as successful programs are founded in healthy caregivers.

BUILD NURSE KNOWLEDGE BASE

- Systematically obtain clinical outcomes data where therapies are delivered.
- Broadly educate leadership on outcomes and strategy around integrative health.

The committee developed a policy that focuses on the safe and effective use of integrative therapies to enhance patient comfort and care. The nursing clinical guidelines promote the use of integrative therapies to help achieve measurable health outcomes that address specific patient symptoms and enhance health and wellbeing.

EFFORTS TO EASE CULTURE CHANGE

Process change was developed and implemented to embed integrative therapies into the nursing practice. The process change provided the opportunity for stakeholders outside the nursing practice to understand and provide input into the on-boarding of new modalities. A checklist was developed to support a transdisciplinary approach and assure a safe and reliable patient experience. (See Table 6.1, Integrative Therapy or Device Assessment Checklist.)

Table 6.1: Integrative Therapy or Device Assessment Checklist

Integrative Therapy or Device Assessment Checklist

Integrative Health Care Advisory Council

Therapy or Device _____

Therapy Category(s)

(See National Center for Complementary & Alternative Medicine—www.nccam.nih.gov)

• Natural Products/Botanicals	• Healing Environment
• Mind/Body	• Manipulative Body Based Practices
• Movement	• Other—explain

Rationale (Narrative):

_____

_____

_____

_____

Symptoms

☐ Nausea/Vomiting ☐ Pain ☐ Sleep ☐ Anxiety ☐ Other _____

Target Population

☐ Adult ☐ Pediatric ☐ Specialty area _____

Evidence/Efficacy

1. Grade from Natural Standard Database (attach)

2. Pertinent Research (attach)

Benefit/Risk assessment, including contraindications:

_____

_____

_____

Hospital Processes Review	Contact Person	Completed	N/A
☐ Clinical Reasoning			
☐ Environmental Services			
☐ Infection Control			
☐ Informatics Technology			
☐ Nursing Senate			
☐ Pharmacy			
☐ Policy Development			
☐ Retail			
☐ Safety			
☐ Spiritual Care			
☐ Supply Chain Management			
☐ Other			

Cost of device/treatment_____

Billable_____

Provided by whom? _____

Estimated time of treatment_____

Implementation

A kick-off event augmented transition into an increased holistic framework. At this event, Mary Jo Kreitzer introduced the principles of integrative nursing, evidence-based outcomes of integrative therapies, and the importance of self-care for caregivers. The conference also featured an integrative healing fair with booths showcasing activities for staff and introducing aromatherapy and acupressure.

In congruence with integrative nursing principles, a focus on the health and wellbeing of the novice integrative nurse was encouraged. In order to provide relationship-based, person-centered holistic care, the nurse must first care for and nourish the self. Jean Watson notes that nurses need to remember and acknowledge that nursing is sacred work (Watson, 2013). Watson's narrative was used in a "Caring Moments" video of nurses that showcased photographs of nurses being present with families; sitting alongside a patient; providing acupressure, aromatherapy; or simply providing a gentle touch. The video is located on the hospital's intranet site, available to all staff.

ALIGNMENT WITH VISION, MISSION, AND NURSING MODEL

An essential aspect of embedding holistic care practices into an organization is alignment with the organization's mission, vision, and values. Sanford Medical Center's mission statement, "Dedicated to the work of health and healing," builds on its vision statement of "Improving the human condition through exceptional care, innovation and discovery." The mission and vision support a holistic approach to care that integrative therapy provides.

The nursing practice was determined to be the principle driver for an integrative therapy initiative that meshes with the organization's mission and vision. Sanford Medical Center is a three-time, designated Magnet hospital positioned in the top 1% of hospitals in the nation for nursing excellence. With a strong and mature nursing practice, potential exists to "impact every patient, every time" with nurses leading an integrative therapy initiative. As a NICHE (Nurses Improving Care for Healthsystem Elders) hospital, integrative therapy meshes well with elder-sensitive care.

Sanford Medical Center's nursing professional practice model is grounded in the science and art of nursing and describes how registered nurses practice, collaborate, communicate, and develop professionally. The model below drives the nursing practice. (See Figure 6.1, Sanford Nursing Professional Practice Model.)

PERSON-CENTERED HOLISTIC CARE

Key to Sanford Medical Center's integrative therapy initiative was the philosophy that person-centered care is fundamental. Person-centered care recognizes the belief that healing involves: knowing the patient as a person; respecting the person's illness

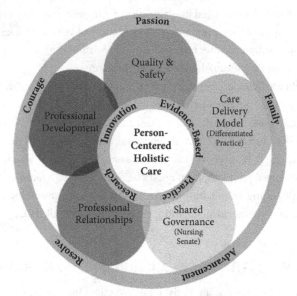

Dedicated to the work of health and healing.

FIGURE 6.1 Sanford Nursing Professional Practice Model

experience, values, and beliefs; and communicating effectively among the interprofessional team regarding customized interventions based on the patient's preferences and needs. At the epicenter of the nursing practice model is person-centered holistic care.

Person-centered care, the fourth core principle of integrative nursing, is exemplified through SMC's nursing practice goal to (1) provide safe, reliable, person-centered care; (2) include patient and family participation in care planning; and (3) recognize the right of every patient and family to have a registered nurse. Evidence-based care is interwoven with patient values and preferences, clinical expertise, and current best evidence (Melnyk & Fineout-Overholt, 2011).

PATIENT FIT

Pivotal to the integrative therapy initiative was establishing a philosophy to promote proper "patient fit." Proper patient fit means tailoring interventions based upon a patient's wants, needs, and preferences while optimizing their health and managing chronic disease. By creating proper patient fit, individuals and family members no longer need to squeeze into a healthcare system limited to conventional care and standardized care plans. Established goals are based upon individual characteristics that improve wellbeing and are realistic and attainable (Waters & Easton, 1999).

Through the nurse's relationship with individuals and families, possible therapies from different disciplines and traditions are identified, prioritized, and integrated to create a person-centered plan of care that supports and honors the whole person. In SMC's nurse-led initiative, interaction with diverse disciplines and perspectives within the health team created a coordinated healthcare experience for the person and his or her family. The nurse collaborates and advocates when treatments are not consistent with the health beliefs of the person. Care is more than symptom-management and diagnosis-driven; it is based on the principles of integrative nursing and designed to meet the whole person's dynamic needs of bodymindspirit.

An educational blueprint was developed to support the nursing practice change. While the organization has traditionally embraced conventional treatments, initial integrative therapies (aromatherapy, acupressure, and guided imagery) were thoughtfully selected and generally known to be safe and widely accepted. Additionally, the concept of self-care first for the nurse and the patients was part of the model (Jones, MacHillivray, Kroll, et al., 2011). The Center for Spirituality and Healing at UMN provided on-site education and consultation via phone or email as questions surfaced. Quarterly conference calls with other organizations provided opportunities to share best practices, review articles, discuss innovative ideas, and critique new evidence.

To help nurses ease into integrative therapy, the practice was framed with concepts from Symptom Management Theory that promote self-care within the symptom experience, symptom management strategies, and symptom status outcomes (Humphreys, Lee & Carrieri-Kohlman, et al., 2008). Symptom management helped the novice integrative nurse identify interventions.

INTEGRATIVE NURSE CHAMPIONS

Patient care departments designated a cadre of nurses interested and vested in integrative therapy to champion the efforts for their department's patient population and serve as ongoing resource experts. The Integrative Nurse Champions attended three train-the-trainer sessions with UMN experts over a four-month timeframe. The eight hours of training per integrative therapy provided a deep foundation for each modality in which didactic and experiential learning occurred. The champions' names and departments are posted on the integrative therapy intranet site as resources for staff.

The Integrative Nurse Champions returned three months later for a review session on the selected integrative therapies. During this interactive session, they practiced and used a criterion checklist specific to each therapy to confirm their knowledge of safety, use, and documentation. The champions were also introduced to the integrative therapy intranet site, resources, and other websites available to support their efforts.

An aromatherapy kit with five essential oils, a carrier oil, inhalers, and labels was provided to each patient care department. Acupressure wristbands were stocked in each department, and a set of laminated three-by-five flashcards of common acupressure sites was provided to each patient care wing. All items are included in the hospital's supply and stocking requisition system for reordering. Selected resource books on aromatherapy and acupressure were recommended to each department director (Gach, 1990; Kolster & Waskowiak, 2003; Price & Price, 2011; Tisserand & Balacs, 1995).

To support competence and confidence, an Aromatherapy Grid (Table 6.2) and an Acupressure Criterion Checklist (Figure 6.2) were created, based on selected essential oils and acupoints, which were linked to common symptoms experienced by patients. Based on patient and symptom fit, the grids can be used to select an acupoint or essential oil.

INTRANET WEBSITE

The SMC integrative therapy intranet site was developed to simplify application of the integrative therapies, to promote user ease, and is available on every computer in the organization with access around the clock to all staff. The intranet site lists the policy,

Table 6.2: Aromatherapy Grid for Symptom Management

Essential Oils	Symptoms				
	Pain	Anxiety or Stress	Insomnia	GI Indications	Other
Lavandula angustifolia (Lavender)	Pain	Anxiety Stress	Insomnia		
Mentha spicata (Spearmint)	Headache, Spasms	Fatigue, Anxiety		Nausea, Vomiting, Indigestion, Flatulence	Colds, Cough
Zingiber officinale (Ginger)	Pain	Fatigue		Nausea, Indigestion	
botanical bergamia (Bergamot)	Pain	Anxiety, Stress, Agitation	Insomnia	Decreased Appetite, Indigestion	
Citrus reticulata (Mandarin)	Pain	Anxiety	Insomnia	Nausea, Indigestion	Hiccups

CRITICAL ELEMENTS	MET	NOT MET
1. Verify patient's interest in receiving acupressure. Note contraindications such as arthritis, fragile skin, pregnancy, or anticoagulants.		
2. Explain the risks/benefits of acupressure.		
3. Identify an appropriate acupressure site for nausea/vomiting.		
4. Identify an appropriate acupressure site for insomnia.		
5. Identify an appropriate acupressure site for headache.		
6. Identify an appropriate acupressure site for pain.		
7. Identify the appropriate acupressure site for anxiety/stress.		
8. Identify the appropriate acupressure site for fatigue.		
9. Identify the appropriate acupressure site to stimulate immune functioning.		
10. Identify the appropriate acupressure site to balance the emotions and calm the spirit.		
11. Identify which site is not to be used during pregnancy.		
12. Instruct patient in self-care and application of acupressure.		
13. Document in EHR on the Integrated Therapy Flow Sheet 1097, the reason, the acupressure site and the pre AND post rating on 0-10 scale.		
14. Demonstrate application of wrist band.		
15. Be aware of resources for acupressure on Integrative Therapy intranet site.		

[ ] PASSED [ ] NEEDS TO REPEAT

NAME_____

VALIDATED BY: _____ DATE: _____

FIGURE 6.2 Acupressure Criterion Checklist

competency criteria checklists, and specific information about aromatherapy, acupressure, and guided imagery. Patient education sheets, written at an appropriate health literacy level, are hyperlinked and may be printed for patient use. Resources, ordering information, and key websites are also on the intranet site.

DOCUMENTATION

Documentation of integrative therapy within the hospital setting is an essential component of care. The Integrative Therapy Nursing Practice Committee developed a template for a basic integrative therapy flow sheet for the electronic health record (EHR). Components of the documentation include: type(s) of integrative therapy, symptom(s) treated, and the patient's subjective symptom rating pre- and post-integrative therapy.

Equally important to the EHR build is the ability to report clinical outcome data. EHR reports summarize the most commonly used integrative therapy for a patient population, the range of symptoms treated, and the patient response. The reports help guide population-specific practice.

Nurses are trained to document on the EHR integrative therapy flow sheet. The nurse documents the type of integrative therapy used, the patient's subjective rating of the symptom on a 0–10 scale prior to the integrative therapy and 30 minutes post-therapy.

INTEGRATIVE HEALTH GO-LIVE FOR NURSES

Each patient care department has regular (quarterly or annual) skills fairs or competency training during which they allot time for updates or new educational topics for the nursing staff. Integrative therapy provided an hour-long, structured training session supporting hospital-wide implementation. This session started with the ringing of a Tibetan singing bowl. Staff found the sound soothing, and singing bowls are now incorporated throughout the hospital to start meetings and to call staff together to the here and now.

NEW EMPLOYEE ORIENTATION

New employee orientation on integrative therapy was developed and includes an hour-long session focusing on self-care strategies and the use of integrative therapy for patient care. The integrative therapy intranet site with resources is introduced (Melnyk & Fineout-Overholt, 2011; Center for Spirituality and Healing, 2013; American Holistic Nurses Association, 2013; National Center for Complementary and Alternative Medicine, 2013; Natural Standard, 2013). Once the nurse begins to work in the patient care department, the Integrative Nurse Champion provides further support.

Evaluation

Nurses and select interdisciplinary staff participating in the integrative therapy training completed a pre-survey to measure their own knowledge and attitudes. The survey asked about their current knowledge, attitudes, and practices regarding integrative health, as well as demographic factors such as years practiced, and their age and gender. A section on patient care asked if they had ever provided aromatherapy, acupressure, guided imagery, or other integrative therapies to a patient, and their level of confidence in using them. The pre-survey asked staff about self-care and if they had ever personally used integrative therapy (Figure 6.3).

Following the sixty-minute training, a post survey queried if knowledge and/or confidence had increased. Each nursing department's responses were summarized and graphed separately. Total responses from all departments were also summarized (Figure 6.4).

The graph below (Figure 6.5) indicates the frequency with which the 616 trained staff who responded to the survey would offer integrative therapy. Seventy-two percent of the nurses indicated that they would offer integrative therapy, at frequencies ranging from every shift to twice a week. This measurement serves as a baseline to determine if integrative therapy use increases or decreases over time.

Nurse confidence using integrative therapy was measured pre- and post-training. Responses indicated that aromatherapy confidence increased by 65% and acupressure confidence increased by 61% following training (Figures 6.6 and 6.7).

Summary

A nursing professional practice model that emphasizes person-centered, holistic care is optimally sustained with solid administrative support, a robust infrastructure, and an emphasis on evidence, quality, and safety. Building blocks discussed for a healthy program include documentation in the electronic health record, easy retrieval of clinical outcomes, online access to resources, and a readiness to involve all stakeholders. Additional considerations include a focus on patient fit, common symptoms, nurse self-care, and cost effectiveness.

Integrative Therapy Pre Survey of Knowledge and Attitudes of Nurses

Dear Nurse: We would be grateful for your responses to this survey of your knowledge, attitudes and practices with regard to what has been called complementary and alternative medicine (CAM) or integrative health care. As stated in a recent NIH document, "CAM practices are those healthcare and medical practices that are not currently an integral part of conventional medicine." We are interested in knowing your current knowledge, attitudes, and practices with regard to integrative health to help us plan and evaluate our program.

Years practiced as RN_____ (write number) **Your Age:**_____**years** (write number)

Your Gender ____Male ____Female

Instructions: Circle or indicate your response

PATIENT CARE:

1. Have you ever provided aromatherapy for a patient?   **YES NO**

2. Have you ever provided acupressure for a patient?   **YES NO**

3. Have you ever provided guided imagery for a patient?   **YES NO**

4. Have you ever provided any other integrative therapies?   **YES NO**

If yes, which therapies_____

5. How confident do you feel providing aromatherapy to a patient?

   Very confident   **Confident**   **Not Confident**

6. How confident do you feel providing acupressure to a patient?

   Very confident   **Confident**   **Not Confident**

7. How confident do you feel providing guided imagery to a patient?

   Very confident   **Confident**   **Not Confident**

SELF CARE:

8. Do you use aromatherapy for yourself?   **YES NO**

9. Do you use acupressure for yourself?   **YES NO**

10. Do you use guided imagery for yourself?   **YES NO**

11. Do you use any other Integrative Therapies?   **YES NO**

If yes, which therapies do you use _____

FIGURE 6.3 Pre-Survey

Integrative Therapy Post-Survey

Instructions: Circle or indicate your response

PATIENT CARE:

1. Following this introduction to Integrative Therapy, how often might you use Integrative Therapy for patient care?

   a. Every shift   b. 2x/week   c. 1x/week   d. 1x/month   e. Other_____

2. How confident do you feel teaching aromatherapy to a patient?

   Very confident   Confident   Not Confident

3. How confident do you feel teaching acupressure to a patient?

   Very confident   Confident   Not Confident

4. What Integrative Therapies do you feel patients might like? _____
   _____

SELF CARE:

5. Following this introduction to Integrative Therapy, are you more likely to use Integrative Therapy for yourself?

   YES   NO

6. Which therapies might you consider?_____
   _____

COMMENTS_____

FIGURE 6.4 Post-Survey

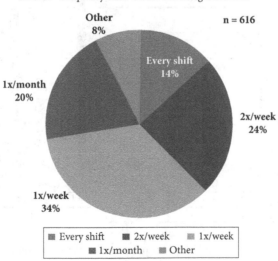

TOTAL - Frequency Staff Would Use Integrative Care

n = 616

- Other 8%
- Every shift 14%
- 2x/week 24%
- 1x/week 34%
- 1x/month 20%

■ Every shift   ■ 2x/week   ■ 1x/week   ■ 1x/month   ■ Other

FIGURE 6.5 Frequency Staff Would Use Integrative Therapy

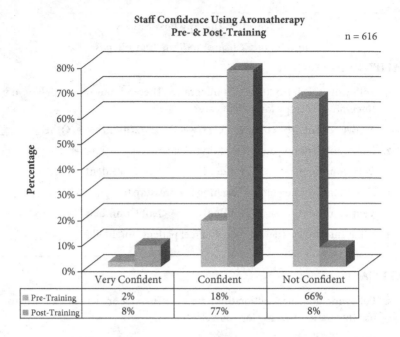

FIGURE 6.6 Staff Confidence Using Aromatherapy for Patients Comparing Pre & Post Training

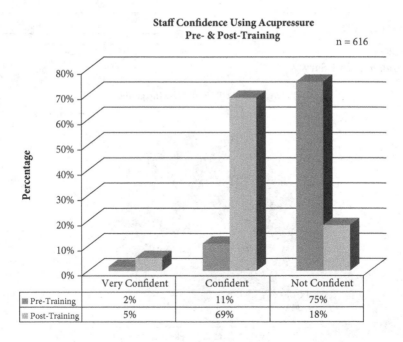

FIGURE 6.7 Staff Confidence Using Acupressure for Patients Comparing Pre & Post Training

SELECTED REFERENCES

American Holistic Nurses Association. Retrieved January 2013 from http://www.ahna.org/.

National Center for Complementary and Alternative Medicine (NCCAM). Retrieved March 2013 from http://nccam.nih.gov/.

Center for Spirituality and Healing at the University of Minnesota. Retrieved March 2013 from http://www.csh.umn.edu/.

Gach, M. R. (1990). *Acupressure's Potent Points: A Guide to Self-Care for Common Ailments.* New York: Bantam Books.

Humphreys, J., Lee, K. A., Carrieri-Kohlman, V., et al. (2008). Theory of symptom management. In Smith, M. J., & Liehr, P. R. (eds.), *Middle Range Theory for Nursing.* 2nd ed. New York: Springer Publishing Co.

Jones, M. C., MacHillivray, S., Kroll, T., Zohoor, A. R., & Connaghan, J. (2011). A thematic analysis of the conceptualization of self-care, self-management and self-management support in the long-term conditions management literature. *Journal of Nursing and Healthcare of Chronic Illness, 3,* 174–185.

Kreitzer, M. J., Mitten, D., Harris, I., & Shandeling, J. (2002). Attitudes toward CAM in medical, nursing, and pharmacy faculty and students: A comparative analysis. *Alternative Therapies in Health and Medicine, 8*(6), 44–53.

Melnyk, B., & Fineout-Overholt, E. (2011). *Evidence-Based Practice in Nursing and Healthcare.* 2nd ed. Philadelphia, PA: Lippincott Williams & Wilkins.

Price, S., & Price, L. (2011). *Aromatherapy for Health Professionals.* 4th ed. New York: Churchill Livingstone.

Watson Caring Science Institute & International Caring Consortium. Retrieved March 2013 from http://www.watsoncaringscience.org.

7

Creating Optimal Healing Environments

TERRI ZBOROWSKY AND MARY JO KREITZER

> *People say the effect is only on the mind. It is no such thing. The effect is on the body, too. Little as we know about the way in which we are affected by form, by color, and light, we do know this, that they have an actual physical effect. Variety of form and brilliancy of color in the objects presented to patients, are actual means of recovery.*
>
> —Florence Nightingale, Notes on Nursing: What It Is
> and What It Is Not (1860), p. 84.

The focus on creating healing environments is not new. The first nurse to document the impact of the built environment on patients was Florence Nightingale. In addition to writing about sanitation, infection rates, and ventilation, she was also very concerned about what many had thought to be merely "aesthetics." Nightingale understood that elements such as color, noise, and light, along with the nurse's presence, significantly contributed to health outcomes. A summary of the themes developed by Nightingale in *Notes on Hospitals* were reported by Dossey (2005):

The hospital will do the patient no harm. Four elements essential for the health of hospitals are:

- Fresh air
- Ample space
- Light
- Subdivision of sick into separate buildings or pavilions

Hospital construction defects that prevent health are:

- Defective means of natural ventilation and warming
- Defective height of wards
- Excessive width of wards between the opposite windows
- Arrangement of the bed along the dead wall

- More than two rows of beds between the opposite windows
- Windows only on one side, or a closed corridor connecting the wards
- Use of absorbent materials for walls and ceilings, and poor washing of hospital floors
- Defective condition of water closets [toilets]
- Defective ward furniture
- Defective accommodation for nursing and discipline
- Defective hospital kitchens
- Defective laundries
- Selection of bad sites and bad local climates for hospitals
- Erecting of hospitals in towns
- Defects of sewerage
- Construction of hospitals without free circulation of external air

Progress in healthcare building design and construction has clearly been made since the mid-1800s; however, many of the concerns identified by Nightingale sadly remain issues today. The designers of contemporary hospitals still grapple with issues of noise, light, cleanliness, and air quality. Nightingale's vision was aspirational and continues to serve as a guide in creating optimal healing environments.

"Optimal Healing Environment" Defined

It is clear from Nightingales' writing that she had a vision for the physical components of a healing environment. The word "healing" comes from the Anglo-Saxon word *hælen*, which means "to make whole." Healing environments are designed to promote harmony or balance of mind, body, and spirit, to reduce anxiety and stress, and to be restorative. The Samueli Institute, a research institute focused on the science of healing, defines an optimal healing environment (OHE) as a place where all aspects of patient care—physical, emotional, spiritual, behavioral, and environmental—are optimized to support and stimulate healing (see Figure 7.1).

As illustrated in Figure 7.1, within an OHE, the attitudes and intentions of all health-care providers and patients are recognized as important. There are opportunities for personal growth and self-care practices that promote wholeness. Healing relationships are cultivated as patients and their families interact with caring and compassionate healthcare providers and staff. Healthy lifestyles are promoted, and patients have options to choose conventional care as well as integrative therapies and healing practices. A culture is created that supports healing through alignment of the organizational vision, mission, resources, and leadership. This culture is supported by a physical environment that embodies design characteristics thought to promote healing, such as nature, light, and color, as well as other design elements that support an optimal

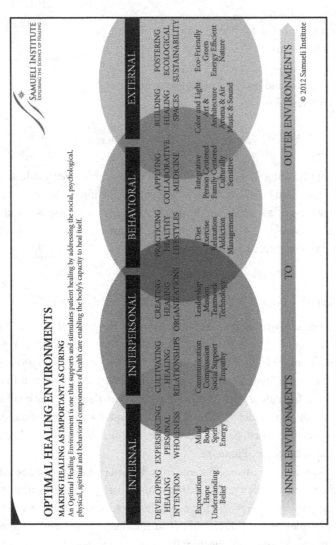

FIGURE 7.1 Samueli Institute Optimal Healing Environment. (Used with permission from Wayne B. Jonas)

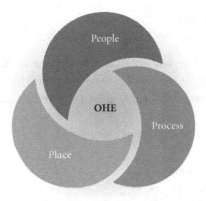

FIGURE 7.2 People, Place and Process: The Role of Place in Creating Optimal Healing Environments. (Zborowsky & Kreitzer, 2009)

healthcare practice, such as the design of a private patient room with zones that support the work of the caregivers, healing of the patient, and amenities for families.

A model developed by the authors of this chapter (Kreitzer & Zborowsky, 2009) and depicted in Figure 7.2 illustrates that an optimal healing environment is created through a deep and dynamic interplay between people, place, process, and culture. In this model, "people" includes the caregivers and support team that surround the patient. The characteristics and competencies of the staff and the knowledge, skills, and attitudes that they embody are some of the most critical elements of an OHE. The "process" element refers to the care processes as well as the leadership processes that support a culture aligned with creating an OHE. Care processes include conventional, integrative, and behavioral interventions. The "place" element focuses on the physical space where care is provided and the geography that surrounds the patient, family, and caregiver. "Place" elements include access to nature, positive distractions, aesthetics, the ambient environment, and ecosystem sustainability.

This model of OHE suggests that, optimally, there is good coherence and alignment between the "people—nurses and patients" who enact "processes—caregiving in the context of patient centered care" in a "place—physical environment" that is designed to maximize positive patient outcomes.

The reality is that much of patient care occurs in old, dysfunctional facilities. Even healthcare facilities built just twenty years ago lack the available space and mechanical systems to function well today, due to changes in building codes, guidelines, and best practice in care models. An inadequate space makes it difficult to attain a truly healing environment, though the elements of the caregiver and the care provided are considered more critical than the physical place or space. Today, there is a better understanding and rigorous research that describes how to choose elements of "place" that support and enable an OHE. The rest of this chapter will focus on these elements.

Research on the Impact of the Designed Environment

There have been three systematic studies on the impact of the healthcare built environment. Rubin, Owens, and Golden (1998) reviewed eighty-four studies and found that the following design features influenced at least one health outcome.

Natural view out of window/access to sunlight
Artificial lighting
Environmental temperature
Environmental humidity
Ventilation systems
Music and/or sound stimulation
Amount, layout, and décor of space
Interior design features such as carpeting selection

Six years later, Ulrich, Zimring, Quan, Joseph, and Choudhary (2004) identified over 600 studies using similar search criteria. They categorized these studies into four outcome areas.

1. Reduce staff stress and fatigue and increase effectiveness in delivering care

Studies in this area included research on improving staff health through environmental measures and increasing staff effectiveness and satisfaction, as well as reducing errors by designing better workplaces.

2. Improve patient safety

Studies in this area focused on reducing infections caused by airborne pathogens, reducing infections with increased hand-washing, reducing infections with single-patient rooms, reducing medication errors, reducing patient falls, and improving patient confidentiality and privacy.

3. Reduce stress and improve outcomes

Studies in this area included reducing noise, improving sleep, reducing spatial disorientation, reducing depression, providing nature and positive distraction, and providing social support and communication with patients.

4. Improve overall healthcare quality

Studies in this area included research on single-patient rooms, reducing length of stay, and increasing patient satisfaction with quality of care.

While the authors included studies that focused on patients and staff, the quality and rigor of the studies varied considerably. Many studies had a small and unique sample size, and therefore the results are not generalizable to a larger population. However, the increase in the volume of articles is notable and indicates growing interest in this discipline.

Four years later, Ulrich and colleagues (2008) conducted another literature review with over 1,200 research articles that met the same criteria. The authors found they were able to expand on the themes found in 2004, as well as add practical recommendations that were supported by these data. Studies were clustered in three content areas.

1. *Patient Safety Issues*: including infections, medical errors, and falls;
2. *Patient Outcomes*: pain, sleep, stress, depression, length of stay, spatial orientation, privacy, communication, social support, and overall satisfaction; and
3. *Staff Outcomes*: injuries, stress, work effectiveness, and work satisfaction.

Ulrich and colleagues concluded that

although many [of these] studies are not well controlled, the strength of evidence is enhanced by the fact that in the case of certain environmental factors, reliable patterns of findings across several studies emerged with respect to outcome influences. Furthermore, these patterns were broadly consistent with predictions based on established knowledge and theory concerning environment and healthcare outcomes. (Ulrich et al., 2008, p. 66)

At the same time as this field of research was growing, many healthcare organizations had taken note of the emerging research in this discipline. Examples of published discussion papers or literature reviews may be found in Table 7.1.

On the basis of these studies, a few conclusions can be reached. First, there appears to be a growing area of scientific inquiry that offers a range of research designs and various methodologies. Some studies are more rigorous than others. This is often the case when doing research *in situ*, during the operation of a healthcare facility. Similarly, in other areas of health science research there appears to be movement towards studies that utilize a mixed-method approach (Creswell, Klassen, Clark, & Smith, 2011). This type of research design appears well suited to the study of the impact of the built environment due to the nature of conducting research in a healthcare setting.

The second conclusion is that, given the Institute of Medicine's reports of the state of healthcare in the United States, along with the patient safety and quality movement promoted by the Institute for Healthcare Improvement, there is merit in the notion that "place" does play a key role, along with the "people" who provide and participate

Table 7.1: List of Published Documents on the Impact of Healthcare Design by Various Healthcare Organizations

Organization	Title	Authors	Year
Institute of Medicine (IOM)	Chapter 6: Work and Workspace Design to Prevent and Mitigate Errors in Keeping Patients Safe: Transforming the Work Environment of Nurses	Committee on the Work Environment for Nurses and Patient Safety, Board of Health Care Services	2004
Agency for Healthcare Research and Quality (AHRQ)	The Hospital Design Environment: What Role Might Funders of Health Services Play?	C. Nelson, T. West & C. Goodman	2005
Military Health System (MHS)	Evidence-Based Design: Application in the MHS	E. Malone, J. R. Mann-Dooks, & J. Strauss	2007
Robert Wood Johnson Foundation (RWJF)	Addressing the Quality and Safety Gap—Part III:The Impact of the Built Environment on Patient Outcomes and the Role of Nurses in Designing Health Care Facilities	RWJF	2007
Agency for Healthcare Research and Quality (AHRQ)	Transforming Hospitals: Designing for Safety and Quality	AHRQ	2007
Institute for Healthcare Improvement (IHI)	Using Evidence-Based Environmental Design to Enhance Safety and Quality	B. L. Sadler, A. Joseph, A. Keller, & B. Rostenberg	2009

in the care in the "processes" of healing. The question remains, can the elements of "place" that have an impact on creating OHEs be isolated in research? Table 7.2 reveals the "place" components of an OHE.

Meeting functional requirements is largely tied to the programming process that occurs during a building project (data gathering and documentation of the types of spaces; sizes of rooms or areas; and any unique needs to be addressed in the facility). Most of this is driven by code and regulations (each state will have adopted certain code standards as well as accessibility standards that need to be adhered to), industry standards, and user needs. Facilities built today must meet a minimum standard set of functional requirements.

Creating an optimal healing environment goes beyond functional requirements. Careful attention must be paid to how the space will be used, often referred to as the "programming" of the space, as well as the aesthetics. During this phase of facilities design, data are gathered on the users' needs within the space. "Users" include patients, families, staff—literally anyone who interacts with the space. Attention is focused on

Table 7.2: Elements of Place: Aspects of the Designed Environment That Impact
People and Process to Enable an OHE

OHE Place Component	Definition
Meets Functional Requirements	Functional requirements are identified during the programming phase of the design process (see Facilities Guidelines Institute for more information). These requirements include patient and staff safety, space for social support, and staff work areas, among others. (www.fgiguidelines.org)
Access to Nature	Actual or visual access to natural settings or designed nature settings. Access to daylight.
Positive Distractions	Includes elements of the design environment that are of a 2-D or 3-D nature; for example, artwork, water features, fireplaces, among others.
Aesthetics	Includes the design elements of color, texture, shape, form and volume; for example, furniture, fabric, and room layout, among others.
Ambient Environment	Includes the elements of artificial light, sound, odor, air temperature, and air quality.
Supports a Sustainable Ecosystem	Includes the economic, social, and ecological impact of the design elements of the building and the impact of any construction.

the physical, psychological, social, and spiritual needs of the users. It is a complex process, often cut short by tight timelines and limited budgets. Decisions made at this juncture heavily drive the selection and manipulation of the elements of the built environment.

In the remainder of this chapter, key design elements will be discussed that have an evidence base linking them to important outcomes in clinical environments. These elements include access to nature, access to daylight, positive distraction, aesthetics, and the ambient environment.

Access to Nature

Human beings relate with nature and other living systems in ways that mutually contribute to health and wellbeing.

—*Kreitzer & Koithan*

"Access to nature" is defined as a connection to the natural environment. This exists on a continuum from gazing through a window, to being fully immersed in a natural environment. As human beings, we are innately drawn to nature. "Biophilia" is defined as the inherent human inclination to affiliate with natural systems and processes. The preferences toward things in nature, while refined through experience and culture, are believed to be the product of biological evolution. The concept, originally proposed by eminent biologist Edward O. Wilson (1984), has grown into a broader framework that increasingly influences the design of the built environment, including hospitals and other healthcare facilities. Biophilic design emphasizes the necessity of maintaining, enhancing, and restoring the beneficial experience of nature and attempts to do so through the use of environmental features that embody characteristics of the natural world, such as color, water, sunlight, plants, natural materials, and exterior views and vistas (Kellert, 2008).

Biophilia has been empirically tested in clinical settings. Exposing patients to nature can produce substantial and clinically important outcomes. Research is strongest in pain reduction. Viewing nature may decrease pain by eliciting positive emotions, reducing stress, and distracting patients from focusing on their pain (Malenbaum, Keefe, Williams, Ulrich, & Somers, 2008; Ulrich et al., 2006; Ulrich et al., 2008). One study compared patients recovering from abdominal surgery with a bedside view of nature (trees) to those in identical rooms with windows overlooking the wall of a brick building (Ulrich, 1984). Patients with the nature view suffered substantially less pain, as indicated by their need for far fewer doses of strong pain medication than their counterparts with the wall view. In addition, the patients exposed to nature had shorter post-surgery stays, better emotional wellbeing, and fewer minor complications such as persistent nausea or headache.

There is emerging research that utilizes a multi-method approach to understanding the effect nature has on patients. Goto, Park, Tsunetsugu, Herrup, and Miyazaki (2013) found that exposure to organized gardens can affect both the mood and the cardiac physiology of elderly individuals. Among the findings, they revealed that the subject's heart rate was significantly lower in the Japanese garden than in the other environments studied; also, the subject's sympathetic function was significantly lower. While this study represents a case study of nineteen subjects living in an assisted-living facility, it provides valuable data of both the psychological and physiological states of the subjects.

Access to Daylight

The mechanism for enabling daylight to play a healing role is different than for nature. The circadian system, or 24-hour "biological clock," regulates cycles of sleep/alertness, body temperature, and hormone production. The circadian system is controlled by light reaching receptors in the retina. Production of melatonin begins when light fades, inducing sleep. Sunlight exposure also increases levels of serotonin, a neurotransmitter known to inhibit pain pathways. For patients, their family members, and staff, particularly those who work nights, it appears that exposure to sunlight is an important OHE component.

Joseph (2006) conducted a literature review of the impact of light on health outcomes. The key findings on the health outcomes of access to light for both patients and staff included:

- Light impacts human health and performance by enabling performance of visual tasks, controlling the body's circadian system, affecting mood and perception, and enabling critical chemical reactions in the body.
- Studies show that higher light levels are linked with better performance of complex visual tasks, and that light requirements increase with age. By controlling the body's circadian system, light impacts outcomes in healthcare settings by reducing depression among patients, decreasing length of stay in hospitals, improving sleep and circadian rhythm, lessening agitation among dementia patients, easing pain, and improving adjustment to night-shift work among staff.
- The presence of windows in the workplace and access to daylight have been linked with increased satisfaction with the work environment.
- Furthermore, exposure to sunlight is critical for vitamin D metabolism in the human body. Light exposure has also been used as a treatment for neonatal hyperbilirubinaemia.

Walch and colleagues (2005) conducted a well-controlled prospective study of the effects of daylight on pain in patients undergoing spinal surgeries, who were admitted postoperatively to rooms either on the bright or the shaded side of a surgical ward. Patients in the bright rooms were exposed to 46% greater sunlight intensity than those assigned to the more shaded rooms. Findings indicated that patients in rooms with more sunlight reported less pain and stress, and they took 22% less analgesic medications, resulting in a 21% reduction in medication costs. The shaded patient rooms and associated heightened pain resulted when a new building was constructed and blocked sunlight from reaching this side of the facility.

The impact of natural light on staff outcomes has also been assessed in several studies (Badia, Myers, Boecker, & Culpeper, 1991; Boyce, Beckstead, Eklund, Strobel, & Rea, 1997; and Figueiro, Rea, Boyce, White, & Kolberg, 2001), and all reported that exposure to short bursts (15 minutes) of bright light between 2,500 and 3,000 lux during the night may have short-term positive effects on brain activity, cognitive performance, subjective alertness, and feelings of wellbeing.

Using a pre-test/post-test quasi-experimental study in two intensive care units, Shepley, Gerbi, Watson, Imgrund, and Sagha-Zadeh (2012) studied the impact of daylight and window views on patient pain levels, length of stay, staff errors, absenteeism, and vacancy rates. Researchers concluded that high levels of natural light and window views may positively affect staff absenteeism and staff vacancy, while factors such as medical errors, patient pain, and length of stay still require additional research. In summary, there is growing evidence that views of nature and light are beneficial for patients as well as staff.

Positive Distractions

A "positive distraction" has been defined as an environmental feature that elicits positive feelings and holds attention without taxing or stressing the individual, thereby blocking worrisome thoughts (Ulrich, 1991). Positive distractions include both two-dimensional and three-dimensional artifacts. According to distraction theory, pain requires considerable conscious attention. If patients become diverted or engrossed in a pleasant distraction such as a nature view or work of art, they have less attention to direct to their pain, and the experienced pain therefore will diminish. The theory predicts that the more engrossing an environmental distraction is, the greater the pain reduction (McCaul & Malott, 1984).

Several well-controlled randomized studies support providing technology (such as video screens and eyeglass displays) to simulate nature in spaces where patients undergo painful procedures and it is not feasible to provide distraction with actual nature. Malenbaum et al. (2008) found that nature simulations with both visual and auditory distraction may be more diverting and engrossing and hence more effective for relieving severe pain. This suggests that patients should not be placed in rooms or treatment spaces that lack nature distraction and contain environmental stressors such as noise, as pain may be exacerbated. Similar findings were reported by Tse, Ng, Chung, and Wong (2002), who found that healthy volunteers in a hospital setting had a higher pain threshold and greater tolerance when they looked at a videotape of nature scenery. Kozarek and colleagues (1997) investigated the effects of seeing and listening to a nature travelogue on patients undergoing painful gastric procedures. Patient reports and nurse observations converged in suggesting that the combination of visual and auditory distraction improved comfort and tolerance for the procedures, as compared to a control condition without distraction. Similarly, Schneider, Ellis, Coombs, Shonkwiler, and Folsom (2003) found that a virtual-reality audiovisual nature distraction (a "walk" through a forest with bird sounds) reduced discomfort and symptomatic distress in female chemotherapy patients. Diette, Lechtzin, Haponik, Devrotes, and Rubin (2003) reported that patients undergoing painful bronchoscopy who were assigned to look at a ceiling-mounted nature scene and listen to nature sounds (moving water, birds) reported less pain than a control group who looked at a blank ceiling during bronchoscopy. Lee and colleagues (2004) conducted a randomized prospective clinical trial on the effects of nature distraction on patients undergoing colonoscopy and reported that that visual distraction alone reduced pain but did not lower the intake of sedative medications. However, a combination of nature scenery with classical music reduced both pain and self-administered sedation during colonoscopy. In reviewing the literature on the use of virtual reality as adjunct analgesic techniques,

Wismeijer and Vingerhoets (2005) concluded that nature exposure may tend to be more diverting and hence pain-reducing if they involve sound as well as visual stimulation and are high in realism and immersion.

Pati and Nanda (2011) utilized a quasi-experimental design to examine pediatric patients' behavior during five distraction conditions, ranging from a slide show to a video with music. All distraction conditions were created on one flat-screen plasma TV monitor mounted on a stand in the waiting areas. Data analysis showed that the introduction of distraction conditions was associated with calmer behavior and less fine and gross movement, suggesting significant calming effects associated with the distraction conditions. Data also suggest that positive distraction conditions are significant attention-grabbers and could be an important contributor to improving the waiting experience for children in hospitals by improving environmental attractiveness.

Based on an extensive body of both scientific studies and anecdotal accounts, Ulrich and Gilpin (2003) recommended that the content of such art include:

- Waterscapes—calm or non-turbulent water
- Landscapes—visual depth or open-foreground trees with broad canopy, savannah landscapes, verdant vegetation, or positive cultural artifacts (such as barns and older houses)
- Flowers—healthy and fresh, familiar gardens with open foreground
- Figurative art—emotionally positive faces, diverse, leisurely

Nanda, Zhu, and Jansen (2012) conducted a systematic review of neuroscience articles on the emotional states of fear, anxiety, and pain to understand how emotional response is linked to the visual characteristics of an image at the level of brain behavior. While there is a paucity of research in this area, they were able to offer implications for practice:

- Viewing images can have a direct impact on emotional processing centers in the brain; thus, art for healthcare facilities must be carefully selected.
- "Restorative" images are defined by content with high valence (positive) and low arousal (calming).
- When viewing novel/unfamiliar images, the brain struggles to create a context and find similar memories, which can be linked to anxiety. This struggle often contributes to create great abstract art by allowing viewers to come up with their own interpretation. For highly vulnerable patients, however, the anxiety related to this process may be more acute, and the primal emotional response can override the higher-level cognitive response. Art should be selected with this tradeoff in mind.
- Fearful expressions on faces can trigger a greater fear response in a viewer than viewing a direct threat; thus, facial expressions should be carefully considered when selecting figurative art.

- The following elements in a visual image should be carefully evaluated and, if possible, avoided in high-stress areas: fearful/angry faces; ambiguous subject matter; high levels of novelty and unfamiliarity; lack of realism; and sharp-edged contours.
- The primal response to images is triggered by a quick evaluative system that rapidly extracts information from an image; this depends on global cues rather than a high level of detail. Form and content relate to global cues and must be addressed together when choosing art.
- Emotional impact must be balanced with aesthetic value in the context of healthcare art.

Aesthetics

Aesthetics in the built environment are impacted by what designers refer to as "design elements and principles." Design elements include color, texture, shape, form, and volume. Design principles, such as rhythm, balance, or contrast, provide guidance on how to manipulate the design elements to create aesthetically appropriate environments. Color is an example of a design element that draws much attention and curiosity.

Color has specific characteristics, including lightness (light vs. dark, or white vs. black), saturation (intense vs. dull), and hue (e.g., red, orange, yellow, green, blue or purple). In a literature review of 3,000 citations focused on the impact of color in healthcare settings, Tofle, Schwarz, Yoon, and Max-Royale (2003) concluded that there were no direct linkages between particular colors and health outcomes. However, they also concluded that there are demonstrable perceptual impressions of color applications that can affect the experience and performance of people in particular environments. For example, the perception of spaciousness was attributed to the brightness or darkness of color and less by its hue (actual color). There are also emotional responses to colors that may be impacted by culturally learned associations or by the physiological and psychological makeup of people. Despite the scarcity of color studies, Bosch, Cama, Edelstein, and Malkin (2012) offer guidelines that may be useful:

- Consider the needs of each specific patient population in the selection of color. In elderly populations, understand how vision changes as the eye ages. Greater contrast and more saturated colors are easier to see than pastel tones.
- Skin color is a vital clinical cue. Each patient zone should have access to natural daylight so that clinicians can assess skin tone properly. Be aware of the effect of the color of walls surrounding a patient.
- Consider religious or symbolic associations with color, including cultural taboos, biases, and nationality, that may be relevant to that particular community.

- Understand how color affects the perception of space—light colors move planes (e.g., walls) forward and dark colors make planes recede.
- Color plays a role in the perception of "clean" and "dirty."
- Consider the effect of lighting on color. Each type of light has a color range itself, and colors look different under different light sources.

Ambient Environment

There are unseen elements in the designed environment, such as artificial light, sound, odor, air temperature, air quality, and sound. Of these elements, the one that has captured considerable attention is sound, as loud noise is well documented as having a negative impact on patient outcomes. Joseph and Ulrich (2007) conducted a literature review to examine how different aspects of sound—noise, speech privacy, speech intelligibility, and music—impact patient and staff outcomes in healthcare settings, and the specific environmental design strategies that can be used to improve the acoustical environment. The authors concluded that hospitals are extremely noisy, and noise levels in most hospitals far exceed recommended guidelines. The high ambient noise levels, as well as peak noise levels, have serious impacts on patient and staff outcomes, ranging from sleep loss and elevated blood pressure among patients, to emotional exhaustion and burnout among staff. Poorly designed acoustical environments can pose a serious threat to patient confidentiality if private conversations between patients and staff or between staff members can be overheard by unintended listeners. At the same time, a poor acoustical environment impedes effective communication between patients and staff and between staff members by rendering speech and auditory signals less intelligible or detectable. This may have serious implications for patient safety. A well-designed acoustical environment is critical in addressing issues related to noise and communication of information.

Solet, Buxton, Ellenbogen, Wang, and Carballiera (2010) exposed twelve sleeping, fully monitored, healthy adults to a series of fourteen hospital sounds, including voices, derived from the recording of an inpatient medical-surgical unit. The sounds were delivered in rising decibel level steps during all stages of sleep at a Harvard Medical School–affiliated sleep laboratory. Results revealed that phone and IV alarms, which are designed to be alerting, were effective in evoking the highest arousal probabilities during the patients' sleep cycles. They also found that intermittent sounds such as staff conversations and voice paging, snoring, and the electric towel dispenser were found to be more alerting than more continuous sounds such as traffic and laundry carts. Trickey, Arnold, Parmar, and Lasky (2012) conducted a prospective observational study comparing sound measures and patient outcomes in a neonatal intensive care unit (NICU) before, during, and after a year-long construction renovation. Researchers found that while the renovation project did not cause substantially louder sound levels, staff perceived important changes in noise and work routines, suggesting that perception of noise may be a mitigating factor in the impact of noise on staff work routine.

Solet et al. (2010) listed a number of strategies that are being used to reduce environmental noise:

- Single-patient bedrooms.
- Installing high-performance, sound-absorbing acoustical ceiling tiles.
- Answering IV alarms promptly and lowering background sound levels so important alarm signals can be easily discerned.
- Reducing telephone ring-tone volume to prevent transmission beyond the patient rooms. Set telephones to stop after a specific number of rings.
- Creating special consulting spaces so voice-based information can be transferred away from open hall areas, yet not far from nursing stations.
- Dimming hall lights at night as a "quiet cue" to limit sleep disruption by staff voices.
- Isolating ice machines from patient areas or dramatically re-engineering them.
- Substituting quieter or low-tech alternatives for automatic hand-towel dispensers (often described as disruptive by patients).
- Installing proper door hardware to limit latch noises.

Conclusion

In recent years there has been much written about the role of healthcare facility design and its impact on patients, family members, and healthcare staff. A lot of this documentation acknowledges the importance that "place" has in optimizing a healing environment. From the days of Nightingale's pie charts, to the scientific rigor of studies funded by Agency for Healthcare Research and Quality (AHRQ), this field is now growing rapidly. Research studies being conducted *in situ* are largely case studies exploring the use of the scientific method and social science methodology. This causes some to question and doubt the validity of this knowledge base. Instead, we must embrace this exploration stage to be ready for innovation to occur, both in uncovering what role the designed environment plays in creating an optimal healing environment, as well as how best to conduct research in this complex area. Nurses are well positioned to be at the forefront of setting this research agenda—much like our visionary forebear, Nightingale, we are now at an important crossroad to inform the future design of healthcare environments, specifically, the creation of OHE.

Case Study Application of Optimal Healing Environments

North Hawaii Community Hospital

North Hawaii Community Hospital (NHCH) embodies the culture of the community in the way it has operationalized the concept of OHE. The footprint of the hospital was aligned so that the front is oriented to the Kohala Mountain and the back to the mountain Mauna Kea. Earl Bakken, one of the founders of the hospital, envisioned that "the hospital itself would be an instrument of healing, rather than a warehouse for sick bodies" (http://www.earlbakken.com). All patient rooms are private and have access to views of nature and fresh air through sliding doors that open to the outside. Art in patients' rooms is culturally and historically meaningful, and can be changed. Hallways are carpeted, and there is minimal overhead paging. Soft music plays in public spaces. Familiar cultural patterns, textures, and colors are used in wallpapers, carpeting, and furniture coverings. Ti plants at all entrances and corners of the building are believed to filter out bad spiritual energy. An interior bamboo garden also offers spiritual protection and represents strength and resilience. All patient rooms have sleep chairs or extra beds for guests to stay over, and there are no limits on the number of visitors or visiting hours. An *ohama* (Hawaiian for "family") room includes a kitchen so that families can prepare special meals. Skylights in halls and windows in the operating rooms were incorporated into the design to enable staff to stay attuned to day/night cycles. In addition to these and many other mechanical, architectural, and engineering adaptations, the hospital embraces a philosophy of blended medicine that encourages the integration of complementary therapies and culturally based healing practices. The vision of NHCH is to be the most healing hospital in the world.

SELECTED REFERENCES

Agency for Healthcare Research and Quality (AHRQ). (2007). Transforming hospitals: Designing for safety and quality. Retrieved October 1, 2012, from http://www.ahrq.gov/qual/transform.htm.

Facilities Guideline Institute. (2010 edition). *Guidelines for Design and Construction of Health Care Facilities*. Chicago: American Society for Healthcare Engineering (ASHE).

Institute of Medicine. (2004). *Transforming the Work Environment of Nurses: Committee on the Work Environment for Nurses and Patient Safety*. Washington, DC: National Academy Press.

Kellert, S. (2008). *Biophilic Design: The Theory, Science, and Practice of Bringing Buildings to Life*. New York: Wiley.

Nanda, U., Zhu, X., & Jansen, B.H. (2012). Image and emotion: From outcomes to brain behavior. *Health Environments Research & Design Journal*, 5(4):40–59.

Shepley, M. M., Gerbi, R. P., Watson, A. E., Imgrund, S., & Sagha-Zadeh, R. (2012). The impact of daylight and views on ICU patients and staff. *Health Environments Research & Design Journal*, 5(2), 46–60.

Solet, J. M., Buxton, O. M., Ellenbogen, J. M., Wang, W., & Carballiera, A. (2010). *Evidence-Based Design Meets Evidence-Based Medicine: The Sound Sleep Study.* Concord, CA: The Center for Health Design.

Trickey, A. W., Arnold, C. C., Parmar, A., & Lasky, R. E. (2012). Sound levels, staff perceptions, and patient outcomes during renovation near the neonatal intensive care unit. *Health Environments Research & Design Journal*, 5(4), 76–87.

Ulrich, R. S., Zimring, C., Zhu, X., DuBose, J. R., Seo, H. B., & Choi, Y. S. (2008). A review of the research literature on evidence-based healthcare design. *Health Environments Research & Design Journal*, 1(3), 61–125.

Wilson, E. O. (1984). *Biophilia: The Human Bond with Other Species.* Cambridge, MA: Harvard University Press.

8

Integrative Nursing Caring Science, Human Caring, and Peace

JEAN WATSON

T his chapter focuses on human caring and peace within the context of integrative nursing principles embedded in a framework of caring science and *caritas* (a Latin word conveying universal caring and love). Nurses' practice of human caring is an emergent quality of whole systems, making new connections between the unitary energetic patterns of worldwide human caring practices and peace in our world. This relationship between human caring and peace represents a fundamental path of consciously attending to the pattern of unity and the human-environmental global-universal field of oneness.

This unitary relationship within integrative principles represents what may be referred to as a quantum world, or even a quantum cosmology. That is, we now know from science and quantum thinking that the mere act of participating in or observing a system causes that system to change its behavior. "Some physicists have postulated that there is something special about consciousness that causes the abstract quantum potentials, described by quantum theory, to 'collapse' into hard physical reality observed in the everyday world" (Vieten, 2012, p. 6). In the world of quantum physics, it is acknowledged that everything is connected with everything else and there is one wholeness of all. The writings of David Bohm address this as well (1980a, 1980b, Bohm & Peat, 1987).

Caring Science: An Integrative Nursing Framework for Caring and Peace

Caring science, as an emerging area of nursing and trans-disciplinary study, grounds this expanded, quantum worldview related to integrative principles and acknowledges a deeper ethic of "belonging" (Levinas, 1969; Watson, 2008), making it explicit that we all belong to the infinity and universal cosmic energetic (quantum) field of the whole. This core integrative principle becomes a fundamental worldview, or even more encompassing, a cosmology, as a starting point for science, integrative principles, and our global society from which we cannot escape. Thus, the ethic of belonging helps us understand that a nurse's conscious acts of human caring have an individual and global effect at the same time. This ethic also is dependent upon evolving human consciousness, whereby we connect with the unitary field of cosmic love (Levinas, 1969).

Consistent with this line of integrative thinking, a 2011 research study on the potential for peace between Israelis and Palestinians affirmed one of the basic integrative principles: that is, caring, health, and peace reflect an ever-changing pattern of creative, adaptive relationships across all dimensions of human experience (Kreitzer & Koithan, 2011). This Israeli national research found that simply teaching Israelis and Palestinians that groups of people are capable of change can have a markedly positive effect on their willingness to compromise. Indeed, the more Israeli Jews believed that groups could change, "the more favorable were their attitudes toward Palestinians—and the more willing they were to make major compromises for the sake of peace. When the researchers repeated this study with Palestinians—both within Israel and the West Bank—they found identical results" (McClure-Stanford, 2011).

This line of thinking is congruent with the emergent quality of whole systems within the framework of integrative nursing principles and caring science, underpinning the dynamics of caring and peace. That is, believing in change can result in concrete connections between two groups, including a change of attitude for adaptive relationships and acknowledging the fundamental unity within and between all beings and their environments.

A 2002 book by David Hawkins, *Power vs. Force*, addressed the evolution of consciousness and notion of shared consciousness; his views are consistent with a caring science ethic of belonging, as well as integrative principles. This view indicates the power of oneness of the human spirit and its relationship to the evolution of consciousness. That is, integrative principles are related to a pure consciousness in the universe, to which we all belong. This points toward options for how to access and manifest caring patterns that affect the whole. This evolution of caring is thought by Hawkins to be a higher consciousness that connects one with a universal life force, the infinite field of cosmos love. There is a connection between caring and love. In the caring science model, everything is connected energetically; thus, the person caring is manifesting universal love, affecting the whole of humanity and contributing to peace in our world.

This unity of consciousness, evolving consciousness framework guides human-environmental energetic healing practices, such as Reiki and Healing Touch. These practices are based upon subtle energy of love, as a high level of consciousness, if not the highest level of cosmic consciousness. The subtle and not-so-subtle connections between caring consciousness and energetic healing practices of love ultimately lead to connections between caring and peace. That is, if one is manifesting an authentically caring consciousness, then one is radiating energy of love and peace into the integrative field of the whole. As Hawkins (2002) noted, if we really understood this basic knowledge, the world as we know it would be irrevocably changed, requiring all practices of politics, war, communications, media, economics, and medicine to transform their patterns of practice.

So, in caring science and the integrative principle model, everything is connected with the infinite, universal, energetic field of cosmic love. Basic human values of loving-kindness, equanimity, compassion, forgiveness, and tolerance, all messages from wisdom and spiritual teachers across time, are embedded in the "faces" of our global community and in the human caring practices throughout the history and tradition of nursing and other health and human service professions.

These global and universal messages and values also are embedded in extant theories, contemporary science, and philosophies guiding human caring and healing for ourselves, others, and our world. For example, the writings of contemporary nursing theorists, such as Martha Rogers, Margaret Newman, Rosemary Parse, Barbara Dossey, and Jean Watson all converge around the same core ontological and epistemological integrative unitary principles. They include:

- A Unity worldview—that is, the view that everything is connected;
- There is one energetic field of human-environment-cosmos oneness;
- Transcendent possibilities for human experiences, while acknowledging we are fully embodied; patterns and processes of relativity of time and space and physicality;
- Unitary worldview acknowledges that, energetically, one's intentional consciousness transcends time and space, and exists beyond the moment, affecting the whole field;
- Evolving consciousness—evolving toward universal cosmic consciousness of love.

National research institutes, such as Fetzer Institute, University of Minnesota's Center for Spirituality and Healing, Institute of Noetic Sciences, Institute of HeartMath, Cleveland Clinic Heart Brain Institute, and the Templeton Foundation, are examples of systems pursuing research models that acknowledge a unitary, integrative worldview. For example, these institutes are pursuing studies that:

- "…emphasize individual and community transformation for self and society, based on principles of wholeness, freedom of spirit, unconditional love; and integration of the inner life of mind and Spirit with the outer life of service and action." (*Fetzer Newsletter*, 2006);
- "[Embody] science and spirit, technology, and dharma." (Klisanen, 2012);
- Explore "big moral and spiritual concepts and questions about human sciences, philosophy and theology, such as altruism, creativity, free will,

generosity, gratitude, intellect, love, prayer, and purpose" (John Templeton Foundation, 2013);
- Research mindfulness, meditation, and practices of healing (Center for Spirituality and Healing, 2013);
- Conduct research and training on health, wellbeing, and consciousness. (HeartMath, 2013).

Unitary, integrative principles are related to the higher-consciousness practices for health and healing. These principles are associated with non-physical domains, such as attitude, intentionality, and consciousness of positive emotions and mental thoughts. They address experiences of gratitude, forgiveness, grace, caring, compassion, and love, including mindful practices of rituals, prayer, and spiritual beliefs of hope and faith.

Conventional medicine does not systematically incorporate non-physical methods of energetic healing. Hawkins (2002) reported that conventional medicine, associated with physical pathology and disease, resides in a lower vibrational field and does not allow for evolution of human consciousness to a higher energetic field. The next turn in integrative nursing principles and medicine is to go beyond exclusive physicality and systematically include consciousness, intentionality, and spirituality for whole-person health, healing, caring, and peace. Integrative nursing principles thus incorporate caring for the individual, the environment and ecosystem, the community, and beyond, as a way of honoring all living things.

Love: The Highest Level of Consciousness

Margaret Newman, a prominent nursing theorist who focused on consciousness and quantum patterns as the context for healing, titled one of her books *Health as Expanding Consciousness* (Newman, 1994). So I pose the question for integrative nursing, related to caring science, the ethic of belonging, and Newman's and Hawkins' theory and research:

What is the highest level of consciousness?
My answer is *love*, which allows for evolution of higher consciousness to what Teilhard de Chardin referred to as the "Omega point"—humans becoming more godlike, connecting with the "infinite field" (de Chardin, 1959, 1964). Chardin posited that our consciousness becomes co-extensive with the universe toward unification (de Chardin, 1964, p. 310).

Ben Okri, prize-winning Nigerian writer, put it this way:

Individual authenticity lies in what we can find that is worth living for. And the only thing worth living for is love. Love of one another. Love for ourselves. Love of our work. Love of our destiny, whatever it may be. Love for our difficulties. Love of life. The love that could free us from the mysterious cycles of suffering. The love that releases us from our self-imprisonment, from our bitterness, our greed, our madness-engendering competiveness. The love that can make us breathe again. Love a great and beautiful cause, a wonderful vision. A great love for another, or for the future. The love that reconciles us to ourselves, to our simple joys, and to our undiscovered repletion. A creative love. A love touched with the sublime. (Okri, 1997, pp. 56–57)

Thus, infinite love is the highest level of consciousness, uniting humanity across continents and time, and is revealed through a reflective integrative nursing context. This relationship is revealed through heart-centered practices that restore the universality of human spirit, common tasks, and connections. Human-to-human, spirit-to-spirit connections, beginning with inner caring and inner peace, facilitate the healing of others and return us to the heart of peace in the world.

As integrative nurses, we know that when we step into the theories and philosophies of human caring and *caritas* (that is, conscious, intentional caring and love) (Watson, 2008, 2012), we step into a deep ethical and life practice that connects us with the heart of our humanity, of healing the whole. It is this unitary consciousness connection that unites humanity across time and space around the world. This expanded worldview raises new questions and offers new connections between personal and planetary transformation related to caring, healing, peace, and the power of love. These core perspectives from caring science and the integrative nursing principles introduce caring as an ethical covenant with humanity.

Within the context of integrative nursing, and an evolved consciousness, we can ask and invite new questions about caring and peace:

What is peace?
What is the origin of peace?
What is inner peace? How do we obtain it?
How do we manifest and sustain human caring and peace in our heart, mind, and daily acts?
Is there a connection between inner peace and outer peace?

These are fundamental yet rhetorical questions that reside within caring science and integrative principles and philosophies. These questions invite us to consider our common tasks as humans in order to sustain human dignity, basic civility, and humanity itself.

Evolving Integrative Human Tasks: Shared Human Pursuits Affecting Our Global Community

An integrative principle underlying shared human tasks for human evolution is realizing that one person's level of humanity is reflected upon the other; thus, what we do and say to ourselves affects others. This concept of shared humanity is identified by Kreitzer and Koithan (2011) in Integrative Principle 6 as "the fundamental unity within and between all beings and their environment." The shared human tasks related to caring and peace include healing our relationship with self and other as the beginning of inner and outer peace. This includes self-acceptance and holding compassion, loving-kindness, forgiveness, and tenderness to oneself first, then opening our hearts to others, even strangers or so-called enemies, and accepting others with loving-kindness and compassion.

More specifically, we can name these common human tasks we share on this journey toward integration. For example, at some level, every human being has the following challenges of being in the world:

- Healing our relationship with ourselves and each other.
- Understanding human suffering—both our own and others'. This includes finding new meanings to transform human suffering and recognizing the shared suffering of the human condition.
- Finding new depth of meaning and purpose in life and all the vicissitudes of the shared human condition of living, change, loss, grief, death, and dying, honoring the enduring human spirit in the midst of impermanence
- Finding personal meaning in the life–death cycle and death itself, as part of the larger sacred circle of infinity
- Coming to terms with our own death and dying
- "Remembering," or awakening to, the deep nature of life and love, and awakening to the ethic of belonging in our infinite field of universal love (Watson, 2008, 2012a).

Integrative nursing is helping to name and awaken to the shared human tasks of life that inform human caring and peaceful actions; such an awakening can help save succeeding generations from non-caring practices, violence, and untold human sorrow, despair, and destruction of humanity and earth itself.

This unified focus brings together principles and practices that invite us to consider our common tasks as humans. It is this consciousness that we seek to sustain human dignity, basic civility, and humanity—peace in action.

When we engage in integrative practices, when we offer our own life, one person to another, finding more conscious, intentional ways to offer gestures of peace to ourselves and others, then we become peace. Through the simple yet profound gestures of daily peace, we change the way we live.

The writer Terry Tempest Williams reminds us that "the eyes of the future are looking right at us and they are praying for us to see beyond our own time" (2001). There are now 7 billion people on this planet, and we have to ask new sacred questions about our survival. Our wisdom traditions from our ancestors and indigenous elders around the world teach us that peace and caring come from within the heart of our humanity, our professions, and our connections across cultures, lifetimes, worlds, words, space, and time. Human cries for love, for human caring and peace, reside within the heart of nursing and healthcare professionals, or we would not be here today.

From this awareness, we now can say that "what we truly love and what we neglect to love affects every aspect in our life." Love and peace are inseparable: I have love, I have peace.

As integrative nursing practitioners, perhaps we have a new role in the world:

> To transform the vision of human health and healing by engaging in service to self and society at a different level, by creating "the energetic field of caritas," through both overt and subtle practices that transmit and affect the field of the whole. We do this one by one and become part of creating a deeper level of humanity by transforming fundamentally what happens in a given caring moment, in a given situation, by experimenting with Being-the-Integrative-Caritas-Field. This is the truly noble work of nursing and healing that transcends the conventional way of thinking...when we proceed and attain this new old level of wisdom...in this line of thinking, there is a connection between caring (as connecting with, sustaining, and deepening our shared humanity) and peace in the world. In these noble integrative caritas (caring and love) practices we become *Bodhisattvas*: those who bless others and who become a blessing to self and others. We actively affect the entire universal field of humanity. (Watson, 2008, p. 48, with slight modifications)

These basic human-heart wisdoms and universal truths are embedded in the faces of our global community and human caring practices across time. Integrative nursing within the context of caring and peace, within the framework of *caritas* and caring science, indeed becomes sacred science (Watson, 2005).

In Levinas's ethics of belonging and ethic of face, he reminds us that the only way we can sustain humanity at this very point in time is through the face-to-face connection. When we look into the face of another person, we are looking into the infinity of human soul, connecting with the infinity of universal love. And there, in this infinite space of universal love, we awaken to our common humanity.

As integrative nursing and nurses, individually and collectively, along with other health and healing practitioners, awaken to our gifts and purpose, we uncover principles that are contributing to the global evolution of human consciousness. With integrative principles and evolving consciousness of humanity, I am hopeful we can evolve toward a moral community of caring and peace for our world.

Summary

Integrative *caritas*-conscious nurses and health professionals represent compassionate caretakers of life's creations, of caring and peace in our world. We can follow the *caritas* path of peace with our individual and collective evolved consciousness in our everyday ways of being.

You are invited to join nurses and others around the globe by signing the International Charter for Human Caring and Peace. Go to www.watsoncaringscience. org, *Caritas Path of Peace*.

SELECTED REFERENCES

Bohm, D., & Peat, F. D. (1987). *Science, Order, and Creativity*. New York: Bantam Books.
Caritas Path of Peace website. Retrieved April 16, 2013, from http://www.watsoncaringscience .org.
Chopra, D. (2005). *Peace Is the Way*. New York: Three Rivers Press.
de Chardin, T. (1964). *The Future of Man*. New York: Harper.
Hawkins, D. (2002). *Power vs. Force*. Carlsbad, CA: Hay House.
Klisanin, D. (2012). *Archetypes of Change in a Digital Age*. IONS Noetic Post, Spring-Summer.
Newman, M. (1994). *Health as Expanding Consciousness*. Philadelphia, PA: F.A. Davis.
Okri, B. (1997). *A Way of Being Free*. London: Phoenix.
Vieten, C. The Noetic Post: IONS.2012, 3(2), 6.
Watson, J. (2005). *Caring Science as Sacred Science*. Philadelphia, PA: F.A. Davis.
Watson, J. (2008). Nursing: *The Philosophy and Science of Caring*. Boulder, CO: University Press of Colorado.
Watson, J. (2012a). *Human Caring Science*. Sudbury, MA: Jones & Bartlett.

9

Informatics and Integrative Healthcare

CONNIE W. DELANEY, BONNIE L. WESTRA, PATRICK J. DEAN,
CHERYL J. LEUNING, AND KAREN A. MONSEN

The triple aims of improving patient care quality, improving patient experience, and reducing costs apply equally to traditional and integrative healthcare professions (Institute for Healthcare Improvement, 2013; Stiefel & Nolan, 2012). Information about the roles, practices, and outcomes of integrative healthcare is critical to the success of integrative nursing within health systems.

Integrative healthcare blends multiple relationship-based caring, healing modalities, and ways of knowing into practice that has long been recognized as effective in advancing human health and wellbeing across multiple care settings. Threads of integrative healthcare are woven within, throughout, and beyond various disciplines in our modern healthcare system. Integrative healthcare practices such as herbal therapies, Reiki, healing touch, aromatherapy, meditation, and guided imagery are grounded in multi-dimensionality and holism and anchored in human relationships that are subjective, personal, aesthetic, and particular to local settings.

Interprofessional health informatics is about managing and processing data (facts in all digital formats from text, audio, and images) and information (facts with attributed meaning), knowledge (synthesis and interpretation of information), and wisdom (applications of facts, meaning, and interpretation). Just as the printing press ushered in a communication revolution and modern society as we know it, the global information technology revolution arising from the objective, empirical world of data and data collection, data management, and processing is ushering in changes in how we interact to deliver healthcare today. "Big Data," information science, and network science are new tools for advancing interprofessional healthcare knowledge and wisdom within dynamic complex systems and social networks (Hey, Tansley, & Tolle, 2009; Silver, 2012). Integrative healthcare, nursing, and all healthcare professions can leverage the benefits of "informatics" to improve information management, support and document care, and capture outcomes.

This chapter explores the intersection of informatics and integrative healthcare and the synergy of possibilities that are rapidly emerging there. This chapter will (a) define informatics, (b) discuss integrative healthcare and its relationship to informatics,

(c) discover exemplars of integrative informatics supporting integrative healthcare and integrative nursing, and (d) imagine the possibilities for integrative nursing practice.

What Is Informatics?

Informatics is a scientific field that draws on information, management, cognitive, organizational, and computer sciences. Informatics tools and methods are used to manage and process data in order to generate information, knowledge, and wisdom. The science of informatics drives disruptive innovation and defines future approaches to information and knowledge management in health research, clinical care, and public health (ANA, 2007; Institute of Medicine (IOM, 2012; Langley & Beasley, 2007) with applications that span the microscopic to the macroscopic dimensions of healthcare and human life.

The microscopic dimension of health informatics is frequently defined as *bioinformatics*, and encompasses the development of new algorithms and statistics used to determine relationships within large datasets; the analysis and interpretation of various types of data, including nucleotide and amino acid sequences, protein domains, and protein structures; and the development and implementation of tools that enable efficient access and management of different types of information. This area of informatics includes genomics, proteomics, and tissue and organ imaging. Biomedical health informatics encompasses data and data standards and data organization in databases to represent clinical care. It addresses appropriate technologies to deliver healthcare services, the art and science of creating clinical documentation systems that support healthcare providers and patients, and effective use of those systems.

The shift toward patient-centric care points to the critical centrality of consumer (patient) health informatics. Consumer health informatics empowers consumers to engage in personal health management practices (PHMP) supported by technology. Health literacy is fundamental for consumers to engage in PHMP and is addressed in Chapter 34. Public health or population health informatics addresses the population/group aggregate and includes surveillance, reporting and health promotion, the environment in which healthcare is provided, as well as information technology in ecology, architecture, climate, and agriculture. Informatics researchers derive new knowledge about the effects of healthcare and the environment on individual and population health using these diverse data sources and types with methods such as data mining, natural language processing, and algorithms (see http://www.amia.org/about-amia/science-informatics, www.AMIA.org).

Knowledge discovery through analysis of "Big Data" from electronic health records (EHRs) and other information systems is key to transforming health and healthcare. Big datasets are increasingly common in many disciplines, as indicated in a recent survey of 1,700 peer reviewers for *Science* magazine (erican Association for the Advancement of Science (AAAS Science Staff, 2011). About 20% of respondents reported that they regularly use datasets that range from over 100 gigabytes to data exceeding 1 terabyte. The science of informatics guides the design of the information infrastructure to capture, store, and reuse data to discover new knowledge. Capturing and storing data that represent integrative healthcare is essential in order to maximize the new methods for discovering knowledge.

The growth of informatics has been driven by the proliferation of information technologies, the explosion of data and information (beyond the limits of human ability to process facts and our capacity to comprehend complex systems), and the exponential technological capacity to both process and store information. National informatics strategic initiatives support definition and implementation of the national information infrastructure. EHRs and consumer health records have been described and are being implemented (see http://www.healthit.gov/newsroom/about-onc http://www.healthit.gov/). The emerging *learning health system* (IOM, 2012) is designed to generate and apply the best evidence for the collaborative healthcare choices of each patient and provider; to drive the process of discovery as a natural outgrowth of patient care; and to ensure innovation, quality, safety, and value in healthcare. The national health research infrastructure is being redesigned based on an informatics framework through the Clinical Translational Science Awards (CTSAs) (see Clinical Translational Science Awards https://www.ctsacentral.org/). The national CTSA transformation addresses the development and implementation of national standards, best practices, and infrastructure support for the full range of translation, from basic discovery to clinical and community-engaged research.

There are specific foci within informatics that are essential to supporting health and the discovery of new knowledge. Data and information structures, databases, terminologies, and knowledge architectures determine what and how healthcare concepts are identified, standardized, and represented in information systems, including the EHR. In addition to capturing and storing healthcare information and knowledge sources, the processes of managing information are key to safe, quality, and effective care. The information infrastructure needed for healthcare includes the type of data, methods of standardizing the data for comparison, and the organization of data to represent information and discover knowledge. The type of data include consumer/patient health needs, services, and outcomes; provider characteristics such as the education, certification, and experience of integrative practitioners; and the environmental context in which care is provided or received.

Two minimum datasets represent nursing and the context of nursing care: the Nursing Minimum Data Set (NMDS) and the Nursing Management Minimum Data Set (NMMDS). These minimum datasets for nursing complement other essential standardized datasets for health information exchange and reuse in clinical data warehouses (Westra, Delaney, Konicek & Keenan, 2008). The NMDS includes sixteen high-level data elements divided into three categories: nursing care, patient or client demographics, and service. Included in the nursing care elements are nursing diagnoses, interventions, and outcomes. The NMMDS is intended to complement the minimum datasets representing care. The NMMDS captures core data describing the environment and nursing care and financial resources. More granular standardized terms, definitions, and codes are needed to implement the minimum datasets in EHRs for clinical documentation. Granular terms can be described as interface terminologies (e.g., Omaha System, NANDA, Nursing Interventions Classification, Nursing Outcomes Classification), which are user-friendly terms that enable healthcare data-capture by humans using computers (ANA, 2013). One of these terminologies, the Omaha System, will be described later.

The American Nurses Association (ANA) also recognizes reference terminologies that can be used for documentation or, more importantly, to link and expand other terminologies. The International Classification of Nursing Practice (ICNP) integrates and expands terms for nursing, while the Systematized Nomenclature of Medicine— Clinical Terms (SNOMED-CT) and the Logical Observation Identifiers Names and Codes (LOINC) are useful across disciplines. SNOMED is a comprehensive terminology of 291,317 coded concepts, terms, and relationships for healthcare documentation and reporting, across the scope of healthcare. Hierarchies of codes within SNOMED CT include clinical findings, procedures, linking concepts, and numerous descriptors that enable precision coding of concepts and relationships (International Health Terminology Standards Development Organization [IHTSDO], 2012). Within the reference terminology of SNOMED CT, the Omaha System is a multidisciplinary ontology for the domain of healthcare (International Health Terminology Standards Development Organisation, 2012; Martin, 2005; Omaha System, 2013).

Integrative Healthcare and Informatics

Integrative healthcare, nursing, and all healthcare professions can leverage the benefits of informatics to improve information management, support and document care, and capture outcomes. Throughout this book, examples have been provided to demonstrate and share ways that integrative nurses use evidence to inform traditional and emerging interventions that support whole person/whole systems healing. Such evidence is the foundation upon which information systems can build assessments, create documentation forms, and generate integrative healthcare data streams. Traditional health has been the focus of development of information infrastructures and processes; integrative healthcare data and processes also need to be examined so that the breadth and depth of informatics can support integrative health practice using diverse modalities in numerous settings. Likewise, the breadth and depth of the integrative health field offers us the opportunity, and challenge, to ensure that informatics supports integrative healthcare and accommodates a variety of communication modalities that engage researchers in use of traditional and emerging data streams, including text, audio, touch, intuition, and energy. The application of workflow processes and human–computer interaction can optimize the way in which integrative health clinicians can easily use the EHRs, decision support and expert systems, and clinical research data management and analysis.

CONTEXT AND CULTURE

Context and culture have major implications for informatics and integrative healthcare. Mutual and reciprocal interactions between contextual and human data, which occur on both personal and organizational levels, influence this interrelationship between informatics and integrative healthcare. Thus, the concept of integration is multidimensional, focusing on the quality of life for clients within the context of everyday living, and considering the multitude of changes that occur in the human health experience. It is especially important to capture context and culture in efforts to understand how health information technology (HIT) can support integrative healthcare globally. For example, are the same questions and datasets relevant for nurses in Namibia and from the United States as they meet health needs in a local community or care setting? Does a dominant perspective privilege one form of knowledge and knowledge acquisition over others? That is, are we only going to consider empirical biomedical knowledge and disregard other useful and relevant ways of knowing so critical to integrative healthcare? It is critical indeed, and should be our hope for nursing and healthcare overall, to learn ways of expressing what we know in a shared language within HIT and to strengthen nurses' skills in being-knowing-doing, thus creating new ways of advancing health and wellbeing in local communities.

EMERGING TECHNOLOGIES

Current healthcare technology relies nearly exclusively on audiovisual data input and output. Emerging technologies contribute to these data streams and offer new modalities for whole person/whole systems healing.

Touch

Contemplate the importance of the largest sensory and expressive organ of the body, the skin. The skin invites a two-way relationship with internal and external environments, in contrast to a unidirectional process of data input represented by sight. For example, consider the old form of fixed-raised Braille for the visually impaired compared to the new "haptic technology." *Haptic technology* is a digital system that translates data into touch-sensitive information, such as the Braille Personal Digital Assistant (PDA). With future designs of transparent computer screens that encircle the body or even conform to typical body morphologies, accurate, consistent, and objective measurements of body surface, wound size, edema, fluid loss, discolorations and rashes, using parallax, ultrasound, and comparative images, could be obtained and recorded in digital format. Future designs of transparent computer screens could support touch to achieve objective assessments and to implement intentional comfort measures embodying nursing presence through massage, reflexology, or a gentle touch on the patient's hand as a direct means of being present to the patient.

Vision

A "knowing look," if captured by the technology support, can be used bidirectionally to convey and receive information between people who have a prior knowledge of shared communication, as is often the case between parent and child, between spouses, between friends, between teacher and student, and between patient and nurse. Nurses are particularly adept at intuitively recognizing signals of unspoken care needs of patients, such as a need for pain alleviation. Informatics innovations may support such a relationship. For example, the development of eye-activated computer tracking in combination with transparent computer screen technology where the eye alone controls activity on the computer screen supports this relationship. While advances in visual magnification have enabled the human eye to passively observe microscopic phenomena remote from the patient, greater patient visibility through a transparent computer could probably reduce patient-to-computer-screen fatigue and distraction. Human-to-human contact, essential for integrative healthcare, will be better maintained through seamless, patient-visible, electronic access to these functions of telehealth technology. This functionality would help nurses and other care providers maintain an uninterrupted visual connection with the patient and support greater freedom of hand–eye coordination to perform necessary actions of direct patient care; in essence an informatics microscope through which the whole person is seen.

Emotions

Examples exist of technological tools and methods used to assess and respond to patient emotions. Consider the experimentation of a Rochester, Minnesota, high school student who programmed a computer for affective human responses using images of peer's facial expressions (Stolle, 2011). The computer electronically compared real-time facial expressions with stored expressions to provide an affective dimension to information interaction. This example of including the emotional communication of body language with digital symbolic language has the potential for comparing user affect with computer interaction for congruity and automatically modifying its reading level to accommodate user ability, or altering the speed of the program when user and computer interaction are incongruent. This is similar to using a biofeedback mechanism, where the computer responds to input of the computer user or healthcare consumer (Goleman, 1997). It is possible to capture other biochemical–electrical interactions, such as detecting galvanic responses of the skin (Luneski, Bamidis, & Hitoglou-Antoniadou, 2008).

Energy

Many emerging technologies show promise in measurement of human energy flow and effectiveness of energy healing modalities. Imagine a future wherein energy fields surrounding patients could be discernible through quantum electrodynamics technology so that the effects of therapeutic touch can also be measured. The reciprocity of touch through haptic technology is a natural fit between patient and nurse. The tactile input of haptic technology could potentially alert the nurse to changes in patient energy fields, including those of an emergent nature that may precede physical manifestations of health changes. Imagine in reflexology an electromechanical stimulator of the feet that could signal the effectiveness of an intervention in affecting patient energy fields, or warn of unseen changes in patient vital signs.

The potential to expand the sensory repertoire of nurses' interactions with patients is addressed at the intersection of informatics and integrative healthcare. Using additional sensory interactions in processing data, such as tactile exchanges on various parts of the body using haptic technology, and using the eye as a computer tracking device, would further support assessments of individual nurse preferences and capabilities regarding human–computer relationships. Research focused on ideal combinations of patient–provider–computer interactions continues to promise the discovery of an optimal balance between informatics and integrative healthcare. Informatics support additionally needs to accommodate a non-contact, remote-tactile experience, such as therapeutic touch, an assessment and intentional intervention related to energy fields (Zahourek, 2009).

TECHNOLOGY AND EVOLUTION

Humans are adapting to the information age by rapidly adopting and adapting to technology solutions that blend and blur the boundaries between people and machines over time and space. Consider supplementing humans with computer-animated androids in the form of greeters, direction providers, and server robots. Informatics and integrative healthcare must consider the ethical dimensions of such technological advances. The intersection of informatics and integrative healthcare invites us to co-define a safe and productive coexistence.

Technorganics

The "technorganic" evolution of endosymbiosis between electrochemical reactions in humans and the electromechanical nature of machines/robots continues at an unrelenting pace, as seen in the implanted medical devices that capture and use bodily generated electrical power. Other examples of this ongoing "technorganic" relationship include assistive devices to which humans are connected, both literally (IV pumps, respirators, Intracorporeal Ventricular Assist Device (IVADs), pacemakers, and artificial hearts), and figuratively (iPads, iPhones, Bluetooth devices, and pagers). This phenomenon is so ubiquitous that there seems to be a need to symbolize a new inclusivity of "I-Thou" (Martin Buber) with "iPad" (Steve Jobs). Consider a new symbol originating from the coined name "PERSO-INFORMATICS," where the "O" symbolizes the basic cellular structure of human life, and the "I" naturally represents informatics. Yes, it does not escape us that computer code, the DNA of computerization, is symbolically represented by zero (0) and one (1), and possibly predicts the writing of new code relationships between the DNA of living cells and inanimate computer code.

Symbiosis

Szczeklik (2012) emphasizes that a symbiosis exists between two separate organisms when their cooperation is mutually beneficial. Though informatics is an inanimate entity, its functionality is analogous to what Szczeklik describes as the process of *endosymbiosis*, in which separate organisms combine over time to form a new entity, perhaps similar to avatars or archetypes. Campbell (1986), in an animate/inanimate perspective similar to that of Szczeklik, maintains that life-preserving periodicity (timeliness) was incorporated into cellular structure as a means to survive our ancestors' prehistoric transition from a marine to a terrestrial environment. Are there implications of this evolution for our current circumstance? Consider the use of genetic coding of computer-generated information into strands of human DNA as a possible means to health; computer-generated personal identifiers living beyond natural lives; consider "cyber-immortality" and learning in high-fidelity simulation laboratories where human physiology is reenacted in an electromechanical avatar resembling the electrochemical environment of human life (Trafton, 2012).

The intersection of integrative healthcare and informatics challenges us to consider the complementary nature of the limits to human cognitive processing ability and the robust computational capacity of current technology (Papadimitriou, 1993). This broader perspective more intimately captures and defines the human linkage with technology, and fosters rigorous discernment of the advantages and disadvantages of technology to humans and integrative healthcare. Integrative nursing offers a perspective of whole person/whole system healing that can humanize and enrich healthcare informatics. We propose that interdependence between integrative healthcare and informatics asks us to protect and be stewards of a relationship between informatics and integrative health with a strategy that benefits humans. Similar to Hamilton's (1964) rule of kinship selection related to human evolution, the cost–benefit equation of the relationship between informatics and integrative healthcare to humans (c) should be greater than the contributory cost (r) of human interaction with informatics and integrative healthcare. In other words, the amalgamation of informatics with integrative health is not an end in itself, but a remarkable means to foster health and evolution of human health and care delivery.

Exemplars of Informatics Supportive of Integrative Healthcare

This section highlights examples of nursing informatics tools that could support integrative nursing. In particular, integrative nurses can use terminologies recognized by the ANA for documenting care congruent with the elements of the NMDS (as previously described; see http://ana.nursingworld.org/npii/terminologies.htm). Other EHR data are also useful, such as those generated by nurses documenting demographic, administrative, and Outcome Assessment Information Set (OASIS) information.

OUTCOME ASSESSMENT INFORMATION SET (OASIS)

The Outcome Assessment Information Set (OASIS) is a homecare assessment tool developed over fifteen years that is valid and reliable for use in home care for adult, non-maternity clients with skilled services. It is a required assessment for home care patients in the United States who receive services funded by the Centers for Medicare and Medicaid Services (CMS). OASIS consists of 101 standard assessment questions, which are differentially completed depending on the reason for the assessment. These items include clinical record items, demographic and patient history, living arrangements and supportive assistance, health status, functional status, and service utilization (Centers for Medicare and Medicaid Services [CMS], 2013).

Applications of OASIS and Administrative Data

A recent study examining the influence of certified wound, ostomy, and continence (WOC) nurses on patient outcomes in home care exemplifies Big Data research that integrates EHR and administrative data (Westra, Bliss, Savik, Hou, & Borchert, 2013). OASIS and other demographic and administrative data were abstracted from the EHRs of 785 home care agencies representing 449,243 episodes of care. Investigators found that agencies with a WOC nurse had significantly better agency-level OASIS outcomes for wounds (pressure ulcers, stasis ulcers, and surgical wounds), incontinence (bowel and bladder), and urinary tract infections. Patients with and without a WOC nurse both had significant improvement in outcomes, except for stasis ulcers; however, the patients with a WOC nurse had more severe problems at admission. This study highlights the role of the WOC nurse as an important contributor to patient improvement, and exemplifies Big Data research in nursing, and the importance of reusing EHR data for knowledge discovery. Further investigation of the reasons for WOC nurse influence could include in-depth examination of WOC nursing interventions, including integrative whole person/whole systems healing modalities. Such study would be facilitated by use of standardized terminologies for documentation.

OMAHA SYSTEM

Implicit within the implementation of an informatics infrastructure for integrative nursing and healthcare is a need for a robust ontology that describes integrative nursing and healthcare and enables data capture. In computer science, Gruber (1993) defined *ontology* as "a specification of a representational vocabulary for a shared domain of discourse." A critical component of health informatics that can facilitate success in nursing and interprofessional practice and education is a shared ontology across the health professions. A shared ontology enables communication about the domains of nursing and healthcare without necessarily operating on a globally shared theory (Gruber, 1993). An ontology provides the necessary foundation for integrative healthcare by formally explicating, defining, and relating concepts (terms) that describe holistic integrative practice.

One multidisciplinary ontology that comprehensively and holistically describes health and healthcare is the Omaha System. It exists in the public domain and is an interface terminology (a terminology that is user-friendly for clinicians) that enables data-capture in EHRs. It provides a knowable, structured, defined problem list and enables rational and relational organization of healthcare concepts for problems, interventions, and outcomes. The concepts are identified by definitions and unique signs and symptoms, and arranged in four domains that reflect a whole-systems-assessment approach: environmental, psychosocial, physiological, and health-related behaviors. Use of the Omaha System ontology together with the SNOMED CT codes for specific integrative modalities to describe patient assessments and integrative care will generate data to enable measurement of integrative healing modalities, patient progress, and healthcare quality leveled with all healthcare interventions across professions.

There are three components of the Omaha System: the Problem Classification Scheme (identifies signs/symptoms of 42 health problems in four domains), the Intervention Scheme (describes interventions relative to the 42 problems in four categories), and the Problem Rating Scale for Outcomes (describes outcomes relative to the 42 problems in three dimensions—knowledge, behavior, and status). Together, these three components enable integrative whole-person assessments and integrative whole-systems-healing approaches and outcomes to be described and quantified, generating data for evaluation and research.

APPLICATIONS OF THE OMAHA SYSTEM

Symptom Assessment and Treatment

Integrative nurses and their patients may seek to use integrative therapies for non-pharmacological relief from the symptoms of pain. A comprehensive pain assessment can be documented using Omaha System signs/symptoms and Problem Rating Scale for Outcomes. The Omaha System signs/symptoms of pain are: expression of discomfort/pain, elevated pulse/respirations/blood pressure, compensated movement/guarding, restless behavior, facial grimaces, and pallor/perspiration. These signs and symptoms can be selected as data points describing patient pain. In addition, the patient's pain status is rated on a scale of 1 (extreme signs and symptoms) to 5 (no signs or symptoms), with parallel ratings for the patient's knowledge ("no knowledge" to "superior knowledge") and behavior ("not appropriate behavior" to "consistently appropriate behavior"). Integrative therapies for pain can be described and documented using the Intervention Scheme. After a course of treatment, this pain assessment can be repeated, to determine whether there is improvement.

Data Visualization and Data Mining

Data visualization and data mining techniques have been successful in demonstrating the effectiveness of interventions for various patient problems. For example, a data-mining study of 651,000 interventions provided by homecare nurses from fifteen agencies showed that patients who received care tailored to their level of need were more likely to improve (Monsen, Westra et al., 2009; Monsen, Westra et al., 2011). In addition, a visualization study of public health nursing interventions over time using streamgraphs found statistically significant differences in intervention approaches between nurses (Monsen, Kim, et al., 2012). These studies could be replicated using data from integrative nursing assessments and care to describe integrative interventions and demonstrate outcomes.

STANDARDIZED TERMINOLOGIES AND CARE PLANS

A study by Gao (2012) investigated the use of standardized terminologies for integrative health. Until recently, integrative healthcare providers have been largely not engaged in the effort to achieve interoperability of health information. Gao asked integrative healthcare practitioners to rate the relevance on a five-point Likert scale for four items and their sub-elements in the Consolidated Continuity Document Architecture (CCDA), which specifies the essential data and format for exchange of health information in the EHR. These included "condition," "medication (prescribed and non-prescribed)," "encounter," and "procedure." All four data elements were rated as relevant by integrative healthcare providers; however, some of the sub-elements were "not relevant." Gao found that no standardized terminologies have been developed to describe integrative healthcare encounters and procedures. However, drugs and herbs were represented in medication terminologies. Gao concluded that the integrative healthcare-specific terms could be included in existing terminologies such as the Omaha System, and would be useful for patient access and sharing of information across both traditional and integrative healthcare practices (Monsen et al., 2012; Gao, 2012).

The implications of the study were that international standardized care plans should be developed for integrative nursing to increase visibility and quality of integrative nursing care. For example, a pain-management care plan for infants and non-verbal and cognitively impaired children includes the Face, Legs, Activity, Cry, Consolability scale (FLACC) and guides treatment options such as swaddling, holding, repositioning, rocking, music, pacifier, feeding, changing diaper, as well as pharmacological treatments (Merkel, 1997; Minnesota Omaha System Users Group, 2013). Such care plans enable consistent data collection and lead to the development of large datasets describing integrative nursing interventions and outcomes. Examples of evidence-based standardized care plans for integrative healthcare for symptoms chapters are available on-line at omahasystemguidelines.org.

PARTNERSHIPS

We encourage partnerships in the Complementary and Alternative Medicine (CAM) Clinical Translational Research (PCCTR) initiative to foster development of translational tools that will contribute to rigorous clinical CAM research and further development of clinical research expertise and leadership at CAM institutions and in the field in general. In addition, two initiatives with the University of Minnesota School of Nursing provide opportunities to advance our capacity to engage in Big Data research to further define integrative healthcare. The Omaha System Partnership for Knowledge Discovery and Health Care Quality has three components:

1. Multidisciplinary scientific teams of researchers with experience in advanced data-analysis and data-mining techniques;
2. affiliate members from many countries who contribute clinical Omaha System data, suggest important clinical questions, and work together with the scientific team on research and evaluation projects; and
3. a warehouse of de-identified clinical Omaha System data including client problems, signs/symptoms, interventions, and knowledge, behavior, and status outcomes.

The Center for Nursing Informatics leads the discovery, application, and cutting-edge thinking for nursing and health informatics scholarship to improve the health of individuals and communities. The Center's purpose is to discover and employ innovative methods of informatics research; use standardized nursing terminologies and essential minimum datasets for knowledge discovery; and apply research methods to clinical and other information systems. This center serves as the home for the NMDS and the NMMDS. These partnerships leverage approaches, tools, and methodologies that will make substantial contributions to the progress of CAM research.

Summary

In summary, we have defined informatics, discussed integrative healthcare and its relationship to informatics, and provided examples of integrative informatics' supporting integrative health. We share a commitment to fostering society's healthy adoption of and alliance with communications and information technologies and informatics. We have invited a conversation, creative practice, and contributions to the evolution of our research and science that boldly represents the healthy synergy between integrative informatics and integrative health.

SELECTED REFERENCES

American Nurses Association (ANA). (2008). Nursing informatics: practice scope and standards of practice. Washington DC, ANA.

Centers for Medicare and Medicaid Services (CMS). (2013). Outcome Assessment Information Set. Available at: http://www.cms.gov/Medicare/Quality-Initiatives-Patient-Assessment-Instruments/OASIS/index.html?redirect=/oasis/.

Institute for Healthcare Improvement (2013). The IHI Triple Aim. Retrieved from http://www.ihi.org/offerings/Initiatives/TripleAim/Pages/default.aspx. Last accessed April 7, 2013.

International Health Terminology Standards Development Organisation. (2012). SNOMED CT User Guide. Retrieved from http://ihtsdo.org/fileadmin/user_upload/doc/download/doc_UserGuide_Current-en-US_INT_20120731.pdf.

Martin, K. S. (2005). *The Omaha System: A Key to Practice, Documentation, and Information Management* (2nd ed.). Omaha, NE: Health Connections Press.

Minnesota Omaha System Users Group. (2013). Evidence-based care plan: Pediatric pain. Available at: http://omahasystemmn.org/Careplans/PeerReviewed/2011-04-09Pediatric%20PainCarePlan.pdf.

Monsen, K. A., Kim, E., Pieczkiewicz, D., Kerr, M. J., Peden-McAlpine, C., & Kesler, V. (2012). Using visualization methods to discover tailoring in nursing intervention data. University of Minnesota School of Nursing Research Day, Minneapolis, MN.

Silver, N. (2012). *The Signal and the Noise: Why So Many Predictions Fail—But Some Don't.* New York: Penguin Press.

Westra, B. L., Delaney, C. W., Konicek, D., & Keenan, G. (2008). Nursing standards to support the electronic health record. *Nursing Outlook*, 56(5), 258–266.

Westra, B. L., Bliss, D. Z., Savik, K., Hou, Y., & Borchert, A. (2013). Effectiveness of wound, ostomy, and continence nurses on agency level wound and incontinence outcomes in home care. *Journal of Wound, Ostomy, & Continence Nursing*, 40(1), 25–53.

II

Optimizing Wellbeing

10

Advancing Wellbeing in People, Organizations, and Communities

MARY JO KREITZER, LOUISE DELAGRAN, AND ANDREA UPTMOR

Wellbeing is a state of being in balance or alignment in the body, mind, and spirit. In this state, we feel contented; connected to purpose, people, and community; peaceful but energized; resilient and safe. In short, we are flourishing.

Wellbeing is not a new concept, but it has been overshadowed by the focus in many healthcare systems around the world on disease and pathogenesis, factors that cause disease. In 1946, the World Health Organization defined *health* as a state of complete physical, mental, and social wellbeing and not merely the absence of disease or infirmity. Over thirty years ago, Aaron Antonovsky (1987), a professor of sociology, coined the term *salutogenesis* to describe an approach that focuses on factors that support human health and wellbeing, rather than on factors that cause disease.

Wellbeing has been the object of study in a broad array of disciplines. Psychology, sociology, public health, and economics have all spawned a variety of theories about the nature of wellbeing and how to measure it, as well as a long list of possible contributing factors. Nowadays, there is general agreement that wellbeing is dependent on a variety of interconnected factors. The Gallup model is typical of this approach.

The Gallup Organization has been studying wellbeing for decades. Working with Gallup, Rath (2010) has identified five elements of wellbeing: career, social, financial, physical, and community. Gallup found that "while these elements are universal across faiths, cultures, and nationalities, people take different paths to increasing their individual wellbeing, and for many people, spirituality drives them in all areas." Rath also reported that while 66% of people are doing well in at least one of these areas, just 7% are thriving in all five. He also noted that if a person is struggling in any one of the domains, it damages overall wellbeing and wears on daily life.

Martin Seligman, the father of the positive psychology movement, writes in the book *Flourish* (2011) that his goal was to shift the focus of psychology from trying to relieve misery to a new goal, the understanding of wellbeing. He describes wellbeing as an active state of exploring what makes life worth living and then building the enabling conditions of such a life. According to Seligman, there is no single measure that captures wellbeing; rather, there are many elements that contribute to it, and the gold standard for measuring wellbeing is flourishing.

Like Seligman, Rath, and others, we believe that different elements contribute to wellbeing. However, the elements in our model differ from others'. We emphasize the fact that wellbeing can be conceptualized and expressed at many levels—at the level of the individual, family, organization or system, and community.

Within the discipline of nursing, wellbeing is a focus that is closely aligned with caring, healing, and wholeness. While health and even the phrase "holistic health" within a nursing lens is understood to encompass "body, mind, and spirit" within a wellbeing paradigm, health is only one of many dimensions impacting wellbeing. There are many other determinants of wellbeing that will be explored in this chapter.

A New Model of Wellbeing

What does a model of wellbeing offer, and what is the value of a new model of wellbeing? Models are often helpful in pointing to what is important—in this case, determinants of wellbeing. The model described in this chapter and developed by Kreitzer (2012) grew out of a belief that the societal transformation needed in the United States and around the world goes well beyond healthcare and needs to encompass not just a shift from disease to health or illness to wellness, but rather a shift to the broader notion of wellbeing that touches every aspect of people's lives and the communities in which they live.

As Kreitzer writes, the role of nurses and other health professionals is to support and maximize *human* and *system* capacity and potential. Simply put, this means that our role is to help people restore and maintain function and capacity in every aspect of their lives and to support them in attaining their full potential. We believe that the dimensions in this model all contribute significantly to flourishing and that they are equally relevant at all levels of a system—individual, family, organization, and community—and also contribute to global environmental wellbeing.

At a personal level, wellbeing is certainly affected by our health, but it is also heavily impacted by other factors illustrated in Figure 10.1, including our sense of purpose and meaning in life, the quality of our relationships, the vitality of the community in which we live, our environment, and our perception of safety and security. When any of these factors is compromised, our personal wellbeing is affected. And these same factors also influence the wellbeing of our organizations and community.

HEALTH

While health is affected by genetics and social determinants, such as the circumstances in which people are born, grow up, live, work, and age, and the systems put in place to deal with illness, the largest determinants of health are lifestyle behaviors and choices.

Wellbeing

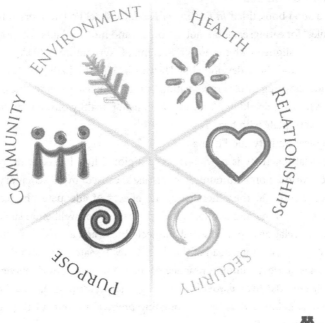

Mary Jo Kreitzer, RN, PhD, FAAN
Director, Center for Spirituality & Healing

UNIVERSITY OF MINNESOTA
Center for Spirituality & Healing

FIGURE 10.1 Kreitzer (2012) Model of Wellbeing. (Used with permission)

It is estimated that 90% of people's health (Clymer et al., 2012) has nothing to do with hospitals, healthcare providers, and drugs per se. Rather, how healthy we are has much more to do with the food we eat, how much we exercise, how we manage our stress, and how much we sleep, as well as our social, environmental, and genetic influences. Social determinants of health are shaped by a broad set of economic and political forces, as well as social policies that are beyond the control of individuals. Lifestyle choices, however, are very much within our control.

Helping people understand the power of "taking charge" of their own health and wellbeing is one of the most important ways to build individual capacity and resilience and help people attain their full health potential. Among other things, individuals need to adopt healthy lifestyle practices, effectively use the healthcare system, and consider a range of therapy options, particularly in the presence of chronic disease. An example of a robust online resource that aims to help people do this can be found at www.takingcharge.csh.umn.edu. In addition to guiding people to information and tools, health coaching is a helpful strategy to empower individuals and motivate behavior change.

Key Healthy Lifestyle Practices

- Diet and Nutrition

  In a 2009 book titled *In Defense of Food*, Michael Pollan offers some simple "rules" for eating: eat food, not too much, and mostly plants. These guidelines are very aligned with the 2010 U.S. Dept. of Agriculture (USDA) recommendations and those developed by Harvard's "Healthy Eating Plate," which include choosing whole grains, eating lean protein like fish and chicken instead of red meat, drinking plenty of water, using healthy oils, and filling almost half your plate with healthy produce.

- Physical Activity and Fitness

  Physical inactivity is now considered a global health risk, with 6%–10% of the world's non-communicable diseases caused by a sedentary lifestyle (Lee, 2012). On the other hand, the effects of adequate physical activity are far-reaching and support other key aspects of wellbeing, such as sleep, healthy relationships and social connectedness, and a sense of purpose (Das, 2012). Dan Buettner, head of the Blue Zones research, has found that centenarians share a common practice of incorporating natural movement into their everyday lives: gardening, walking, and performing manual housework become habits that encourage ongoing physical movement throughout the day (2009).

- Sleep

  Sleep can be thought of as a time of refreshment, a necessary activity whose function is twofold: to process information from the previous day and prepare the body and mind for the next. Most research agrees that adults require seven to eight hours of sleep each night to receive maximum benefits. Too little or too much sleep has been associated with health conditions such as colon cancer (Thompson, 2011), obesity, and diabetes, as well as an increased risk of death (Rath, 2010). Just as sleep influences other aspects of wellbeing, it is also affected by factors illustrated in Kreitzer's model: for example, a survey of over 3,000 people found associations between strained familial relationships or low social/emotional support and insufficient sleep (Ailshire, 2012), suggesting that cultivating strong relationships can support healthy sleeping patterns.

- Emotions and Attitudes

  The well-established link between emotions and physical health has encouraged ongoing research into the benefits of positivity. Barbara Fredrickson's research suggests that positive emotions both expand one's perspective and enhance creativity as well as build up lasting resources, such as emotional resilience, in addition to undoing the negative cardiovascular effects of stress. She recommends cultivating positive emotions by practicing gratitude, connecting with others and with nature, and "savoring" goodness—in other words, applying awareness and appreciation of the positive things one encounters in life (Fredrickson, 2009).

- Mindfulness

Mindfulness, the practice of paying attention with a nonjudgmental attitude, is an integral component of enhancing wellbeing. While Buddhist practitioners have suggested the positive effects of mindfulness for thousands of years, recent research also shows that mindful awareness can help people enhance their wellbeing in a variety of ways. Lilian Cheung, co-author of *Savor: Mindful Eating, Mindful Life,* has found that mindful eating has the potential to reduce the risk for obesity (2010), while Richard Davidson's functional magnetic resonance imaging (fMRI) scans of meditators have shown that mindfulness can improve immune function (Davidson et al., 2003), reduce the inflammatory response caused by stress (Rosenkranz et al., 2012), and improve attention (Lutz et al., 2009).

- Healthy Habits

According to Roy Baumeister, people spend at least a fifth of their day resisting desires, and this depletes their limited stock of willpower, leaving them susceptible to unhealthy choices (Baumeister, 2011). One way to combat this is to consciously develop positive health habits that automate your behavior—for example, making it a habit to exercise before dinner. A similar strategy is to pre-commit to actions in advance, which helps us keep our long-term health goals in mind and overcome our short-term desires. Better yet is making that commitment public. You can also reinforce desired behaviors with rewards, such as a short social break when you resist the urge to snack in the afternoon.

COMMUNITY

The community we live in has an impact on our individual wellbeing in many ways—our health, safety, and education being just a few examples. Key to this is the infrastructure of the community, including housing, transportation, schools, and parks, along with equitable access to these community resources.

While the impact of community infrastructure and equity on individual wellbeing is obvious, the role of our social connections, otherwise known as *social capital*, is equally important. Social networks allow us to accomplish what we cannot on our own, whether it is raising money for a good cause or simply passing information along quickly. They have value not just for members of the network but for the organization or community as a whole. Vibrant social networks contribute to the public good in the form of increased social trust, lower crime rates, better public health, reduced political corruption, and increased altruism and charity, to mention just a few benefits (Helliwell, 2005).

Because we are part of these social networks, we can also influence them, and through them, the wellbeing of others. As Christakis points out, "The ubiquity of human connection means that each of us has a much bigger impact on others than we can see. When we take better care of ourselves, so do many other people. When we practice random acts of kindness, they spread to dozens or even hundreds of other people" (Christakis, 2009, p. 302). So we should be conscious about the behavior we are modeling in our social networks and choose to act in ways that increase the trust, reciprocity, and altruism in our organization or community. We should also actively involve ourselves by volunteering, voting, contributing to fund-raising events, and helping others. In addition to contributing to the community, research indicates that individuals benefit personally from altruistic acts, experiencing an elevation in mood (Rath, 2012).

Because our social connections play a large role in our health and wellbeing, we also need to help those who are struggling with their social connections. As Christakis writes: "To reduce crime, we need to optimize the kinds of connections potential criminals have...to make smoking-cessation and weight-loss interventions more effective, we need to involve family, friends, and even friends of friends" (Christakis, 2009, p. 302).

PURPOSE

A key message in this area of wellbeing is that "purpose matters," probably more than people realize. Purpose can guide life decisions, influence behavior, shape goals, offer a sense of direction, and create meaning. Its presence can induce episodes of "flow," an optimal state of being in which one's creative and intellectual limits are challenged but not stretched beyond one's ability (Nakamura, 2009). There is abundant evidence that purpose is directly related to both health and happiness, and whether or not we have clarity about our sense of purpose and live out our purpose in our lives will have a major impact on our wellbeing.

Likewise, a lack of purpose can have ramifications for our physical health: research at the Rush Alzheimer's Disease Center in Chicago has shown that the risk of Alzheimer's increases when a person does not have a sense of purpose, and people with purpose are less likely to develop impairments in their daily living and mobility disabilities (Boyle, 2010, 2012). A significant amount of research on purpose has been conducted in Japan, where the concept of *ikigai*, or a "reason for being," is prevalent in the culture. These studies link strong purpose to long life and a decreased risk for cardiovascular disease (Tanno et al., 2009; Kim et al., 2012).

Richard Leider, a nationally ranked coach and purpose expert, has found that a sense of purpose can be clarified and nurtured through two key practices: contemplation and activation. Reflective exercises, such as meditation and journaling, enable us to access a broader perspective, which allows us to contemplate our values, gifts, and passions in life. The activation process is a synchronizing of our inner life with the outer reality, which creates a sense of vitality, wholeness, and meaning (Leider, 2010).

RELATIONSHIPS

It has now been well documented that "Isolation is fatal." In fact, loneliness and isolation are risk factors for disease that are comparable in impact to obesity and hypertension. If personal lives are devoid of positive relationships, it also detracts from joy, meaning, and ultimately wellbeing. Recent research suggests that loneliness predicts depression and fatigue in cancer patients (Jaremka, 2012), high blood pressure (Hawkley, 2010), and a 50% increased mortality risk (Holt-Lunstad, 2010). Likewise, strong relationships provide support that can act as a buffer against the negative effects of stress, leading to a longer, healthier life. Research on healthy communities around the world, called Blue Zones, estimates that committing to a life partner can add three years to one's life expectancy (Buettner, 2009).

Gallup research has found that thriving people spend about six hours per day being social—this time includes interactions with friends, colleagues, and family—and spending fewer hours results in less daily satisfaction. In addition, it is the quality of the relationships, not the quantity, that matters—having three or four close friendships equates to higher engagement at work, better health, and an increased sense of wellbeing (Rath, 2010).

Our model maintains the powerful influence our relationships have on our overall wellbeing and also acknowledges that the cultivation of relationships is not a passive act. Interpersonal relationships can only thrive, and thus exert a positive influence on personal wellbeing, when they are tended to with gratitude, compassion, deep listening, and forgiveness.

ENVIRONMENT

When we reflect on ways that a poor environment could adversely impact our wellbeing, it is easy to think of three things: air, water, and toxins. It is critical to ensure that our home and work environments are healthy and that we are not exposed to hazards. We also need to consider our global environment and take steps to protect our natural resources from contamination and depletion. One approach is the Natural Step Framework from Sweden, which has been used by numerous businesses, government agencies, nonprofits, and individuals around the world to become environmentally responsible (and save money). Within healthcare, the Healthcare Without Harm coalition sets similar goals, working to transform the healthcare sector so it is no longer a source of harm to people and the environment.

Another important factor in environmental wellbeing is access to nature. There is a preponderance of evidence that "Nature heals." Being in nature, or even viewing scenes of nature, reduces anger, fear, and stress and increases pleasant feelings. Exposure to nature not only makes you feel better emotionally, it contributes to your physical wellbeing—reducing blood pressure, heart rate, muscle tension, and the production of stress hormones. Roger Ulrich's pioneering research in this area has been supported by researchers around the world (Ulrich, 1984; Largo-Wight, 2011). Even a simple plant in a room can have a significant impact on stress and anxiety, according to research done in hospitals, offices, and schools (Park, 2009; Bringslimark, 2008).

One of the most intriguing areas of current research is the impact of nature on general wellbeing. In one study, 95% of those interviewed said their mood improved after spending time outside, changing from depressed or anxious to calmer and more balanced (Mind, 2007). Other studies show that spending time in nature or viewing scenes of nature is associated with a positive mood (Kim, 2010) and psychological wellbeing, meaningfulness, and vitality (Cervinka, 2012). Furthermore, spending time in nature or viewing nature scenes increases our ability to take on new mental tasks and pay attention (Berman, 2008; Meyer, 2009; Bowler, 2010).

SAFETY AND SECURITY

In both our personal and our work lives, "Fear incapacitates." People can have excellent physical health and a strong purpose in life, but if they live in fear, their sense of safety and security and overall wellbeing is eroded.

Fear is a basic survival mechanism that triggers our bodies to respond to a threatening stimulus with a fight-or-flight response. As such, it is an essential part of keeping us safe. However, people who live in constant fear, whether from real dangers in their environment or threats they only perceive, can become incapacitated. Once the fear pathways are ramped up, the brain short-circuits more rational processing paths and reacts immediately with a flood of stress hormones. When the brain is in this overactive state, it tends to remember mostly negative events. To someone in chronic fear, the world looks scary, and their memories confirm that.

This not only impacts thinking and decision-making in negative ways, it has real physical repercussions. Living under constant threat weakens the immune system and can cause cardiovascular damage, decreased fertility, gastrointestinal problems such as ulcers and irritable bowel syndrome, damage to certain parts of the brain (such as the hippocampus), and impaired formation of long-term memories. Other symptoms include fatigue, clinical depression, accelerated aging, and even premature death (Sapolsky, 1998). So whether dangers are real or perceived, they impact mental and physical wellbeing. Fear also diminishes joy and creativity and makes human flourishing impossible.

As individuals we can address our perceived fears. We can work to realistically assess threats and put into perspective the hype often created by TV stations and newspapers. We can reverse overactive fear responses by deliberately shifting to positive emotions and practicing mindfulness-based stress-reduction techniques.

Application of Wellbeing

AT THE INDIVIDUAL LEVEL

Matt Sanford was paralyzed from the waist down after a devastating car accident and is dependent on a wheelchair. But he credits that accident with his discovery of the importance of body awareness in creating a conscious and compassionate life. In his current life as a yoga teacher and inspirational speaker, he feels a great sense of purpose and connection, focusing on the positive task of "transforming trauma, loss and disability into hope and potential."

Kaitlin moved to Washington, D.C., after graduating from college. Although she had a job that paid fairly well, and her physical health was excellent, Kaitlin was miserable. She was working long hours but not finding her work meaningful. She wasn't making social connections at work and didn't know many other people in D.C. She noticed that she was getting irritable about small things at work, then ruminating on them and blaming herself. One day she found herself screaming with rage and frustration when she spilled a little tea on the hem of her skirt and realized that she needed to do something to find more positivity and balance in her life.

AT THE ORGANIZATIONAL LEVEL

The data-mining corporation Google has utilized its own rigorous research process to uncover the key to a successful company: an innovative workplace culture that prioritizes employee satisfaction and wellbeing. Recognizing that the best way to cultivate a strong, vibrant organization is to nudge individual employees into making healthier choices, Google offers its workers three free meals each day—organic, chef-prepared food on smaller plates to discourage overeating. Treadmill desks are available so that employees can "walk" while they work, and the company offers free garden space and bicycles to boost company health and morale. Relationships and strong social connections are valued at Google as well: managers personally greet new hires with a warm hello, and the lunchroom tables are long to encourage socializing and conversation. The result is a company whose impressive growth and innovation continually earns it the award of Best Company to Work For in America.

AT THE COMMUNITY LEVEL

Beginning in 2009, Albert Lea, a small Minnesotan city of 18,000 residents, took part in a Blue Zones Vitality Project that focused on Dan Buettner's methods for improving wellbeing and increasing longevity in communities. The transformation included encouraging local restaurants and grocery stores to serve healthier foods, coaching residents about life purpose, creating more bicycle- and foot-friendly commuter routes, and increasing healthy options offered by workplace vending machines. The results of this pilot project emphasize the inextricable nature of the individual and the community in which he or she lives: Buettner estimates that Albert Lea residents increased their life expectancy about three years each as a result of community-based change. The financial impact is significant as well, reducing absenteeism by key employers by 21% and decreasing healthcare costs of city employees by 40% (www.bluezones.com).

Ideas for Wellbeing in Organizations

HEALTH

When people have the resources they need to take charge of their own health, the organizations in which they exist also flourish. Businesses can cut healthcare costs and sick leaves by ensuring that their employees work in an environment that encourages health at the individual level. As exemplified by Google, companies that provide access to healthy foods, stress-management resources, and a positive work environment may find that the benefits of these resources extend far beyond the individual employee.

COMMUNITY

Social networks play a large role in organizational culture and productivity. Individuals and leaders in organizations should act in ways that increase the trust, reciprocity, and altruism in the organizational networks. Individuals also need to be aware of their significant influence on others in their networks and choose the behaviors they want to model.

PURPOSE

Purpose is also important at the organizational level. When an organization does not have clarity of purpose, it impacts work flows, productivity, employee engagement and morale, and ultimately, the wellbeing of the organization, including the financial bottom line.

RELATIONSHIPS

The quality and nature of relationships has an impact at an organizational level. If there are poor relationships among employees or between employees and leadership, effectiveness and efficiency may be compromised. Employees who believe their managers care about them on a personal level are also more likely to excel at work, take less sick time, and are less likely to switch jobs (Rath, 2010). Nurturing key relationships and building strong partnerships is a key factor in promoting organizational wellbeing and success.

ENVIRONMENT

It is clearly beneficial to spend time outdoors, especially where there is vegetation or water. Organizations are likely to see employee wellbeing and productivity increase if they provide access to green space. Adding plants and scenes of nature has the potential to contribute to employee focus and efficiency.

SECURITY

Fear impacts thinking and decision-making in negative ways and can severely impact performance. Organizations can work to reduce fear by building networks of trust and reciprocity. Deep listening and honest communication help create an environment that feels safe and secure for everyone.

Summary

While the focus of healthcare in the United States and around the world has been predominantly on disease, there is a growing understanding that we need to shift our attention and resources to health promotion, prevention, and the cultivation of wellbeing. The current strategy in most healthcare systems is costly and does not produce human flourishing.

A comprehensive wellbeing approach includes a focus on health as well as other factors, such as purpose, relationships, community, safety and security, and the environment. An integrative nursing, whole person/whole systems approach is aligned with advancing wellbeing at multiple levels, including people, organizations, and communities.

SELECTED REFERENCES

Antonovsky, A. (1987). *Unraveling the Mystery of Health—How People Manage Stress and Stay Well*. San Francisco, CA: Jossey-Bass.

Buettner, D. (2009). *Blue Zones: Lessons for Living Longer from the People Who've Lived the Longest.* Washington, DC: National Geographic Society.

Diener, E., & Seligman, M. (2009). Beyond money. In *The Science of Well-being: The Collected Works of Ed Diener.* New York: Springer.

Frederickson, B. (2009). *Positivity.* New York: Three Rivers Press.

Helliwell, J., & Putnam, R. (2005). The social context of wellbeing. In Huppert, F., Baylis, N., Keverne, B. (eds.), *The Science of Well-being.* Oxford, UK: Oxford University Press.

Nakamura, J., & Csikszentmihalyi, M. (2009). Flow theory and research. In Snyder, C. R., Lopez, S. J. (eds.), *Handbook of Positive Psychology* (pp. 195–206). Oxford, UK: Oxford University Press.

Pollan, M. (2009). *In Defense of Food: An Eater's Manifesto.* New York: Penguin Books.

Rath, T., & Harter, J. (2010). *Wellbeing: The Five Essential Elements.* New York: Gallup Press.

Tay, L., & Diener, E. (2011). Needs and subjective wellbeing around the world. *Journal of Personality & Social Psychology, 101*(2), 354.

Wiseman, J., & Brasher, K. (2008). Community wellbeing in an unwell world: Trends, challenges, and possibilities. *Journal of Public Health Policy, 29,* 353–366.

World Health Organization. (1946). Preamble to the constitution of the World Health Organization as adopted by the International Health Conference, New York, June 19–22, 1946, signed on July 22, 1946, by the representatives of 61 States (Official Records of the World Health Organization, no. 2, p. 100) and entered into force on April 7, 1948.

11

Facilitating Lifestyle Choice and Change

JUDITH AUFENTHIE

Obesity, hypertension, diabetes, and heart disease are on the rise (WHO, 2013). Individuals are experiencing an increased amount of stress. The perception of not having enough time to take care of ourselves and still live up to the expectations of the world around us can often be paralyzing. Media continually remind us of how easy it is to eat healthy foods, improve our physical fitness, and buy the latest exercise equipment. And yet, behaviors are difficult to change. Even healthcare professionals struggle with self-care, adopting healthy lifestyles, and pursuing activities that promote health and wellbeing (Letvak, Ruhm, & Gupta, 2012). We have been taught the pathophysiology of disease; ways to support the body, mind, and spirit to facilitate our own health and wellbeing; and we still make choices that lead us down the path of imbalance and "dis-ease." Despite a plethora of adequate information, research suggests that nurses still do not take care of themselves (Mokdad et al., 2003).

The term *self-care* originated in the 1960s with the advent of social movements and consumerism. These movements were concerned with the issues of autonomy, self-determination, and independence in both health and illness. Self-care is now concerned with development and use of personal health practices and coping skills, decision-making, consulting others, and using one's own resources to manage one's health and wellbeing. Choosing behaviors that balance the effects of emotional and physical stress (i.e., eating healthy foods, exercising daily, getting seven to nine hours of sleep, relaxation practices, abstaining from unhealthy behaviors, and pursuing creative outlets) all involve making choices. We believe that the health of people has far more to do with their lifestyle choices and daily decisions than anything else. Self-care is not about indulgent, self-pampering behaviors; it is about becoming educated in the optimal ways of becoming or staying healthy and following through with those choices consistently to maintain our wellbeing.

Health and wellness education is available from many sources. Using evidence-based sources is important to ensure that one is getting reliable, safe information. Therefore, many educational institutions and corporate employers are offering more resources that help people take charge of their health and wellbeing.

Self-care is a matter of giving oneself permission to take the time, to make the commitment, and to negotiate the roadblocks. Caring for oneself and creating life balance allows one to be fully present. Hans Selye (1978), the father of stress management, suggests that there are two keys to managing stress. The first is "knowing thyself," which involves listening to the body's signs of personal stress through self-reflection and self-awareness. The second key to stress management is to add some variety to your life.

Self-knowledge is a fundamental component of self-care. Self-knowing increases our capacity for emotional maturity, healthy interpersonal relationships, and empathy (Goleman, 1997). Effective self-care means that individuals possess the skills and knowledge to manage their own stress, articulate their personal needs and values, and balance the demands of life with their physical and emotional health and wellbeing.

This chapter provides an understanding of how choices are an "inside job." Recent psychoneuroimmunology literature suggests how choices, including self-care and lifestyle behavioral choices are made, and the connection between perceptions, thoughts, beliefs, and choice. While this process seems effortless at times and extremely difficult at others, it is multifaceted and physiologically based. Because of its complexity, this process can be very difficult to define and understand in its entirety. A brief overview of how the brain, hormones, and neurotransmitters direct or play a part in making decisions and choices makes it easier to understand the foundation of behavioral changes.

The Brain and Behavioral Change

Making choices and decisions, although seemingly effortless for some, is actually a very complicated process that involves many chemical compounds and interactions, brain and bodily responses, as well as thoughts, feelings, and behaviors. While they may seem like very conscious activities, there are a myriad of unconscious underpinnings that occur each and every time a choice or decision is made.

BIOLOGICAL FACTORS

The prefrontal cortex, which is the part of the frontal lobe lying in front of the motor area, is closely linked to the limbic system. Besides apparently being involved in thinking about the future, making plans, and taking action, the limbic system also appears to be involved in the same dopamine pathways as the ventral tegmental area and plays a part in pleasure and addiction like the limbic system (Boeree, 2009).

The limbic system is a complex set of structures that includes the hypothalamus, the hippocampus, the amygdala, and several other nearby areas. It sets the mind's emotional tone, filters external events through internal states (creates emotional coloring), tags events as internally important, stores highly charged emotional memories, modulates motivation, controls appetite and sleep cycles, promotes bonding, directly processes the sense of smell, and modulates libido, according to Dr. Daniel Amen, in *Change Your Brain, Change Your Life* (1998). Thus, the limbic system appears to be primarily responsible for our emotional life and has a lot to do with the formation of memories. Emotionally directed behaviors are unconsciously controlled by the limbic system, and the choices we make regarding how to behave are also affected by the input and activity of the limbic system. Decision-making involves the orchestration of multiple neural structures and cognitive systems. Research has shown that areas such as the amygdala, insula, hippocampus, and areas of the prefrontal cortex are all involved in various aspects of decision-making (Guptaa, 2011).

The hypothalamus is one of the busiest parts of the brain. It sends instructions to the rest of the body in two ways: the first of which is to the autonomic nervous system. This allows the hypothalamus to have ultimate control of all the sympathetic and parasympathetic functions. The other way the hypothalamus controls things is via the pituitary gland, which in turn pumps hormones called *releasing factors* into the bloodstream.

The hippocampus consists of two "horns" that curve back from the amygdala. This structure appears to be very important in converting things that are "in your mind" at the moment into things that you will remember for the long run.

The brain, coupled with the remainder of the body, forms extremely complex interactions that create a state where actions are planned, internal commands are created, and then actions are executed. This complexity not only has a neurobiological basis but also involves intentions, thoughts, choices, and decisions. Thus, when choices are made and behaviors implemented, it is much more difficult to change them than pictured in the "just do it" campaigns promulgated by current media.

NEUROTRANSMITTERS AND HORMONES

The structures of the nervous system do not act alone in creating the physiological environment of decision and change. Neurotransmitters and hormones affect the function of the structure through complex mechanisms that eventually affect decision-making.

A *hormone*, by definition, is a compound produced by an endocrine gland and released into the bloodstream, where it can find its target cells at some distance from its actual site of release. A *neurotransmitter*, on the other hand, is a compound released from a nerve terminal. When an electrical impulse travels to the end of a nerve cell, it stimulates the terminal of this cell to secrete a chemical-signaling molecule at a special junction between nerve cells called a *synapse*. These nerve terminals are in direct opposition with their target cells to ensure rapid and specific delivery of the signal. Both target cells possess receptors for the signaling molecule and may produce identical biochemical responses. Therefore, the release mechanism determines whether a given molecule is a neurotransmitter or a hormone. For example, when released by the adrenal gland, adrenaline is a hormone that signals the blood vessels to dilate and the heart rate to increase, preparing for flight or fight. Alternatively, adrenaline is a neurotransmitter when it is released from a stimulated presynaptic nerve cell and acts on its neighboring postsynaptic cell to regulate attention, mental focus, arousal, and cognition.

Dopamine

Dopamine is a neurotransmitter that helps control the brain's reward and pleasure centers. Dopamine also helps regulate movement and emotional responses, and it enables us not only to see rewards, but to take action to move toward them (Hall, 2011). Dopamine is broadly distributed throughout the body. When present in the frontal lobe, the decision-making, memory, and reward systems are activated.

Serotonin

Serotonin is a neurotransmitter that regulates signal intensity. Serotonin changes how efficiently neurons communicate with each other, making signals "louder" or "softer." Most often, it accompanies other transmitters, changing a neuron's response to that particular signal. Because of this, it is used by all kinds of nerve cells all over the body. Furthermore, serotonin levels can dramatically alter our behavior. Levels that are too high can lead to sedation, whereas low levels are associated with debilitating psychiatric conditions and sudden infant death syndrome (SIDS). When serotonin is found in the brainstem, it plays a role in sleep as well as behavioral restraint. It helps to give us pause when making decisions and plays an important role in regulating social responses when found in the frontal cortex. Derived from amino acid proteins, 80%–90% of the body's serotonin resides in the intestinal tract, where it does its part to aid in digestion. The rest resides in the central nervous system, activating responses that alter our mood, feelings of hunger, and anger (Hall, 2011).

Norepinephrine

Norepinephrine (NE) is a catecholamine with multiple roles, including functioning as a hormone and neurotransmitter. When released in the brain from the locus ceruleus as a neurotransmitter, it plays a role in alertness, attention, arousal, and memory, as well as activation of the reward system. As a stress hormone, NE stimulates the sympathetic nervous system to activate the flight-or-fight response.

It is evident that the connection between the neurological system and behaviors is a complex series of events. Despite the complexity of decision-making, recent work in the field of cognitive neuroscience has begun to explain the component processes underlying decision-making and to localize the processes in the brain. In the last decade, this cognitive neuroscience research has begun to uncover links between the physical structures, hormones, and neurotransmitters in the decision-making process. The amygdala appears to have an inner connection with the frontal cortex (Guptaa,

2011). Limbic and cortical dopaminergic projections have been implicated in reward and addiction (Schultz, 2002; Wise, 2002). There is also some work supporting a role for prefrontal serotonin in reinforcement-driven learning and deciding (Clarke, 2004; Rogers, 1999, 2003). These are only a few examples of the work that is now available on the connection between the mind, body, and decision-making process and the complex mechanisms that bring behaviors, thoughts, and intentions to the forefront. And it is that very complexity that makes it difficult to change our decisions. Most decisions are made unconsciously. Jim Nightengale (2008), author of *Think Smart—Act Smart* states that we make decisions simply without thinking much about the process.

PSYCHOLOGICAL AND BEHAVIORAL FACTORS

In addition to biological factors, numerous psychological and behavioral factors influence decision-making. Our thoughts, beliefs, experiences, and perceptions influence what choices we make. Understanding these factors influences the integrative nurse's ability to effect behavioral change.

Past experiences (Juliusson, Karlsson, & Garling, 2005); cognitive biases (Stanovich & West, 2008); age and individual differences (de Bruin, 2007); belief in personal relevance (Acevedo & Krueger, 2004); as well as thoughts, beliefs, experiences and perceptions, all influence the choices people make. A thorough assessment of each of these factors is key when trying to understand and modify lifestyle choice and behavioral decisions. For example, even though most people know the physical side effects of smoking, most smokers enjoy smoking. They choose to continue smoking for any number of reasons. Once the "cost" tips the scale, motivation changes and then becomes a factor in their choice to quit.

Thoughts

A thought is an energetic creation that is stimulated in one's mind. It contains no emotion in its initial state. Thoughts may be stimulated from the chemical reactions in the brain and body, a feeling, an emotional interaction, or a connection to a belief. Nevertheless, in its pure state, it is only energy. Our minds are an incredibly powerful tool, and we only use a small portion of them every day. Our thoughts play a significant role in how we view the world, and the positive and negative thoughts we carry with us can be the foundation for all sorts of things in our lives, both positive and negative. We can control our thoughts, and therefore we can control whether our thoughts are positive or negative, a catalyst for living a positive, happy life or a life of doom and gloom.

Dale Carnegie (1968) said that what you think about is what makes you happy, not the things you have, where you live, who you are, or what you do for a living. Are our thoughts ones that encourage us to act positively, to look forward with eager anticipation of the joys ahead, and even to embrace the challenges of life as positive learning steps? Or, do our thoughts paralyze us with fears of the future, fears of failure, and an expectation that life will turn out difficult, scary, and doomed? Of course, most of us find ourselves somewhere in between on most days, swinging to the extremes at times of stress or exhilaration. Yet, it is true to say that *how* we think about ourselves is fundamental to how we view our lives and make our life choices.

Beliefs

"Our beliefs have the power to change the flow of events in the universe—literally to interrupt and redirect time, matter, and space, and the events that occur within them" (Braden, 2008, p. 15). Therefore, when we focus on what we want to become and on taking care of ourselves, we are better able to attain a higher level of wellbeing. Our thoughts affect our feelings, which then affect our life choices. For example, if we feel like a failure, our actions will encourage and anticipate failure. We will attempt little that is new and challenging, and it can even leave us open to others' treating us badly as they reflect the poor opinion we have of ourselves. Alternatively, envisioning success encourages us to approach a task with confidence, a "can do" attitude that is met by those around us with reciprocal acceptance and belief that success is just around the corner. Therefore it is important to transform those negative aspects into positive ones that focus on health and wellbeing.

In the field of "New Biology," (Epigenetics, the link between the mind and matter and the effect on our lives), Lipton (2005) has examined the processes by which cells receive information, proposing that genes and DNA alone do not control our biology; rather, DNA may be influenced by signals from outside the cell, including the energetic messages emanating from our positive and negative thoughts. A belief is accumulated thought forms, created from learned and lived experiences, behaviors, and emotion that occur in the current lifetime, or passed on from generations through genetic material. Beliefs may be stored in the mind, cells, genetic material, and body and are composed of energy (thought) that has taken on another other form in the mind-body through a connection with the cellular, genetic material (Lipton, 2005).

> Men often become what they believe themselves to be. If I believe I cannot do something, it makes me incapable of doing it. But when I believe I can, and then I acquire the ability to do it even if I didn't have it in the beginning. (Mahatma Gandhi)

Experiences

Researchers have shown that past experience really does help when we have to make complex decisions based on uncertain or confusing information (Biotechnology and Biological Sciences Research Council, 2009). The human brain's plasticity, its ability to actually change its internal structure, has been well documented. In addition, recent advances note that the circuitry in the cortices is changed by our past experiences (Marik, 2010). That is to say, when we are confronted with a situation that is not very clear, or for which we have insufficient information to make a clear decision, the experiences from our past jump to mind and help the brain categorize the situation, finding resolutions for complex dilemmas.

One of the main tasks that the brain has to perform on a regular basis is to assign meaning and clarification to the sensory data it collects from our five senses (sight, smell, hearing, touch, and taste). However, these data are naturally unclear and uncertain. Therefore, the cortices involved in the process need to be on high alert at all times (Li, 2009). Also very important is our ability to discern between visual stimuli that look relatively the same. "What we have found is that learning from past experience actually rewires our brains so that we can categorize the things we are looking at, and respond appropriately to them in any context" (Kourtzi, as cited by ScienceDaily, 2009). When the brain is "wired" and categorized by past experiences it is better able to choose appropriate behaviors and actions when making decisions.

Perceptions

All decisions require perceptual processes to extract information from the external world that can be used to help develop an answer to a problem. Perception is a process consisting of sequential steps that begins with the environment and leads to a conscious awareness of that stimulus. Recognition follows awareness with interpretation or meaning-making, which then typically results in some form of action. This process is continual; not a great deal of time is spent actually thinking about the *process* that occurs as you move throughout your world (Humphreys et al., 2008).

Perception may also come via intuitive knowing, a potent wisdom not mediated by the linear mind, which aids with decisions (Orloff, 2012). Intuition can be a hunch, a dream, a "knowing," specific guidance, or a warning of danger. During troubled times, intuition is a voice in the wilderness to get you through, and when things are good, it will help them stay that way. Intuition can actually be perceived physically as a "gut feeling." Although cutting-edge science associates this with a separate "brain" in the gut called the *enteric nervous system*, a network of neurons that learn and store information, others have linked this intuitive capacity to the basal ganglia, a part of the brain that informs us something is not right and we had better act on it (Orloff, 2009).

Motivation

Motivation is a basic drive for all of our actions. *Motivation* refers to the dynamic of our behavior, which involves our needs, desires, and ambitions in life. Our motives for achievement can range from biological needs to satisfying desires or winning in competitive endeavors (Rabideau, 2005). Motivation is important because it affects our lives every day. All of our behaviors and actions are influenced by our inner drive to succeed. It is easy to say or think about what you are going to do, but actually doing what you say takes commitment. In addition, taking action once is not difficult; anyone can motivate themselves to get to the gym to work out one time. But being able to consistently take action is the challenge for most people.

Lifestyle Choice and Decision-Making

Lifestyle choices, including self-care, result from numerous habitual activities that are unique to each individual. These choices lend consistency to activities, behavior, coping, motivation, and thought processes. Lifestyle choices define the way individuals live. Choices fueled by feelings include: How hungry am I? Will I exercise today? Who are my friends and support people? Emotions, preferences, perceptions, beliefs, and thoughts all inform our decision-making processes.

In general, the decision-making process begins with the perception and recognition of cues or evidence, followed by an evaluation of these pieces of information. As common sense and psychological research suggest, our decisions are based, at least in part, on *plausible scenarios* that we construct (Damasio, 1994). These plausible futures are themselves influenced by our *past experiences* (Conway, 2000). Not only do past experiences directly impact the emotional state during decision-making, but past experiences also represent an important source of information to construct anticipations that will influence the immediate emotion and the decision process (Lowenstein, 2003).

Decision-making models tend to consider past experiences as a stored piece of information that is or is not being accessed (Wilson, 2003). However, contemporary work on *autobiographical memory* (i.e., the memory of our past experiences) suggests that a past experience is not directly accessed, but rather that its different aspects (e.g., episodic aspects, emotional aspects) are stored separately (Conway, 2000).

The voluntary retrieval of an experience is, therefore, a *reconstructive process* requiring activation and integration of different memories, all of which requires significant cognitive resources. An important contribution of this line of research has been to demonstrate that the very same processes and sources of autobiographical information are used to reconstruct past experiences as well as to construct representations of plausible future experiences (Conway, 2000; Wheeler, 1997). Thus, change is as much informed by our past and present as by our desires for the future.

Getting from Here to There: Wellbeing and Change

While there are numerous theoretical perspectives about individual change, the one that has been the most cited when considering lifestyle and health-behavioral change is the Transtheoretical Model of Change (Prochaska & DiClemente, 1983; Prochaska & Velicer, 1997).

The Transtheoretical Model is an integrative model of behavior change that combines key constructs from other theories. The model describes how people modify a problematic behavior or acquire a positive behavior. It has been very influential in guiding the design of behavioral change interventions during the last three decades (Littell, 2002).

The central organizing construct of the model is the "stages of change" theory. The model also includes a series of independent variables, the processes of change, which include ten cognitive and behavioral activities that facilitate change and a series of intermediate outcome measures, including the decisional balance inventory, self-efficacy or situational temptations scale, and behavior measures. The Transtheoretical Model is a model of intentional change. The specific focus is on behavior change, and the key constructs are dynamic variables (i.e., open to modification), whereas more static variables such as gender and past history are included only as moderator variables. In addition, the model primarily focuses on the decision-making of the individual while other approaches to health promotion focus on social or biological influences on behavior. The model (Figure 11.1) has been applied to a wide variety of problem behaviors; however, it is most commonly utilized in smoking and alcohol cessation.

The model cites five stages necessary for long-term behavioral change. *Precontemplation* is the stage when the person is not considering a change and will not for at least the next six months. Someone in this stage has no thoughts about changing and does not perceive their behavior as damaging or harmful in any way; perhaps this individual is a smoker who enjoys smoking. As this smoker progresses to the *contemplation* stage, he or she begins to be aware of the side effects as well as cost and actually considers stopping somewhere in the future. The *preparation* stage occurs when this smoker may begin to cut back on their smoking. Perhaps he or she begins to look into methods of smoking cessation or talk to others who have quit, gathering information.

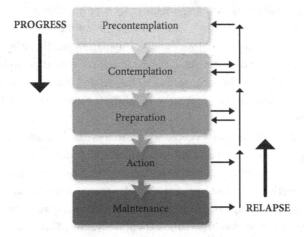

FIGURE 11.1 Di Clemente and Prochaska's Transtheoretical Model of Change (http://www.addictioninfo.org/articles/11/1/Stages-of-Change-Model/Page1.html)

Progressing to the *action* phase, the smoker modifies his or her environment; perhaps smoking only in the garage at home or smoking only at night. He or she might make an appointment with a primary care provider to enlist the help of medication. The *maintenance* stage is where the individual continues to focus on becoming a nonsmoker and may utilize self-talk, encouragement from family and friends, or other behavioral or pharmacological methods to sustain the behavioral change.

FACILITATING CHANGE: THE ROLE OF THE INTEGRATIVE NURSE

Wellness is an active, multifactorial process of becoming aware of and making choices toward a more successful existence. Human beings, inseparable from the environment, are complex living wholes that are continually developing and evolving; we never arrive at a point where there is no possibility of improvement. We are by nature continuously seeking more information, ever-changing patterns of creative, adaptive relationships across the dimensions of human experience. We are constantly assessing and considering a variety of options through our thoughts, beliefs, senses, perceptions, and outcomes of our behaviors. As we become more self-reflective and self-aware, we become more successful at creating personal optimal wellness.

The integrative nurse supports the wellbeing journey by addressing patient activation. An activated person is one who understands the role he or she has in managing health and the knowledge and skills to move forward. Clinical as well as behavioral support that is respectful of the individual's preferences and motivation is necessary for optimal outcomes.

Individuals who are overwhelmed by their diagnosis and have experienced failure in the past are among those who require the most support. They need understanding to help them move forward slowly, one small step at a time, overcoming their fears and experiencing successes in self-care and self-management. The integrative nurse is mindful that activation does not entail passive receipt of education and information, the typical method of addressing needed health-related behavioral change. Rather, strategies that engage, explore, motivate, and innovate more reliably elicit growth and transformation.

Hibbard (2004) claimed that people with chronic health conditions who receive coaching tailored to their level of health activation displayed significant improvements in clinical outcomes and experienced fewer hospitalizations and visits to the emergency room than those coached using traditional methods. Specific coaching strategies are described in later chapters, as are other motivational and activation activities to encourage health promotion change. The Patient Activation Measure (PAM) offers one method to measure patient engagement and help to determine patient activation as an immediate outcome in the behavioral change process (Hibbard et al., 2004).

Conclusion

Given nursing's current focus on promoting health and wellbeing in addition to patient safety and quality of care, it is imperative to empower our patients to seek optimal wellbeing on their self-care journey. By meeting our clients where they are, determining where they want to go, and utilizing the foundational principles of integrative nursing, the nurse is better able to assist the patient in this journey. Healthcare providers who use therapeutic presence as the basis of patient relationships will use the following: active listening, sitting down to meet people on their level, turning negative thoughts into statements of possibility, and helping the patient create achievable outcomes. Providers with therapeutic presence are those who will creatively partner with patients to achieve higher levels of wellbeing.

Self-care is critical to the health and wellbeing of the nation. The integrative nurse fosters lifestyles that prevent disease, promote health, support vibrant relationships, and assure human flourishing and wellbeing; in other words, a central component of integrative nursing practice is self-care.

SELECTED REFERENCES

Braden, G. (2008). *The spontaneous Healing of belief: Shattering the Paradigm of False Beliefs.* New York: Hay House.

Biotechnology and Biological Sciences Research Council (2009, May 15). Past Experience Is Invaluable For Complex Decision Making, Brain Research Shows. *ScienceDaily.* Retrieved August 6, 2013, from http://www.sciencedaily.com/releases/2009/05/090513130930.htm

Conway, M., & Pleydell-Pearce, C. (2000). The construction of autobiographical memories in the self-memory system. *Psychological Review, 107*(2), 261–288.

Guptaa, R., Kosicka, T. R., Becharap, A., & Tranela, D. (2011). The amygdala and decision making. *Neuropsychologia, 49*(4), 760–766.

Hibbard, J. (2005). Weighing the past and the future in decision making. *European Journal of Cognitive Psychology, 17*(4), 561–575.

Lipton, B. H. (2005). *The Biology of Belief: Unleashing the Power of Unconsciousness, Matter and Miracles.* Carlsbad, CA: Hay House.

Prochaska, J. O., & Di Clemente, C. C. (1983). Stages and processes of self-change of smoking: Toward an integrative model of change. *Journal of Consulting & Clinical Psychology, 51,* 390–395.

Prochaska, J. O., & Velicer, W. F. (1997). The Transtheoretical Model of health behavior change. *American Journal of Health Promotion, 12,* 38–48.

Rabideau, S. (2005, Nov.). Effects of achievement motivation on behavior. Retrieved from Personality Research: http://www.personalityresearch.org/papers/rabideau.htm

Rogers, R. D., Owen, A. M., Middleton, H. C., & Williams, E. J. (1999). Choosing between small likely rewards and large, unlikely rewards activates inferior and orbital prefrontal cortex. *Journal of Neuroscience, 20*(19), 9029–9038.

Selye, H. (1978). *The Stress of Life.* New York: McGraw-Hill.

12

Movement and Integrative Nursing

SUSAN MASEMER, MARY FARRELL, JAYSON KING, AND MATTHEW KOITHAN

P hysical activity—and movement—is a core component of a healthy lifestyle and wellbeing. Although physical activity is highly effective, it is often underutilized. A recent survey indicated that almost two-thirds of patients would be more interested in exercise if advised to do it by their healthcare provider and given additional resources (American College of Sports Medicine [ACSM], 2009). However, only four out of ten providers typically mention exercise or provide resources: citing lack of knowledge, skill, and time to implement these health-promotion and disease-prevention strategies (Jonas & Phillips, 2009).

Physical Activity as an Effective Whole-Person Intervention

Physical activity and improved fitness allows the body to better regulate all of its physiological functions and avoid or manage many healthcare conditions and injuries. Furthermore, "fitness activities" contribute to overall wellbeing and enhanced functional ability. While it is important to remember that exercise alone does not ensure optimal wellbeing, it is a vital part of our "bodymindspirit" prescription (Emmons, 2005; Seaward, 2012).

Lack of physical activity is a modifiable risk factor for a wide variety of chronic diseases, including cardiovascular disease, diabetes, certain cancers, depression, and obesity (Bouchard & Katzmarzyk, 2010; Durstine, 2009). An active lifestyle contributes to numerous physiological changes (e.g., increased strength, endurance, balance, and bone density, and decreased resting blood pressure and heart rate) by promoting increased energy stores in muscle, the growth of fatigue-resistant muscle fibers, increased capillary density, and increased mitochondrial enzymatic activity (Coffey, 2007; Farrell, 2012; Powers, 2009). Thus, physical activity helps the body become resistant to the downstream bodymindspirit of fatigue (Barry, 2008; Coffey, 2007).

Creating an Effective Activity Plan

Although there are different ways to encourage patients to increase physical activity and achieve fitness goals, partnering with the patient is always recommended as the most effective approach. Methods include structured exercise programs or a routine that incrementally increases activities of daily living (ADLs), thereby increasing physical activity. Regardless of the approach, the individual's current fitness level, availability of resources, health concerns, and readiness should be considered. In addition, the American Medical Association (AMA)/ACSM (2010) has promulgated standard recommendations for health-related fitness, suggesting that all programs include resistance, endurance, and flexibility exercises. Persons with health or physical challenges, or those who have not recently engaged in regular physical activity, may require adaptations to these recommendations and should be referred to qualified medical fitness experts.

PROGRAMMING OPTIONS

A traditional, structured exercise routine may be preferable for individuals who need to schedule their daily activities with some degree of certainty, plan and evaluate their progress, and track fitness changes. A more flexible approach incorporates exercise into ADLs. Over the course of the day, minutes of exercise accumulate, resulting in equivalent health benefits (Murphy, Blair, & Murtagh, 2009). Though this method may seem random, it appeals to many people, allowing for ongoing exercise without the need to set aside blocks of time that are difficult to schedule.

As a person's awareness of exercise and movement increases, activities become intentional. When using this more flexible approach to exercise, the question becomes how much activity should be recommended. The easiest metric to track is number of steps per day, using a pedometer, accelerometer, web-based tool, or smartphone application. To advance and progress, patients should be advised to measure their steps for one week and add ten percent per week, with the ultimate goal of 10,000 steps or more per day (Tudor-Locke, 2010).

When describing a more structured exercise program, the Frequency, Intensity, Time and Type (FITT) principle is often used. FITT indicates the recommendations for four major components that should be addressed in any exercise program: (1) frequency (days/week); (2) intensity (percent of maximal effort/light, moderate, vigorous); (3) time (duration/volume); and (4) type (Aerobic/Endurance—cycling, running, swimming; and Anaerobic/Resistance—free weights, weight machines, resistance bands). Progression should be incremental; 10% increase per week in no more than one of these categories each week (Whaley et al., 2006).

PROGRAM TYPES

Cardiovascular or "aerobic" exercise occurs when large-muscle groups are used in a rhythmic manner for a sustained period of time. Examples include walking, bicycling, swimming, dancing, jogging, and aerobic classes. The ACSM (2010) recommends 20–60 minutes of moderate-to-vigorous (40%–85% maximal effort) exercise 3–5 days each week for an accumulation of at least 150 minutes each week for healthy adults. To promote weight loss, ACSM recommends a minimum of 300 minutes each week of moderate-intensity exercise or 150 minutes of vigorous exercise.

Resistance exercise increases the strength of muscles and bones, as well as enhances muscle tone, coordination, and balance. Examples include weight training, resistance bands, kettle bells, and exercises using body weight for resistance. Resistance training should performed at least 2–3 days each week, targeting each of the major muscle groups with 48 hours of rest between training sessions (ACSM, 2010). Typically, a range of 6–12 exercises are included in each session, using 2–3sets of 8–12 repetitions to increase strength, mass, and endurance. Adjustments are made based on desired results; if emphasizing strength, intensity is increased and repetitions decreased; if emphasizing endurance, intensity is decreased and repetitions increased.

Flexibility exercise encourages gentle, full range of motion, causing the joints and tendons to become more flexible over time, reducing muscle tension, and providing protection from various injuries. Examples include gentle stretching exercises, yoga, Pilates and *tai chi*. The mind–body connection of these exercises greatly enhances their value: research links participation in activities such as yoga with a reduction in symptoms of anxiety and depression and improvement in overall wellbeing (Brown, 2005). ACSM (2010) recommends stretching a minimum of 2–3 days each week for at least 10 minutes at a time, using four or more repetitions for each major muscle (ACSM, 2010).

The Use of Exercise in Chronic Conditions

The benefits of physical activity for the prevention and management of chronic conditions have gained increasing attention from the research community (ACSM, 2010). Many of these conditions contribute to rising healthcare costs, negatively impacting our community and social fabric. Furthermore, these conditions negatively affect personal functioning, quality of life, and social relationships (Durstine & Moore, 2003; Hacker, 2009). Conditions that are particularly responsive to physical activity are discussed next.

CARDIOVASCULAR HEALTH

Cardiovascular disease continues to be the leading cause of death for both men and women in the United States (American Heart Association, 2013). Physical activity aids in the prevention and treatment of heart disease, stroke, hypertension, and peripheral arterial disease, as a result of improved heart function, blood vessel health and dilation, enhanced blood circulation, and reductions in blood viscosity and blood pressure (Durstine & Moore, 2003; Durstine, 2009; Rankovic, 2012). Recent studies have shown that being physically active can reduce the risk of death from cardiovascular disease by up to 50% (Washburton et al., 2010). Physical activity is also highly effective for secondary prevention; 1600 kilocalories' expenditure of energy per week has been shown to halt the progression of Coronary Artery Disease (CAD), and 2200 kcal per week is associated with plaque reduction in patients with heart disease (Washburton, Nicol, & Bredin, 2006). Exercise can also improve an individual's emotions, mental status, and outlook by reducing depressive feelings (Pinto, 2013).

ACSM (2010) suggests that a thorough risk-evaluation be completed before a patient begins any exercise program. Generally, individuals with diagnosed cardiovascular disease begin training at a lower intensity for short durations, but are encouraged to exercise more frequently for fitness and health progression—for instance, low-intensity exercise, such as casual walking, for 5–15 minutes, as tolerated by symptoms, up to four times each day (ACSM, 2010). As their fitness improves, the duration and intensity can be gradually increased (ACSM, 2010; Durstine, 2009).

DIABETES

Physical activity is highly effective in the prevention and management of Type II diabetes due to improved glucose utilization, insulin regulation, metabolic activity, and weight management (ACSM 2010; McArdle, Katch, & Katch, 2010). Washburton, Nicol, and Bredin (2006) reported that aerobic or resistance exercise reduced the risk of Type II diabetes as well as other associated risk factors; for every 500 kcals in energy expended, a 6% reduction in Type II diabetes risk can be expected. Additionally, proper diet and exercise can reduce the need for medications (ACSM, 2010). Guidelines suggest exercising 5–7 days a week at 50%–80% of maximal effort for 20–60 minutes to promote healthy weight. Endurance training is suggested for fat loss; however, resistance exercise is still encouraged and is similar to resistance-training guidelines for healthy populations (ACSM, 2010).

OSTEOPOROSIS

Approximately 10 million people live with osteoporosis: 80% are women (National Osteoporosis Foundation, 2002). Osteoporosis can be largely prevented with lifestyle changes (including exercise) and treatment (McClung, 1994). Weight-bearing physical activities (e.g., jumping, fast walking, or jogging) and resistance training are recommended because of their positive impact on bone mineral density when performed at least three days per week for 30–60 minutes (ACSM, 2010; DHHS, 2008; Durstine & Moore, 2003). Exercises with flexion and twisting of the spine should be avoided for individuals with reduced bone mass (ACSM, 2010).

CANCER

Increased physical activity appears to be beneficial for the prevention of certain cancers (breast and colon), as well as for improvements in functional capacity, mental wellbeing, and quality of life during treatment and recovery phases (National Cancer Institute [NCI], 2012). Physical activity has been shown to improve patients' quality of life as well as ameliorate their symptoms (e.g., nausea, lymphedema, fatigue, orthopedic-related concerns, anxiety and depression) (Courneya, Segal, Gelmon, et al., 2007; Courneya, Segal, Mackey, et al., 2007; Hayes et al., 2013; Monga et al., 2007). However, exercise recommendations need to take into the account the extent of the cancer and its treatment and should be planned by professionals so that variations can be considered. Guidelines suggest endurance training 3–5 days each week and resistance training 2–3 days each week (ACSM, 2010). Flexibility training should also be added. Intensity should begin at about 40%–60% of maximal effort with approximately 20–60 minutes of aerobic exercise with resistance training (ACSM, 2010).

CHRONIC PAIN

Chronic pain contributes to social, emotional, physical, and economic losses and accounts for over $100 billion in treatment-related costs and lost work productivity (American Academy of Pain Medicine, 2013). Functional decline often accompanies chronic pain; physical activity frequently ceases due to temporary increases in pain and/or fear of re-injury. This leads to a vicious de-conditioning cycle of inactivity, weight gain, increased pain, and further functional decline (Gaskin & Richard, 2012).

Once pain has become a chronic condition, passive conservative (i.e., pharmacotherapeutics) and active conservative treatments are often recommended. Consistent with integrative nursing principles, active conservative treatments are preferred due to their improved safety, fewer side effects, and, often, reduced overall healthcare costs. Physical activity, along with meditation, healthy sleep practices, good nutrition, and stress management, fall under the category of "active conservative" treatment, a self-care strategy. Adopting a more flexible "as tolerated" daily exercise program can help those with chronic pain build endorphins, reduce stress, and preserve function (Tracy, 2002). ACSM (2010) recommends endurance training 3–5 days each week and resistance exercise 2–3 days each week, with emphasis on flexibility and range of motion. Low-impact endurance exercise, such as swimming, is often preferred. Since the intensity and duration of exercise may be limited by pain symptoms, low intensity and short bouts are recommended to start, slowly increasing the frequency and duration as tolerated.

CHRONIC OBSTRUCTIVE PULMONARY DISEASE

Chronic obstructive pulmonary disease (COPD), including asthma, emphysema, and chronic bronchitis, benefits from exercise by increasing the person's fitness and conditioning and decreasing the inflammatory response of tissues in some patients (Durstine, 2009; Pleger, 2009). Yet, response is individual, and each person's exercise tolerance should be carefully monitored, because exercise may exaggerate the inflammatory response following exercise in some individuals (Mojtaba, 2011; Pleger, 2009). Guidelines for those with moderate to severe COPD focus on aerobic training and allow for intensities of 60%–80% maximal effort, 3–5 days each week. When duration and intensity must be limited, multiple short bouts of training (total 30 minutes) are often suggested. Guidelines for those with mild COPD and well-controlled asthma are similar to that of healthy populations, with greater emphasis on the warm-up period, which reduces bronchoconstriction (McKenzie, 1994).

The Psychosocial Effects of Exercise

Research has shown that multiple forms of exercise can also have a positive effect on mental and emotional health. Ikenouchi-Sugita (2013) found that subjects who exercise regularly, even daily walking, experience fewer depressive feelings and exhibit better social adaptation. Consistent participation in physical activity (especially endurance training) has also been shown to improve acute and chronic mental health conditions (Silveira, 2013). Blumenthal et al. (1999) reported that physical activity was more effective than Zoloft in managing depressive symptoms. Emmons (2005) claimed that exercise has the ability to alter brain chemistry by enhancing levels of serotonin, dopamine, norepinephrine, endorphins, and enkephalins, pointing to its possible effectiveness as a viable intervention for chronic depression.

Regular exercise also supports improved mental wellbeing in healthy populations by encouraging the development of self-esteem and confidence, particularly around the ability to perform daily tasks. Preliminary research indicates that resistance exercise and mind–body forms of exercise (e.g., yoga, tai chi, qigong) may also provide mental health benefits, although more research is needed to identify an exact "dose response" and identification of psychosocial and mental health contributions (Emmons, 2005).

Exercise Across the Lifespan

Exercise needs and programs should vary across the lifespan. Children at particular risk for obesity and its accompanying chronic conditions should be encouraged to engage in 60 minutes of activity each day. This includes moderate to vigorous aerobic activity and bone and muscle strengthening activities at least 3–4 days per week (ACSM, 2010). The integrative nurse, working within a family context,

can encourage parents to set a positive example, be positive about physical activity, and make it fun: this can include involving the child with sports and using
age-appropriate games. Fostering this positive family relationship with exercise will
pay off in dividends throughout the child's lifetime as well as the parents'. A child
exposed to multiple exercise options (e.g., tai chi, yoga, sports, solo activities) will
adopt lifelong practices and engagement with exercise, the benefits of which will
manifest for decades to come.

Healthy women are encouraged to exercise throughout their pregnancies unless
medically contraindicated (American College of Obstetricians and Gynecologists,
2009; ACSM, 2010). The benefits of exercise in pregnancy are well documented and
include reduction in backaches; prevention and/or treatment of gestational diabetes;
and improvement in energy, mood, posture, and quality of sleep (Dempsey, 2005;
Nascimento, 2012). Generally, exercise should be low-impact, moderate aerobic training three days a week for 30–60 minutes with low to moderate resistance training.
Duration and intensity should be moderated based on stage of pregnancy as well as
the mother's previous physical activity levels. Exercises should be appropriate (i.e.,
low-impact, not performed in a prone position, without extreme range of motion)
(ACSM, 2010).

Advancing age is no reason to discontinue activity, and, in fact, physical inactivity
is a risk factor in and of itself. The goals of exercise in a senior population are to (a) reduce health risks, (b) engage in favorite activities, and (c) remain independent for
as long as possible. Exercise variety is critical; resistance and endurance training in a
long-term program provide more cardiovascular health benefits than endurance training alone (Sousa, 2013). Additionally, regular moderate physical activity can help manage stress, improve mood, and reduce feelings of depression (Sousa, 2013). Studies also
suggest that exercise can improve or maintain some aspects of cognitive function, such
as the ability to shift quickly between tasks, plan an activity, and ignore irrelevant information (Sakurai, 2012).

Promoting Physical Activity

The ACSM (2010) recommends that "more should be done to address physical activity
and exercise in healthcare settings," urging all healthcare providers to make exercise
consultation a regular, important part of their interaction with every patient at every
visit (www.exerciseismedicine.org; last accessed March 25, 2013). This means that discussions about physical activity are part of the patient's "vital signs," assessed at every
visit and as part of patient-discharge instructions. As part of routine integrative nursing care, exercise has the potential to be the most effective instant happiness-booster
of all activities (Biddle, Fox, & Boutcher, 2000). Thus, exercise takes a prominent place
in the world of integrative nursing, with profound effects on the patient's health and
wellbeing.

The "Four Ms" are an easy way for the practitioner to remember how to assist patients beginning a program of regular physical activity (http://exerciseismedicine.org/)

- **Mention.** Sixty-five percent of patients would be more interested in exercising if so advised by their provider and given resources. Yet exercise is currently discussed in only four of ten visits (ACSM, 2009). Providers identify time as a major barrier, but a meaningful dialogue can be initiated in as little as two minutes.
- **Motivate.** Recognize that change is difficult. When a cardiologist tells a patient to "change or die," only one in seven patients is able to respond adequately (Keegan & Lahey, 2009). This statistic does not imply that the other six patients do not care; it simply illustrates that change is difficult. Understanding the basics of behavioral change and engaging the patient is central to success. In addition, when you recognize your patient's need for autonomy, connection, and meaningful achievement, your "change talk" becomes more consequential. A certified health & wellness coach may also be an appropriate referral to assist your patient (see http://www.wellcoachesschool.com/index.cfm?page=selfCoachingCourses, last accessed March 19, 2013).
- **Model.** It is vital that you "walk the talk" and model healthy behavior. Being a role model inspires your patients, increases your credibility, and improves your own health. Sharing your own struggles, obstacles, motivators, and successes vastly enhances the impact by making it personal.

In addition, exercise as part of the provider's self-care regimen is vital. Understanding and knowing about physical activity is not enough. The work of the integrative nurse demands her or his full presence, and there must be re-energizing, renewal, and rest to thrive in this work. As activity is so clearly a part of our wellbeing, the wise integrative nurse weaves exercise and movement it into his or her daily routine, balancing the type of work with a selected workout routine. For example, an inpatient nurse may do better with activities that restore calm and peace, such as yoga, tai chi, or swimming. For those who sit for prolonged periods, a more active routine may be preferred. Considerations also include how you engage in the activity (solo or group), where the activity takes place (outdoors or indoors), and when (structured times or small bits woven into the day).

- **Multiply.** When it comes to motivating people to exercise, "going it alone" is neither desirable nor practical. Create a team approach, identifying resources and referring them to credentialed experts who are equipped to handle special needs. Having a good support network of friends and family may also help to keep us on the right track.

THE PROFESSIONAL EXERCISE TEAM

When working with vulnerable populations, integrative nurses often find themselves in need of consultants or collaborators who can assist with exercise recommendations. Professionals you might consider include the following:

- *Exercise physiologists* have graduate degrees in exercise physiology and the knowledge to work with clients who have a variety of health concerns, as well as with athletes at all levels.
- *Professional exercise specialists* have completed a degree in an exercise-related field and are certified by an accredited organization such as the American College of Sports Medicine (ACSM), the National Academy of Sports Medicine (NASM), the American Council on Exercise (ACE), or the National Strength and Conditioning Association (NCSA). Be certain to ask for references when working with an exercise specialist (www.exerciseasmedicine. org; last accessed on March 18, 2013).
- *Personal trainers* are usually certified by one of the national organizations previously identified. Their education and affiliations should be commensurate with the patients' conditions, needs, and desires.
- *Health and wellness coaches* are certified professionals who can help build confidence and motivation, as well as provide support and accountability as patients move towards their activity goals. Look for certification through organizations such as WellCoaches in conjunction with ACSM, and credentialing through the International Coaching Federation.
- *Physical therapists* are licensed professionals who work with persons who have sustained disabilities, impairments, or limitations, to improve their overall physical function. Physical therapists restore function, improve mobility, and decrease pain with the goal of reestablishing a patient's prior functional level.

Patient Engagement

While knowledge about exercise and its importance is valuable, patient engagement is imperative. The key to patient engagement is meeting them "where they are," the importance of which cannot be overstated. Unless the patient is engaged, the chance of achieving sustainable change is nil. In his seminal work about behavioral change and lifestyle modification, Prochaska (1984) proposes several stages, with attendant intervention strategies.

- **Pre-contemplation.** Pre-contemplators fall under the category of "I can't" or "I won't." Employ these strategies appropriately:

- *"I won't."* This is not the time to say "Just do it." Patients who say "I won't" benefit from additional information about the benefits of exercise. They can be encouraged to list their reasons for wanting to exercise and weigh these benefits against the consequences of staying sedentary.
- *"I can't."* These patients need extra support when beginning to gain confidence in their exercise skills and fitness abilities. Discussing the benefits of starting gradually will be valuable here, as will identifying who will serve as support for the patient.
- **Contemplation.** At this stage, participants are beginning to say "I might," noting their intention to start exercise. While they may be more aware of the benefits of change, there continue to be barriers to action, such as ambivalence about change. Delaying or stalling tactics are common. Strategies for this stage include identifying compelling reasons for them to become physically active and measuring/recording the individual's physical abilities across multiple exercise modes, such as muscular and cardiovascular endurance, strength, flexibility, balance, and coordination. Identifying real and pseudo barriers is also helpful, refuting the ones that are imagined and constructing feasible, focused goals (e.g., getting information about a water-exercise class, or finding a walking buddy). The patient may also not be aware of gentler exercises that focus on the mind–body connection such as yoga or tai chi.
- **Preparation.** People at this stage are ready to start taking action, stating "I will." They take small steps that can help them make regular activity a part of their lives, such as telling their friends and family that they want to become active. At this stage, the integrative nurse can suggest coping strategies in anticipation of problematic situations (e.g., join a mall-walking group or investigate membership at a community center).
- **Action.** People at this stage ("I am") have become physically active within the last six months and need to work hard to keep moving ahead. Learning how to strengthen their commitment to change and fight urges to slip back is central. At this stage, the integrative nurse can suggest tracking their progress or using reward systems.
- **Maintenance.** After more than six months of exercise, those who are still engaged are saying "I still am!" Physical activity has become a habit. To encourage maintenance of healthy lifestyle, integrative nurses can teach individuals how to recognize lapses, prevent boredom by variety, and mentor others in their physical activity journey.

EXERCISE READINESS RISK-ASSESSMENT

Before recommending a physical activity regimen, initial risk-readiness and risk-screening should be completed using the Physical Activity Readiness Questionnaire

(PAR-Q). The PAR-Q questionnaire focuses on symptoms of heart disease while identifying musculoskeletal problems that should be evaluated prior to participation in an exercise program (www.exerciseasmedicine.org). If your patient answers *No* to all of the PAR-Q questions, independent physical activity may be warranted.

If your patient answered *Yes* to any of the PAR-Q questions, independent or monitored physical activity may still be possible, but a more thorough assessment of physical health and history should be completed to identify any contraindications and allow for proper risk-stratification. Contraindications for exercise, both relative and absolute, for specific populations can be found in the *ACSM Guidelines for Exercise Testing and Prescription* (2010). This will determine if it is safe for the individuals to exercise on their own and enable the health professional to prescribe a safe exercise protocol based on the FITT principle. When in doubt, refer to a qualified clinical exercise professional.

Conclusion

Throughout this chapter, we have focused on the impact that physical activity has on overall health and wellbeing. Understanding basic exercise strategies as well as mastering the skills of engagement leading to sustainable action will contribute to promote health and wellbeing in various patient populations. Yet promoting exercise in others does not satisfy the call to integrative nursing. Integrative nurses should also be concerned about weaving a lifetime of physical activity and movement into their own lives as they travel their own path towards bodymindspirit wellbeing and flourishing.

SELECTED REFERENCES

American College of Sports Medicine. (2010). *ACSM Guidelines for Exercise Testing and Prescription*. 8th ed. Philadelphia, PA: Lippincott Williams & Wilkins.

Durstine, J., Moore, G., Painter, P., & Roberts, S. (2009). *ACSM's Exercise Management for Persons with Chronic Diseases and Disabilities*. American College of Sports Medicine.

Hacker, E. (2009). Exercise and the quality of life: Strengthening the connections. *Clinical Journal of Oncology Nursing, 3*(1), 32–39.

Jonas, S., & Phillips, E. M. (eds.) (2009). American College of Sports Medicine. *Exercise Is Medicine™: A Clinician's Guide to Exercise Prescription*. Philadelphia, PA: Lippincott Williams & Wilkins.

Murphy, M., Blair, S., & Murtagh, S. (2009). Accumulated versus continuous exercise for health benefit: A review of empirical studies. *Sports Medicine, 39*(1), 29–43.

Powers, S., & Howley, E. (2009). *Exercise Physiology: Theory and Application to Fitness and Performance*. New York: McGraw-Hill.

Prochaska, J. O., & DiClemente, C. C. (1984). *The Transtheoretical Approach: Crossing the Traditional Boundaries of Therapy*. Melbourne, FL: Krieger Publishing.

Ribisl, P. M. (2001). Exercise: The unfilled prescription. *American Journal of Medicine and Sports, 3*, 13–21.

Seaward, B. (2012). *Managing Stress: Principles and Strategies for Health and Well-being.* 7th ed. Burlington, MA: Jones & Bartlett Learning LLC.

Whaley, M., Brubaker, P., Otto, R., et al. (2006). *ACSM's Guidelines for Exercise Testing and Prescription.* Philadelphia, PA: Lippincott, Williams & Wilkins.

13

Nutrition and Integrative Nursing

LAURA SANDQUIST AND LAURIE KUBES

Florence Nightingale, the founder of modern nursing, emphasized the importance of creating a healing environment in order to "put the patient in the best possible position for nature to act upon him" (Light, 1997, p. 33). The environment of a patient not only includes the external factors such as temperature and lighting, but also the inner environment of the patient's body, including thoughts and physiology. This chapter focuses on creating an optimal healing environment for a patient's inner physiology through an integrative-nursing perspective on nutrition.

Food Is Information

Consistent with complex systems science, food can be viewed as "information" that informs the internal human web-like system, affecting the physiological processes that are constantly occurring in the body and leading to expressions of sickness or health (C. Denton, personal communication, 2011; Hyman, 2012; Koithan, Bell, Neimeyer, & Pincus, 2012; Lamb, 2010). If an individual has a poor diet, his or her internal environment is impoverished, receiving too little or improper information to fuel the many decisional pathways that occur physiologically. On the other hand, if an individual has a healthy and balanced diet that provides good information, they have within them greater potential for an optimal healing environment that promotes health and healing. Since food communicates with the body to inform all of its various functions, nutrition is central to promoting health and wellbeing (Bland, 2010). As it follows the laws of a complex system, it is unknown exactly how and to what degree the food will affect a person biologically, socially, psychologically, or spiritually. What is certain is that food can and will have affects on our wellbeing.

Food is ingested several times a day, every day. The impact of such frequent input must not be downplayed when considering the effect of food on the health of an individual. If the food (information) going into the body is poor, the functioning of the body will be less than optimal, no matter what else is altered in the external environment. While there may be a degree of compensation, eventually, with a continual influx of poor information, the negative effects will become apparent biologically, psychologically, and spiritually (Bland et al., 2004; Emmons, Bourgerie, Denton, & Kacher, 2012; Hyman, 2009; Hyman, 2012).

Biologically, intake of poor food choices creates a destructive inner environment that eventually leads to severe physiological dysfunction, including disorders such as diabetes, heart attacks, strokes, and cancers (Bland, 2010). However, before these conditions are present, nondescript and troubling symptoms are often apparent, including: fatigue, gastrointestinal issues, joint pains, skin rashes, and headaches. Warning signs such as these signal a less-than-optimal internal environment, suggesting that the information coming into the body needs to change to prevent chronic illness (Bland, 2010). Ignoring these warning signs or masking them with medications does not solve the underlying issue of poor system information causing inflammation, eventually leading to chronic disease (Hyman, 2010). Furthermore, the emerging science of epigenetics suggests that genetic expression can be altered with the input of the right nutritional information and the right environment. While a person may have genetic susceptibility to biological conditions like heart disease or cancer, these genes can actually be turned on and off with the right environment, with food being central to the creation of that right internal environment (Bland, 1999; Hyman, 2012; Jones & Quinn, 2010).

While food most obviously nourishes the physical body, the psychological and spiritual effects of foods are equally important. Serotonin and dopamine, chemicals needed for a healthy emotional state, are both produced from nutrients in food (Emmons et al., 2012). Poor food choices, with subsequent lack of adequate nutrients, can lead to psychological symptoms like depression, anxiety, agitation, low energy, inattention, and hyperactivity (Emmons et al., 2012; Hyman, 2009). An integrative nurse considers the psychological impact of food in his or her holistic assessment. Furthermore, just as humans thrive in an environment of love and health, food that is grown with love and care is thought to express a thriving positive energy. Similarly, products from animals raised in poor conditions may express a negative energy. The integrative nurse acknowledges the importance of the energy of food and how that energy impacts the person who consumes it, not only biologically but psychologically and spiritually as well. An integrative and holistic nursing perspective on nutrition can be challenging to maintain, as many of the concepts oppose mainstream attitudes about food and call attention to several ethical concerns.

Food Ethics: In Search of Whole-Person/Whole-Systems Wellbeing

Nutrition from an integrative, holistic nursing perspective questions many of the common food and nutrition practices prevalent in American culture today. While we are fortunate to live in a time where food is abundant and cheap, the production and quality of our food is increasingly coming under scrutiny, and its role in overall human and planetary wellbeing questioned.

The production of genetically modified organisms (GMOs) is a science that has been used to modify foods by altering their DNA through the insertion of a modified gene or a gene from another organism using the techniques of genetic engineering. The United States is the top producer of genetically modified (GM) crops, which include canola, corn, soybeans, and cotton (Rosenthal, 2008). It is estimated that 70% of the foods in grocery stores in the United States and Canada contain GMOs (Rosenthal, 2008). According to reports from the Union of Concerned Scientists, food safety experts have identified several potential problems with GMOs, including introducing toxins or allergens into previously safe foods and increasing toxins to dangerous levels (Rosenthal, 2008). Altering the information found in food raises the logical question of how doing so affects the health of the human body, which depends on high-quality information from that very food to inform its function. Interestingly, GMOs do not require labeling in the United States, although foods labeled "organic" cannot be GM (Rosenthal, 2008). With the increasing consumer knowledge regarding the way food is being produced and the effects of mass production on our health, organic food sales have increased by nearly 20% since 1990 (Winter & Davis, 2006). Though not yet widely accepted as necessary for improving nutritional quality of foods, surveys indicate that American consumers purchase organic foods due to the perceived benefits to nutrition and health (Winter & Davis, 2006). This rise in consumer interest in organic products, often despite a higher product cost, may reveal a shift back toward foods grown as nature intended them to be: whole, non-processed, without GMOs, and full of healthy nutrients.

Additionally, food production practices such as refinement, chemical additives, and the use of antibiotics decrease the quality of foods available today. Foremost on the list of foods that cause symptoms and promote illness are refined sugars, the two main culprits being sucrose and high-fructose corn syrup (Gaby, 2011). Excessive consumption of these refined sugars has been linked to rising rates of obesity, type 2 diabetes, hypertension, heart disease, fatigue, and depression, among other diseases (Gaby, 2011). More than 2,700 chemicals are now being added to our foods intentionally, including additives in food categories such as bleaching, buffering, coloring, flavoring, preservatives, sweeteners, and stabilizers (Gaby, 2011). Furthermore, the routine feeding of antibiotics to animals poses a threat to human health, given that laboratory findings of antibiotics in the meat we eat is thought to contribute to the rise in antibiotic-resistant bacteria (Gaby, 2011).

In his ground-breaking work *Food Rules*, Pollan (2009) describes how the diets of the animals we eat affect the nutritional quality of the food they produce, noting that food such as meat, milk, or eggs from animals with access to green grass contains healthier fats and higher amounts of vitamins and antioxidants. Additionally, Pollan emphasizes the emerging research findings that food grown in soils rich in organic matter and without chemical fertilizers have higher levels of antioxidants, flavonoids, vitamins, and minerals, and have little or no residue from synthetic pesticides or pharmaceuticals. With increasing evidence in this area, buying organically grown, local produce whenever possible is proposed as one of the best ways to ensure that one ingests wholesome, nutrient-rich products (Hyman, 2012; Gaby, 2011).

Locally grown organic food also promotes a connectedness to the earth and nourishes not only the body physically, emotionally, and spiritually, but the local community and surrounding environment as well. Nature provides certain foods at a specific times of the year in certain regions for specific reasons. Often, these foods provide the information necessary to prepare the body for a change in season and to optimize function in that climate (Rosenthal, 2008). Not only does this method provide the nutrition for the body that nature intended, but it also supports the local economy and farmers who choose to take the more complicated path to providing organic foods. The rise and growth of Community Supported Agriculture (CSA) operations promotes the consumption of locally grown foods and offers an example of collective wellbeing. In this model, all members of the community benefit, both human and non-human. The inherent risk of farming is shared between farmer and community: individual membership fees cover farmers' costs and wages, members enjoy readily available, seasonal, local products, and farmers have guaranteed markets for their goods, creating more time for them to nurture the land and tend to animals and crops with careful attention (Tegtmeier & Duffy, 2005).

Overall, an integrative nursing nutrition perspective takes into account the origin of food as well as the process that brought the food to the table, including the effects of food production on the environment and the use of sustainable farming methods. An integrative nurse can assist people in making positive choices when obtaining food and advocate that these choices be easily accessible and affordable to populations of all socioeconomic classes and locations. Integrative nutrition from a nursing perspective calls for a new cultural attitude about food that emphasizes relationships; relationships between the people and food, the people who share the food, and the people who create and eat the food. The entire experience of food can be pleasurable physically, mentally, socially, and spiritually when people become conscious of and connected to their food choices. Good food makes people smile, can change their physical health, and brings joy and sweetness to life in a mindful way. Therefore, food choice cannot be ignored when addressing individual and societal health and disease concerns.

Food as Cause of Inflammation and Disease

Nature designed whole foods to deliver perfect nutrition; however, current food production practices greatly disrupt this design. The addition of chemicals, along with refining, processing, and genetic modification, removes many of the core nutrients, resulting in poor-quality foods that no longer communicate and provide for the body in the same way as foods occurring in their natural state (Emmons et al., 2012). When poor-quality foods are consistently ingested and the body cannot interpret the information from these foods, immune barriers are weakened over time, and the immune system may begin to attack the food as a threatening invader (Kharrazian, 2010). When the immune system becomes overstimulated and out of balance from reacting to inappropriate stimuli (like poor-quality food), misdirected inflammation occurs (Kharrazian, 2010). Inflammation, combined with compromised immune barriers, leads to a wide array of symptoms including various presentations of pain, digestive issues, mood problems, and skin eruptions (Roundtree, 2010). Persistent ingestion of foods that cause inflammatory reactions perpetuates disease and is destructive to wellbeing (Roundtree, 2010). For any health condition, decreasing inflammation in the body through identification and elimination of poor-quality food and the resulting food intolerances and allergies will help correct the underlying dysfunction: inflammation (Roundtree, 2010).

The integrative nurse always considers the possibility of food allergies and intolerances when evaluating nutritional status. A true food allergy is the immediate, anaphylactic response to a food. A food intolerance is a reaction that occurs over hours to days, with symptoms that are chronic, fluctuating, low-grade, and do not produce an anaphylactic immune response (Gaby, 2011; Manahan, 2003). Food intolerances often develop with excessive and prolonged exposure to food that creates an immune response (Manahan, 2003). Environmental pollutants, along with poor-quality food containing additives and genetic modification, contribute to the increasing number of food allergies and sensitivities (Gaby, 2011). A simple way to test for food intolerance is by following an elimination diet, in which the potential culprit foods are removed from the diet for at least two weeks and then slowly added back in one at a time every three days while monitoring for reactions (Denton, 2012). Another way to detect food sensitivities is to have a blood test by a healthcare provider familiar with diagnosing food sensitivities (Gaby, 2011; Manahan, 2003). Either way, individual food allergies and intolerances should always be considered when discussing nutrition from an integrative nursing perspective. Referral to a holistic healthcare provider or nutritionist who routinely works with food intolerances may be appropriate, because they can be very difficult to pinpoint (Denton, 2012). Food intolerances are a common cause of physical, mental, and behavioral symptoms and diseases due to the immune response and resulting inflammation; failing to recognize food intolerances can lead to distressing symptoms and further disease (Kharrazian, 2010). It is crucial to address the potential for food intolerances when applying an integrative-nursing nutrition perspective (Gaby, 2011).

Food as Medicine

Just as poor-quality foods can instigate disease, high-quality foods can be used as medicine. Foods from nature provide the body with the right information to function properly and prevent inflammation and autoimmune reactivity by triggering proper enzymatic reactions, providing the correct nutrients, and getting rid of toxic free radicals (Gaby, 2011). Whole, real, fresh food that is cooked at home and ingested regularly is the most potent medicine for wellbeing (Hyman, 2012). Integrative nurses focus on using nutrition to address the cause of disease by optimizing the innate and intelligent physiological reactions within the body. Proper nutrition must be included in the treatment plan for any symptom or disease. As the first and most important prevention strategy, nutrition should also be optimized in individuals who are considered to be "healthy" and without symptoms in order to maximize their wellness potential and promote health. Unfortunately, many biomedical providers, including nurses, are poorly informed about nutrition and lack an effective approach for promoting optimal nutrition. Furthermore, a survey assessing nutrition training in U.S. medical schools revealed only 30% of medical schools required a nutrition course, and that, on average, medical students receive fewer than 25 hours of nutrition instruction throughout medical school training (Adams, Lindell, Kohlmeier, & Zeisel, 2006). This is unfortunate, considering that scientific research and clinical experience have shown that nutritional modifications and therapies are frequently effective for preventing and treating a wide variety of symptoms and illnesses without serious side effects (Gaby, 2011). Often, patients who are given a nutritional program to follow actually report a positive side-effect profile, including more energy, a better mood, fewer cravings, increased mental concentration, and fewer aches and pains (Gaby, 2011). Interestingly, in a drastic contrast with biomedicine, most traditional healing systems incorporate a strong foundation of nutrition in their philosophies.

Food choices are the primary considerations in the treatment plans of traditional medicine systems. Indian Ayurveda believes that one's *Rasa*, or "plasma," contains all nutrients from digested food, which in turn nourishes all the body's tissues, organs, and systems (Lad, 1984). If imbalance occurs, dietary adjustments are first-line treatments aimed at restoring balance and health. Traditional Chinese medicine (TCM) proposes that the human body consists of the five elements of metal, earth, wood, water, and fire, and when these elements are out of balance, disease results (Potenza & Mechanick, 2009). The use of food therapy and natural herbs in TCM is a mainstay of treatment aimed at realigning the elements, thereby treating disease. Bitter melon is one example of a popular herb that has been used by practitioners of TCM for more than 600 years to treat various disease states, including type 2 diabetes (Potenza & Mechanick, 2009). As a rule, the current biomedical approach to healthcare does not include nutrition prescriptions as a first-line treatment. Instead, clinical guidelines focus on medication and/or surgical treatment protocols to address disease- or symptom-management

(Jones, Bland, & Quinn, 2010). Utilizing food as a means of addressing underlying physiological imbalances, thus eliminating the serious side effects of pharmaceuticals, offers a model of care with great potential and little risk (Gaby, 2011).

Intelligent Nutrition

Integrative nursing assumes that the body can be healed if placed in the proper environment; thus, integrative nursing assumes that the body is intelligently designed and has the innate capacity to heal itself if given the proper environment. It can also be assumed that things that exist naturally in the environment are also intelligently designed. Therefore, it would be reasonable and logical to believe that naturally occurring foods were intended to be paired or ingested with the intelligently designed human body. Unfortunately, as discussed earlier, many of the foods found in grocery stores in this modern age of convenience are full of added chemicals, processed, genetically modified, and refined, providing poor information for the human body (Hyman, 2012). As integrative nutrition from a nursing perspective is explored, intelligent nutrition emerges as the underlying theme for making healthy food choices.

A "post-modern" approach to eating intelligently goes back to the wisdom of our ancestors who lived from the land. They certainly did not focus on counting calories and recommended daily allowances (RDAs). Instead, they learned to listen to and trust their own bodies and instincts, which told them to eat foods found in nature, in their natural form. They also ate food that was local, in season, and grown naturally (Rosenthal, 2008). Their food was intelligently designed to inform their bodies how to function optimally. There were no additives, genetic modification, or processing. Intelligent nutrition is about rethinking how and what we eat and going back to what is natural and simple.

Nutrition is a complicated and frustrating topic for both the providers who lack holistic nutrition knowledge and patients seeking counsel on what to eat. Patients are confused due to contradicting recommendations found online and in thousands of drastically varying diet plans (Hyman, 2010). The wise integrative nurse will begin by focusing on recommending the ingestion of foods that were intelligently designed (occur in nature) and the avoidance of those that have been manipulated, processed, or genetically modified. The focus does not need to be on counting calories but rather on nutrient-rich foods full of good information because the quality of food matters more than the quantity eaten (Hyman, 2012). While dietary recommendations should be individualized, there are basic principles that can be applied broadly. In general, consumption of a variety of whole, unprocessed foods that are free of additives and grown without the use of pesticides, herbicides, and other toxic agricultural chemicals is recommended (Gaby, 2011). This approach is very similar to the well-known Mediterranean diet and includes an abundance of plant foods such as vegetables, fruits, nuts, and seeds along with healthy fats such as extra-virgin olive oil, olives, avocados, omega-3 fats, and modest amounts of lean animal protein (Hyman, 2012). To summarize simply, Michael Pollan (2009, p. 1) states it best: "Eat food. Not too much. Mostly plants."

Vegetables and fruits are the most important of the intelligently designed foods because they contain copious amounts of vitamins, minerals, carotenoids, phytochemicals, and fiber, which are anti-inflammatory and provide important information to the body for functioning (Gaby, 2011). Additionally, they are alkaline, which balances the pH level of the body (Hyman, 2010). Trending toward acidity (low pH) results in increased inflammation and disease, while a body that trends toward an alkaline state (higher pH) will support a balanced immune system and decreased inflammation (Hyman, 2010). The "standard American diet" (SAD) of fried and processed foods causes the body to be more acidic; fruits and vegetables are part of the antidote (Hyman, 2010). An important note here is that while corn and potatoes are often staple vegetables of the American diet, the focus should shift from eating these to eating a variety of green and colorful vegetables (Hyman, 2012). Shifts like these away from common cultural norms can be difficult, especially when they challenge established eating patterns and habits.

The integrative nurse understands that people are at different levels of readiness when striving to make intelligent nutrition choices. Some patients may need to begin with one step, such as eliminating sugared drinks from their diet. Once that is mastered, a second step can be identified and tackled. Whatever the individual circumstances, the patients should be met where they are at and encouraged and guided as they lead the way at their own pace. Changing years of eating habits and creating lasting lifestyle change does not happen overnight and can be overwhelming. The ultimate goal is not to "arrive" at perfect nutrition, but to continue to learn and grow toward making healthy choices. With the integrative nurse as an advocate and guide, the patient can arrive at his or her own individualized plan for intelligent nutrition.

Unique Body: Unique Nutrition

A general principle understood across all integrative disciplines is that every patient must be considered as an individual. Effective nutritional treatment will vary from person to person, based on individual needs. For instance, the symptom of fatigue for one person may be best addressed by decreasing the consumption of refined sugars in order to decrease high post-prandial blood sugars, while another person may require B_{12} replacement to correct a deficiency. While the basic principle of eating a variety of good foods from nature remains the same for all, physiologies, lifestyles, experiences, and preferences vary widely, decreasing the effectiveness of one generic diet or food guideline as an option for society as a whole. Discussing changes in nutrition from a holistic perspective requires consideration of the physical, social, mental, and emotional factors that contribute to why and how a person eats. It is a complex and gentle art to coach an individual through this complicated maze to discover his or her own nutritional plan.

TELLING VERSUS COACHING

Conversations about changing behavior are difficult. Lack of motivation is often viewed as an obstacle to change that cannot be overcome (Rollnick, Miller, & Butler, 2008). Motivational interviewing in the form of coaching can uncover the reason behind the lack of motivation, allowing one to move forward toward lasting change. Motivational interviewing (MI) involves deep listening, identifying the person's true motivation for change, and empowering that individual toward change (Rollnick et al., 2008). Through the use of these principles, the patient is able to identify what it will mean to have a better level of nutrition, which goes deeper than a goal of losing weight or getting rid of bothersome symptoms. Identified reasons may include being able to stay alive longer to watch their grandchildren grow, or to resume a hobby. If there isn't a clear, deep reason motivating the change, the likelihood of its lasting declines sharply. Another powerful coaching principle to internalize is that the patient must identify and verbalize their own reasons and methods regarding how they will follow through on a nutritional plan. "We tend to believe what we hear ourselves say," is a potent statement toward facilitating lasting behavior change (Rollnick et al., 2008, p. 8). Individuals will come to a place of change through the integrative nurse listening and asking questions that guide them to come up with their own solutions and ideas. Realizing that just telling an individual which nutritional changes to make does not facilitate change is the first step in promoting lasting lifestyle change.

LIFESTYLE CHANGE

When it comes to nutrition, "diet" is a term that is better left out of the discussion when helping patients optimize what they eat. Diets are temporary solutions, while a lifestyle change is lasting and more likely to be effective. Most diets deprive people of food, making them feel hungry, dissatisfied, and irritable. On the other hand, a lifestyle change focuses on all of the delicious and satisfying foods that CAN be eaten. Fortunately, once people begin to try new foods and consistently eat natural and nutritious foods, they will crave even more of these high-quality foods and discover new things they never tried before when stuck in their old nutrition routine. Overall, the change has to be sustainable for the individual and fit in with their lifestyle in order to withstand the test of time and provide optimal health benefits.

THE RULE OF 90/10

When it comes to making sustainable nutritional modifications, the tendency to "give up" when one is not perfect can be overwhelming. Rosenthal (2008) proposed a 90/10 approach, where 90% of the time you choose foods that are good for you, and 10% of the time you eat whatever you feel like eating. Rosenthal explains that having fear and guilt about eating is unhealthy and results in failure. Using a 90/10 approach, the "all or nothing" attitude is eliminated, allowing for flexible options 10% of the time. When a poor food choice is made, the integrative nurse encourages the patient to acknowledge the situation, learn from it, and continue to move forward. Allowing for human error from time to time assists in keeping the majority of nutrition choices positive and assists with fear and guilt elimination. To further a positive mental experience when making nutritional changes, the principles of mindful eating can be added to the 90/10 rule.

MINDFUL EATING

The principle of mindful eating empowers people to trust themselves with food choices by becoming aware of which foods make them feel well and energized and paying attention to the foods that do not. Jon Kabat-Zinn (1990) describes the core of mindfulness practice as "knowing what you are doing while you are doing it." Many people have become accustomed to eating a certain way but have never paid attention to what they are eating and how it makes them feel physically and emotionally. In the fast-paced, high-stress American culture, most food is eaten on the run or while multitasking. Changing this pattern of behavior and our relationship to food is a challenge. The integrative nurse can assist individuals in becoming more aware of their automatic behaviors surrounding their eating, thoughts, and feelings about food and the many social customs linked to how, why, and what they eat through exploring the art of mindfulness in relation to food (Kabat-Zinn, 1990). Mindful eating assists us in acknowledging that food affects us physically, mentally, emotionally, and spiritually, by encouraging us to slow down and pay attention to what we're eating and how it makes us feel.

Summary

The most important thing an integrative nurse can do when addressing nutrition is empower patients to optimize their wellbeing through food choices. Emphasizing the importance of personal power over food choices and the potential effects on health is critical. Patients need to be aware that there isn't a pill to fix poor food choices, and that they hold the key to unlocking lasting behavior change. Maximizing wellness through nutrition is completely dependent upon the patient's individual motivation and commitment. If the motivation is not present, identifying a deeper reason for wanting to change that aligns with the patient's values can assist in personal transformation. Acknowledging how challenging it is to make nutritional change while promoting patient self-awareness and providing ongoing encouragement is central to an integrative nursing nutrition approach. Finally, integrative nurses must care for themselves and serve as examples by providing their own body with optimal healing information from wholesome, natural foods that make their hearts sing the praises of eating intelligently for wholeness and wellbeing.

SELECTED REFERENCES

Bland, J. S. (2010). Environmental inputs. In D. S. Jones (ed.), *Textbook of Functional Medicine* (pp. 123–128). Gig Harbor, WA: Institute of Functional Medicine.

Emmons, H., Bourgerie, S., Denton, C., & Kacher, S. (2012). *The Chemistry of Joy Workbook.* Oakland, CA: New Harbinger Publications.

Gaby, A. R. (2011). *Nutritional Medicine.* Concord, NH: Fritz Perlberg Publishing.

Hyman, M. (2010). Clinical approaches to environmental inputs. In D. S. Jones (ed.), *Textbook of Functional Medicine* (pp. 347–387). Gig Harbor, WA: Institute of Functional Medicine.

Hyman, M. (2012). *The Blood Sugar Solution.* New York: Little, Brown and Company.

Koithan, M., Bell, I. R., Niemeyer, K., & Pincus, D. (2012). A complex systems science perspective for whole systems of complementary and alternative medicine research. *Forschende Komplementarmedizin, 19*(suppl 1), 7–14. doi:0.1159/000335181

Lamb, J. J. (2010). Homeostasis: A dynamic balance. In D. S. Jones (ed.), *Textbook of Functional Medicine* (pp. 93–96). Gig Harbor, WA: Institute of Functional Medicine.

Pollan, M. (2009). *Food Rules: An Eater's Manual.* New York: Penguin Group.

Rosenthal, J. (2008). *Integrative Nutrition.* New York: Integrative Nutrition Publishing.

Roundtree, R. (2010). Immune imbalances and inflammation. In D. S. Jones (ed.), *Textbook of Functional Medicine* (pp. 299–326). Gig Harbor, WA: Institute of Functional Medicine.

14

Health Coaching: A Partnership on the Journey to Wellbeing

JANE ANDERSON

Wellbeing is supported by health, purpose, and body, mind, and spirit balance. A healthy lifestyle has physical, psychological, emotional, and spiritual dimensions, all part of the dynamic of being human. For those who struggle with a health issue, or just want to learn to take care of any part of their health, this could be intimidating and overwhelming. A professional partner can facilitate this health journey and accompany you on the path. Health coaching is one such partnership.

Two-thirds of healthcare costs are driven by our daily choices (Institute of Medicine, 2006). Yet, understanding, adopting, and sustaining a healthy lifestyle can be a complex endeavor. Furthermore, behavior change is difficult to contemplate and just as hard to initiate and maintain. Doing this on your own can be difficult, given that no single approach is clinically adequate for all issues and situations (Prochaska, 1994). Therefore, professionals equipped with various methods that support behavioral change can create dynamic partnerships to move a person toward a satisfying and healthy lifestyle (Duke Integrative Medicine, 2013).

It is more difficult to change behavior and attitudes when the focus is placed on what is wrong and what is not working, rather than on what is going well. Health coaching is an effective process that facilitates disease prevention and health management because it focuses on a person's unique strengths and life experience. Health coaching is a new, evolving professional role wherein the coach and the client partner to meet the needs of people actively seeking to improve their wellbeing in the midst of complex and often confusing healthcare options (Center for Spirituality and Healing, University of Minnesota [CSpH/UM], 2013).

Within that relationship, the health coach presumes that the person is intrinsically healthy, whole, wise, and the ultimate expert in his or her healing journey (CSpH/UM, 2013). Moore and Tschannen-Moran (2010) further define health coaching as a way of being that creates an environment through conversation, which facilitates the process by which a person can move toward desired goals in a fulfilling manner. "Health coaching is a vehicle that assists people seeking to attain a higher level of both physical and mental wellbeing" (p. 3). Thus, this process is evolutionary and client-centered; the client fully participates as the director of his or her treatment process. The coach's role is as facilitator and guide, assisting the client to achieve his or her goals.

Health coaches assume that a person is not ill or faulty in any way, regardless of the way that other healthcare disciplines might view them. Coaches co-participate with the person using an active, collegial, and balanced relationship. Through discovery, the coach and client build a path toward health, although accountability and responsibility for outcomes rests with the client. The process uses goals created by the client as the framework for success.

Self-exploration and healing transformation occur with attendant acquisition of new knowledge, skills, and attitudes. A personalized health plan focused on balance and personal growth, as well as physical, emotional, and spiritual issues, guides the interactive process during which tools and self-care practice are developed. When clients, often vulnerable and with complex health-related issues, face our current fragmented healthcare system, a health coach can play an integral role by supporting and understanding the client's unique healthcare needs and desires. Coaches can help clients understand the system and the meaning and implications of the various treatment recommendations.

Health coaches are members of the integrated healthcare team, supporting the client in a collaborative, interprofessional, and co-created environment. Although health coaches can provide a separate service and support system, they often will work with a client and other care providers to facilitate and support communication within the interprofessional team, communicating unique needs and helping to empower the client to make decisions that are critical to achieving long-term health and wellbeing.

Health coaching is particularly popular among organizations and employers as an approach to fostering employee heath; to promote the health, efficiency, and productivity of the individual as well as the corporate entity; and to curtail soaring healthcare costs. Insurance-based programs and employee health-coaching programs support weight loss, exercise, smoking cessation, lifestyle interventions, and stress-management strategies.

Coaching: Defining the Scope of Practice

Health coaching, and the integrative nurse's role in this specialty arena, is an emerging practice discipline. Credentialing and certification, the processes that non-governmental authorities use to grant recognition to an individual who has met specified qualifications and competencies in a defined area of practice, are currently being defined and promulgated through various institutions and healthcare organizations (American Holistic Nurses Certification Corporation, 2012).

The National Consortium for Credentialing Health and Wellness Coaches (NCCHWC) is a group of 75 participating organizations and individuals founded in 2009. Their vision is to "transform the health care system in America by integrating health and wellness coaches; addressing health issues with a whole-person orientation; focusing on prevention and wellness; and facilitating personal engagement and empowerment for all ages, levels of socioeconomic status, and cultures" (NCCHWC, 2013). They are currently working to (a) develop standards for the new role of professional coaches in health and wellness; (b) support the integration of basic coaching core competencies into professional practice; and (c) advance research in health and wellness coaching (NCCHWC, 2013). This interprofessional organization of health coaches identifies values and beliefs consistent with the principles of integrative nursing and integrative approaches to healthcare, including a commitment to self-care, empowerment, patient-centeredness, and reflective practice.

TYPES OF COACHING

Health coaches join a lengthy list of coaching specialties. The International Coach Federation (ICF) defines coaching as:

> partnering with individuals in a thought-provoking and creative process that inspires them to maximize their personal and professional potential. Professional coaches provide an ongoing partnership designed to help clients produce fulfilling results in their personal and professional lives. Coaches help people improve their performance and enhance the quality of their lives. Coaches are trained to listen, to observe and to customize their approach to individual needs. The coach's job is to provide support to enhance the skills, resources, and creativity that the client already has. (2012, p. 1)

The International Coaching Community (ICC) identifies several types of coaching (Table 14.1).

The IFC offers credentialing in three areas of coaching: (a) the Associate Certified Coach (ACC), which requires IFC-accredited training and 100 hours of coaching experience; (b) the Professional Certified Coach (PCC), requiring ICF-accredited training and 750 hours of experience; and (c) the Master Certified Coach (MCC), which requires ICF-accredited training and 2,500 hours of coaching experience (www.coachfederation.org). The ICF's rigorous credentialing process demonstrates the coach's commitment to attaining the knowledge, skills, and abilities as set forth in practice standards and applied in the clinical environment. There is currently no legal requirement for certification or credentialing for a health coach to practice, yet there are competencies, standards, and credentialing that will be further defined in subsequent parts of this chapter.

Table 14.1: Types of Coaches

Executive Coach	Coaching for top-level management to improve strategic decision-making and leadership.
Business Coach	Coaching people to work on professional issues, often working with managers inside a company, may also coach teams within a business.
Team Coach	Coaching business teams, to help teams to give their best, helping them to work smoothly and effectively.
Life Coach	Coaching that deals with the client's life in all its dimensions—personal and professional, health and relationships.
Career Coach	Coaching that specializes in helping a client find a job, change careers, or get back into the job market after a break from work.
Sports Coach	A coach who knows the game, motivates the player and builds their skills in their chosen sport.

Source: International Coaching Community. (2013). What are the different types of coaching? Available at: www.internationalcoachingcommunity.com/en/faq-what-is-coaching. Accessed April 10, 2013.

Professional Nurse Coaching

"Nurse coaching is a role that speaks to the heart of nursing... It's about interactions with clients in a skilled, purposeful and results-oriented way. This structured, relationship-centered approach by registered nurses promotes achievement of client goals" (Dossey, 2012). A professional nurse coach is defined as a registered nurse who integrates coaching competencies into any setting or specialty area of practice to facilitate a process of change or development that assists individuals or groups to realize their potential (Hess et al., 2013). Identifying the American Nurses Association's (ANA) Scope and Standards for Nursing Practice as a framework for professional nurse coaching practice, Hess et al. (2013) identify eighty-nine nurse coach competency statements, further defining the relationship between the practice of professional nursing and the role of the specialty nurse coach.

Trust is an essential element in establishing the coaching relationship that supports the healing process. Annually, polls place nurses as one of the most trusted professions; nurses are considered to be honest, ethical, and the most trusted professionals (Gallup, 2012). "People connect with nurses and trust them to do the right thing" (Daley, 2012, p. 1). Relationship-centered care is another key element to coaching success, a perfect fit with professional nursing's commitment to placing the patient at the center of healthcare services. Nurse coaches use behavioral-based coaching to help clients make informed choices and take ownership of their health, while receiving healthcare support. Professional nursing education addresses patient education, decision-making, choice, and health promotion.

Nurses have the ability to perform the role of the nurse coach within their current scope of practice, using skills they have acquired through their educational process, and they are perfectly placed to assume this role in a transformed healthcare environment

(Hess et al. 2013). A nurse learns from the very beginning of his or her education and training to view each individual at any age from a holistic or integrative perspective, seeing a person as "bodymindspirit." Nurses are also educated about evidence-based or evidence-informed practice. Evidenced-based coaching with industry best practice is more powerful, more accurate, more efficacious, and safer.

Therefore, nurses already use coaching skills across the varied settings within which they currently work as they counsel patients and promote health and wellbeing. However, nurses who intend to perform the role of an independent nurse coach outside typical employment in organizations or institutions would benefit from additional specialty education that is offered through certificate or advanced-practice education programs. These programs provide additional knowledge and skills that support the nurse coach in independent practice, leadership, and other areas not typically offered in traditional registered nurse curricula.

PROFESSIONAL COACHING COMPETENCIES

Coaching in all its forms shares key values, including listening, presence of the coach, remaining present and/or future-focused, holding the client in the highest regard, and helping the client process his or her own skills. Coaching core competencies are well defined; the American Holistic Nurses Credentialing Corporation (AHNCC) recently developed Nurse Coach competencies, which align with these traditional coaching values as well as the values and competencies of professional nursing (Table 14.2).

These competency statements emphasize the differences between coaching and other types of therapy and counseling. Health coaching is not psychological therapy; traditional psychotherapy deals with the impact of past events on a person's wellbeing. A therapist is trained to elicit that information and help the client understand how assigned meanings influence current health challenges and opportunities. Therapy may focus on pathology and diagnoses, established using the Diagnostic and Statistical Manual of Mental Disorders IV (DSM IV), and recommend a directive treatment plan. In contrast, the coaching relationship develops a co-created partnership focused on specific goals to improve lifestyle or attain goals associated with resilience, healing, and wellbeing.

While a person's past certainly provides a context within which anyone approaches a change in health behaviors, the coach does not interpret the meaning of this experience or provide counseling to change a person's interpretation or perspective of it. Rather, the coach actively listens to the person, aware that past experiences are part of everyone's current experience, and will encourage the client to identify how the past may inform the present. However, the coach does not delve into that impact, choosing instead to focus on the present with forward thinking, supporting movement in

Table 14.2: ICF Coach and Nurse Coach Competencies

ICF Core Competencies	Nurse Coach Core Competencies
Meeting the ethical guidelines and professional standards	Understands and effectively discusses with the client the ethical guidelines and specific parameters of the nurse coaching relationship
Establishing the coaching agreement	Co-creates with the client an agreement that identifies the role of the nurse coach and the role of the client
Establishing trust and intimacy with the client	Co-creates a relationship between the nurse coach and client that promotes trust and intimacy
Coaching presence	Becomes fully present to self and client prior to collecting data pertinent to the coaching interaction
Active listening	Clarifies the client's issues and concerns and/or opportunities for change based on a whole person assessment, confirms the client's issues and/or opportunities with client
Powerful questioning	Explores through powerful questions and feedback, multiple sources of information to assist the client to become aware of areas for coaching
Direct communication	Clarifies the client's issues and concerns and/or opportunities for change based on a whole-person assessment, confirms the client's issues and/or opportunities with client
Creating awareness	Facilitates the client's process of self-discovery related to establishment of the client's goals
Designing actions	Assists the client to identify strategies to attain goals
Planning and goal setting	Determines the need for, and refers to, other professionals and services as appropriate. Creates with the client an action plan with clearly defined steps and anticipated results, explores obstacles and responses to obstacles
Managing progress and accountability	Adjusts plan as desired by client

Sources: International Coach Federation. (2012). ICF Core Competencies. Available at: http://www.coachfederation.org/icfcredentials/core-competencies/. Last accessed April 18, 2013.

Hess, D., Dossey, B., Southard, M. E., Luck, S., Gulino Schaub, B., & Bark, L. The Art and Science of Nurse Coaching. Silver Springs, MD: Nursebooks/ANA. 2013.

the client. Furthermore, health coaches do not diagnose clinical dysfunction, although they may work collaboratively with or refer to a counselor or psychologist when necessary.

Consider the following case. A client comes into your coaching practice, experiencing difficulty losing weight. He has not discussed or processed this with anyone. During your sessions, you identify, through listening and clarifying, that this person has also recently gone through a divorce and was in an emotionally abusive marriage for fifteen years. You immediately recognize that this is a multifactorial issue, acknowledging that stress plays a part in this weight problem and that this need could be addressed through an integrative health coaching session. Yet, you also know that there could be other core concerns contributing to weight gain and stress; concerns that a therapist trained in grief, loss, and relationships could better address. While you agree to see this man to facilitate development of his skills in stress reduction, you also refer him to a therapist/counselor whom you will work with collaboratively to address his needs.

Coaching is not "mentoring." Mentoring is focused on succession training wherein an older or wiser mentor offers answers for the less experienced person. A mentor may show a new employee or student the culture and rules of a new workplace or school. The relationship has a power differential (expert to novice), although friendships often develop during the mentoring process. In contrast, a coach co-creates a plan for change with a person who already possesses the knowledge and solutions necessary to address his or her own problems, again reinforcing the core concept of coaching that the client is the expert.

There are times when coaching seems to be consistent with case management or care coordination. However, case managers/care coordinators organize services for an individual client for the purposes of directing the client's health experience, procuring and recommending vetted services or approaches to care, or navigating the complexity of the healthcare system. In some cases, care coordination is used to manage costs and improve quality outcomes. Coaching, in contrast, focuses on the coach–client relationship and attempts to move the client in a direction toward a specific goal that is revealed through personal discovery and self-identification. Goals are set in relationship, but ultimately coaching goals and therapies are determined by the client, rather than the expert provider. Consider another case. A client with a health history of long-term HIV infection, substance abuse, and poverty comes to your practice to seek support through health coaching. She tells you that she is trying to improve her overall quality of life by adopting a healthier diet, regular exercise, and greater financial stability. As a health coach, you agree to meet with her, and together you identify ways to support daily walks in a safe environment and menu plans to incorporate fruits and vegetables that she has access to. In addition, you collaborate with a case manager who can help arrange meetings to discuss increased disability payments, referrals and access to food items and food banks, safe housing, and social services.

While counselors, mentors, case managers and others may choose to become a health coach with appropriate education and credentialing, nurses are uniquely positioned to facilitate health and wellbeing using an integrative and holistic approach to coaching because of their education and focus on bodymindspirit. Nursing practice emphasizes behavior change that promotes wellbeing, while preventing disease and its complications, supporting the client to achieve his or her goals to live life more fully. Effective nurse coaches integrate their extensive knowledge of evidence-informed multiple modalities and strategies for health and healing to support their clients.

Principles and Processes Used in Health Coaching

The multiple organizations and credentialing bodies associated with health coaching may take different approaches, yet share many core philosophical concepts and guiding principles.

HEALTH COACHING PRINCIPLES

Health coaching is client-centered, assuming a whole person/whole system approach to being-knowing-doing. The coach–client relationship is a partnership that facilitates greater understanding of the client's health and wellness. This relationship, grounded in mutual respect, safety, and trust, allows the client an opportunity for vulnerability, growth, and transformation. The facilitated healthcare plan is personalized, addressing physical, mental, emotional, and spiritual issues. The coach will be self-aware, understanding his or her own life experiences and patterns and how they may impact the coaching relationship.

The "Four Pillars" support the foundation for a healthy and supportive coach–client relationship (Lawson, 2012).

Mindful presence. Mindful presence entails full attentiveness with the client during the coaching experience, sitting in an accepting and non-judgmental way. Using the skills of listening deeply, the coach practices empathy that "primes the pump," enabling an ability to hear beyond what is being spoken. The client should know and feel that you are there, that you are fully present in the moment and are not distracted by other thoughts or activities. This process can even occur on the phone, a method that many coaches use for their practice. "Presence" is known and communicated through the intention that the coach sets for each and every session. A way to prepare for this could be just a simple moment of silence, naming your intention either to yourself or to the client. Alternatively, the integrative nurse coach could engage in a meditation alone or with the client. This centers the coach and/or client and brings you into the experience and away from a busy outside world.

Authentic communication. Open, honest communication that honors and respects both the coach and the client and the relationship that is developed is an essential component of the interaction. Coaching communication begins with deep listening and awareness of body language; the coach wants to really hear what the client is saying. Curious inquiry and reflection encourages dynamic communication in which needs can be explored and understood (Lawson, 2012). A coach may ask the client, "I heard you say you feel that others don't hear you speak at work, am I hearing this correctly?" This allows clients to modify their communication if what they hear back is not what they intended to say. Silence is also a powerful communication technique that can be used very effectively to allow clients to reach deep into themselves for thoughts and words.

Self-awareness. The client and the coach are most effective when they practice self-awareness. The coach's self-awareness will allow them to practice with their authentic self, addressing any issues, biases, and strengths that may alter or inform the coach–client relationship. This is also true for the client; often a goal of coaching is to facilitate this self-understanding. A coach and/or the client could use self-reflective time, taking a walk to be silent with themselves, engaging in journaling, or meditating to facilitate awareness.

Sacred space. The client should always feel that the relationship is sacred; the space created is physically and emotionally safe and intentional, with clear boundaries. Although the coach often provides the space, the client should be encouraged to bring personal items that facilitate comfort. This space should be quiet, private, and decorated to be a healing environment (Sternberg, 2010). The space should be entered with intention, which can be created by a short centering exercise. It is imperative that this space hold what happens during a coaching session and the client trusts that what occurs stays in that space.

Personal transformation occurs during the health coaching experience. Transformation is the process whereby the client is reviewing the current concern or situation, moving through a process of change, and "arriving" on the other side. As they move along the trajectory of change, each person chooses what to carry with him and what to leave behind. This process could occur in one session, or over a period of weeks, months, or even years; each person's journey is uniquely theirs. Transformation can be uncomfortable, as it has its own time, yet the rewards of discovery, wisdom, and moving forward to create a new story are many.

HEALTH COACHING STRATEGIES

Behavior change is a key component of the coach–client relationship and a common goal associated with the coaching plan of action. Determining where a client may be in his or her process is an essential starting point. Prochaska's behavior change model, "Changing for Good," is commonly used to frame the change process. As previously discussed, key components of the model include: (a) Precontemplation–the "I won't" or "I can't" phase; (b) Contemplation—the "I might" phase; (c) Preparation—the "I will" phase; (d) Action—the "I am" phase; (e) Maintenance—the "I still am" phase; and (f) Termination—the phase when the client and coach feel that there is an end to the issue. Termination is truly a rare occurrence in a coaching environment, as most people are more likely to remain in "maintenance" throughout most of their life. There is value in each phase of this process; the coach facilitates awareness of these phases, increasing self-awareness of the client, while gently guiding and facilitating the client's movement forward.

"Nonviolent communication" (NVC), the language of empathy, is a key component of a coach's skill mix and enhances connection and honest understanding between people. This form of communication, first defined by Rosenberg (2003), supports deep, compassionate listening. "Violent communication" is easily defined as the bully who uses blame, insults, put-downs, moralistic judgment, demands, and denial of responsibility. NVC is coaching with compassion, taking responsibility for our own feelings and helping the client do the same, and sharing power in communication. When clients are honored in this way, they feel safe and often will begin to engage in this form of communication to support other relationships in their lives.

"Motivational interviewing" (MI) is a client-centered communication strategy that is used to prompt change by exploring and resolving ambivalence while activating the clients' own motivation and adherence to goals (Rollnick, 2008). The goal of MI is to encourage change talk and discourage resistance talk. There are four general principles associated with MI: (a) expressing empathy, (b) identifying discrepancy, (c) rolling with resistance, and (d) supporting self-efficacy. This is a powerful interviewing technique used not only by health coaches, but by other healthcare professionals as a way to truly understand the client's experience (Moore & Tschannen-Moran, 2010). Questions often used in MI include: (a) What would you like to see different about your current situation? (b) What will be the good things that will happen if you change this behavior? (c) What would your life look like in three years if you changed this behavior? (Sobell, 2008).

"Appreciative inquiry" (AI) is a philosophy and an approach that identifies, appreciates, and amplifies strengths, thereby supporting people to move beyond problem-solving to resolution and life change (Moore & Tschannen-Moran, 2010). Inherent in this process is valuing, esteeming, prizing, and honoring (or appreciating!) the client. Questions used in an AI approach could include: (a) Can you identify a time in your life when you felt engaged in life? (b) Tell me about a time when you felt particularly healthy. (c) What skills do you have that help you feel particularly effective in your roles as a mother/father/teacher/student? Basically, AI asks the person to think about and identify skills surrounding a positive experience, or a time when they felt particularly powerful and accomplished. AI is purposeful communication that uses positive messages to acknowledge their strengths and imagine possibilities in order for clients to rise above their problems (Moore & Tschannen-Moran, 2010).

Storytelling is a way to facilitate compassionate communication, learning about and taking in account the client's interests, curiosities, and desires, which is core to a client-centered relationship. While there are many techniques and skills that a health coach may be taught and use in a health coaching relationship with a client, authentic listening is inherent in each. Storytelling is a universal skill, an opportunity to be open to the paths that clients wish to take and the experiences that they believe to be important. It is an opportunity for appreciation of another's experiences, bringing clarity to both the client's and coach's understanding. Using reflection, repeating back to the client what is heard, strengthens understanding. "I hear you say you love walking in the woods for stress reduction, is this how it is for you?" Reframing, or saying the same thing in a new way—perhaps in a more positive light—may give the client a new lens through which to view something. "It seems your boss is short-tempered with you, and I hear you say with others as well. Could this mean that your boss is under a lot of stress and it is not your performance that is at issue here?" By listening to stories, the coach hears in a non-judgmental, respectful way and the client feels able to convey his or her feelings as well as the events that are shaping the present.

Art and other aesthetic modalities can unlock stories, meaning, and creativity in clients, helping them explore and understand themselves in new ways. Vibrant colors on paper, a collage of photos and pictures, textures, and shapes can all expand the awareness of the clients' experiences (Haltiwanger, Rojo, & Funk, 2011). Lastly, but far from the end of a long list of techniques or resources, is the enneagram. The enneagram is a powerful and dynamic personality system that describes nine distinct and fundamentally different patterns of thinking, feeling, and acting. Each of the nine patterns represents a basic proposition or belief about a person's personality or motivating force, what a person may need for survival or satisfaction in life. This system gives the client a look into how they direct their attention and use their energies to focus in the world (Daniels & Price, 2000).

Educational Opportunities

Given the current healthcare environment and the emphasis on healthy lifestyles, health promotion, and increased access to health coaches, there are increasing opportunities for education and training. Some programs are specific to interprofessional health coaching, others are specific to nursing, and still others incorporate coaching concepts and techniques into advanced degree programs. Most, but not all, of the programs require some form of healthcare background. Table 14.3 provides a variety of programs to explore, although it is not intended to be an exhaustive list of available programs.

Integrative Health Coaching Models

As the field of health coaching matures, models of practice continue to emerge. Corporate environments, such as insurance, healthcare, and large corporate structures, have incorporated health coaches into their organizations to improve employees'

Table 14.3: Educational Programs for Health Coaching

Coaching Program	Website
Bark Coaching Institute: holistic coach training for health professionals	www.barkcoaching.com
California Institute for Integral Studies: MA in Integrative Health Studies, including wellness coaching	www.ciss.edu/Academics/Graduate_Programs/Integrative_Health_Studies.html
Duke Integrative Medicine: Integrative Health Coach professional training	www.dukeintegrativemedicine.org
Integrative Nurse Coach Certificate Program (INCCP)	www.integrativenursecoach.com
National Institute of Whole Health: whole health coaching	www.wholehealtheducation.com
Tai Sophia: health and wellness coaching certificate	www.tai.edu
University of Minnesota Center for Spirituality and Healing: integrative therapies and healing practices—health coaching	www.csh.umn.edu

health and wellbeing as well as their job satisfaction and productivity. Health insurance companies provide coaching to enrollees to decrease the incidence and prevalence of chronic conditions and to increase cost savings for both the client and the company.

Both conventional healthcare environments (academic health sciences centers, community hospitals, and private practices) as well as integrative healthcare clinics are beginning to incorporate health coaching as an essential part of the client experience. Coaching is used as a complement to other services to help the client better understand his or her own health and wellness and as an opportunity to understand and integrate other healthcare modalities into a person's health journey.

Therefore, practice models that encompass the role of the employed health coach as well as the independent or consulting practitioner are being developed. In an independent practice, the coach sees clients on a one-on-one basis or perhaps in a group environment. Coaches in independent practice have many local, national, and international resources available to them to better understand the challenges and opportunities of developing their own business models.

Conclusions

Health coaching is a new and emerging field that continues to identify competencies, educational requirements, credentialing, and practice models. Yet fundamental values and beliefs, principles, and intervention strategies clearly align health coaching with an integrative approach to healthcare. Nursing as a discipline, and integrative nurses in particular, are uniquely situated to assume the role of professional health coach in a transformed healthcare environment because of our educational background, professional role and scope of practice, and inherent trust that we bring to the provider–patient relationship. Integrative nursing principles and the integrative nurse's commitment to meet the client wherever his or she is, to honor and respect their perspective, to hold their trust in sacred space, and to work collaboratively toward whole person/whole system wellbeing form the basis of integrative nurse coaching practice.

SELECTED REFERENCES

American Holistic Nurses Credentialing Corporation. (2013). Professional Nurse Coach Handbook. Available at: http://www.ahncc.org/certification/nursecoachnchwnc.html. Accessed April 10, 2013.

Hess, D., Dossey, B., Southard, M. E., Luck, S., Gulino Schaub, B., & Bark, L. (2013). *The Art and Science of Nurse Coaching.* Silver Springs, MD: American Nurses Publishing.

International Coach Federation. (2012). *ICF Core Competencies.* Available at: http://www. coachfederation.org/icfcredentials/core-competencies/. Last accessed 4/18/13.

International Coach Federation. (2012). What is a coach? Available at: http://www. coachfederation.or/clients/coaching-faqs/. Accessed October 20, 2012.

International Coaching Community. (2013). What are the different types of coaching? Available at: www.internationalcoachingcommunity.com/en/faq-what-is-coaching. Accessed April 10, 2013.

Moore, M., & Tschannen-Moran, B. (2010). *Coaching Psychology Manual.* Baltimore, MD: WellCoaches Corporation.

National Consortium for Credentialing Health Coaches. (2013). Our vision, mission and plan. Available at: www.ncchwc.org. Accessed April 10, 2013.

Prochaska, J. O., Norcross, J. C., & DiClemente, C. O. (1994). *Changing for Good.* New York: HarperCollins.

Rosenberg, M. (2003). *Nonviolent Communication: A Language of Life.* Encinitas, CA: PuddleDancer Press.

Rollnick, S., Miller, R., & Butler, C. (2008). *Motivational Interviewing in Health Care.* New York: Guilford Press.

III

Symptom Management and Integrative Nursing

15

Integrative Nursing and Symptom Management

DEBBIE RINGDAHL

Integration is the cornerstone of nursing as a discipline and practice; it guides our thinking, our actions, our relationships. (Chapter 1).

The six principles of integrative nursing described in Chapter 1 refocus the meaning of nursing practice by shaping priorities based on the dynamic and complex nature of the healing process. Ultimately, integrative nursing practice occurs through nursing actions that create outcomes of health and wellbeing and improve quality of life. In other words, integrative nursing care is holism in action, moving beyond being to knowing and doing.

The integrative nurse is mindful of the role that these fundamental principles play in sustaining health, translating and synthesizing these principles into an appropriate plan of care. In this section, integrative nursing practice with individuals will be operationalized using the six principles to manage nine common symptoms: stress, nausea, sleep disturbance, anxiety, mood disturbances, fatigue, pain, cognitive impairment, and spiritual distress. Although symptom relief is often the primary focus of nursing interventions when working with individual clients, the integrative nurse considers the whole person when developing a plan of care. In reviewing the case exemplar below, consider how the principles of integrative nursing are reflected in the nursing actions that support whole person and whole systems healing.

Operationalizing the Principles of Integrative Nursing

1. Human beings are inseparable from their environments.
2. Human beings have the innate capacity for health and wellbeing.
3. Nature has healing and restorative properties that contribute to health and wellbeing.

Case Scenario

IR, an 82-year-old Caucasian male, was admitted to the medical unit after several days of a full body rash, body aches, and low-grade fever. Several hours after admission, his condition worsened and a spinal tap confirmed a diagnosis of meningeal encephalitis. Anti-herpetic and antibiotic drug therapies were initiated. By then, IR was hallucinating, agitated, and unaware of his surroundings. The family met with the medical team (composed of primary care, infectious disease, and neurology) to discuss treatment options and decided to support a do not resuscitate (DNR) status. A diagnosis of West Nile encephalitis was confirmed the next day, and intravenous drug therapy was discontinued. After two days, IR's condition started to improve and the physicians were "cautiously optimistic" he would survive. After ten days of steady improvement, IR was transferred to a nursing home for rehabilitation and was discharged home eight weeks later with resolution of most West Nile-related problems.

Integrative Nursing Care

The hospital nursing staff used an integrative nursing approach to support the health and wellbeing of IR. They were actively engaged in managing the physiological and psychological sequelae of meningeal encephalitis while also attending to the larger healing context. Intravenous hydration was maintained, but antibiotics and anti-herpetic medications were discontinued after the West Nile encephalitis diagnosis was confirmed. Due to concern that narcotic use would produce further nervous system compromise, the medical staff prescribed neurotin, ibuprofen, and acetaminophen for pain and fever. Nursing care included ongoing assessment and treatment for his severe headache pain, body aches, dizziness, confusion, and agitation, by focusing on his comfort through timely administration of pain medications and the use of warm/cold compresses, position changes, massage therapy, and Reiki. IR was also having difficulty sleeping, eating, and drinking. They worked together with the family to discuss strategies to improve his nighttime sleep, which included frequent position changes, extra pillows, human presence, and Reiki. A small bed was moved into the room so his wife and daughter could sleep in the room at night, taking turns sitting with IR when he was agitated. The nursing staff worked with the dietician and family to provide food and beverages that were selected by the patient. As IR's condition began to improve, they collaborated with physical therapy, occupational therapy, chaplain visits, physicians, and family to support his bodymindspirit recovery through a caring and therapeutic presence, adaptive physical rehabilitation, and selected integrative therapies (Reiki and massage therapy).

4. Integrative nursing is person-centered and relationship-based.
5. Integrative nursing practice is informed by evidence and uses the full range of therapeutic modalities to support/augment the healing process, moving from least intensive/invasive to more, depending on need and context.
6. Integrative nursing focuses on the health and wellbeing of caregivers as well as those they serve.

The limitations of the biomedical model are particularly evident in this case exemplar: there is no medical treatment or "cure" for West Nile encephalitis. In spite of this, IR survived a serious illness and is on his way to regaining a high quality of life. What contributed to his health and wellbeing? Was it good nursing care, good medical care, the love and support of friends and family, or all of the above? What qualities existed in the nursing care that reflect integrative nursing? How did the nursing staff assess and care for the bodymindspirit of IR and support his health and wellbeing?

First, assessments were developed in the context of the whole person and environment. By asking the question "How is his bodymindspirit doing as a whole?" the immediate need for physical stabilization shifted to a nursing plan of care that addressed IR's needs as a biopyschosocialspiritual being. Throughout his hospital stay, IR's condition was assessed on multiple levels of organization, from his body's physiological response to encephalopathy to other environmental influences, including his physical environment and relationships with providers and family members. Stated simply, the nursing staff identified the critical role comfort and family presence played in creating a healing environment (Principle 1).

Secondly, the nurses tended to the bodymindspirit of IR by assessing his need for comfort, emotional support, and pain relief, prioritizing his care based on those needs while maintaining physiological support for his body. Nursing care included position changes, the use of warm and cold compresses, and ongoing nursing presence and therapeutic touch. By attending to and supporting all dimensions of his experience (bodymindspirit), they were assisting IR in accessing his innate capacity for health and wellbeing (Principle 2). Their plan of care also included the development of a trusting relationship with IR and his family. They demonstrated person-centered and relationship-based nursing care through their caring presence and effective communication between and among all those involved with his care (Principle 4). Lastly, they integrated a variety of therapies that further supported the healing process, moving from least to more invasive (Principle 5). In addition to the physiological interventions (e.g., IV fluids, nutritional supplementation, anti-inflammatory medications) necessary to support the neurological system, they provided Reiki and massage therapy, which are especially effective in reducing pain and anxiety.

Principle 5 is particularly salient when proposing an integrative approach to symptom management because it requires the nurse to consolidate or "integrate" a plethora of knowledge and nursing skills. Moving from least to more invasive requires an understanding of complex adaptive systems, nature as a tool for healing, and relationship-based and person-centered care (Principles 1–4), representing the critical evaluation process that occurs from moment to moment during the course of providing care. Ongoing assessment of IR's physical and psychological state guided nursing action. Without a medical treatment to "cure" the infection, nursing care was focused on supporting the healing process. The need to balance "intensive care interventions" that support and maintain the physiological system while addressing priorities of pain reduction, sleep restoration, comfort, and emotional support was paramount. Therefore, ongoing IV therapy and nutritional supplementation optimized the physiological environment for healing. To assure that neurological support was maximized, alternatives to pharmacological pain and anxiety management (massage and Reiki) were identified as more appropriate (Birocco, Guillame, Storto, Ritorto, Catino, et al., 2011; Bronfort, Nilsson, Haas, Evans, Goldsmith, Assendelft, & Bouter, 2004; Fazzino, Griffin, McNulty, & Fitzpatrick, 2010; Harris & Richards, 2010; Lee, 2008; Richeson, Spross, Lutz, & Peng, 2010; Toms, 2011).

The nursing staff also focused on the health and wellbeing of the caregivers by providing them with support and resources (Principle 6). While the family actively participated in IR's care, they were simultaneously being "cared for" by the nursing staff.

Core Competencies of Integrative Nursing

Translating the work of integrative healing and caring into tangible nursing skills, "core competencies," and measurable outcomes is challenging. Nursing, like other healthcare disciplines, uses a basic process, grounded in critical thinking and diagnostic reasoning, that assesses, identifies core strengths (resources) and areas for improvement, names problems, identifies interventions, and evaluates outcomes. Developing new models of nursing care requires new language and/or creating new definitions for old language. What kind of nursing assessment represents integrative practice? How does an integrative nurse assess each clinical problem and identify priorities? What are the "core competencies" that represent integrative nursing practice?

ASSESSMENT

Integrative nursing assessments must occur within a context, and this requires a larger and more dynamic view of health and wellbeing. Assessments generated by healthcare's biomedical model primarily focus on the cause and effect that are necessary to understand in order to diagnose and treat disease. Engel's biopsychosocial model

(1977) added the psychological and social components to this model, and complex systems science (CSS) further expands this perspective by proposing how complex adaptive systems (CAS) generate a dynamic context in which health and wellbeing reside (Koithan, Bell, Niemeyer, & Pincus, 2012). A CAS is characterized by complex information exchange and nonlinear patterns of evolution and change. This means that integrative nursing assessment must simultaneously attend to physiological systems and their interactions with the whole person. For the nurses providing care to IR in the case scenario above: what does bodymindspirit assessment look like?

Body: Central nervous system viral infection with profound neurological compromise for 82-year-old client, including severe pain and hallucinations, need for stabilization of multiple body systems and pain reduction.

Mind: Altered consciousness, limited awareness of surroundings, cognitive impairment, need for emotional support, therapeutic touch, anxiety reduction.

Spirit: Confused state, unclear connection to self and others, need for spiritual care in form best understood by IR and family.

This assessment generates a whole picture that guides nursing care priorities and selected integrative interventions. Enlarging the assessment to include bodymindspirit not only more clearly identifies each component part, it also expands "treatment" options. The dynamic nature of healing requires ongoing assessment by asking additional questions that focus on adaptation and change:

- How are these systems working with the whole person?
- Are there compensations going on?
- How is IR adapting to these system changes?
- How can nursing care best support this intrinsic healing process?
- What kind of nursing care places IR in the best place to heal?

Practicing as an integrative nurse may require abandoning some of the interview techniques supported in many healthcare settings. It can be challenging to engage in data collection without using a well-defined script, but gaining access to relevant information is not achieved by going through a checklist. The integrative nurse conducts a health assessment by presence and intention: this dynamic interaction focuses on process, not outcome. Whether practicing as an advanced practice nurse in a primary care clinic or a staff nurse working on an oncology unit, a nurse generates an integrative nursing assessment through partnership, presence, and deep listening.

Increasingly, nursing practice includes the use of assessment tools to evaluate and "grade" specific problems, such as pain, anxiety, nausea, fatigue, depression, stress, cognition, and sleep. For example, the Beck Depression Inventory may be used to evaluate risk for postpartum depression, with the resultant score guiding priorities and interventions. The symptom chapters that follow include a variety of assessment tools used to measure these symptoms and score responses to treatments. These tools serve as a starting point in collecting data about a particular problem and are easily used in conjunction with a more comprehensive approach. Assessment tools are also used to evaluate outcomes and guide clinical decision-making for integrative nursing. As noted by Quinn in Chapter 24, assessment is "inherently interconnected" with the intervention, and using a linear tool for measurement may not fully capture this dynamic process.

The decision to shift to a more intensive/invasive plan of care occurs through ongoing data collection of bodymindspirit from multiple sources, including intuitive ways of knowing. Nurses utilize multiple methods when taking in information, including those beyond the five senses. These different "ways of knowing" include verbal, auditory, tactile, and visual cues, as well as previous personal and professional experiences that offer the nurse distinctive ways of receiving and understanding information. At some point in every nurse's career, there is a moment when he or she becomes distinctly aware of a deep understanding and sense of what is happening or needed with a patient, regardless of any objective signs or symptoms. Fundamental to developing unique "ways of knowing" and intuition is for the nurse to develop an awareness of when these moments arise and learn to trust what their inner voice is saying about the patient and their needs. Nurses use all of these forms of "knowing" and data gathering interchangeably and many times do this unconsciously (Buckingham & Adams, 2000).

PRIORITY-SETTING AND PLANNING CARE

Care for each patient should consider all therapeutic modalities that support healing, starting with the least invasive. As noted in the scenario above, non-pharmacological options such as position changes, hot and cold compresses, massage, and Reiki were used to provide IR comfort and reduce his pain and anxiety. At the very same time, more invasive physiological measures (intravenous therapy and nutritional supplementation) were deemed necessary because IR was unable to take anything by mouth, and essential hydration is required for optimal healing to occur.

The least invasive modalities are those that can be safely administered and for which there is evidence supporting their effectiveness in symptom management. In the case presented, IR's age and neurological status placed him at risk for an unfavorable response to medication: anti-anxiety and sleep medications among the elderly can result in confusion, dizziness, hallucinations, and increased fall risk (Neutel, Skurtveit, & Berg, 2012) and in the neurologically compromised patient can further depress function (Scott, Gray, Martin, & Mitchell, 2012). In other cases, the use of medication may be contraindicated due to pregnancy, allergy, and/or polypharmacy risks. Safety of administration and minimal side effects of non-pharmacological therapies provide a compelling rationale for starting with the least invasive modalities with the elderly, pregnant woman, and children.

In the symptom chapters that follow, an intervention hierarchy composed of five tiers is used to guide and organize nursing actions. This format suggests how integrative nurses move from least to most invasive/intensive when managing a specific symptom. Tier one represents the least invasive interventions with minimal healthcare interactions (self-care), and tier five interventions require healthcare provider interactions and are considered the most invasive. Tiers two, three, and four are on a continuum of decreasing self-care and increasing healthcare provider involvement. Each clinical circumstance determines which tier of "engagement" is utilized by an integrative nurse. For example, dietary changes, acupressure, aromatherapy, and ginger would be recommended for a pregnant woman experiencing morning sickness (tiers 1–2), whereas a woman with hyperemesis needs pharmacological therapy and IV hydration (tier 5).

INTEGRATIVE SYMPTOM MANAGEMENT

Florence Nightingale's invitation to "put the patient in the best condition for nature to act upon him" places symptom management within the context of whole-systems healing. In fact, the purpose of nursing interventions aimed at symptom relief is to support and facilitate whole-person healing. Without first attending to the most immediate human needs, from adequate sleep to pain relief, the healing process is easily stymied. The nine common symptoms discussed in the following chapters—stress, nausea, sleep disturbance, anxiety, mood disturbances, fatigue, pain, cognitive impairment, and spiritual distress—provide opportunities to support healing on multiple levels. Altering these potential impediments to healing supports a healthy reorganization of bodymindspirit. Integrative nursing management of fatigue, for example, may initially include nutritional support in order to increase stamina, shifting to energy therapies and/or yoga to further support health, wellbeing, and spiritual growth.

The principles of integrative nursing support assessment and management of these common health problems using a range of approaches and evidence-based healing modalities. Biomedical management of symptoms frequently begins with a pharmacological intervention intended to suppress symptoms and "fix" the problem. Integrative nursing offers an alternative by shifting the focus from curing to healing. This shift also changes the nature of problem solving and prioritizing; integrative nursing practice may shift priorities to focus on anxiety reduction or pain relief rather than on performing physical tasks. This does not imply that biomedical interventions are discarded but rather that they are introduced when that level of supportive intervention is warranted. Intervention priorities are constantly realigned to best support healing; surgical and medical interventions are introduced when less invasive interventions are not effective and/or emergent conditions require a more invasive approach.

Management of physical and emotional discomfort has emerged as a focus within integrative nursing practice, with evidence that stress reduction and relaxation play a significant role in promoting overall health and wellbeing, in addition to managing specific symptoms. The relaxation response (Benson, 1975) is the physiological counterpart to the stress response, resulting in lowered blood pressure, heart rate, respiration, and muscle tension. In many ways, activities that invoke this response serve as an antidote to stress. In addition to physiological changes associated with the relaxation response, an altered state of consciousness emerges, accompanied by feelings of wellbeing and calm, which can also influence the experience of pain.

Nursing has been at the forefront of providing high-quality hands-on care that mitigates stress and promotes relaxation. Many "old" nursing skills, such as giving bed baths and back rubs, have long provided avenues for human connection, comfort, and support (Ruffin, 2011). The introduction of touch therapies into clinical practice not only adds another dimension to hands-on care but it also invites a reconceptualization of intentional touch. An enlarging body of literature supports the use of touch therapies such as stress reduction and relaxation techniques. The majority of studies focus on specific touch modalities, but there is also evidence that intentional, tactile touch intervention reduces stress indicators (Henricson, Ersson, Maatta, Segesten, & Berglund, 2008). In a study undertaken to measure the psychophysiological effects of the nonverbal communication of compassion, loving-kindness meditation and touch were associated with decreased stress and increased relaxation and peacefulness (Kemper & Shaltout, 2011). Researchers investigating the effect of gentle touch on people with mental health disorders or psychological stress found reduction in stress, anxiety, and depression and increases in relaxation and ability to cope (Weze, Leathard, Grange, Tiplady, & Stevens, 2007).

The emerging skills of an integrative nurse are not merely the "add-on" of integrative therapies, but reflect a practice philosophy that supports the integration of both old and new nursing skills into practice. Therapeutic presence, caring, and touch can be incorporated into any clinical encounter. The use of aromatherapy, Reiki, Healing Touch, guided imagery, music, and other modalities also provide avenues for connection, comfort, and support that convey presence and caring. A "caring moment" (Watson, 2008) may emerge between a nurse and client while administering chemotherapy or using guided imagery to manage pain. Integrative nursing translates into a "both/and" model of care, where any and all nursing interventions have the potential to promote healing of bodymindspirit. This increase in integrative health modalities has expanded the repertoire of treatment options; at the same time, nurses are reminded that very simple methods such as touch, comfort, and presence have therapeutic value and healing potential.

A patient experiencing anxiety before gallbladder surgery represents a culmination of a long chain of dynamic and complex events resulting in a hospitalization for a surgical intervention, the presumed endpoint, or "cure." In this case, the role of the integrative health nurse may be to engage in a myriad of whole-person interventions that promote the healing process by reducing anxiety. All interventions also add complexity to the system, bringing new information, change, and adaptation. Interventions to reduce anxiety are not just geared towards suppressing anxiety or fixing the problem, but adding more information that provides future guidance to a system in its continual search for health and wellbeing. A nursing intervention that focuses on anxiety reduction by using massage, aromatherapy, or music therapy may be the beginning point in supporting balance, providing tools for stress reduction, and encouraging self-care.

The most sustainable healthcare practices are those practiced as self-care by each individual. The anxiety of a pre-operative patient may set into motion a heightened awareness of the bodymindspirit connection and lead to a series of self-care strategies that fundamentally shift this person's health and wellbeing. Ultimately, a major goal of integrative nursing is to teach self-care. Translating integrative nursing skills into self-care practices and supporting autonomy and empowerment in the healing process are the natural consequences of integrative nursing practice. Practicing self-care as an integrative nurse is also essential to working authentically and effectively in supporting the healing of others. The use of integrative therapies to reduce nursing burnout is a good example of extending healing practices into nursing self-care (Cuneo, Cooper, Drew, Naoum-Heffernan, Sherman, & Walz, 2011).

Integrative Therapies

The National Center for Complementary and Alternative Therapies (NCCAM, 2011a) has organized the large number of integrative therapies, identified as *complementary* or *alternative*, into defined categories of intervention. An extensive listing of integrative therapies along with their descriptions and scientific evidence regarding their efficacy is located on the NCCAM website (http://nccam.nih.gov/health/whatiscam#types). Although the full range of potential integrative therapies is too extensive for these chapters to cover, their effective use to manage specific symptoms will be described in the following chapters, applying a stratified or tiered approach based on intervention intensity.

Nurses use the full complement of interventions as supported by evidence. Some of the integrative therapy modalities used today have their origins in nursing practice and others in ancient and indigenous healing traditions. For example, Therapeutic Touch and Healing Touch were developed by nurses and incorporated into direct care by assessment of the energy field and treatment through learning techniques for "energy field disturbance" (NANDA, 2011). Providing a "massage" to patients before bedtime or in conjunction with bathing was once routine nursing care (Ruffin, 2011). Aromatherapy has been accepted as part of nursing in Switzerland, Germany, Australia, Canada, and the United Kingdom for many years (Halcon, 2010). Other hands-on integrative modalities such as Reiki (Ringdahl, 2010), reflexology (Gunnarsdottir, 2010), and acupressure (Weiss-Farnan, 2010) represent healing traditions that were developed centuries ago in Japan and China.

Other integrative modalities, originating from mind-body practice and scholarship, have also found a place in integrative nursing practice. Meditation, mindfulness-based stress reduction (MBSR), compassion-based cognitive therapy (CBCT), guided imagery, self hypnosis, and deep breathing are all practices that are well suited to incorporation into direct nursing care (Fitzgerald & Langevin, 2010; Kreitzer & Reilly-Spong, 2010; Pestka & Cutsall, 2010). Significant scholarship exists that supports the use of these modalities for reducing pain, anxiety, and stress and supporting the relaxation response (Astin, Shapiro, Eisenberg, & Forys, 2003). Within the context of nursing practice, innumerable occasions exist in which patient wellbeing can be enhanced through stress reduction and relaxation techniques. Additionally, integrative nurses can support and teach self-care through cultivation of health coaching skills (Hess et al., 2013).

The range of skills that exist within the nursing role supports multiple avenues for integrative therapy use. From inserting an IV and administering chemotherapy, to preparing someone for surgery or providing labor support, integrative nursing interventions support the human potential for natural healing. Research on integrative therapies is rich with narratives and favorable outcomes that accompany integrative therapy use for a myriad of clinical conditions that can be implemented in a variety of clinical settings (Anderson & Taylor, 2011; Bell, 2010; Coakley & Duffy, 2010; Fazzino et al., 2010; Hardwick, Pulido, & Adelson, 2012; Hellstrom & Willman, 2011; Kemper, Bulla, Krueger, Ott, McCool, & Gardiner, 2011). Direct nursing care is a natural fit for the use of integrative therapies. The integrative nurse uses all skills, all ways of knowing, and all healing modalities to support health and wellness.

Many professional organizations and state boards of nursing have developed statements that provide parameters for integrative therapy use by nurses, reinforcing the notion that integrative nursing care is often accompanied by the use of specific integrative modalities. The American Holistic Nurses Association's (AHNA, 2012) scope and standards for holistic nursing claim that both conventional and complementary or alternative therapies fall within the scope of nursing practice. Additional support for the use of complementary and alternative therapies by nurses is provided by professional nursing organizations such as Hospice and Palliative Nurses Association (HPNA, 2011), Oncology Nursing Society (ONS, 2009), and the Society of Pediatric Nurses (SPN, 2006).

In addition, over half of the state boards of nursing that regulate nursing practice have developed statements on the use of integrative therapies by nurses (Sparber,

2001). "It is becoming clear that Boards of Nursing understand that the very nature of nursing lends itself to a framework that welcomes these non-invasive complementary practices" (p. 1). These statements define and support the integration of these therapies into nursing work environments. For example, the Minnesota Board of Nursing (2010) provides a list of twelve parameters for integrative therapy use among nurses. It is worth noting that statements emanating from the state boards of nursing are not pro-scriptive, but rather provide general guidelines granting nurses the authority to prac-tice integrative therapies within the context of safe nursing practice. Responsibilities such as ensuring that she or he "personally possesses specialized nursing knowledge, judgment and skill and current competence to perform the act with reasonable skill and safety…" still lie with the individual nurse choosing to use these various therapies (Minnesota Board of Nursing, 2010, p. 1). Moving forward, it remains paramount that scopes of practice provide safety parameters without compromising the creative and intuitive nature of integrative nursing practice.

Challenges and Opportunities for Integrative Nursing

The profession of nursing is increasingly challenged to retain "high touch" skills in a "high tech" environment. Nursing scholarship suggests that the role of healer is to create a healing environment, which occurs through the intention of the healthcare provider: "We can become midwives to this process of healing, creating and being safe, sacred space into which the healing might emerge. We can, literally, become the healing environment" (Quinn, 1992, p. 28). The metaphor of touch easily translates into a care paradigm that illustrates the role of caregiver as an instrument of heal-ing. Research suggests that recipients of touch therapies frequently experience an integration of body, mind, and spirit that promotes feelings of wellbeing (Engebretson & Wardell, 2002).

While touch therapies are particularly congruent with integrative nursing prac-tice and are linked to decreased pain, stress, and anxiety, many barriers exist to the hands-on work of nursing. Time constraints and delegation of direct care to nurs-ing assistants with acute and long-term-care facilities reduce opportunities for human touch of all kinds, from the touch that accompanies routine nursing care, to massage, acupressure, reflexology, and energy touch therapies. Consequently, these modalities are often offered by volunteers and/or licensed therapists through a nurse and physician referral system. Yet, evidence supports a shift to greater nursing engagement in touch therapies, including informal application in all clinical encounters (Ringdahl, 2010).

Additional challenges, including leadership and autonomy, also exist within the context of integrative nursing. Integrative medicine does not guide practice of inte-grative nursing but rather coexists within a context of cooperative, interprofessional practice. Integrative nursing, based on identified principles and core competencies that foster autonomy and leadership, addresses different but related human needs. In fact, the conventional definition of autonomy may not accurately reflect the interdependence and relational imperative that guides nursing practice (Watson, 1990).

Operationalizing integrative nursing principles requires "pragmatic idealism," a task well suited to a profession invested in both the art and the science of healing. Foundational and evolving nursing theory combine with traditional as well as emerging knowledge, skills, and abilities to create a solid base for practice-leadership in integrative health. In addition to the formal and informal role that nurses play in supporting the health and wellbeing of their patients, advanced education in integrative health contributes to greater nursing expertise and leadership in innovative health models (Edwardson, 2010; Zaccagnini & White, 2013). As integrative health gains more acceptance and prominence in our healthcare system, it is vital that nursing take leadership in developing innovative models of integrative care in a variety of settings.

Summary

Mobilizing theory into an action plan is one of the challenges that exist in any integrative practice. For example, how does a nurse practice the science of caring and relationship-based care? There is not a singular formula or process that promises good health, but there are basic tenets that support the healing process and are used by integrative nurses in creating an integrative clinical practice. Weaving these foundational principles of being-knowing-doing into nursing practice generates a care model that expands the practice of nursing, making the whole greater than its individual parts.

Metaphorically, one could view symptoms as the consequence of an inadequate "root system" that yields a poorly nourished "plant." Tending to the plant naturally brings forth the diversity and complexity that exist in the cultivation of health, contributing long-term to a stronger root system. Interconnectedness exists between all parts of this system, from the physical environment, to the bodymindspirit of the client, to the one providing care. Therefore, symptoms should be viewed as coexisting and interacting in this interconnected network. Assessment of a sleep disturbance may reveal that the underlying cause is rooted in spiritual distress.

Each chapter in this section will provide an integrative approach for the individual symptoms: describing how the integrative nursing principles inform patient care, including assessment, priority setting, and interventions. A tiered approach based on the principle of least to more invasive/intensive, as well as evidence supporting the use of various therapies to treat the specific symptom, is provided, but an exhaustive description of each therapy is beyond the scope of this work. Instead, this section offers the integrative nurse a vision of integrative nursing in action.

SELECTED REFERENCES

Astin, J. A., Shapiro, S. L., Eisenberg, D. M., & Forys, K. L. (2003). Mind-body medicine: State of the science, implications for practice. *Journal of the American Board of Family Medicine*, *16*(2), 131–147.

Benson, H. (1975). *The Relaxation Response*. New York: William Marrow.

Buckingham, C., & Adams, A. (2000). Classifying clinical decision making: Interpreting nursing intuition, heuristics and medical diagnosis. *Journal of Advanced Nursing*, *32*(4), 990–998.

Edwardson, S. (2010). Doctor of nursing practice—Integrative health and healing as challenge. *Alternative Therapies*, *16*(5), 32–33.

Koithan, M., Bell, I. R., Niemeyer, K., & Pincus, D. (2012). A complex systems science perspective for whole systems of CAM research. *Forschende Komplementarmedizin und Klassische Naturheilkunde*, *19*(Suppl 1). 7–14. doi:10.1159/000335181.

Quinn, J. F. (1992). Holding sacred space: The nurse as healing environment. *Holistic Nursing Practice*, *6*, 26–36.

Ringdahl, D. (2010). Reiki. In Snyder, M., and Lindquist, R. (Eds.), *Complementary/Alternative Therapies in Nursing*. 6th ed. (pp. 271–286). New York: Springer Publishing Company.

Sparber, A. (2001). State board of nursing and scope of practice of registered nurses performing complementary therapies. *OJIN* (*The Online Journal of Issues in Nursing*), *6*(3). Available at: www.nursingworld.org/MainMenuCategories/ANAMarketplace/ANAPeriodicals/OJIN/TableofContents/Volume62001/No3Sept01?Articleprevioustopic/ComplementaryTherpiesReport.

Weze, C., Leathard, H. L., Grange, J., Tiplady, P., & Stevens, G. (2007). Healing by gentle touch ameliorates stress and other symptoms in people suffering with mental health disorders or psychological stress. *Evidence Based Complementary Alternative Medicine*, *4*(1), 115–123.

Zaccagnini, M., & White, K. (2014). *The Doctor of Nursing Practice Essentials*. 2nd ed. Burlington, MA: Jones & Barlett Learning.

16

Integrative Nursing Management of Stress

RUTH LINDQUIST, DAWN R. WITT, AND LYNETTE CRANE

S tress is ubiquitous in the modern age. Daily life stressors are woven into the fabric of life. Human beings are also surrounded by environmental stresses such as noise and pollution. Stress is simply a part of the human condition. Acute or chronic stress can be unpleasant and can have serious health effects. As stress is unavoidable, strategies to manage stress to reduce the toll on health and quality of life are sought.

Integrative therapies, by their nature, provide a buffer and a healthy alternative to the stresses of life. In this chapter, the concept of stress is described and defined, and integrative therapies and strategies that integrative nurses can use to effectively combat stress are identified. A case example illustrating the successful employment of integrative therapies is offered for self-care and integrative nursing practice.

Historical Underpinnings: The Stress of life

Stress, as a concept, appeared in published literature early in the twentieth century and has evolved over time. Enumerable definitions of stress exist and are wide-ranging. Walter Cannon (1927) identified stress as a whole-body response, coining the well-known term "the fight or flight syndrome." Subsequently, Hans Selye (1976), an endocrinologist and one of the most prolific writers in the field of stress and stress management, defined stress as a non-specific physiological reaction to harmful stimulation. Selye also acknowledged that, while most humans have experienced stress, the nature of stress is difficult to capture, define, and fully characterize, since there is great variability in people's responses to stress.

Stress has historically been viewed as a stimulus, a response, or both. One may or may not be aware of stress and its effects on one's health and wellbeing. Although the stress response is often considered to be an exaggerated, biologically programmed physiological response to stimulation, it has an enormous subjective component affected by our psychology, history, experience, and conditioning. When first studied, the term "stress" denoted both the causes and effects experienced. Now, however, *stressor* denotes the provoking stimuli of the *stress response* experienced. For example, one might view one's work as stressful or causing stress; or, one may respond to one's environment as causing stress and view it as stressful. Thus, the target of the intervention may be the environmental stimulus, the way we perceive the stimulus, or our response to the stimulus. Recently, a genetic component to sensitivity and response was identified (National Institute on Alcohol Abuse and Alchoholism (NIAAA)/National Institutes of Health (NIH), 2010). This finding may have important implications for treating individuals and understanding vulnerability to stress-related disorders.

Stress-related symptoms can be psychological, physiological, spiritual, or a combination, manifested within the whole. The body's stress response is commonly experienced as an unpleasant awareness that "all is not well" or that "something is wrong." Although it may be viewed as a generalized response of the whole person, it is helpful to understand and examine stress by systems and associated symptom patterns.

The "stress response" is characterized by sensations of a pounding, racing heart, dry mouth, and altered vision and attention as the sympathetic nervous system is activated. This may be accompanied by an awareness of feelings such as alarm, fright, fatigue, dread, or "dis-ease." Stress is generally considered a negative experience; however, classic work in the field suggests that an accumulation of stimulation, even by positive events and circumstances, can create demands on the human organism that can cause feelings of psychological stress, overload, and physical illness (Holmes & Rahe, 1967).

MODELS OF STRESS

There are numerous conceptual models, including Lazarus and Folkman's theory of stress and coping (1984a/1984b). This model is used to explore psychological stress and posits that stress is a process that changes over time and is largely contextual, mirroring the experience of the person with his or her environment. Lazarus and Folkman (1984a) define stress as a situation that is assessed based on the personal significance it has for one's life. The effects of stress can be measured by one's ability to cope with the demands of that stressor. There is a high rate of variability in people's reactions to stress, depending upon whether they feel equipped to manage the stressor. The processes of cognitive appraisal and coping are vital to mediating the demands of stress.

Effects of Stress on Health

The relevance of the stress response to health is significant. Indeed, stress has been implicated in the development and progression of many, if not most human illnesses (Cohen, Janicki-Deverts, & Miller, 2007). Stress has also been implicated in the pathogenesis of cardiovascular disease (Rozanski, Blumenthal & Kaplan, 1999). In the

INTERHEART study, a 52-country study with over 30,000 patients, chronic stress was second only to smoking as a predictor of cardiac mortality (Rosengren et al., 2004).

Untoward cardiac effects may be manifested by increases in blood pressure and heart rate as well as wear and tear on the vascular system. *Takotsubo syndrome* is suspected to be largely stress-induced and is characterized by the stunning of the myocardium (the heart muscle ballons and decreases in function), generating symptoms mimicking a heart attack (Kurisu et al., 2003). Although the syndrome may result in death, the symptoms are generally self-limiting and resolve in days to weeks. The search for the etiology or cause of this syndrome has led back to a stress stimulus—psychological or physiological (Sharkey et al., 2005; Wittstein et al., 2005).

Stress is a risk factor for depression, upper respiratory infections, and delayed wound healing (Cohen, 2007). Stress has also been associated with markers of biological aging (Epel et al., 2004). Researchers suggest that stress may affect cancer progression or a person's susceptibility to cancer due to changes observed in the immune system function (Segerstrom & Miller, 2004; Thaker et al., 2006), although a *direct* relationship between psychological stress and the development of cancer has not been scientifically demonstrated (Garssen, 2004).

As integrative nurses, we find that stress is ubiquitous and commonly found within individuals, families, caregivers, patients, and families in ICU or surgery, and surrounding commonly experienced events such as childbirth, job changes, marriage, or divorce. While assessing the effects of stress on an individual, the integrative nurse views the system processes in context of the whole person and integrates the associated evidence manifested in human system parts.

An Integrative Nursing Approach to Stress

The six principles of integrative nursing are naturally woven into practice when we are considering the effects of stress on health and wellbeing. While biomedicine often treats symptoms of stress without treating the "root cause" of the stress condition or source, integrative nurses holistically assess stress and manage or alleviate symptoms through a wide range of interventions and the use of healing relationships. Consider the following case scenario.

Case Scenario

An 83-year-old retired professor entered a large teaching hospital for a genito-urinary procedure. He became anxious while being transferred to the renal unit on a gurney, since the hospital and events surrounding his health condition were so foreign to him, and he noticed new heart palpitations. Upon

arrival on the unit, he was diagnosed with atrial fibrillation. He was transferred to the cardiac step-down unit where his electrolytes were examined and
corrected without change in his atrial fibrillation; efforts to pharmacologically
convert his rhythm to normal sinus rhythm failed. He was transferred to the
coronary care unit for an elective electro-cardioversion procedure.Integrative
nursing care

Environmental manipulation: The integrative nurse closed the door of the
room, dimmed the lights, drew the shades, and made the room dim and
quiet. She moved about the room slowly and confidently to prepare the
room and the patient for the cardiac procedure.

Presence: As the integrative nurse prepared him for the
electro-cardioversion, a procedure in which paddles would be placed on his
chest to pass current through his heart, the nurse stayed by the patient's
side, sat on the side of the bed, and was still and therapeutically present
with and for him.

Therapeutic listening: The integrative nurse attentively and carefully listened to him with good eye contact as he described his experience of entering
the strange hospital environment, his unfamiliarity with the hospital environment, and his anxiety when he was being transferred for a procedure that
he knew little about. She listened quietly and carefully, acknowledging, nod-
ding, valuing, and accepting his thoughts and expressed fears. She assured
him that she would remain with him during the procedure. She assured him
that the doctors were competent, highly respected, well-trained, and caring.

Touch: The integrative nurse gently touched the patient's forearm and
lifted it gently to take the patient's blood pressure. At that moment, the
patient's heart rate alarm sounded at the desk outside the room and a
rhythm strip was generated. The patient's heart rate momentarily slowed
from an irregular [atrial fibrillation] rhythm, rate of 80–100, to a bradycardia
(rate of 40–50), and then converted to a normal sinus rhythm. No further
treatment of his rhythm was required.

Aspects of the caring, therapeutic relationship engendered by the integrative nurse include environmental management, presence, listening,
and touch to foster healing and positive health outcomes. We know that a
carefully designed and considered, non-distracting healing environment is
conducive to stress reduction (Kreitzer, 2010). In the process of assessing the
individual, the integrative nurse builds a foundation for the intervention by
initiating a caring and healing relationship and environment (Principle 4).
This foundation is a significant and virtually indistinguishable aspect of the
intervention and vital to the achievement and outcomes of healing, health,
and wellbeing.

Recognizing the inseparability of the person from his environment, the integrative nurse closed the door and made the room dim and quiet. She moved

slowly and confidently to prepare the room and the patient for the cardiac procedure (Principle 1). By actively listening (Watanuki, Tracy, & Lindquist, 2010) with "real presence" (Penque & Snyder, 2010), this nurse established an authentic "encounter" with this patient as they shared the experience (Principle 4).

While she prepared this patient for electro-cardioversion (an intervention that was necessary to sustain his physical body), the integrative nurse recognized that nursing interventions, including touch, could reduce the stress experienced with these types of procedures. Intentional touch that is thoughtful and timely may add to the connection between the integrative nurse and the individual; the intervention and interventionist effects are virtually inseparable and used by expert integrative nurses to establish a foundation for healing (Principles 2 and 5).

Selye (1976) himself identified nursing as one of the most stressful professions. The stress of caregiving for nurses can be manifested in their psychological and physiological responses—similar to the responses experienced by their patients. Strategies to deal with stress, such as self-care techniques, informal support, psychotherapy, education, and setting of realistic goals, can all be used to offset and manage the effects of stress for the integrative nurse (Badger, 2001). Therefore, following the procedure, the integrative nurse debriefed with the interdisciplinary team of colleagues working in the unit to provide closure and as an act of self-care (Principle 6).

REFLECTION

While used for purposes of stress reduction, the various interventions in this case study may improve overall health, wellbeing, and quality of life. Fortunately, there is a wide variety of choices of interventions from which to select. The nurse must engage the patients to learn their perspective on the effects of stress in their lives and tailor the intervention to suit their preferences and needs. These interventions may include the removal of the stressor from the individual's biophysiological environment; cognitive approaches to the processing of stressful stimuli received by the mind or senses; strategies that alter the body's response to stressful stimuli; education to better understand the individual's response to stress and the health outcomes that are affected by it; or integrative therapies that are used to "buffer" the stress. Thus, the approach to intervention may include strategies that attenuate the stress response or alleviate the health effects of stress.

Together, the nurse and patient consider what steps to take and what interventions are acceptable and effective in achieving stress reduction. The choice of therapy rests on time-frame, severity, the acute or chronic nature of the stress or stressor, and therapy preference as negotiated with the individual who is seeking care. Some interventions may require delivery by providers who have specialized training, or interventions may require that the patient is trained and certified in self-administration or trained to practice the intervention agreed on in the plan. For example, the nurse and patient may agree that acupuncture may relieve tension headaches. Unless the nurse has certification in acupuncture therapy, the individual may require a referral for treatment or training in the recommended practice. Therapies of increasing intensity may be introduced and added to the therapeutic plan to achieve and sustain stress relief. Although it is laudable when an individual feels immediate stress relief after an integrative treatment session, the goal of treatment is to make the relief long-lasting.

Assessing Stress

PHYSIOLOGICAL INDICATORS

Most commonly, physiological indicators of stress include increased blood pressure, rapid and shallow breathing, increased heart rate, sweating, increased respiratory rate, pupil dilation, cold and clammy hands, shaking or tremors, muscle tension, constipation or diarrhea, irritability, and changes in appetite.

BIOPHYSIOLOGICAL MEASURES

It is theorized that the adverse effects of stress on health may be mediated by the chronic or acute activation of the neuroendocrine system, producing higher cortisol and catecholamine levels (Young & Breslau, 2004; Ruiz, Fullerton, Brown, & Schoolfield, 2001) or suppression of the protective immune system (Burns, Drayson, Ring, & Carroll, 2002). Thus, measurements of activity of those systems is part of clinical or research interest in studies of stress response, including catecholamines (e.g., epinephrine, norepinephrine) and cortisol. Inflammation is also affected by stress; thus, measures include inflammatory cytokines (Cohen, Doyle, & Skoner, 1999) and high-sensitivity C-reactive protein (Inoue, Kobayashi, & Yokoyama, 2004). The shortening of telomeres in response to stress is an intriguing field; the significance is that the length of telomeres is irreversible and associated with life length. In this field, the length of telomeres has been shown to shorten in persons undergoing substantial stress (Epel et al., 2004). Salivary measures may include salivary alpha-amylase (Nater & Rohleder, 2009), or salivary cortisol (Pawlow & Jones, 2002).

PSYCHOLOGICAL AND PSYCHOSOCIAL MEASURES

Perhaps the most widely used method to measure stress is self-report. Measures may be used to assess perceptions of stress at baseline (before intervention is initiated) and immediately post-intervention, in addition to follow-up periods as relevant to the condition treated. The Perceived Stress Scale is one of the most commonly used self-report instruments to assess stress; it is currently available in 4-, 10-, and 14-item versions (Cohen, 2012). Other measures of psychological and psychosocial response are reviewed elsewhere (Cohen, 2012a).

Behavioral Indicators

The effects of stress can manifest as behavioral changes, including decreased adherence to medical regimens, and distraction that contributes to risk, neglect of self-care, or engagement in risky behaviors. Poor or unhealthy behaviors such as excessive smoking, drinking, or drug use may be evidence of stress, as individuals seek temporary relief in the "dulling" or removal of stress. Sleep patterns may be altered and the quality, and quantity of sleep may be affected as measured by tools such as the Pittsburgh Sleep Quality Index (Buysse et al., 1988).

Events

Measuring demanding events that persons encounter has been an approach to understanding and predicting the potential stress "load" and risk of illness. The Holmes-Rahe Life Stress Inventory (Holmes & Rahe, 1967) was one of the early attempts to measure cumulative life stress. This classic scale is no longer state of the art. Cohen (2000) provides a survey of additional self-report stress tools. When using these tools, be sure that they comprehensively cover the events experienced by the population and are culturally appropriate.

Cognitive Measurements

Humans have memory that is designed to be protective; however, incidents that cause stress are remembered and oftentimes avoided due to the recurrence of unpleasant emotions such as fear, anxiety, or helplessness (Rosellini & Seligman, 1975; Young & Breslau, 2004). When individuals are stressed, attention, learning, and normal thought patterns may be disrupted. Assessment of cognitive changes goes beyond the scope of this chapter, but the effects of stress on cognitive processes ought to be noted by the integrative nurse, since such effects may affect the individual's attentiveness to instruction, learning, and response to interventions employed.

Integrative Stress Interventions

As previously described, integrative nurses use a full range of evidence-based interventions (Table 16.1), implementing them in a step-wise, sequentially "tiered" fashion of increasing intensity (Table 16.2) based on assessment findings, patient needs and preferences, and available resources. The integrative nurse also considers whether the stress should be addressed by short-term or long-term approaches.

Table 16.1: Evidence Illustrating Support for Selected Complementary Therapies Used for Treatment of Stress

Therapy	Source	Technique	Findings
Multi-faceted lifestyle intervention (diet, exercise, stress mgmt, & social support)	Daubenmeir et al. (2007)	Three-month lifestyle change intervention addressing diet, exercise, stress management, and social support.	Those who increased exercise time and reduced intake of dietary fat indicated lower perceived stress levels.
Hypnosis	Butler et al. (2005)	Forty-four children received hypnosis while undergoing a genitourinary radiological procedure.	Hypnosis resulted in lower distress levels, overall decrease in difficulty of conducting the procedure, and shortened procedure time.
	VandeVusse et al. (2010)	Thirty-minute recording of relaxing, affirming hypnotic suggestions played to female volunteers	Reduced heart and respiratory rates and heart rate variability, and reduced tension and anxiety
Exercise	Blumenthal et al. (2005)	Aerobic exercise training for 35 minutes, 3 times per week for 16 weeks, comprising weekly 1.5-hour stress management training	Exercise resulted in a decrease in emotional distress and improvement in cardiovascular risk markers.
	Blumenthal et al. (1997)	Four-month program of exercise training or stress management for patients with ischemic heart disease.	"Stress management was associated with a relative risk of 0.26 compared with controls."
Biofeedback	Cutshall et al. (2011)	15 computer-guided biofeedback sessions for nurses 30 minutes per session, four times a week, for four weeks.	Improvement in stress management, as measured by SF-36 vitality subscale
	Lemaire et al. (2011)	A 28-day biofeedback /stress management program for physicians including self-generated positive emotion, rhythmic breathing, and use of a biofeedback device.	Mean stress scores declined at 28 days and were maintained for 56 days post-intervention.
Mindfulness-Based Stress Reduction (MBSR)	Carlson et al. (2003)	Eight-week standard MBSR program for patients with breast and prostate cancer.	Significant improvements were demonstrated in symptoms of stress, sleep, and quality of life.
	Carmody & Baer (2008)	Eight-week home practice of MBSR.	Decrease in stress symptoms and increase in mindfulness and wellbeing.
	Gross et al. (2010)	Eight-week standard MBSR program for patients receiving solid organ transplants.	Improvement in quality-of-life measures, improved anxiety, depression, and sleep.

(continued)

Table 16.1: (Continued)

Therapy	Source	Technique	Findings
Meditation	Schneider et al. (2005)	Transcendental Meditation (TM) 1- to 1.5-hr session of personal instruction, plus three follow-up sessions for African-Americans with stage I or II hypertension. Participants practiced on their own, at home, for one year.	TM significantly decreased diastolic BP and showed a trend for a reduction in systolic BP.
Massage	Field et al. (1999)	Massage therapy for stress in prenatal period; 20 min. massage therapy sessions given 2 times/week for 5 weeks.	Massage reduced anxiety, improved sleep, improved mood, and decreased back pain. Fewer complications reported during labor and delivery; infants had fewer postnatal complications.
	Hayes & Cox (1999)	Five-minute foot massage for patients in critical care.	Significant decreases in blood pressure, respiration, and heart rate were observed during the foot massage intervention.
	Cady & Jones (1997)	Fifteen-minute chair massage conducted as part of worksite stress reduction program.	Significant reduction in SBP and DBP after receiving the massage.
	Field et al. (1996a)	15 min of massage was given to 1- to 3–month-old infants born to depressed adolescent mothers for 2 days per week for a 6-week period.	Infants had greater decreases in urinary cortisol, gained more weight, showed greater improvement on sociability, emotionality, "soothability," and temperament.
Energy Therapies	Cuneo et al. (2011)	Reiki instruction was given to registered nurses for self use, and the Perceived Stress Scale tool was administered before and 3 weeks after Reiki self-practice.	Practicing Reiki resulted in reduced perceived stress levels.
	Maville et al., (2008)	Effect of 30-minute Healing Touch (HT) session was tested using stress perception and biological correlates.	Changes in all measures except muscle tension were observed (State–Trait Anxiety Inventory, heart rate, blood pressure, skin conductance, skin temperature) during HT.
	Cox & Hayes (1999)	Therapeutic Touch (TT) administered by TT practitioner/nurse in ICU and CCU.	TT was useful in enhancing sleep and relaxation in critically ill patients.

Cognitive-Behavioral	Hammerfald et al. (2006)	Cognitive-behavioral stress management (CBSM) training comprising 10 hrs of cognitive restructuring, problem-solving, self-instruction, and progressive muscle relaxation.	The cognitive-behavioral stress management group showed significantly reduced cortisol stress responses.
Music	Nilsson (2009)	Patients who had a coronary artery bypass graft or aortic valve replacement were exposed to 30 minutes of uninterrupted bed rest with music and then 30 minutes of bed rest; or alternatively, 60 minutes of uninterrupted bed rest the day after procedure.	After 30 minutes of bed rest, there was a significant decrease in cortisol levels.
	Nilsson & Rawal (2005)	Patients undergoing hernia surgery were exposed to music both during surgery and postoperatively.	Those in the intraoperative group reported a decrease in postoperative pain, and the postoperative group reported less anxiety, pain, and morphine consumption.
Humor	Bennett, Zeller, Rosenberg, & McCann (2003) Berk & Tan (2008)	Thirty-three women viewed a humorous video.	Stress decreased for subjects in the humor group; natural killer cell activity was improved.
Yoga	Hartfiel et al. (2011)	Six-week workplace program of Dru Yoga: 1 hr/wk	Mood, wellbeing, and self-confidence [resilience] during stressful situations improved.
	Smith et al. (2007)	Ten weekly sessions of hatha yoga for community-dwelling subjects	Stress, anxiety, and quality of life scores improved over time.
Progressive Muscle Relaxation	Pawlow & Jones (2002)	Two sessions of acute relaxation training provided on two separate occasions	Brief relaxation training led to significantly lower salivary cortisol, heart rate, state anxiety, and perceived stress.
Aromatherapy	Seo (2009)	Aroma essential oil inhalation	Stress levels lower; salivary IgA significantly lower than controls.
Breathing	Parati et al. (2002)	Music-guided slow breathing in normal subjects.	Acute effects on cardiovascular parameters and baroreflex sensitivity.

Table 16.2: Interventions for Stress Management

Level of Intensity	Integrative Therapy Approach
Tier 1 Interventions	Dietary Therapies • Vitamins • Probiotics • Supplements Mind-Body Therapies • Controlled/coached breathing • Guided imagery • Music • Prayer •Journaling • Positive self-talk/cognitive restructuring Basic Foundational Integrative Nursing Therapies • Touch • Therapeutic listening, presence • Environmental manipulation • Intentional social support (support/self-help groups) • Humor • Distraction • Education
Tier 2 Interventions	Natural Products • Aromatherapy Energy Therapies • Biofeedback • Stress management (e.g., progressive muscle relaxation) Mind-Body Therapies • Animal-assisted therapy Movement Therapies • Walking, jogging • Yoga, chi gong, tai chi
Tier 3 Interventions	Mind-Body Therapies • Hypnosis • Cognitive behavioral [stress management] therapy • MBSR, meditation Manipulative Therapies • Massage • Reflexology Energy Therapies • Reiki • Healing/therapeutic touch • Acupuncture
Tier 4 Interventions	Whole Systems • Traditional Chinese Medicine • Herbal therapies
Tier 5 Interventions	Pharmacological Therapies

Short-term approaches (e.g., breathing, massage, biofeedback, aromatherapy, or humor) may be used to relieve acute stress encountered by individuals. The regulation of and focus on breathing as a strategy to alleviate stress can be used effectively by individuals alone or in conjunction with other therapies. Slow, deep, and regular breaths effectively reduce respiratory rate and may reduce blood pressure and heart rate. In addition to the physiological effects, deep breathing may serve as a distraction and may give persons a sense of control over the situation.

If the stressful circumstances or response persists, longer-term approaches may be implemented over time (e.g., mindfulness-based stress reduction, meditation, cognitive-behavioral stress management, or yoga). For example, for those in states of chronic stress, yoga as an integrative approach may provide a foundation of literal and figurative "flexibility" and sense of coherence or wholeness to combat stress. Alternatively, mindfulness-based stress reduction (MBSR) techniques can be used to learn how to "respond" to stress rather than "react" to it (Kabat-Zinn, 1990).

Kabat-Zinn described the stress reaction as the involuntary human interaction with one's environment, which can be tempered by thoughtful, conscious efforts to respond in such a way as to reduce the excessive activation of the mind and body, and the response of the autonomic nervous system. MBSR is utilized to cultivate a moment-to-moment, non-judgmental awareness that is fostered by paying attention: attention for the sake of awareness. Mindfulness is not a process whereby one seeks to "attain" anything; rather, it is a non-deliberate practice that explores living in the present. In a meta-analysis that included only a few small studies due to issues of quality or relevance, Grossman et al. (2004) found that, overall, "mindfulness training might enhance general features of coping with distress and disability in everyday life, as well as under more extraordinary conditions of serious disorder or stress" (Grossman et al., p. 39).

Other techniques build new patterns and retrain patients in how to view the stressful encounters. Positive self-talk is one technique (Mayo Clinic Staff, 2011); cognitive restructuring is another (Bryant, Harvey, Dang, Sackville, & Basten, 1998). Massage is a popular, commonly used therapy to alleviate the accumulation of bodily stress, and there is good evidence that it produces a reduction in stress-related measures in the short term (Moraska et al., 2010). Massage can be used for a wide range of patient populations, including infants (Field et al., 1996), women prenatally (Field et al., 1999), and patients in critical care settings (Hayes & Cox, 1999). Changing diet and eating right may reduce stress (Daubenmeir et al., 2007). The use of humor may also alleviate stress (Bennett, Zeller, Rosenberg, & McCann, 2003).

Hypnosis, progressive relaxation, yoga, exercise (walking), support groups, and animal relationships may also be helpful, although evidence indicating an immediate, if short-lived, response to integrative therapies is much stronger than evidence supporting longer-term effects. For children undergoing radiological procedures, hypnosis has been demonstrated to be safe and effective in decreasing levels of distress and the difficulty of conducting the procedure as well as shortening procedure times (Butler et al., 2005). Cutshall et al. (2011) and Lemaire et al. (2011) demonstrated reduced stress in populations of nurses and doctors after completion of biofeedback training. While these therapies are not entirely representative of the integrative therapies available, these are a sampling of the modalities that can be incorporated into integrative nursing care. Once again, the foundation of the integrative nursing encounter is a therapeutic relationship based on essential actions of active or therapeutic listening, reflecting back, presence, and touch.

Outcome Evaluation

To determine the potential health benefits and efficacy of integrative interventions delivered, it is important to assess carefully selected measures before initiating intervention and following intervention. Information gleaned from such assessments is often useful feedback for the individual cared for, as well as data for the integrative nurse. Data can be used to determine whether the intervention was successful; whether the intervention should be terminated, continued, or modified; or whether a new intervention ought to be considered as an add-on or replacement. It is important to schedule follow-up, or establish a means to monitor and support the practice of integrative therapies, and depending on the therapy, to assess the success of the intervention in achieving the use for which it was intended.

Summary

This chapter provides a foundation for understanding stress and the stress response in contemporary society, grounded in our historic roots of survival. An approach to integrative nursing, with the promise of combating stress and improving health, has been provided. Beyond diseases caused by stress, our wellbeing depends on our responses to a changing world and our everyday health choices—behavioral and psychological.

SELECTED REFERENCES

Burns, V. E., Drayson, M., Ring, C., & Carroll, D. (2002). Perceived stress and psychological wellbeing are associated with antibody status after meningitis C conjugate vaccination. *Psychosomatic Medicine, 64*(6), 963–970.

Cohen, S., Janicki-Deverts, D., & Miller, G. E. (2007). Psychological stress and disease. *JAMA, 298*, 1685–1687.

Folkman, S., Lazarus, R. S., Dunkel-Schetter, C., DeLongis, A., & Gruen, R. (1986). The dynamics of a stressful encounter: Cognitive appraisal, coping and encounter outcomes. *Journal of Personality & Social Psychology, 50*, 992–1003.

Grossman, P., Niemann, L., Schmidt, S., & Walach, H. (2004). Mindfulness-based stress reduction and health benefits. A meta-analysis. *Journal of Psychosomatic Research, 57*(1), 35–43.

Kabat-Zinn J. (1990). *Full Catastrophe Living: Using the Wisdom of Your Body and Mind to Face Stress, Pain and Illness.* New York: Delacorte.

Kreitzer, M. J., & Zborowsky, T. (2010). Creating optimal healing environments. In M. Snyder & R. Lindquist, (Eds.), *Alternative/Complementary Therapies in Nursing*, 6th ed. (pp. 321–333). New York: Springer.

Neilsen, N. R., Kristensen, T. S., Schnohr, P., & Gronbaek, M. (2008). Psychological stress and cause-specific mortality among men and women: Results from a prospective cohort study. *American Journal of Epidemiology, 168*, 481–491.

Penque, S., & Snyder, M. (2010). Presence. In M. Snyder & R. Lindquist (Eds.), *Alternative/ Complementary Therapies in Nursing*, 6th ed. (pp. 35–46). New York: Springer.

Selye, H. (1976). *Stress in Health and Disease*. Reading, MA: Butterworths.

Watanuki, S., Tracy, M., & Lindquist, R. (2010). Therapeutic listening. In M. Snyder & R. Lindquist (Eds.), *Alternative/Complementary Therapies in Nursing*, 6th ed. (pp. 47–59). New York: Springer.

17

Integrative Nursing Management of Nausea

SUSANNE M. CUTSHALL AND LISA M. VAN GETSON

Recently, there has been a renewed interest by nursing practice in the management of nausea and vomiting. The physiological mechanisms involved in the process of causing nausea and vomiting are better understood. Pharmacological agents are being used in combination with integrative modalities in the treatment and ongoing management of nausea and vomiting. Most episodes of nausea and vomiting are preventable, or at least manageable. Nurses trained in integrative nursing practice play an important role in patient education and assisting the patient in the treatment and management of nausea. This chapter provides an overview of integrative nursing assessment and management of nausea.

Background and Significance of Nausea

Nausea and the often-subsequent vomiting are common symptoms with medical illness and can be caused by a wide variety of physical and chemical conditions, including pregnancy, chemotherapy, surgery, and other conditions and illnesses, such as viral gastroenteritis. Certain medications can cause nausea and vomiting, including anesthesia commonly used for surgery (Acalovschi, 2002; Watcha, 2002). These unpleasant and debilitating symptoms can prolong recovery times, increase medical costs, lead to serious complications, and affect quality of life and satisfaction with overall medical care. Severe nausea with vomiting can lead to dehydration, aspiration pneumonia, malnutrition, metabolic disturbances, and surgical site disruptions. Unpleasant experiences with nausea may also contribute to future anticipatory nausea and anxiety (Acalovschi, 2002; Bloechl-Daum et al., 2006).

Nausea can be described as the feeling of being "sick to the stomach" or the sensation that is associated with the urge to vomit. Nausea and vomiting are basic human reflexes that protect us against absorption of toxins and other stimuli. Nausea is often linked with vomiting; however, they are separate experiences that are assessed differently. Nausea is a subjective, unpleasant, wavelike experience and sensation in the back of the throat or epigastrium that can be associated with flushing, tachycardia, pallor, and the awareness of an urge to vomit. Vomiting is the actual physical contraction of the abdominal muscles that results in forceful expulsion of stomach contents. Sometimes there is the contraction without expulsion of gastric contents, as with retching or the "dry heaves" (Garret et al., 2003). Vomiting can be differentiated from retching, regurgitation, or rumination.

Retching, also called the dry heaves, involves the same physiological mechanism as vomiting, but occurs against a closed glottis (Acalovschi, 2002). There is no expulsion of gastric contents. *Regurgitation* is the return of small amounts of food or secretions to the hypopharynx. This may be related to a mechanical obstruction of the esophagus, gastroesophageal reflux disease, or esophageal motility disorders. *Rumination* is similar to regurgitation; however, the small amount of completely swallowed food is returned to the hypopharynx and often reswallowed. Rumination is not associated with nausea (American Society for Health-System Pharmacists (ASHP) therapeutic guidelines, 1999).

There are four classifications of nausea and vomiting. Each classification identifies the underlying cause and the time at which nausea occurs (Garret et al., 2003).

- *Acute*: Nausea and vomiting occurring within 24 hours of taking a medication or other trigger.
- *Delayed*: Nausea and vomiting that occurs more than 24 hours after taking a medication or being exposed to a trigger.
- *Anticipatory*: Nausea and vomiting that occurs in anticipation of a treatment or specific trigger.
- *Chronic*: Persistent, long-term nausea and vomiting.

PATHOPHYSIOLOGY OF NAUSEA

Stimulation of the nucleus of neurons located in the medulla oblongata, the vomiting center, initiates the vomiting reflex. The vomiting center can be directly or indirectly activated or stimulated by signals from: (a) the cerebral cortex (stimulated by anticipation, fear, or memory); (b) sensory organs (stimulated by sights, smells, or tastes); (c) the vestibular apparatus of the inner ear (associated with motion sickness); and (d) indirect stimuli that activate the chemoreceptor trigger zone (CTZ). The CTZ, a highly vascular cerebral area lacking a true blood–brain barrier, can react directly to substances (neurotransmitters) in the blood, by signals in the stomach and small intestines that travel along vagal afferent nerves, or by the direct action of emetogenic compounds that are carried in the blood (anticancer drugs, opioids, ipecac) (Garret et al., 2003, p. 32). This reaction is a natural way for the body to initiate the vomiting cascade so that the harmful substances can be expelled (Figure 17.1). Many antiemetic medications work in the body by blocking one or more of these receptor triggers for nausea (Garrett et al., 2003).

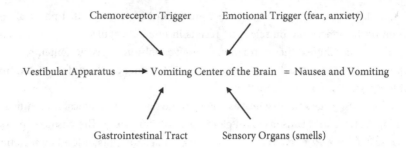

FIGURE 17.1 The Emetic Response—Multiple Stimuli and Complexity

PREVALENCE OF NAUSEA

Symptoms of nausea and vomiting are all too familiar to most nurses. Because most episodes of nausea and vomiting are preventable, integrative nursing should understand various types of nausea and its prevention and management.

Chemotherapy-Related Nausea

Nausea and vomiting continue to be among the most distressing adverse effects of chemotherapy. Advances in antiemetic medications and chemotherapy medications have helped reduce nausea in this population. Research indicates that, with the implementation of antiemetic medication protocols during chemotherapy treatment, the incidence of nausea has decreased by at least 50% (Liau et al., 2005; Neymark & Crott, 2005).

Nausea in this population is multifaceted. Chemotherapeutic agents themselves have different nausea potentials, ranging from 1 (least) to 5 (greatest) (Garret et al., 2003). Additional risk factors include an age younger than 50, being female (potentially from the influence of hormones), having a history of motion sickness, a history of pregnancy-related nausea, and associated nausea previously with chemotherapy. Anticipatory nausea may occur before the beginning of a new cycle of chemotherapy in response to previous experience of nausea and usually happens around 12 hours before the administration of chemotherapy. Acute nausea occurs within the first 24 hours after administration of chemotherapy. Delayed nausea usually begins at least 24 hours after the administration of chemotherapy and may last up to 120 hours after administration. Breakthrough nausea may also occur despite preventative therapy (Garret et al., 2003).

Postoperative Nausea

Postoperative nausea and vomiting continue to be a problem in post-anesthesia settings, occurring in 20% to 30% of all surgical patients. Yet, the incidence can be as high as 70% to 80% among patients with predetermined risk factors (Acalovschi, 2002;

Watcha, 2002). Acute postoperative nausea occurs within 24 hours of receiving anesthesia. A wide range of stimuli can contribute to postoperative nausea and vomiting, including the chemical anesthetics and opioids that directly stimulate the vomiting center. Other direct stimuli may occur to the vomiting center before, during, and after surgery and may include sensory input (visual, olfactory, and pain) and stimulation of the vestibular apparatus. The gastrointestinal tract can be stimulated by nitrous oxide directly and activate the vomiting center (Garret et al., 2003). Because of the wide range of stimuli to nausea, prevention of postoperative nausea can be difficult. Risk factors for nausea can be different preoperatively, intraoperatively, and postoperatively (Table 17.1).

Pregnancy-Related Nausea

Pregnancy-related nausea and vomiting are common, reported to occur in 70% to 90% of pregnancies (ACOG, 2004). Rising estrogen and progesterone levels and maternal serum prostaglandin E2 levels during pregnancy are implicated as causes of nausea. The onset can occur shortly after the first missed menstrual period (4 to 6 weeks' gestation) and may be the first signal of possible pregnancy. Symptoms typically peak by 8 to 12 weeks and begin to resolve around the 20th week. Nausea with or without vomiting occurs especially in the morning but can last all day. The prognosis for mother and baby is generally good. However, if pregnancy-related nausea and vomiting are not characteristic of morning sickness, other potential serious conditions (e.g., hyperemesis gravidarum) need to be considered. This disorder has an estimated incidence of 0.5%–2% of all live births (ACOG, 2004).

Table 17.1: Risk Factors for Nausea

Preoperative	Intraoperative	Postoperative
Higher in adults than children	Laparoscopic procedures	Unrelieved pain
Higher in women than in men	Surgery: Plastic, ophthalmic, orthopedic shoulder, gynecological, and ear, nose, and throat	Opioid used to manage pain
History of motion sickness	Longer procedures with general anesthesia	Sudden motion or change in body position
History of postoperative nausea	Gastric distention	Premature oral intake
Greater for obese patients and those with delayed gastric emptying	Some medications used in association with anesthesia (e.g., atropine, propofol)	Hypotension
Decreased with a history of smoking		

Other Causes of Nausea

There are many additional causes of nausea (e.g., medications, medical conditions, and specific procedures). Drugs may initiate gastric irritation and cause nausea, including non-steroidal anti-inflammatory drugs (NSAIDs), selective serotonin reuptake inhibitors (SSRIs), and antibiotics. Some medications directly stimulate the vomiting center in the brain, such as digoxin, morphine, alcohol, ipecac, and anti-cancer medications. Motion and inner ear disorders can cause nausea by directly stimulating the vomiting center. Other stimuli of the olfactory, visual, vestibular, and psychogenic systems may induce nausea.

An Integrative Nursing Approach to Nausea

The six principles of integrative nursing are naturally woven into practice when we are considering the effects of stress on health and wellbeing. While allopathic medicine often treats symptoms of stress without treating the "root cause" of the stress condition or source, integrative nurses holistically assess stress and manage or alleviate symptoms through a wide range of interventions and the use of healing relationships. Consider the following case scenario.

Integrative nurses focus on the whole person, the complexity of personal systems, and the systems in which they care for patients. Integrative nurses take into account the whole picture of health and illness, even when managing individual symptoms (Principle 1). In the case of nausea, an integrative nurse utilizes a relationship-based approach to engage in a full assessment of all aspects of potential causes of nausea, potential patient concerns and distress, and all potential interventions that could be utilized. These interventions can be planned in partnership with the patient with

Case Scenario

Carol is a 60-year-old woman who has a history of noteworthy nausea with vomiting during recovery from surgeries. She has been admitted to a cardiac medical floor awaiting cardiac bypass surgery. The integrative nurse introduces herself to Carol and asks her what her concerns are with surgery and if she has any questions. Carol expresses concerns about her previous experience with nausea after her hysterectomy surgery. This nausea and vomiting was so severe that she had to stay extra days in the hospital as a result of dehydration. The medications she took were somewhat helpful, but she was still miserable. She is concerned because she could not get herself moving after that surgery due to nausea and knows how important early ambulation is after heart surgery.

Integrative nursing care

The nurse listens intentionally to Carol's concerns about her nausea. Together they discuss Carol's past experience with nausea, including when the nausea occurred, what she utilized during this time for management of the nausea, and her wish to utilize some self-care techniques. The nurse also lets the anesthesia staff know about Carol's apprehension about her experiences with nausea in the past. The anesthesiologist is able to discuss with Carol the potential to use some preventative medications that are sometimes utilized with patients who have a history of nausea. Carol's goal is to keep her nausea to a minimum so that she will be able to get up and moving after surgery and get back home when expected and without a delay. This goal is communicated in the medical record, and the integrative nurse relays this goal to the medical team on rounds. As the integrative nurse discusses this goal with Carol, they also discuss non-pharmacological approaches to nausea. Carol is familiar with some dietary suggestions for nausea because, for her previous surgery and nausea, she was given crackers and some carbonated beverages to drink. Carol is open to exploring other options this time. The integrative nurse discusses and provides information on dietary guidelines for managing nausea. The nurse also discusses therapies such as aromatherapy and self-acupressure for nausea. The nurse gives Carol a sample of essential oils (ginger and spearmint) on a cotton ball to try and also demonstrates how to provide acupressure to the P6 point on the wrist. The nurse notes in the record that Carol would be open to acupuncture and massage therapy to manage her nausea after surgery.

respect to their narrative of nausea, preferences, interests, and ability to carry out self-care interventions (Principle 4). Integrative nursing practice is informed by multiple sources of evidence. Expert nurses use all forms of evidence (empirical, personal, clinical) when selecting an intervention for their patients. Integrative nurses proceed from least invasive and least disruptive to more invasive treatments with the intent of supporting the natural healing process. Integrative therapies are being increasingly utilized in healthcare settings and by patients to help manage nausea symptoms; in this case, the integrative nurse offered Carol options including aromatherapy, massage, acupuncture, and acupressure (Principle 5).

This example shows how the integrative nurse provided a space for relationship-based care and guidance related to a concern regarding nausea. The integrative nurse was present and listened to the narrative story and elicited a full picture of this health concern. The nurse offered reassurance and resources and worked within the medical system to communicate the patient's goal for management of nausea (Principles 1, 4).

She allowed the patient to be an active partner in the planning of her care and respected her wisdom and choices for treatments for self-care (Principle 2).

Assessing Nausea

Nurses play an important role in identifying nausea and vomiting, using a variety of assessment tools and a patient-centered approach. An effective assessment tool can help engage patients in the process of evaluating treatment experiences, monitoring, and individualization of their own care. Integrative nurses collaborate with clients to co-create a healing team in order to move the whole system forward. With attentive presence and listening by the integrative nurse and engagement of the patient, a collaborative plan to manage nausea can be developed.

Assessment often begins by establishing a trusting relationship during an initial history, allowing time for reflection by both practitioner and patient. Useful assessment of nausea and vomiting requires more than just an account of its presence. To develop useful integrative interventions, the assessment must be comprehensive and requires a clear sense of the patient's whole symptom experience. An important initial assessment includes question such as:

- When did these symptoms first occur, and what else was happening at this time?
- Could symptoms present for less than a week be due to conditions that are separate from those causing symptoms over weeks, months, or years?
- Is the nausea an acute condition, or has there been chronic nausea and vomiting?
- What has been tried thus far for managing the nausea?
- Are there other associated symptoms—such as vomiting, abdominal or chest pain, light-headedness, cough, or hematemesis—that would prompt immediate therapy or attention?

The four characteristics of nausea that should typically be assessed are its duration, frequency, severity, and associated distress. For duration, ask when the person started to experience nausea and the number of hours that nausea was experienced during a specific time frame. Frequency is measured as the number of nausea episodes during a specific time frame. Severity is typically rated and recorded using a categorical rating scale, such as a Likert-type scale (e.g., none [0], mild [1], moderate [2], or severe [4]); a visual analogue scale (i.e., anchored or non-anchored); or a numerical rating scale (e.g., on a scale of 0 to 10, with 10 being the most severe). Alternatively, nausea can be graded according to severity and influence on fluid and food intake, as illustrated in Table 17.2.

Table 17.2: Nausea Severity Scale

Grade 1	Mild nausea that does not lead to altered eating, or mild vomiting (one episode per day).
Grade 2	Nausea leading to reduced food intake, not weight loss, or 2–5 episodes of vomiting in a 24-hour period. May require IV fluids to prevent dehydration.
Grade 3	Nausea that leads to inadequate food and fluid intake, or > 6 episodes of vomiting in a 24-hour period. May require IV fluids to prevent or reverse dehydration and tube feeding.
Grade 4	Nausea and vomiting with life-threatening consequences.

Distress is assessed by examining how much subjective discomfort there is or how upsetting the nausea is to the person. This is not always included, but integrative nursing might consider this factor to be the most important measure for patients. Likert-type scales ranging from *none* to *severe distress or discomfort* may be used. Other tools address distress by assessing how the patient perceives the symptoms as having an impact on daily functioning and quality of life.

Other factors, such as the meaning of an illness and other life events, may have an influence on a patient's perceived distress. The duration of symptoms can also influence the perceived distress.

NAUSEA MEASURES

The subjective nature of nausea and multiple possible causes and ways to assess nausea make it sometimes the most difficult symptom for care providers to measure and provide adequate treatments for. Research discussions indicate that nausea has a stronger negative impact on quality of life than vomiting (Bloechl-Daum et al., 2006). Integrative nurses can be assisted by using an instrument that facilitates assessment of this symptom. Wood and colleagues (2011) identified more than twenty instruments. Several tools evaluated nausea specifically in the oncology population. Three tools that may be particularly helpful because of their specific context and use of multiple sources of information:

- The Morrow Assessment of Nausea and Emesis, with questions about pretreatment nausea
- The Multinational Association of Supportive Care in Cancer (MASCC) Antiemesis Tool, which addresses both acute and delayed nausea
- The Behavioral Observation Tool, which assesses the patient's experience as well as patient's behaviors (Wood et al., 2011)

Integrative Nausea Interventions

Integrative nurses can have an impact on a patient's sense of wellbeing and quality of life by collaboratively crafting a plan to address nausea symptoms, thereby reducing its length and severity, and enabling the patients to maintain normal life functions, including caring for themselves and others and engaging in productive work and home lives. Failure to effectively prevent and treat nausea and vomiting lengthens hospital stays; potentially increases medical complications such as malnutrition, dehydration, electrolyte imbalances; and contributes to physical and mental stress.

The integrative nurse uses all the information available and then assesses resources for treatment and interventions to assist a patient with the management of nausea and vomiting. He/she then determines the appropriate type of intervention based on symptom intensity, patient preferences, and current patient condition using the least invasive strategy possible to address the symptom and assure that the person is in the best condition for healing (Table 17.3).

Nutritional, integrative, and pharmacological strategies are often needed in combination to help prevent and manage nausea of all causes. Integrative nurses have several integrative strategies that offer some relief from nausea, such as mind–body modalities, acupressure, or aromatherapy. Many of the strategies can be taught directly to patients and family members as ongoing coping and treatment methods. Other integrative therapies may require referral to other practitioners that are trained in certain modalities such as acupuncture, massage, or music therapy. However, if the nausea and vomiting are accompanied by: (a) pain or a severe headache; (b) inability to keep liquids down for 8 hours or inability to eat or drink anything for 12 hours; (c) signs or symptoms of dehydration (i.e., excessive thirst, dry mouth, infrequent urination, dark-colored urine, and weakness, dizziness, or light-headedness upon standing); or (d) emesis that contains or looks like blood, resembles coffee grounds, or is green in color, the person should be encouraged to seek immediate medical attention (see the Mayo Clinic website at http://www.mayoclinic.com/health/nausea/MY00572).

NUTRITIONAL INTERVENTIONS

Experts recommend dietary interventions, depending on the cause of the nausea, to minimize nausea and vomiting, although there is limited evidence of the efficacy of these interventions. However, if a bowel obstruction or ileus is suspected, dietary intake should be limited. In general, dietary interventions include smaller portions, frequent small meals, reducing aromas from food and other stimuli, and avoiding foods that are spicy, fatty, or salty (Polovich et al., 2005). If the patient vomits, fluids by mouth are recommended to maintain hydration, although milk products should be avoided. Sipping liquids slowly throughout the day may also help. When the vomiting stops, broth and unbuttered whole-grain toast are recommended. If the patient keeps these

Table 17.3: Interventions for Nausea

Level of Intensity	Integrative Therapy Approach
Tier 1 Interventions	Dietary Therapies: • Avoid milk products • Small, frequent meals • Avoid spicy, fatty, salty foods Mind–Body Therapies: • Deep breathing • Guided imagery • Progressive relaxation Natural Products: • Ginger
Tier 2 Interventions	Dietary Therapies: • Liquids to avoid dehydration if vomiting • Limit intake to easy-to-digest foods Natural Products: • Aromatherapy Energy Therapies: • Acupressure (wrist bands) Movement Therapies: • Yoga
Tier 3 Interventions	Mind–Body Therapies: • Hypnosis and/or self-hypnosis • Music therapy Manipulative Therapies: • Massage • Reflexology Energy Therapies: • Acupuncture • Reiki • Healing/therapeutic touch
Tier 4 Interventions	Whole systems: • TCM • Homeopathic remedies
Tier 5 Interventions	Pharmacological Therapies: IV therapy/hydration and nutritional supplements

down, graduate to brown rice, potatoes, soups, steamed vegetables, or yogurt. Taking an antiemetic an hour before eating may also be helpful. Cleaning the patient's teeth and mouth regularly can help reduce aftertaste (Duke, 2008).

Examples of foods that are easy to chew, swallow, and digest include dry foods like toast, crackers, and pretzels; bland foods; hard candies such as peppermint or lemon drops; yogurt; hot cereals or broth; boiled or baked chicken without skins; and clear liquids. The literature has identified some foods that can help prevent nausea, such as ginger and peppermint (Duke, 2008). Ginger is a perennial plant native to Asia that is now widely cultivated in the tropics. There are multiple studies on ginger's nausea-soothing abilities.

HERBAL MEDICINES

Herbal medicines reflect some of the first attempts to improve the human condition through the use of plant or parts of plants including flowers, leaves, bark, fruit, seeds, stems and roots for their potential therapeutic properties. Ginger and peppermint used as aromatherapy are common biologically-based modalities used for nausea and vomiting.

Ginger (*Zingiber officinale*) is used in China to treat a variety of gastrointestinal problems, including nausea and vomiting. Ginger has spasmolytic, carminative, and absorbent effects (Ernst & Pittler, 2000). The compound 8-gingerol enhances gastrointestinal transport in animal models and antagonizes ileal 5-HT_3-receptors (Yamahara et al., 1989, 1990). The recommended dose for prophylaxis of postoperative nausea and vomiting (PONV) is 1 gram of powdered ginger root given preoperatively. Much of the data suggesting the antiemetic effect of ginger have come from small studies that had questionable designs. Ernst and Pittler (2000) performed a meta-analysis of randomized controlled trials of ginger for nausea and vomiting, concluding that ginger was more effective than placebo and as efficacious as metoclopramide. A study of women undergoing gynecological laparoscopy found no benefit, however, from the administration of ginger in doses equivalent to 1g to 2g of powdered ginger (Eberhart et al., 2003).

Aromatherapy uses the inhaled scent of essential oils from flowers, herbs, and trees to promote health and wellbeing or physiological effects in the body. Several studies have produced promising results. Peppermint, a digestive aid, is considered one of the most effective essential oils for curbing nausea. Other oils used for their action on the digestive tract are chamomile, damask rose, fennel, and lavender.

Peppermint essential oil has a long history of use as a folk remedy. The primary active constituents are menthol and menthone. Orally administered peppermint oil has been studied for relief of flatulence, colic pain, and symptoms of irritable bowel syndrome (Sommerville et al., 1984). In animal models, peppermint oil decreases the gut's contractile response to histamine, serotonin, acetylcholine, and substance P (Hills & Aaronson, 1991). There are fewer studies on the ability of olfactory administration of peppermint oil to relieve nausea and vomiting. Tate (1997) reported a slight reduction in nausea and need for antiemetic medicines, as well as increased tolerance of anesthesia in the peppermint oil treated group when using peppermint oil prior to gynecological surgery. A recent systematic literature review by Lau et al. (2012) reviewed five studies of use of essential oils for nausea. The authors concluded that existing evidence (*n* = 5 articles) is encouraging, but further well-designed studies are need to confirm the effectiveness of essential oils in treating nausea and vomiting.

Isopropyl alcohol (70%), used as two or three inhalations from a standard alcohol wipe, has been used as aromatherapy to reduce nausea (Merritt et al., 2002). Langevin and Brown (1997) suggested a positive role for isopropyl alcohol as a cost-effective means of treating postoperative nausea and vomiting (PONV) in a study of 15 patients undergoing elective surgery. In a quasi-experimental study, Merritt et al. (2002) compared isopropyl alcohol with standard antiemetic treatment for PONV in 111 day-surgery patients, concluding that isopropyl alcohol was therapeutically equivalent to and considerably less costly than standard treatment. Further research is needed to determine the duration of action, dose, and most effective mode of inhalation.

MIND–BODY THERAPIES

Mind-body modalities include a number of practices such as guided imagery, progressive muscle-relaxation, self-hypnosis, meditation and deep-breathing exercises, music therapy, and yoga. These modalities may be considered relaxation techniques and can be considered helpful in relieving nausea caused by chemotherapy or other triggers.

Studies utilizing guided imagery and relaxation techniques have indicated that these techniques have been able to lessen the nausea caused by some chemotherapy drugs (Lerman et al., 1990; Molassiotis et al., 2002; Mundy et al., 1993). A study utilizing guided imagery and relaxation with 96 breast cancer patients indicated that those who utilized these techniques were more relaxed during chemotherapy and had a better quality of life, concluding that relaxation and guided imagery were "simple, inexpensive, and beneficial" for patients undergoing chemotherapy (Walker et al., 1999).

Deep breathing that focuses attention on the sensations of breathing, including rhythm and the rise and fall of the chest, is often used during progressive muscle-relaxation practices. In a pilot study of patients undergoing chemotherapy, Molassiotis and colleagues (2002) found that the experimental group receiving progressive muscle-relaxation had less duration and intensity of nausea. In another study, by Yoo et al. (2005), progressive muscle-relaxation and guided imagery for breast cancer patients found that those who received the training had less anticipatory nausea and post-chemotherapy nausea.

Hypnosis is a behavioral mind–body intervention process that involves focusing one's attention on thoughts or images unrelated to a source of distress (nausea and vomiting). The patient is guided to relax through a meditation-like state with suggestions of pleasant locations and or activities and states of calmness and wellbeing. Evidence suggests that self-hypnosis is effective in reducing the incidence of chemotherapy-induced and anticipatory nausea and vomiting and postsurgical nausea and vomiting in adults and children (Jacknow et al., 1994; Marchioro et al., 2000; Mundy et al., 1993; Richardson et al., 2007).

There are several meditation techniques used to relieve chemotherapy-related nausea and vomiting. However, there is no published evidence validating its effectiveness for nausea and vomiting. Although one unpublished dissertation suggests benefits from the use of a simple meditation intervention for anticipatory nausea, more studies are needed (Shapiro, 2011).

Simple paced deep-breathing can engage the relaxation response and is utilized in many meditative practice and relaxation exercises as a beginning focus. A study by Jokerst et al. (1999) suggests that slow, deep breathing can help control motion sickness, but again, more studies are needed on the effects of paced breathing for the treatment of nausea.

Music specialists often use music therapy with other behavioral techniques to engage the relaxation response. To date, research regarding the therapeutic effects of music therapy has been small and is limited to special groups (Tipton et al., 2007). Ezzone et al. (1998) found that listening to music helped relieve nausea and vomiting in individuals receiving cancer treatment. A study by Karagozoglu et al. (2012) found that music therapy and visual imagery had a positive effect on chemotherapy-induced anxiety, nausea, and vomiting.

Yoga may help individuals with cancer treatment by helping to relieve treatment-associated symptoms such as nausea, but further research is needed. A study of the effects of an integrated yoga program on chemotherapy-induced nausea and vomiting in 62 breast cancer patients utilized the Morrow Assessment of Nausea and Emesis scale (Raghavendra et al., 2007). The results of this study showed a noteworthy decrease in nausea frequency and intensity compared to the control group. There was also a meaningful decrease in anticipatory nausea and vomiting compared to the control group. The authors concluded that stress-reduction interventions such as yoga complement conventional antiemetic treatments (Raghavendra et al., 2007).

Energy-Based Therapies

Several energetic modalities open or balance these energy pathways in attempts to reduce nausea and vomiting. Acupressure and acupuncture are among those most commonly utilized for this purpose.

Stimulating the P6 (Pericardium 6) acupressure point has been shown to reduce postoperative nausea and vomiting (Lee & Done, 2004). The P6 acupressure point is located two finger-breadths above the first wrist crease (toward the elbow) in the center of the wrist between the tendons (Figure 17.2). Although it appears to be more effective in preventing vomiting than in reducing nausea, studies have shown that applying pressure to the P6 point can alleviate nausea in cases of motion sickness, morning sickness, surgery recovery, radiation, and chemotherapy (Lee & Done, 2004; Roscoe et al., 2009). In several trials, researchers used elastic wrist bands that apply pressure with plastic disks. A study by Dibble et al. (2007) of women undergoing chemotherapy for breast cancer found that acupressure applied to an acupuncture point with a wrist device was value-added by reducing the amount and intensity of delayed nausea and vomiting in addition to pharmaceutical management (Dibble et al., 2007).

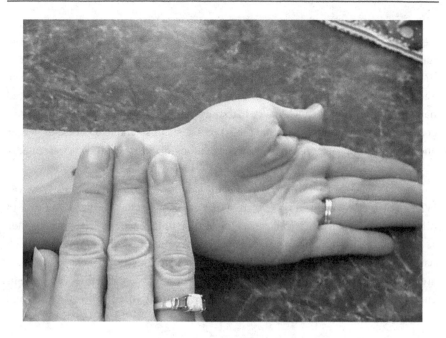

FIGURE 17.2 P6 Acupressure Point

In a Cochrane Review, Lee and Fan (2011) concluded that there was evidence for use of acupressure at the P6 acupoint to prevent postoperative nausea and vomiting.

Acupuncture is used to relieve nausea and vomiting, with several clinical trials evaluating the effectiveness of different acupuncture methods on nausea and vomiting caused by chemotherapy, surgery, and morning sickness (Streitberger et al., 2006). A study of patients treated with chemotherapy for ovarian cancer found that acupuncture and vitamin B₆ together gave more relief from vomiting than acupuncture or vitamin B₆ alone (You et al., 2009). Enblom et al. (2011) studied acupuncture for nausea and vomiting in patients undergoing radiation therapy, finding that those who received either true acupuncture or sham acupuncture developed less nausea and vomiting than those in the standard care group.

Reiki may help some cancer patients with pain management, relaxation, and side effects of treatment like nausea and stomach upset, although there is no evidence supporting its use and effectiveness for nausea. Danhauer et al. (2008) reported that Healing Touch performed on adult acute leukemia patients led to suggestive short-term improvements in fatigue and nausea.

Manipulative Therapies

Manipulative and body-based practices (e.g., massage and reflexology) focus primarily on interventions that affect the structures and systems of the body, such as the bones and joints, soft tissues, and circulatory system and lymphatic system.

Studies of the effect of massage on nausea symptoms in individuals receiving cancer treatment have reported promising results, but more evidence is needed. In a small, randomized study of massage in patients undergoing chemotherapy for breast cancer, the results indicated that massage lowered the incidence of nausea (Billhult et al., 2007). Tactile massage is recommended as adjunct therapy for severe pregnancy-induced nausea and vomiting (ACOG, 2004). In a study of foot reflexology for patients undergoing chemotherapy ($n = 34$), Yang (2005) reported considerable decrease in nausea and vomiting in the experimental group, concluding that further study is warranted.

Whole Medical Systems

Whole (alternative) medical systems are systems of care that have evolved over time in different cultures and apart from conventional allopathic practices. These may include several indigenous healing methods from Eastern and Western cultures. Although nausea has not been specifically studied, some specific Chinese herbal combinations are utilized for nausea and vomiting. In addition, homeopathic remedies (e.g., arsenicum album, ipecacuanha, and *nux vomica*) are currently used to treat nausea and vomiting.

PHARMACOLOGICAL INTERVENTIONS

Pharmacological interventions for nausea and vomiting are based on the type of nausea and/or vomiting and the potential causes. There is a range of options for prevention, management, and treatment of nausea and vomiting when conditions warrant their use. Antiemesis practice guidelines by the National Comprehensive Cancer Center (2007) "support the use of benzodiazepines such as alprazolam and lorazepam for anticipatory nausea and vomiting." In addition, "a 5-HT3 receptor antagonist such as granisetron and ondansetron or dolasetron; a corticosteroid such as dexamethasone; and aprepitant and a benzodiazepine are recommended for acute nausea and vomiting associated with moderately and highly emetogenic chemotherapy" (Tipton et al., 2007).

PATIENT SELF-CARE INTERVENTIONS

Engaging and coaching the patient in self-care interventions for nausea or anticipated nausea is invaluable and often utilized by integrative nurses. By engaging in self-care techniques, patients may feel a better sense of control over their symptoms. Several relaxation therapies (deep breathing, visualization, and meditation practices) can be taught to help them ease symptoms and cope with nausea. Encouraging patients to listen to music of their choice may also be beneficial. Family members can also be engaged in the planning by discussing some simple massage techniques for hands and feet and acupressure techniques with the P6 point. Safe use of aromatherapy can be discussed and oils sampled to determine which are pleasant.

Summary

Nausea is a common symptom associated with a wide variety of conditions that can be very unpleasant and debilitating and can lead to serious complications and increased healthcare cost. The integrative nurse is in the position to have an impact on the patient's experience of nausea, using whole-person/whole-systems assessment and interventions while considering evidence, safety, and patient preference when planning care. While the evidence for integrative therapies effective in the treatment of nausea and vomiting is growing, additional research and practice evaluations are needed.

SELECTED REFERENCES

Acalovschi, I. (2002). Postoperative nausea and vomiting. *Current Anaesthesia Critical Care, 13,* 37–43.

ASHP (1999). Therapeutic guidelines on the pharmacological management of nausea and vomiting in adult and pediatric patients receiving chemotherapy or radiation therapy or undergoing surgery. *American Journal of Health-System Pharmacy, 56,* 20–64. Retrieved April 8, 2012, from www.ashp.org/bestpractices.

Bloechl-Daum, B., Deuson, R. R., Marvos, P., et al. (2006). Delayed nausea and vomiting continue to reduce patient's quality of life after highly and moderately emetogenic chemotherapy despite antiemetic treatment. *Journal of Clinical Oncology, 24*(2), 4472–4478.

Duke, J. (2008). *The Green Pharmacy Guide to Healing Foods.* New York: Rodale.

Ernst, E., Pittler, & M. H. (2000). Efficacy of ginger for nausea and vomiting: A systematic review of randomized controlled trials. *British Journal of Anaesthesiology, 84,* 367–371.

Garrett, K., Tsuruta, K., Walker, S., Jackson, S., & Sweat, M. (2003). Managing nausea and vomiting. *Critical Care Nurse, 23*(1), 31–52.

Lau, P. L., & Salihan, N. (2012). A brief review of current scientific evidence involving aromatherapy use for nausea and vomiting. *Journal of Alternative and Complementary Medicine, 18*(6), 534–540.

Lee, A., & Fan, L. T. Y. (2011). P6 acupoint prevents post operative nausea and vomiting with few side effects. *Cochrane Summaries, 2.* Retrieved April 17, 2013, from http://summaries.cochrane.org/CD003281/p6-acupoint-stimulation-prevents-postoperative-nausea-and-vomiting-with-few-side-effects.

Walker, L. G., Walker, M. B., Ogston, K., Heys, S. D., Ah-See, A. K., Miller, I. D., et al. (1999, April). Psychological, clinical and pathological effects of relaxation training and guided imagery during primary chemotherapy. *British Journal of Cancer, 80*(1–2), 262–268.

Wood, J. M., Chapman, K., & Eilers, J. (2011). Tools for assessing nausea, vomiting and retching. *Cancer Nursing, 34*(1), 14–24.

18

Integrative Nursing Management of Sleep

NORMA G. CUELLAR

One-third of our life is spent in sleep. The importance of sleep, either too little or too much, is increasingly recognized as a contributor to health outcomes across the lifespan. The amount of time spent sleeping may be predisposed by genetics, environment, and cultural influences. According to the National Sleep Foundation, most adults sleep an average of seven hours per night, with 33.3% sleeping less (National Sleep Foundation [NSF], 2010). Up to 62% report having sleep problems at least twice per week, resulting in daytime sleepiness, which negatively affects daytime functioning in 43% of adults (Center for Disease Control, 2011).

Sleep problems result in increased dollars in national healthcare costs. Direct costs include visits to healthcare providers, hospital admissions, and pharmacological or sleep treatments. Indirect costs may include lost days of work related to sleep disorders, complications of the sleep disorder, and comorbid conditions that impact health outcomes (e.g., motor vehicle accidents, work-related accidents, hypertension, obesity, cancer, mental health disorders, etc.). Medicare payments alone for polysomnography increased from $62 million in 2001 to $235 million in 2009 (Office of Inspector General, 2010). Persons with sleep-disordered breathing (SDB) have 20% higher healthcare costs when symptoms of daytime sleepiness, insomnia, and insufficient sleep are reported (Kapur & Friedman, 2002; Kapur et al., 2002). The lost work performance in persons with insomnia is equivalent to 11.3 days of work per year, with an estimated loss of $2,280 per employee, an estimate of $63.2 billion dollars lost per year due to insomnia (Kessler et al., 2011).

What Is Sleep?

Sleep is a neurobiological need with a circadian cycle that includes both sleep and wakefulness. The transition from sleep to wakefulness is measured by cortical activity. Sleep is identified by (a) brain wave activity using electro-encephalogram (EEG), (b) eye movements using electro-oculography (EOG), and (c) muscle tone using electromyography (EMG). These measurements distinguish sleep from coma and anesthesia and can be measured with polysomnography (PSG) (Landis, 2011).

Sleep architecture follows a pattern of alternating REM (rapid eye movement) and NREM (non-rapid eye movement) sleep throughout a typical night. During sleep, phases are identified as "stages of sleep," previously known as the "four stages of sleep" or REM vs. non-REM (NREM) sleep. Stages three and four of NREM sleep are now combined into a single stage of sleep referred to as "deep sleep." The cycle through these stages occurs every 90 minutes; time spent in REM sleep increases throughout the night. The sleep-wake cycle is a complicated neurobiological response to maintain arousal of the cortex of the brain, involving a cascade of neurotransmitters, neuro-peptides, and primary signaling mechanisms (Arrigoni & Fuller, 2012; Bianchi, 2012). Characteristics of REM and NREM sleep are identified in Table 18.1.

CONSEQUENCES OF POOR SLEEP

Lack of sleep is reported as a restriction of sleep, an interruption of sleep, or frag-mented sleep. While one night of sleep loss results in short-term sleepiness, habitual sleep restriction (up to two hours/night) leads to chronic sleepiness, which is linked with increasing morbidity and mortality in obesity, diabetes, cardiovascular disease, depression, substance abuse, and cognitive performance (Buxton & Marcelli, 2010; Knutson, Spiegel, Penev, & Van Cauter, 2007; Sabanayagam & Shankar, 2010; Tucker, Marquie, Folkard, Ansiau, & Esquirol, 2012; Kronholm et al., 2011; Park et al., 2012).

Table 18.1: Characteristics of NREM and REM Sleep

Non-REM Sleep (75% of sleep time)	REM Sleep (25% of sleep time)
Stage 1 (N1) Transitional state between being awake and falling asleep Light sleep lasting a few minutes	Surge of sympathetic activity resulting in an increase in pulse, blood pressure, and body temperature Provides energy to brain and body
Stage 2 (N2) Onset of sleep Most of sleep time is in this stage Sleeper becomes disengaged from surroundings Breathing and heart rate are regular Body temperature drops (so sleeping in a cool room is helpful)	Muscle atonia: body becomes immobile and relaxed, as muscles are turned off Brain is active and dreams occur: resembles waking period Eyes dart back and forth
Stage 3 (N3) Slow Wave Sleep Deepest and most restorative sleep Blood pressure drops Breathing becomes slower Muscles are relaxed Blood supply to muscles increases Tissue growth and repair occurs Energy is restored Hormones are released	

In addition, quality and quantity of work is diminished in sleepy employees. Davis (2012) reported that 28% of respondents in a recent survey missed work, social events and activities, and had increased workplace errors because of poor sleep. As well, 22% of people who were late for work said it was because of sleepiness. Daytime sleepiness interferes with concentration and handling stress in 68% of adults (NSP, 2005).

More importantly, 51% of adults report they drive when drowsy, resulting in 100,000 car crashes annually. The National Department of Transportation estimates drowsy driving to be responsible for over 1,000 fatalities and 40,000 nonfatal injuries annually in the United States (National Highway Traffic Safety Administration, 2011). The dangers posed by drowsy driving are found to be as great as those of drunk driving (Blazejewski et al., 2012). Lack of sleep has been correlated not only with motor vehicle accidents but with industrial disasters and occupational errors.

Healthcare providers who get less sleep and work long hours are more likely to make errors in judgment and decision-making processes, resulting in detrimental outcomes for patients (Lombardi et al., 2012; Tucker et al., 2012; Wehrens, Hampton, Kerkhofs, & Skene, 2012; Wright, Bogan, & Wyatt, 2012). Studies of nurses have also shown that long shifts (12 hours or more) cause insufficient sleep. If nurses are scheduled for long hours consistently, the lack of sleep places not only the patients' health at risk but nurses' health as well (Rogers, Hwang, Scott, Aiken, & Dinges, 2004). When rotating shifts, sleepiness is associated with alcohol use, caffeine, poorer health status, poor hygiene, use of sleep aids, and low job satisfaction (Dorrian et al., 2011).

Sleep Requirements

It is difficult to distinguish between "normal" and "abnormal" sleep. Sleep requirements over the lifespan are based on maturational and chronological changes in the body systems as well as the environment, culture, genetics, and racial/ethnic and sociocultural issues (Baldwin, 2011; Minarik, 2011). A health-disparity issue exists when comparing sleep among different populations. The 2010 Sleep in America poll focused on racial and ethnic differences of sleep (NSP, 2010). Whites are more likely to be assessed and diagnosed for sleep problems by the healthcare provider than any other ethnic or racial cohort.

Sleep problems in women may be more prevalent due to hormonal changes over the lifespan (Nordin, Knutsson, Sundbom, & Stegmayr, 2005). The 2007 Sleep in America poll found that women's sleep was affected by menstruation, pregnancy, post-partum status, perimenopause, and postmenopause (National Sleep Foundation, 2007). Women have also a higher likelihood of interrupted sleep throughout the lifespan based on societal norms for caregiving of young children and parents (Burgard & Huges, 2010).

Factors that affect sleep include normative values, roles, expectations, education, work patterns, living arrangements, and parenting styles (related to children's sleep patterns). In summation, sleep requirements vary across the lifespan—newborns sleep approximately two-thirds of the day, children and adolescents require up to twelve hours of sleep per night, and adults sleep seven to eight hours each night, with older adults needing 6.5 hours a day (Redeker, 2011; Ohayon, Carskadon, Guilleminault, & Vitiello, 2004). Sleep disorders fall into four main categories: (a) problems with falling and staying asleep, (b) problems with staying awake or sleeping at inappropriate times, (c) problems with adhering to a regular sleep schedule, i.e. excessive sleep times, and (d) abnormal behaviors associated with sleep.

An Integrative Nursing Approach to Sleep

An integrative, comprehensive approach to improved sleep health outcomes advances the health and wellbeing of persons, families, and communities. Sleep wellness should be the focus for all healthcare providers in order to maintain optimal health and prevent the development of sleep problems. Goals of a good sleep intervention should be subjectively stated by the patient, with the intention that they have improved and restorative sleep. It is important to refer a patient to a sleep specialist if it is suspected that a sleep problem or a disorder exists.

Integrative nurses recognize that the complexity of a person's life and circumstances often affects his or her day-to-day patterns, including sleep. This is particularly true for women who are trying to balance children, aging parents, homes, and jobs. By carefully listening to the patient's story and conducting a complete sleep history, the nurse focuses on a multitude of factors that might play a role in interrupted or poor sleep, rather than immediately assuming that altered sleep requires a more intensive assessment and laboratory testing (Principles 1 & 2). The integrative nurse begins her recommendations by talking with Mrs. Little about ways that nature reminds our bodies about the rhythms of life (the setting sun, the cool breezes of the evening, the

Case Scenario

Mrs. Little is a 43-year-old married woman who has teenage children and is caring for her mother in her home. She is a product of the "sandwiched generation." She comes to the integrative nurse with complaints of feeling tired and having problems sleeping. She reports her children are involved in various activities, and they come and go. Her mother, while fairly independent, often awakens her when she gets up during the night. Her husband often keeps her up at night while watching TV in their bedroom. She estimates that, on the average, she is sleeping about six hours a night, but that sleep is often interrupted.

Integrative Nursing Care

The integrative nurse listens carefully to Mrs. Little's concerns about her sleep disruptions. During the assessment, the integrative nurse determines Mrs. Little's sleep history, conducts a physical assessment, and inquires about any medical conditions that may be causing sleep problems. After determining that Mrs. Little does not have physical problems (e.g., hypertension, diabetes, etc.), the integrative nurse discusses different ways to improve sleep based on improving her sleep hygiene, and environmental modifications. She suggests that Mrs. Little try lowering the lights as evening progresses, cooling the temperatures of the living and then bedroom areas, and decreasing use of electronic devices to evoke the tendencies found in nature that slow the body rhythms. They discuss what Mrs. Little typically eats and drinks throughout the day, with recommendations to switch from iced tea beginning at noon each day. Recognizing that televisions or any equipment in the bedroom (cell phones, clocks with lights) can often disrupt sleep patterns, they talk about alternatives that include taking a warm bath with low lights or candles while her husband watches that last television program. The nurse talks to her about sleep disruptions during the night, recommending that if she does awaken that she might think about having a small snack and returning to bed as quickly as possible without turning on the lights. Together, they decide to try these suggestions before any further evaluation or treatment, including sleep remedies.

softening of sounds) and the way that nature signals it is time to rest and restore ourselves (Principle 3). Recommendations also include methods to alter stimulants during the day (caffeine) or in the bedroom at night (artificial lighting), preferring to remove barriers to sleep rather than adding medications or natural products that induce sleep (Principle 5). The integrative nurse recognizes how important Mrs. Little's relationships are, recommending ways to minimize the disruption (light snack, keeping the lights off if rising) if her mother or children waken her during the night (Principle 4). This example shows how the integrative nurse provided care that recognizes the uniqueness of the individual, offering specific ways Mrs. Little could alter her environment to encourage rest, relaxation, and peaceful sleep.

Assessment of Sleep

An integrative approach to a sleep assessment can improve health outcomes related to not only sleep but other comorbidities. While doing a physical assessment, the integrative nurse should be sensitive to the cues that the patient may not be getting sleep, including symptoms of fatigue, anxiety, and depression. Healthcare providers should be aware of the adverse consequences of poor sleep and the effects on health outcomes, although sleep disorders often go undiagnosed or mistreated. Components of an integrated sleep assessment include a sleep history with a medication review, physical examination and laboratory/diagnostic findings.

SLEEP HISTORY

Patients who have sleep problems will complain about poor sleep quality, disrupted or fragmented sleep, frequent awakenings during the night, short sleep duration, or sleep episodes throughout the day. Any of these complaints requires further assessment (Ward, 2011). Healthcare providers may also ask about assistive devices used for sleep as well as sleep and lifestyle habits.

Many healthcare providers use the BEARS instrument (Bedtimes problems, Excessive sleepiness, Awakenings, Regularity of sleep, and Sleep-disordered breathing) to organize a thorough sleep assessment with both pediatric and adult populations (Lee & Ward, 2005). The physical exam will provide information about other medical or psychiatric health conditions that may interfere with sleep.

Many medications may have side effects that result in sleep problems, so patients should be queried about antidepressants, steroids, stimulants, and beta blockers as well as over-the-counter medications that can affect sleep patterns. Psychiatric conditions are often treated with medications that affect sleep or exacerbate symptoms of sleep disturbances, such as dopamine antagonists in restless leg syndrome (RLS) (Cuellar, 2012).

PHYSICAL EXAM

A good physical exam should include information about the patient's general health, including any physical and mental health conditions that can impact sleep. Also, health conditions that are identified with sleep problems (e.g., heart disease, hypertension, congestive heart failure, diabetes, Parkinson's disease, pain, depression, or anxiety) should be a red flag that a sleep problem may exist. Any patient with obesity should also be considered at high risk for a sleep disorder (e.g., obstructive sleep apnea) and head, neck, and oral cavity should be carefully examined.

LABORATORY/DIAGNOSTIC FINDINGS

Laboratory findings rule out any condition that can be treated that may cause sleep problems, including electrolyte imbalances, thyroid disease, or diabetes. An electrocardiography may provide information on an enlarged heart or dysrhythmias that may be seen in sleep disorders. Pulmonary function tests may identify measures of oxygenation when identifying sleep-disordered breathing.

SLEEP MEASURES

Sleep measures (subjective and objective) may be used to evaluate patterns of sleep. Subjective sleep measures include self-reports using a sleep diary, or questionnaires that identify sleep patterns. A sleep diary is used to accurately describe a variety of sleep patterns (e.g., time the individual went to sleep, time in bed, number of awakenings, time of awakenings) established over time that can provide the healthcare provider sleep characteristics of the patient. A variety of questionnaires are also available and can facilitate identification of sleep disorders in both children and adults. These questionnaires are often in English, and translation to other languages poses limitations in non-English speaking populations. Questionnaires are available for general sleep problems as well as for specific sleep disorders (e.g., sleep apnea, RLS, insomnia). Objective sleep measures include polysomnography (PSG), actigraphy, multiple sleep latency test, maintenance of wakefulness test, and the suggested immobility test (SIT). A description of these measures can be found in Table 18.2.

Table 18.2: Objective Measures of Sleep

Polysomnography (PSG)	• Gold standard for sleep measurement done in a sleep laboratory • Measures EEG, EOG, and EMG to determine phases of sleep and sleep patterns • Measures obtained: airflow, respiratory rate, and oxygen saturations are measured coinciding with an electrocardiogram, leg movements, seizure activity and other physiological variables are obtained • Diagnose sleep-related breathing disorder, narcolepsy, periodic limb movements in sleep, nocturnal seizures • Is not required for all sleep disorders
Actigraphy	• An electronic accelerometer used to record motion • Reliable and valid sleep measure to estimate sleep patterns • Worn on the wrist or legs • Records over several nights at a reasonable cost
The Multiple Sleep Latency Test (MSLT)	• Determines the propensity to fall asleep during the day (narcolepsy) as well as a measure of daytime sleepiness
The Maintenance of Wakefulness Test (MWT)	• Measures daytime sleepiness and the ability to stay awake in a quiet, non-stimulating environment.
Suggested Immobilization Test (SIT)	• Measures activity and discomfort while the patient with RLS sits in an inclined position with legs elevated; used to diagnose RLS

Integrative Sleep Interventions

Integrative healthcare provides a comprehensive approach to advance the health and wellbeing of patients, families, and communities by improving sleep health outcomes. Sleep wellness should be the focus for all healthcare providers in order to maintain optimal health and wellbeing.

Sleep health is not measured by hours of sleep. Priority care should be given to patients who have other comorbid conditions and complain of sleep disruption, as the two can aggravate each other with escalating symptoms. Also, anyone with mental health issues and sleep problems may present unique issues related to treatment. Sleep is often disrupted as we age and should not be minimized. Specific interventions to improve sleep may vary depending on the degree of sleep disruption and the condition of the patient, but sleep disorders should be approached using the least intensive and invasive treatment appropriate to the situation (Table 18.3).

First-line interventions include independent activities that will improve sleep. Sleep hygiene (Table 18.4) and environmental changes that mimic natural light/dark and day/night patterning are the first steps in treating sleep complaints.

In addition, mindfulness meditation has been shown to improve biomarkers of stress and has been effective in the treatment of sleep problems across the lifespan (Brand, Holsboer-Trachsler, Naranjo, & Schmidt, 2012; Gross et al., 2011; Ong, Shapiro, & Manber, 2009; Ong & Manber, 2011; Yook et al., 2008). Yoga improves the stimulatory effect on the nervous system, increasing circulation and enhancing relaxation and sleep through deep breathing (Kudesia & Bianchi, 2012; Afonso et al., 2012; Taibi & Vitiello, 2011). Evidence indicates that aromatherapy improves quality of sleep in cardiac patients (Moeini, Khadibi, Bekhradi, Mahmoudian, & Nazari, 2010) and healthy individuals across the lifespan (Field et al., 2008; O'Flaherty et al., 2012; Lee & Lee, 2006; Moeini et al., 2010). Lavender is one botanical agent that has been used to promote sleep. More recently, studies have shown that lavender may in fact improve sleepiness and quality of sleep (Hirokawa, Nishimoto, & Taniguchi, 2012).

If these interventions do not result in improved quality of sleep, the integrative nurse may consider a variety of natural products or herbs, including valerian (*Valeriana officinalis*), hops (*Humulus lupulus*), chamomile (*Chamaemelum nobile*), lemon balm (*Melissa officinalis*), skullcap (*Scutellaria baicalensis*), Indian pipe (*Monotropa uniflora*), and snake root (*Ageratina adenophora*). Other nutritional supplements that have been shown to help sleep include tryptophan, 5-Hydroxytryptophan (5-HTP), magnesium, and vitamin K. Caution should always be used when recommending any of these natural products because of their potential interactions with other medications or alcohol.

While melatonin and valerian are often cited to remedy sleep alterations, they have not been shown to be effective in clinical trials. Melatonin, often referred to as an herbal supplement, is perhaps one of the most common over-the-counter medications

Table 18.3: Interventions for Sleep

Level of Intensity	Integrative Therapy Approach
Tier 1 Interventions	**Basic Foundational Integrative Nursing Therapies** • Sleep hygiene measures **Environmental Modifications** • Lowering lights as the evening progresses • Reducing artificial stimuli • Cooling the environment **Mind-Body Therapies** • Meditation (Mindfulness and others) • Reiki **Movement Therapies** • Yoga **Natural Products** • Aromatherapy
Tier 2 Interventions	**Natural Products/Herbs** • Valerian (*Valeriana officinalis*) • Hops (*Humulus lupulus*) • Chamomile (*Chamaemelum nobile*) • Melatonin • Lemon Balm (*Melissa officinalis*) • Skullcap (*Scutellaria baicalensis*) • Indian Pipe (*Monotropa uniflora*) • Snake Root (*Ageratina adenophora*) • Suan Zao Ren Tang (SZRT) **Natural Products/Supplements** • Tryptophan • 5-Hydroxytryptophan (5-HTP) • Magnesium **Mind/Body Therapies** • Cognitive Behavior Therapy • Music Therapy • Self-Hypnosis • Biofeedback **Energy Therapies** • Therapeutic Touch **Movement Therapies** • Qi Gong • Tai Chi
Tier 3 Interventions	**Mind-Body Therapies** • Hypnosis **Manipulative Therapies** • Massage • Osteopathy • Craniosacral Therapy • Reflexology **Energy Therapies** • Acupuncture/Pressure • Light Therapy **Over-the-Counter Medications** • Diphenhydramine (Benadryl)
Tier 4 Interventions	**Whole Systems** • Chinese Medicine • Ayurvedic Medicine • Naturopathy • Homeopathy

Table 18.3: (Continued)

Level of Intensity	Integrative Therapy Approach
Tier 5 Interventions	**Pharmacological Therapies** • Benzodiazepines • Non-benzodiazepines • Melatonin Receptor Agonists • Hypnotics • Barbiturates • Anti-depressants • GABA-A Receptors **Sleep Lab and Sleep Studies**

Table 18.4: Sleep Hygiene Recommendations

Go to bed when sleepy.	If you lie in bed for longer than 30 minutes without going to sleep, get up and then come back to bed later.
Develop your own sleep rituals.	Do the same thing every night before you go to bed to signal your body that you are preparing to sleep.
Don't take your worries to bed.	If you worry, set a time in your day to worry and then quit worrying. "I am going to do all my worrying from 6 p.m. to 8 p.m., and then I am going to let it go!"
Eat a light snack before bedtime.	Light snack: warm milk, bananas, turkey—foods that may induce sleep. No heavy meals or spicy food before bedtime.
Avoid caffeine, nicotine, and alcohol at least 4–6 hours before bedtime.	Avoid these foods completely if you have problems with sleep. Alcohol may induce sleep, but it disrupts sleep architecture, fragmenting patterns throughout the night.
Get up and go to bed at the same time every night, including weekends.	Set your body to a schedule and do not disrupt it.
Do not nap if you have trouble sleeping at night.	Napping may cause sleep disruptions during the night.
Determine the best time to exercise for you.	Rigorous exercise should be done early in the day. Refrain from exercising right before bedtime if you cannot sleep.
Use the bed for sex and sleep only.	Condition your mind that the bed is a time for the Two S's. Do not watch TV, eat, or read in bed.
Make your sleep environment comfortable.	Make sure your bedroom is dark, quiet, and cool. The mattress should be in good condition, the sleep area is clean, the linen is clean. Use earplugs or eye shades if needed.
Before going to bed, try relaxation techniques.	Hot bath, deep breathing, yoga, or meditation may help induce sleepiness.
Do not watch the clock.	Get up if you are in bed for longer than 30 minutes and unable to sleep. If possible, remove clocks from the room.
Sleep on your side if you snore.	Lying on your back can occlude your airway, thereby causing snoring and decreasing oxygenation, interrupting sleep.
Avoid sleeping pills and other sedatives.	Long-term use is addictive. Some medications may actually disrupt sleep architecture.
Lose weight if your BMI is >25.	Being overweight may cause difficulty in breathing, thereby interrupting sleep.

used for sleep. Melatonin is an endogenous neurohormone produced by the pineal gland. Studies have shown that melatonin may reset the "circadian clock" and is helpful in persons who do shift work or who travel and cross time zones when the sleep–wake cycle has been disturbed. However, Buscemi et al. (2006) cited no evidence that melatonin had any effect on improving sleep latency or sleep restriction from jet lag or shift work in a recent meta-analysis. The long-term effects of the use of melatonin for disrupted sleep have not been reported (Bellon, 2006).

Valerian is a common herb used to treat anxiety and improve sleep widely used in Europe. However, several systematic reviews consistently report that valerian has not been effective in treating sleep disorders (Bent, Padula, Moore, Patterson, & Mehling, 2006; Stevinson & Ernst, 2000; Taibi, Landis, Petry, & Vitiello, 2007). These findings may be due to the dosage variations (800 mg. or less in clinical trials, versus up to 2000 mg/day in traditional settings) or length of trials. Recently, studies have reported decreased daytime sleepiness in a study of individuals with RLS (Cuellar & Ratcliffe, 2009) and improved sleep quality for patients in ICU (Chen, Chao, Lu, Shiung, & Chao, 2012).

Passionflower and chamomile are two herbs that are often used with other supplements to promote relaxation and sleep (Krenn, 2002). Short-term benefits of sleep quality were reported in healthy adults who used passionflower in a tea (Ngan & Conduit, 2011). In Chinese medicine, the herbal supplement *suan zao ren tang* (SZRT) was shown to improve sleep quality in postmenopausal women (Yeh, Arnold, Chen, & Lai, 2011).

Overall, studies of massage therapy show positive results on sleep quality and sleep time (Castro-Sanchez et al., 2011; MacCune, 2010; Oliveira, Hachul, Tufik, & Bittencourt, 2011). Li et al. (2011) reported benefits from the use of reflexology to improve sleep quality in postpartum women. A meta-analysis examining the use of reflexology on sleep ($n = 18$), fatigue ($n = 15$), and pain ($n = 11$) reported that reflexology is a safe intervention that is effective for the treatment of sleep, fatigue, and pain (Lee, Han, Chung, Kim, & Choi, 2011).

There are mixed results linking acupuncture and traditional Chinese medicine to sleep improvements. A 2011 overview of ten systematic reviews from 2003 to 2010 examined the use of acupuncture for insomnia (Ernst, Lee, & Choi, 2011). Despite the fact that some of the studies found positive associations between acupuncture and insomnia, the overall review could not assume the same findings because many of the studies were of poor methodological quality. However, Reza et al. (2010) reported that older adults with insomnia residing in a long-term care facility showed improvement in symptoms with acupressure at the Shenmen Point (indexed at HT7) at five weeks and post-treatment.

Pharmacological interventions are reserved for ongoing, unremitting sleep disturbances. These agents require ongoing reevaluation and monitoring because of their complications and side effects as well as their addictive properties.

Evaluation of Sleep Outcomes

Symptoms of sleep disorders should be reevaluated within one to three months of any intervention. Baseline data should be compared following treatment, and include laboratory values, sleep diaries, and self-reports of sleep. The healthcare provider should never assume that the sleep problem has been resolved, because patients often do not understand the impact of sleep on health outcomes. In older adults, sleep complaints are often ignored; McCoy (2007) reported that sleep complaints are only discussed 19% of the time during a healthcare provider's visit.

Summary

This chapter provides a foundation of understanding for facilitating restful, high-quality sleep. Often underemphasized, adequate sleep is a necessary component of a healthy lifestyle. Sleep problems have been linked to a wide variety of chronic illnesses, workplace safety issues, and increased healthcare costs. The integrative approach considers all of the factors associated with poor sleep and individually structures an intervention plan that mitigates impediments to sleep (light, noise, stimulants) and modifies the environment so as to encourage sleep (cool environment, sleep routines). These are interventions that may be overlooked yet are relatively easy to use. Individual and collective wellbeing depends on a well-rested population, something that is difficult to achieve in the overly stimulating, constantly-in-contact world that we live in.

SELECTED REFERENCES

Arrigoni, E., & Fuller, P. (2012). An overview of sleep: Physiology and neuroanatomy. In T. Barkoukis, J. Matheson, R. Ferber, & K. Doghramji (Eds.), *Therapy in Sleep Medicine* (1st ed., pp. 43–61). Philadelphia, PA: Elsevier Saunders.

Brand, S., Holsboer-Trachsler, E., Naranjo, J. R., & Schmidt, S. (2012). Influence of mindfulness practice on cortisol and sleep in long-term and short-term meditators. *Neuropsychobiology*, 65(3), 109–118. doi:10.1159/000330362

Castro-Sanchez, A. M., Mataran-Penarrocha, G. A., Granero-Molina, J., Aguilera-Manrique, G., Quesada-Rubio, J. M., & Moreno-Lorenzo, C. (2011). Benefits of massage-myofascial release therapy on pain, anxiety, quality of sleep, depression, and quality of life in patients with fibromyalgia. *Evidence-Based Complementary and Alternative Medicine: ECAM, 2011*, 561753. doi:10.1155/2011/561753

Ernst, E., Lee, M. S., & Choi, T. Y. (2011). Acupuncture for insomnia? An overview of systematic reviews. *European Journal of General Practice*, 17(2), 116–123. doi:10.3109/13814788.2011.568475

Knutson, K. L., Spiegel, K., Penev, P., & Van Cauter, E. (2007). The metabolic consequences of sleep deprivation [*see comment*]. *Sleep Medicine Reviews*, 11(3), 163–178.

Landis, C. A. (2011). Physiological and behavioral aspects of sleep. In N. Redeker & G. Phillips-McEnanym (Eds.), *Sleep Disorders and Sleep Promotion in Nursing Practice* (pp. 1–18). New York: Springer.

Minarik, P. (2011). Gender and sleep. In N. Redeker, & G. McEnany (Eds.), *Sleep Disorders and Sleep Promotion in Nursing Practice* (1st ed., pp. 33–42). New York: Springer Publishing Company.

Ong, J., & Sholtes, D. (2010). A mindfulness-based approach to the treatment of insomnia. *Journal of Clinical Psychology, 66*(11), 1175–1184.

Taibi, D. M., Landis, C. A., Petry, H., & Vitiello, M. V. (2007). A systematic review of valerian as a sleep aid: Safe but not effective. *Sleep Medicine Reviews, 11*(3), 209–230.

Ward, T. (2011). Conducting a sleep assessment. In N. Redeker, & G. McEnany (Eds.), *Sleep Disorders and Sleep Promotion in Nursing Practice* (pp. 53–72). New York: Springer Publishing Company.

19

Integrative Nursing Management of Anxiety

LINDA L. CHLAN AND MELINDA BORS

Anxiety is a state marked by apprehension, agitation, increased motor tension or activity, autonomic arousal, and fearful withdrawal (McCartney & Boland, 1994). The Psychology Lexicon (www.psychology-lexicon.com) defines *state anxiety* as a sense of apprehension and fear often marked by physical symptoms (such as sweating, tension, and increased heart rate). Anxiety can express itself in various ways, including having trouble falling asleep; dwelling on a particular situation and finding it difficult to think of something else; feeling tense, restless, jittery, dizzy, and sweaty; having trouble concentrating; appetite changes; being overly vigilant and startling easily; having a feeling of impending disaster, as if "something bad is going to happen;" or feeling depressed (anxiety can mask depression). Anxiety is an emotional response to a threat or danger (DeMarco et al., 2011). State anxiety is that which changes readily and is amenable to intervention. Contrastingly, *trait anxiety* refers to a personality characteristic that manifests itself as a more or less constant feeling of dread or uneasiness.

Anxiety can be experienced in any situation and in any setting in which there is a perceived threat or danger. Therefore, it is not possible to report incidence statistics. From a psychiatric perspective, *generalized anxiety disorder* (GAD) is characterized by persistent and uncontrollable worry (for more than six months) and includes symptoms such as restlessness, fatigue, difficulty concentrating, and somatic signs (heart palpitations, muscular tension, dizziness, respiratory distress, sweating, hyperthermia) (American Psychiatric Association, 2000). The lifetime prevalence of GAD is approximately 5% (American Psychiatric Association). This chapter will focus on how a nurse practicing from the viewpoint of integrative nursing can empower persons to self-manage their anxiety or implement integrative interventions to ameliorate anxiety.

It is important for integrative nurses to manage anxiety or provide self-care strategies for patients, as there are physiological and psychological consequences of sustained anxiety in various adult populations. Persistent anxiety symptoms that do not meet the criteria for GAD are still associated with serious negative consequences, such as sleep disturbances, interferences with daily activities, and distress (Thorp et al., 2009, p. 105). In the elderly, anxiety symptoms are associated with medical illnesses, such as coronary heart disease, self-reported mobility limitations, and higher levels of healthcare utilization. Evidence implicates anxiety in the development of heart disease in both men and women (Tacon et al., 2003). Distress-induced atherosclerosis and endothelial dysfunction support the hypothesis that anxiety plays a role in the onset of coronary heart disease.

Anxiety experienced with diagnostic or screening procedures can hamper successful completion of the exam, increase the length of the exam, or induce undue distress in patients, thus affecting future compliance with screening adherence recommendations. Medications such as benzodiazepines and opioids are typically administered in these situations, but these agents can cause serious side effects, including respiratory depression and delayed recovery after the procedure. Approaching anxiety from an integrative nursing perspective can play a central role in reducing the amount of medication needed to safely and successfully complete screening and diagnostic procedures, such as colonoscopy screening and needle-biopsy procedures.

This chapter will present information on assessment tools for anxiety, including both self-report instruments and physiological correlates of anxiety with both indirect markers and direct biomarkers. A review of current research will be discussed, highlighting specific therapies and modalities that a nurse may choose to implement to manage anxiety or promote anxiety self-management in selected patient populations. The processes a nurse practicing from an integrative perspective can implement to optimize the health and wellbeing of persons by selecting appropriate interventions to manage anxiety will be addressed.

An Integrative Nursing Approach to Anxiety

The principles of integrative nursing inform the care of persons experiencing anxiety and its effects on their health and wellbeing. When working with anxious patients, the integrative nurse seeks interventions that offer long-term calming solutions and ways to mitigate returning bouts of anxiety through self-care and self-management. Consider the following case scenario.

Case Scenario

Martha Collins is a 74-year-old woman who is being followed in an outpatient pulmonary clinic for the management of her pulmonary fibrosis. Mrs. Collins's pulmonary function tests are severely compromised, and she is required to be on supplemental oxygen therapy with activity. She tells the clinician that she sometimes gets anxious about going out in public and taking part in some of her favorite interests, such as going to church or to the semi-annual quilting retreat. Upon further questioning, the clinician learns that Mrs. Collins's anxiety is related to how she perceives others might view her because of her need for supplemental oxygen therapy. She states that she knows this is an irrational source of anxiety as it should not matter to her what others think, and she wishes she could just "get over it." She confides that she is not sure how to best manage these feelings of anxiety.

Integrative Nursing Care

After listening to Mrs. Collins describe her anxiety, the clinician validates her feelings and reassures her that it is not irrational for her to be experiencing symptoms of anxiety. After mentally reviewing some of the integrative interventions for managing symptoms of anxiety, the clinician rules out the movement-based therapies, as performing these interventions will require Mrs. Collins to use her portable oxygen unit and thus might create increased feelings of anxiety.

After reviewing some of the literature on integrative interventions, the clinician concludes that mind/body-based therapies are non-invasive and suggests that meditation might prove beneficial to Mrs. Collins. The clinician asks her if she is familiar with what resources are near her home. Mrs. Collins replies that a Yoga Soul Center near her home offers classes in meditation without the yoga movements. She is particularly interested in a class that is offered outside on a patio surrounded by a beautiful garden. Since it is early spring, she thinks that this is a perfect setting to begin trying a new way to manage her anxiety. She says that she has a few books at home on meditation that she has been meaning to read, but has not yet gotten around to doing so. Mrs. Collins seems eager to explore this as a possibility, but states that she would first like to learn more about meditation and what it entails.

Mrs. Collins and the clinician formulate a plan for her to familiarize herself with meditation and decide if it is something that she would be comfortable trying. Her follow-up clinic appointment is in one month, which will give her enough time to read through some of her books on meditation. She will also stop by the Yoga Soul Center and speak to some of the meditation instructors about the classes that they offer and how much they cost. At her follow-up visit, the clinician will review with Mrs. Collins what she has learned about meditation and will assess her comfort level in moving forward with meditation program. The clinician will check in with Ms. Collins at future visits to determine if she was able to initiate a meditation program and to assess its effectiveness in reducing her symptoms of anxiety.

The first step when helping someone manage their anxiety is to take inventory, helping the patient identify potential sources of anxiety (Principle 4). Often, sources of anxiety can be found within the person's environment; listening to their fears, concerns, and interpretations facilitates understanding of the person–environment interplay in the anxiety (Principle 1). Once the assessment has uncovered possible sources of stress and the patient's goals for treatment, interventions should be tailored to individual patient preferences and abilities; one size does not fit all! In this case, movement therapies, often found effective in reducing anxiety, are excluded from the plan of care, given Mrs. Collins' oxygen requirements and the limitations that this would impose on the intervention (Principle 4).

Working to identify an amenable solution, the integrative nurse and Mrs. Collins identified a number of plausible interventions and modalities that have been linked to reduced anxiety, selecting meditation as a beginning place for self-management. Mrs. Collins is interested in this type of therapy, stating that this meets her needs and her preferences, while the nurse knows that there is evidence supporting its use (Principle 5). The nurse also takes the time to discuss why Mrs. Collins might be particularly drawn to outdoor classes, noting that nature offers a calming exterior environment that is mirrored internally (Principle 3). During follow-up visits, the integrative nurse will use her time to coach Mrs. Collins to practice anxiety self-management by recognizing the triggers that increase anxiety throughout her day. The nurse encourages Mrs. Collins to keep a diary, noting what specific activities, meditations, and setting are most effective for anxiety self-management and what does not seem to alleviate her anxiety (Principle 2).

Assessment of Anxiety

Because there are both physiological and psychological components to the experience of anxiety, it is important to consider anxiety as a whole-person/whole-system phenomenon when completing an anxiety assessment. A comprehensive approach helps the integrative nurse appropriately plan and implement interventions and determine the effectiveness of those interventions. A complicating factor in reviewing the literature is that anxiety is interrelated with other symptoms, such as stress, distress, dyspnea, and pain, which can make assessment a challenge. For example, depression and anxiety are frequently co-occurring symptoms in many patient populations such as women with a cancer diagnosis; women with both depression and anxiety are more likely to use integrative interventions (Eschiti, 2008). Likewise, perceived tension can be manifested physiologically in some persons as a feeling of anxiety.

Thus, it is critically important to select appropriate assessment methods and measures. First, there needs to be a clear definition of terms and a clear conceptualization of anxiety. This section will highlight some of the more commonly used measurement instruments and variables, including self-report (which is crucial to a patient-centered approach), physiological indicators, and biomarkers.

PSYCHOLOGICAL MEASURES

Self-report of anxiety includes a number of paper and pencil instruments with which individuals report their current feelings or how they usually feel. Many of the self-report instruments consist of a certain number of items with a specific response format, such as a Likert scale, that requires the respondent to indicate his/her response using a 4- or 5-point scale ranging from "not at all" to "very much so." A higher score is indicative of higher anxiety levels.

One self-report anxiety instrument is the Spielberger State-Trait Anxiety Inventory (STAI). It is one of the most widely used anxiety assessment instruments in research and practice; it contains both state and trait scales. "State anxiety" refers to how one feels as the present moment, while "trait anxiety" refers to how one generally feels. State anxiety is thought to be amenable to intervention, whereas trait anxiety is a personality trait that contributes to how an individual experiences and perceives anxiety. The STAI is a copyrighted instrument that is available for purchase, including translation in several languages; a shortened version is available to reduce respondent burden (at www.mindgarden.com).

While the Spielberger STAI may be one of the most widely used self-report anxiety assessment instruments, the Hamilton Anxiety Rating Scale (HAM-A) was one of the first rating scales to measure the severity of anxiety symptoms (1959). It is still widely used today and is available in the public domain in English, Cantonese, French, and Spanish. The HAM-A consists of fourteen items reflecting mental agitation and psychological distress, as well as physical complaints related to anxiety. Each item is scored on a scale of 0 (not present) to 4 (severe); higher scores are indicative of moderate to severe anxiety.

An instrument used frequently with persons who are acutely ill is the Hospital Anxiety and Depression Scale (HADS). The HADS was specifically developed to detect both depression and anxiety, as these two symptoms are common in persons with physical health problems requiring hospitalization. The HADS consists of fourteen items; half of the items measure anxiety and the other half depression on a 0–3 response scale (Snaith, 2003). The Copenhagen Institute of Mental Health owns the copyright to this instrument, which is available for purchase.

The Anxiety Control Questionnaire (AxCQ) is a thirty-item scale that measures an individual's perceived control over anxiety-related events (Gould et al., 2010). The AxCQ utilizes a Likert scale with options ranging from strongly disagree (0) to strongly agree (5); higher scores indicate greater perceived control over anxiety (Rapee, Craske, Brown, & Barlow, 1996). This instrument could be applicable for measuring responses to anxiety self-management interventions that enhance personal control. The AxCQ is in the public domain and freely accessible (at http://www.psy.mq.edu.au/CEH/ACQ.html).

Single-item response scales are also popular in measuring changes in perceived anxiety levels. These instruments include the Numeric Rating Scale (NRS) and the Visual Analog Scale (VAS). The NRS is usually on a scale of 0 (no anxiety) to 10 (highest anxiety ever). Respondents provide an answer either verbally or by marking a specific number in response to "how anxious are you feeling right now?" Likewise, the VAS captures the current anxiety level and can be presented vertically or horizontally on a 100-millimeter scale. Respondents indicate their current level of anxiety, from 0 (no anxiety) at the bottom or left anchor, to 100 (most anxiety ever) at the top or right side anchor. The anxiety score is derived from the distance from the zero end/mark to the placement of the respondent's mark, using a ruler to measure the distance in millimeters. These single-item scales can be used when response burden and energy levels are an issue with participants, or when a quick response is needed for a clinical situation. Given the single item contained in each of these scales, the NRS and VAS represent a single domain, so the reliability of these types of measures will be lower than that of anxiety instruments that contain more individual items to determine anxiety.

General Recommendations for the Selection of a Self-Report Instrument

When selecting a self-report instrument, the integrative nurse needs to carefully consider the reasons for choosing a particular instrument, as well as his or her conceptualization of anxiety. Some helpful questions include: (1) Do you want to get an idea of how an individual usually feels or perceives anxiety? (2) What is the respondent's capacity (cognitive and energetic) to complete a lengthy instrument? Is there a shorter version of a lengthy instrument available? (3) What is the respondent's reading level and ability to understand? The answers to these general questions will influence the quality and quantity of responses. The quality of the obtained data is crucial to implementing evidence-based interventions to manage anxiety and in conveying the effectiveness of these modalities to clinicians.

Of particular note, the psychological measures described in this chapter are not specific for chronic anxiety (GAD). Additional information about measures that can be used in this population (e.g., Symptom Checklist-90 anxiety sub-scale and the Beck Anxiety Inventory) can be obtained elsewhere for purchase (see www.pearsonassessments.com/tests/htm).

PHYSIOLOGICAL MEASURES

Indirect physiological indicators of anxiety include heart rate, blood pressure, heart rate variability, respiratory rate, oxygen saturation, skin temperature, galvanic skin response, skin conductance, and muscle tension. Like psychological measures, these measures require careful selection and justification for their use in anxiety management or intervention research. Careful attention needs to be given to the apparatus and devices used to obtain values on these parameters. All are prone to measurement errors that need to be considered in protocols that pay careful attention to sensitivity and specificity of any measuring device and the values obtained.

BIOMARKERS

A *biomarker* is a biochemical or molecular parameter associated with the presence and/or severity of a specific disease state (Marcantonio et al., 2006). Biomarkers can be measured with physical examination, laboratory assay, or imaging (Marcantonio et al., 2006). A biomarker can serve as a risk marker for disease, serve as a disease marker, or be an end product of disease. Biomarkers associated with anxiety could be used to understand the effect of anxiety on the development of disease. However, biomarkers are expensive to obtain, and expertise is needed for their interpretation. Thus, appropriate understanding, rationale, timing and frequency of sample collection, and personnel are needed when considering biomarkers in research studies or for any clinical setting to promote anxiety management. Careful thought needs to go into any measurement protocols that plan to include biomarkers. It is beyond the scope of this chapter to provide extensive information on biomarkers associated with anxiety and anxiety-reduction interventions. Resources are available to the interested reader (see www.biomarkers.org).

Several biomarkers found in serum and urine have been used in anxiety-reduction intervention research, including cortisol, blood glucose, prolactin, and catecholamines such as epinephrine and norepinephrine. Many of these biomarkers are associated with the stress response, which is interrelated with anxiety, and are markers of hypothalamic-pituitary-adrenal (HPA) axis activation.

Clinical Decision-Making for Anxiety Symptom Management

Once the integrative nurse collects the appropriate biopsychosocial measures that indicate the degree of distress anxiety is causing, she/he can develop a plan either with or for a patient, based on his/her preferences and current medical condition. First, the integrative nurse will need to consider the physiological status of any patient for whom anxiety management interventions may be suggested. Patient safety and acceptability are of the utmost importance. For example, a patient hospitalized for an acute illness may have a needle phobia. For this patient, acupuncture would not be an acceptable intervention, given the use of needles to deliver the treatment. Likewise, meditation may conflict with some individuals' religious beliefs and preferences.

Nurses working in acute care or critical care hospital settings as well as home health and public health, should review the medication administration record, noting any medications that have the potential to alter heart rate, respiratory rate, or blood pressure. Many of the interventions used to manage anxiety can also promote relaxation, sleep, and alterations in cardiovascular status, which is why the nurse needs to have an in-depth understanding of all medications, their actions, and potential side effects (Freeman et al., 2010).

Integrative Anxiety Interventions

The integrative nurse makes full use of a range of interventions based on the evidence supporting their use for anxiety self-management. Interventions should be based on an individual patient's needs and preferences, offering the least intensive intervention required to support the person's healing journey (Principle 5). Integrative therapies (alone or in conjunction with biomedical strategies) offer ways to manage transient, situation- or experience-specific anxiety. When determining which therapies to try, a multi-disciplinary patient-centered approach is necessary. A review of selected evidence-based integrative therapies for anxiety symptom management is summarized in Table 19.1 and presented below.

Table 19.1: Interventions for Anxiety

Level of Intensity	Integrative Therapy Approach
Tier 1 Interventions	**Mind–Body Therapies** • Deep breathing • Music therapy • Art therapy • Prayer **Manipulative Therapies** • Self-massage **Movement Therapies** • Yoga • General exercise
Tier 2 Interventions	**Mind–Body Therapies** • Progressive relaxation • Meditation **Natural Products** • Aromatherapy **Energy Therapies** • Healing touch **Movement Therapies** • Yoga • Qi Gong
Tier 3 Interventions	**Mind-body Therapies** • Meditation **Manipulative Therapies** • Massage • Reflexology **Energy Therapies** • Touch therapies (healing/therapeutic) by practitioner • Acupuncture • Acupressure
Tier 4 Interventions	**Natural Products** • Kava
Tier 5 Interventions	**Pharmacological Therapies**

SELF-CARE INTERVENTIONS

Music has been systematically shown to decrease anxiety in various medical conditions and settings and has been used as a healing modality for many centuries (Bittman et al., 2001). It is generally thought of as a cost-effective approach without adverse effects and used for a variety of reasons, including social wellbeing and improved quality of life. Chang and Chen (2005) demonstrated the positive effects of music therapy when used for anxiety management in women undergoing a caesarean birth. When compared with a control group, participants treated with music therapy had significantly lower levels of anxiety during the final phase of the intraoperative period. In a pre- and post-test study examining relaxation and anxiety among patients undergoing mechanical ventilation in the ICU, Chlan (1998) found that patients who received music intervention reported significantly less anxiety than those in the control group. A recent Cochrane Review indicated that music intervention is effective in reducing anxiety and promoting relaxation in mechanically ventilated patients, although the findings generally are based on small sample sizes (Bradt, Dileo, & Grocke, 2010). Of the various integrative modalities, music appears to have the strongest evidence to support its use in the management of anxiety.

Some data suggest that intercessory prayers, the petition to God or a higher deity on behalf of another, may help reduce the anxiety for the individual who is being prayed for. In one randomized study that enrolled volunteers to either pray for others, to be prayed for, or to participate as part of the control group, individuals in both the prayed-for group and the group that was performing the prayers had improved anxiety levels after twelve weeks of praying fifteen minutes daily (O'Laoire, 1997). These data suggest that those doing the praying were as much benefitted from the prayers as the individuals for whom they were praying. Prayer is not recommended as the sole therapy for individuals with serious medical concerns, and a multidisciplinary approach is suggested for the treatment of individuals requesting to be prayed for (Narayanasamy & Narayanasamy, 2008).

Meditation, another commonly used integrative therapy, has been shown to help individuals reduce symptoms related to anxiety and stress. Many forms of meditation are in existence, and its definition is very broad and varied, although generally thought of as a state of being deliberately freed from conscious thoughts (Huynh et al., 2007). Although the evidence supporting the use of meditation for anxiety is not as robust as it is for music, Arias et al. (2006) found that meditation offers benefits when used for the management of non-psychotic mood disorders and a variety of anxiety disorders. There continues to be a lack of data to determine which types of meditation work best and in what conditions.

Aromatherapy is the delivery of essential oils to the body. Aromatic oils are typically mixed with a "carrier" oils (e.g., vegetable oil) and are applied to the skin, sprayed in the air, or directly inhaled. The two most commonly used essential oils in the management of anxiety are lavender and rosemary. In a pre-test, post-test designed study examining female patients with chronic renal failure on hemodialysis, the researchers found that lavender oil significantly decreased anxiety levels compared to the natural smell of the room in which they were receiving treatment. The researchers concluded that lavender may be beneficial in alleviating feelings of anxiety (Itai et al., 2000). In a quasi-experimental trial consisting of junior nursing students, the experimental group was given a combination of lavender, rosemary, pepper, and Clary-Sage aromas delivered by an aroma lamp. Participants receiving the intervention reported lower levels of anxiety and perceived stress (Park & Lee, 2004). Although these results are promising, more rigorous research is needed in order to make specific recommendations for the use of aromatherapy in anxiety management.

Yoga is an ancient practice of relaxation and exercise with roots in Indian philosophy and has been described as the union of the mind, body, and soul. There are various schools of yoga practice including Hatha yoga, Karma yoga, Bhakti yoga, and Raja yoga. Yoga classes last, on average, 30–90 minutes, and expert yogis suggest that the most remarkable benefits arise after years, or even decades, of practice (Telles & Naveen, 1997). A study by Rao et al. (2009) on the anxiolytic effects of yoga in breast cancer outpatients revealed that those receiving the intervention demonstrated an overall significant decrease in self-reported state anxiety compared to those receiving simply supportive therapy without a yoga component. Another randomized controlled trial consisting of a sample of 114 college students showed that yoga, when used with imagery, was associated with increased scores of self-reported relaxation levels (Khasky & Smith, 1999). Although it is difficult to design rigorous research protocols for the study of yoga, the evidence appears to be in favor of using yoga in the management of symptoms related to anxiety.

Qigong, a therapy from the traditional Chinese medicine (TCM) tradition, is commonly practiced in China for general health maintenance. It encompasses a series of breathing and movement exercises, which are thought to induce a relaxation response by influencing the flow of *qi*, body energy. A randomized controlled trial showed that hospital staff who participated in a qigong program lasting six weeks reported decreased levels of stress when compared to a control group (Griffith et al., 2008). To date, however, there are not enough scientific data to make recommendations supporting the use of qigong in the management of anxiety.

PROVIDER-DIRECTED INTERVENTIONS

Massage is a broad category inclusive of various techniques. Most types of massage involve varying amounts of pressure, fixed or moving, applied to the muscles and connective tissues of the client (Bost & Wallis, 2006). A study researching the effect of a weekly fifteen-minute massage in nurses showed that participants who received the intervention had significantly decreased anxiety scores compared to those who did not

(Bost & Wallis). In a study of patients in the postoperative recovery period following coronary artery bypass graft surgery, Hattan et al. (2002) found a significant difference in calmness between those receiving massage therapy and those in the control group, with the massage group exhibiting a greater degree of calmness. Although numerous studies have shown positive effects of massage therapy, the exact mechanisms involved remain unknown.

Reflexology consists of the placement of manual pressure to areas of the feet that correspond with other areas of the body, based on a system of zones or reflex areas (Gunnarsdottir & Jonsdottir, 2007). Some evidence suggests that reflexology alleviates anxiety, although the exact mechanism in not understood. A randomized, controlled trial found that individuals undergoing coronary artery bypass graft surgery who received reflexology had significantly lower anxiety scores and systolic blood pressure when compared to a control group not receiving the intervention (Gunnarsdottir & Jonsdottir, 2007). Further research is needed to recommend the use of reflexology in the management of anxiety, as there is very little evidence that supports this modality.

As one of the founding pillars of TCM, acupuncture utilizes needles to manipulate the body's *qi*, or energy. Chinese healers have identified roughly 360 acupuncture points along fourteen meridians, or lines, on the human body. The specific points treated depend on the symptoms experienced by the individuals; a combination of several specific acupoints and needle techniques may be used to restore the meridian(s) and *qi* to its optimal functioning (Bresler & Kroening, 1976). Acupressure uses the application and pressure of hands on these points instead of needles. Although numerous studies have tested acupuncture for symptom palliation, there is extremely limited evidence suggesting that these therapies might be beneficial for the treatment of anxiety (Jorm et al., 2004). One study reported that anxiety levels in elderly individuals who received acupressure while being transported to the hospital via ambulance experienced less anxiety than those in the control group (Mora et al., 2007).

Touch therapies are a complex system of energy-based therapies based on the practitioner's use of focused intent and the placement of hands in various formations either on the body or above it. It involves the movement of the hands through the client's energy field to influence and promote the circulation of energy (Eisenber et al., 1998). Touch sessions generally last 20 to 30 minutes, and, although a series of sessions is recommended, no data yet exist on a specific recommended dose. In a mixed methods study, Wilkinson et al. (2002) reported a significant reduction in stress levels after two healing touch sessions with themes of relaxation being identified in the qualitative analysis; specific reductions in anxiety ratings were not examined.

Guided imagery may help individuals relax and concentrate on images associated with personal issues they are presently battling (Halpin et al., 2002). Practitioners of guided imagery may choose to help clients find answers to their problem by objectively guiding them to explore their inner resources, although compact discs and DVDs can also be used to assist individuals with self-directed guided imagery. In a study examining preoperative anxiety and postoperative pain among individuals undergoing cardiac surgery, Halpin et al. (2002) found that participants who completed the guided imagery program had, on average, shorter in-hospital length-of-stay, decreased direct pharmacy costs, and decreased direct pain-management costs, with no difference in patient satisfaction compared to those who did not participate in the program.

NATURAL PRODUCTS

Kava, a derivative from kava-kava (*Piper methysticum*), a bush-type plant from the South Pacific regions of the world, has historically been used to elicit a calming effect in humans. Research, including clinical trials and meta-analyses, has shown a moderate benefit when used for anxiety with dosages varying from 50mg–400mg/daily (Pittler & Ernst, 2003). A pre- and post-test study on anxiety in menopausal women revealed that those taking kava-kava experienced greater resolution of anxiety symptoms at six months than those who did not (De Leo et al., 2000). There is concern that kava has been associated with abnormal liver-function tests and in some cases even hepatic cirrhosis; therefore, it should be used with caution and should not be used in individuals with known hepatic conditions, or women who are pregnant or breastfeeding (Clough et al., 2003). Clinicians recommending kava, and individuals taking kava, should use it with caution and be aware of its adverse effects. Clinicians should assess what other medications an individual may be taking and monitor for potential toxicities related to metabolizing multiple medications via the hepatic system.

Because there is a lack of strong, empirical evidence supporting the efficacy of some integrative therapies for anxiety management in particular, Kienle et al. (2011) recommend carefully assessing the evidence prior to recommending integrative modalities, by asking the following questions:

- Does the therapy adhere to the criteria of professional treatment and medical professionalism?
- Does this patient value this type of integrative therapy? Is there demand for this therapy?
- What is the conceptual framework of the therapy and how does it theoretically relieve the symptom of anxiety? Is there theoretical plausibility?
- Has the therapy been researched as a whole and in real-life conditions or settings? What are the results from these studies?

Outcome Evaluation

Evaluating the effectiveness of an integrative therapy can be a complex process; outcome evaluation depends on a patient's healthcare goals as well as his or her personal belief systems. To best meet the patient's needs, a pluralistic approach to care is needed in conjunction with open and honest dialogue between patient and clinician, as perceived treatment effects are frequently based on values and beliefs; it is not uncommon for patients to make decisions about using integrative therapies based on anecdotal information (Verhoef et al., 2007). Therefore, when patient care is the primary focus, the evaluation of the effectiveness of integrative therapies and the methods used will vary based on patient values, the nature and context of the illness, symptom severity and perception, and the goals of treatment (Verhoef et al., 2007). At times, psychological or physiological measures may be required; at other times, patient descriptions of experience and anecdotal accounts of symptom relief may be more appropriate. However evaluated, follow-up and ongoing evaluation of outcomes is an essential part of care.

Summary

Anxiety is a state marked by apprehension, agitation, increased motor tension or activity, autonomic arousal, and fearful withdrawal (McCartney & Boland, 1994). Anxiety is an emotional response to any threat or danger (DeMarco et al., 2011) that can be experienced in any situation and in any setting. We have reviewed a number of modalities the integrative nurse can suggest to patients to self-manage anxiety or to implement in a healthcare setting to reduce anxiety. A selection of instruments that consider both self-report and biophysiological markers have been suggested to measure change or amelioration of anxiety with any number of integrative modalities. The integrative nurse is advised to carefully consider the evidence, safety, and any contraindications in patient condition or personal preferences prior to implementing or suggesting integrative therapies for anxiety symptom management. While the evidence base is growing, additional research is needed to advance the science and demonstrated benefits of these modalities in practice for anxiety symptom management.

SELECTED REFERENCES

American Psychiatric Association. (2000). *Diagnostic and Statistical Manual of Mental Disorders, Fourth Edition, Text Revision (DSM-IV-TR)*. Arlington, VA: American Psychiatric Association.

Arias, A. J., Steinberg, K., Banga, A., & Trestman, R. L. (2006). Systematic review of the efficacy of meditation techniques as treatments for medical illness. *Journal of Alternative & Complementary Medicine, 12*(8), 817–832.

Bradt, J., Dileo, C., & Grocke, D. (2010) Music interventions for mechanically ventilated patients. *Cochrane Database of Systematic Reviews.* Accessed April 9, 2012; (12):CD006902.

DeMarco, J., Alexander, J., Nehrenz, G., & Gallagher, L. (2011). The benefit of music for the reduction of stress and anxiety in patients undergoing elective cosmetic surgery. *Music and Medicine, 4*(1), 44–48.

Gunnarsdottir, T. J., Jonsdottir, H. (2007). Does the experimental design capture the effects of complementary therapy? A study using reflexology for patient undergoing coronary artery bypass graft surgery. *Journal of Clinical Nursing, 16*(4), 777–785.

Halpin, L. S., Speir, A. M., CapoBianco, P., & Barnett, S.D. (2002). Guided imagery in cardiac surgery. *Outcomes Management, 6*(3), 132–137.

Jorm, A. F., Christensen, H., Griffiths, K. M., Parslow, R. A., Rodgers, B., & Blewitt, K. A. (2004). Effectiveness of complementary and self-help treatments for anxiety disorders. *Medical Journal of Australia, 181*(7 Suppl), S29–46.

Kienle, G. S., Albonico, H., Fischer, L., et al. (2011). Complementary therapy systems and their integrative evaluation. *Explore, 7*(3), 175–187.

Pittler, M. H., & Ernst, E. (2003). Kava extract for treating anxiety. *Cochrane Database of Systematic Reviews*, (1):CD003383. doi:10.1002/14651858

Thorp, S., Ayers, C., Nuevo, R., Stoddard, J., Sorrell, J., & Wetherell, J. (2009). Meta-analysis comparing different behavior treatments for late-life anxiety. *American Journal of Geriatric Psychiatry, 17*(2), 105–115.

20

Integrative Nursing Management of Depressed Mood

MERRIE J. KAAS, GISLI KRISTOFERSSON, AND SUE TOWEY

Humans associate feelings with mood. Most of us "feel a mood" when we think about an experience; our moods are often dependent on our lived experience. Some of us can readily label our moods, while some of us have a difficult time describing them. Labels such as anxious, sad, calm, cheerful, blah, energetic, mellow, morose, relaxed, and even "okay" are used to describe our moods. Moods fluctuate and most of us have a wide range of moods, expressing them in a variety of ways. Some people have rapid fluctuations in mood; for others, moods vary less often. For some, moods can be the cause of creativity, and for others, of thoughts of death. There is no "normal" mood, yet to the extent that conventional biomedical taxonomies determine the normalcy or pathology of our moods, moods are treated as an illness or a symptom, almost separately from the personal context in which they occur.

Integrative mental health nursing is founded on the principles of whole-person, relationship-based care provided within the personal, lived context and the use of the best range of therapies to support the individual's health and healing. The integrative mental health nurse conceptualizes mood as a whole-system response to the relationship between the individual and the environment. The focus of this chapter is the application of integrative mental health nursing principles to one type of mood disturbance, that which we traditionally call the "depressed" mood. It is depressed mood, or depression, that has exacted and will continue to exact huge costs on healthcare systems globally and the quality of life individually. Depression is projected to be the second leading cause of disability in the world by 2020, outranked only by ischemic heart disease, which depression will overtake as the leading cause of disability in the world by 2030 (Mathers & Loncar, 2006).

What Is Depressed Mood?

We often say we feel "depressed," but do we really have symptoms of a depressive illness caused by neurotransmitter imbalance, or depletion or the blocked flow of *prana* or *qi*?

Or, is our depressive mood an intermittent experience brought on by a personal experience of tragedy or loss? In a recent U.S. government report, about one in ten adults report significant depressive symptoms (Centers for Disease Control [CDC], 2010a). Absenteeism from work and lost productivity, mortality costs from depression-related suicides, and $26 billion in direct treatment costs add up to over $83 billion to the U.S. economy, rivaling the costs of AIDS and cardiovascular illness (Mental Health in America, 2013). Suicide is the tenth leading cause of death in the United States, with more than 105 suicides each day resulting in an estimated $34.6 billion in combined work loss and medical costs (CDC, 2010b).

Major depressive disorder, commonly called depression, is considered a psychiatric illness in the *Diagnostic and Statistical Manual of Mental Disorders, Fourth Edition, Text Revision* (DSM-IV-TR) category of "mood disorders" (2000). Major depressive disorder is a common disorder with a lifetime prevalence of between 15%–25%, with a higher prevalence in women than men, middle-aged adults than older adults and younger adults, single than married adults, and in adults with chronic illness. Depression can occur as a single disease or coexist with other psychiatric and medical maladies. For example, there is a higher risk of depression in persons with substance abuse problems, Parkinson's disease, and various types of cancers and brain traumas. Major depressive disorder may also be confused with an extended grief response, anxiety, and other medical illnesses, such as congestive heart failure. Mood disturbances can include both depressed moods alone, or depressed moods alternating with manic moods (DSM-IV-TR, 2000).

Symptoms of major depression include sad and/or depressed mood, diminished interest or pleasure, weight changes (both gain and loss), significant changes in sleep patterns, psychomotor slowing or agitation, fatigue and loss of energy, diminished concentration, feelings of worthlessness or guilt, and recurrent thoughts of death or suicide (DSM-IV-TR, 2000). In the conventional biomedical taxonomy, depression is characterized by number and length of these depressive moods and the impact of these depressed moods on social and physical function and quality of life (DSM-IV-TR, 2000). Mental health practitioners make the diagnosis based on patient interviews, standardized assessment tools, and medical tests to rule out medical causes such as cancers, thyroid disease, and nutritional depletion.

There is a variety of theoretical models hypothesizing the causes of depression. In conventional biomedicine, biological factors thought to be associated with depression are the imbalance or depletion of specific neurotransmitters (serotonin, norepinephrine, dopamine), neuroendocrine dysregulation (especially the hypothalamus-adrenal-thyroid axis), abnormalities or changes in the circadian rhythm, neuroimmune dysregulation, adverse effects of prescribed medications, nutritional depletion, substance abuse, genetic factors, changes in life events, and environmental stress, along with personality and cognitive factors, which impact an individual's self-esteem (Sadock & Sadock, 2003). Traditional Chinese medicine

(TCM) addresses the link between the body, mind, and spirit and treats patterns of illness, rather than symptoms of illness. These patterns describe how an illness begins, what may cause it to progress, and how this illness/pattern impacts other body systems. For example, patterns related to depression might include "blood stagnation," "liver fire," "heart *yin* deficiency," and "liver *qi* stagnation" (see http://www.yinyanghouse.com retrieved March 9, 2013), although Flaws & Lake (2001) report that depressed mood is associated with kidney *qi* and *yang* essence deficiency. Ayurvedic medicine also characterizes "dis-ease" as something that affects the whole human system, not an aberration in one organ or chemical component, and treats it with practical techniques that promote the wellness of the mind, spirit, and body. In an Ayurvedic framework, depression is thought to be caused by the loss of self-consciousness, an imbalance in one's constitutional type (*Vata, Pitta,* or *Kapha*), failing to act or think in ways that support a healthy lifestyle, and environmental influences, including human interactions and chemical toxins (Brooks, 2002). The question is, which model is correct? The best answer may well be an integrative model of mental health.

An Integrative Nursing Approach to Depressed Mood

Given the growing prevalence of depression that is quickly contributing to disability worldwide (Kessler, 2012), and a growing interest in alternatives to conventional psychotherapy and psychopharmacological treatment for depression (Su & Li, 2011), a new model is needed for the prevention, assessment, and treatment of this enormously costly illness, one that considers a more "bodymindspirit" approach to mental health and illness. Integrative mental health nursing incorporates evidence-informed traditional and non-traditional approaches in the assessment and treatment of depressive symptoms and promotion of wellbeing. Using the following case study, we will approach our work with Barbara S. from an integrated mental health nursing perspective.

Assessing Depressed Mood

Integrative Nursing Principles 1, 2, and 3 guided the PMHNP's assessment of Barbara's depressed mood. Barbara's depressed mood was informed by a biomedical approach (a clinical interview, physical assessment, and laboratory studies) to describe the symptoms and possible causes of her depressed mood, as well as an integrative approach to assess the situating of the depressed mood in the whole of Barbara's life. Taking into account that human beings are inseparable from their environment, the PMHNP's assessment considered Barbara's personal definition of

Case Scenario

Barbara S. is a 36-year-old, Caucasian, married woman without children, with a history of depression, anxiety, and eating disorder. Barbara was referred to a prescribing psychiatric/mental health nurse practitioner (PMHNP) by a psychologist for an integrative assessment and treatment plan for her depressed mood.

Barbara reports low energy and motivation, poor concentration, and a history of depression with coexisting anxiety and past panic attacks, feelings of depersonalization, worry, rumination, social anxiety, and poor sleep patterns. She denies psychoses or overt paranoia, although she is "cautious" in sharing her history and treatment preferences. Barbara's poor nutritional eating patterns include restriction from food all day and then eating in the evening, choosing carbohydrates, fats (primarily pizza), and sugars. Her exercise patterns (walking) are erratic and dependent on her energy level, although she knows exercise is beneficial to having a more positive mood. Barbara has worked in her family creative art business since she was young. During childhood, her parents were absent due to long work hours, so she ate alone most days and developed anxiety and fears around eating patterns and mealtime routines. She describes her depressed mood as related to a history of childhood emotional neglect. Barbara finds relief from her depressive symptoms and anxiety through her painting. Although Barbara has been working with a psychologist, she finds it difficult to verbally express her emotions through traditional talk therapy. Barbara describes her five-year marriage as "supportive." She also describes a rich non-traditional spiritual life that she finds comforting.

Over the years, Barbara has taken a variety of psychotropic medications for her depression and anxiety, including selective serotonin reuptake inhibitors, anticonvulsants, mood stabilizers, and benzodiazepines, all with no significant lasting benefit. She is currently taking a small dose of Seroquel (quetiapine) for sleep. Barbara is also taking a multivitamin with extra calcium and vitamin B. Barbara brought her latest physical exam results from her primary care provider to the consultation. Barbara's lab assessments are within normal limits, except her vitamin D level is 15. Barbara states that she prefers to try "non-allopathic" interventions at this point.

her mental health and physical wellbeing, the impact of the depressed mood on Barbara's bodymindspirit, and the purpose of the depressed mood in Barbara's life. Given that all people have the innate capacity for health and healing, the PMHNP addressed Barbara's goals for her health and mental health, including but not limited to diminished or ameliorated depressed moods. When the PMHNP discussed

Barbara's practices to rebalance her health and mental health, she explored previous routines to feel grounded, such as walking outside, positive self-talk, meditative and spiritual practices, and her painting (Principle 3). If the PMHNP was an expert in Ayurvedic medicine or traditional Chinese medicine or could refer Barbara to a qualified practitioner, further assessment could determine the possible relationships between the patterns of her depression and anxiety and other body systems, and clarify symptoms of her depressed mood in light of her basic constitution (Principle 1). Lake (2009) describes both conventional and non-conventional methods for assessing depressed mood that have been validated by Western medicine. Types of assessments used in an integrated approach are summarized in Table 20.1.

Once a thorough assessment has been completed, a plan can be made to promote Barbara's health and management of her depressed mood and anxiety. The psychiatric/mental health nurse practitioner works with Barbara to help her regain balance on all levels—physical, mental, emotional, and spiritual. Ultimately, the goal is for Barbara to learn self-care practices to manage her moods independently or partner with her health/mental health care provider.

Integrative Depressed Mood Interventions

When developing a plan with Barbara to manage her depressed mood and anxiety, it is important to incorporate the practices that support her own innate healing capacity (Principle 2), in addition to the full range of evidence-informed interventions, moving to more intensive/intrusive treatments from least intensive/intrusive (Principle 5). Keeping in mind the safety and side effect profile of all the potential interventions means that the integrative mental health nurse needs to carefully weigh the benefits of each potential intervention against the possible risks and costs, while also considering the principle of least to more invasive/intensive. In addition, integrative mental health nurses need to alert individuals in their care to this same issue, ensuring that they make informed decisions based on an accurate assessment of safety and risk information for all interventions. Barbara came to the PMHNP requesting interventions that were more "natural," holistic, and "non-allopathic," yet she was taking an antipsychotic medication, quetiapine, which was effective in helping her sleep. The PMHNP reviewed Barbara's current self-care practices and her use of quetiapine for sleep in light of the risks and benefits of other approaches for treating Barbara's depressed mood.

There are many approaches for addressing depressed mood, some of which are supported by clinical evidence, sometimes dating back hundreds of years, but without support of the scientific evidence that accompanies pharmaceutical approaches. The reasons for this lack of evidence include limited amount of research for integrative approaches as well as inherent biases against these complementary approaches, many

Table 20.1: Integrative Assessment Options for Barbara's Depressed Mood

Assessment	Purpose
Structured clinical interview with presence and intention	Identify the characteristics of depressed mood, length, and quality, self-harm and suicidal risk Medical history Spiritual issues Family and social history, which might be contributing or protective factors. Interview assessments that characterize the severity of depressive symptoms for a comparison to the diagnostic criteria found in the DSM-IV-TR: • Beck Depression Inventory • Hamilton Rating Scale for Anxiety • Patient Health Questionnaire (PHQ-9). Determine quality of and satisfaction with life and activities that bring life meaning. Assess normal mood fluctuations and acceptable variance. Obtain sleep and nutritional history and current patterns.
Laboratory screening tests for possible causes of or indicators of depressed mood	Laboratory findings that may suggest underlying medical causes of depressed mood: • Thyroid studies • Blood glucose • Serum electrolytes • Liver and renal studies • Complete blood counts • Serum iron levels Genetic tests to determine potential causes and successful pharmacological treatment.
Traditional Chinese medicine	Constitutional assessment to clarify symptoms: • Fire • Water • Earth • Metal and wood types Observation and physical assessment to determine the blockage of *qi* (Flaws & Lake, 2001)
Ayurvedic medicine	Constitutional assessment for mind/body types to clarify symptoms (Emmons, 2006). • Vata • Pitta • Kapha
Energy-information assessment	Electroencephalography (EEG), Qualitative EEG (qEEG), or Auditory Evoked Response (AER) to determine differences in brain electrical activity and/or organic causes of depressed mood (Lake, 2007).

of which are not easily understood by biomedical practitioners (Fønnebø et al., 2007). Yet people stand to gain directly from establishing the effectiveness of many of these interventions, in part due to their less invasive, less expensive nature and yet more enduring outcomes.

In working with Barbara to develop a personal plan to help her manage her depressive symptoms, the integrative nurse understood it was important to support the

Table 20.2: Intervention Options for Barbara's Depressed Mood

Level of Intensity	Integrative Therapy Approach
Tier 1 Interventions	**Dietary Therapies** • Avoid caffeine, alcohol, drugs • Functional nutrition (consultation) **Mind–Body Therapies** • Guided imagery • Meditation • Music (playing piano and singing) • Art (painting) **Spirituality (continue current practice)**
Tier 2 Interventions	**Natural Products** • Aromatherapy **Natural Products/Supplements** • Omega 3 (2000mg concentrated fish oil) • Vitamin D (4000 IU/day, continue with multivitamin with extra B_6 and B_{12}) **Movement Therapies** • Yoga (once a week to start) • Exercise (continue walking 2–3 times a week) • Tai chi **Mind-Body Therapies** • Mindfulness interventions
Tier 3 Interventions	**Light Therapy** • Psychotherapy (continue with psychologist) **Mind–Body Therapies** • Music therapy **Energy Therapies** • Reiki
Tier 4 Interventions	**Natural Products** • Rhodiola rosea **Whole Systems** • Homeopathic medicine • Traditional Chinese medicine (herbal, acupuncture) • Ayurvedic medicine
Tier 5 Interventions	**Psychotropic Medications (continue with quetiapine 25mg–50mg for sleep)** **Natural Products/Herbs** • St. John's Wort **Amino Acid Derivatives** • S-adenosyl methionine (SAMe). • 5-Hydroxytryptophan (5HTP) **Electroconvulsive Therapy (ECT)** **Transcranial Magnetic Stimulation (TMS)**

activities that currently worked well for Barbara (Principle 4). A five-tier framework based on levels of intrusiveness is a place to begin. Table 20.2 provides a summary of some key evidence-informed approaches that could be used to manage Barbara's depressed mood and anxiety. The interventions in bold are the ones Barbara chose and will be described in more detail.

TIER 1 INTERVENTIONS

Together with the PMHNP, Barbara developed a plan that started with the least intrusive approaches available. These strategies engage people independently without professional input. These interventions are relatively safe for most people using a common-sense approach such as reading the directions on the bottle of a supplement or stopping an activity if it causes emotional or physical pain.

An initial place to start with Barbara is to address her nutritional status and dietary habits. Functional nutrition is closely related to the field of functional medicine, which "addresses the underlying causes of disease, using a systems-oriented approach and engaging both patient and practitioner in a therapeutic partnership" (Institute for Functional Medicine, n.d.). We all have the experience of different foods' affecting our mood and functioning in certain ways, and in the rapidly growing field of functional nutrition, dietary changes are used to address general wellbeing. Caffeine is a clear example; it remains a well-documented fact that caffeine can contribute to mental health problems, as is evidenced by the presence of caffeine-induced anxiety disorder in the DSM-IV-TR (2000). As in Barbara's case, excessive consumption of refined sugars can affect insulin levels and blood glucose to the extent that a fairly immediate effect on mood and energy is felt.

When dealing with mood disorders, the functional nutritionist uses data about the effect of particular foods on mood and functioning. During the initial appointment, the PMHNP recommended increased intake of fruits, vegetables, and grains in Barbara's limited diet. Barbara also agreed to a consultation with a functional nutritionist for a thorough nutritional assessment and potential dietary adjustments and supplementation to improve her overall health and mood (Emmons, Bourgerie, Denton, & Kacher, 2012). Barbara was also referred to many excellent resources and websites, including http://www.functionalmedicine.org to learn about the impact food can have on mood and function.

There is growing evidence for the use of guided imagery and other relaxation techniques in the treatment of depression and anxiety. Unfortunately, the variation among types of guided imagery and relaxation methods used in research makes it difficult to compare across studies; inconsistent data makes meta-analysis difficult (Jorm, Morgan, & Hetrick, 2008). Yet guided imagery was a good fit for Barbara as it is minimally intrusive and a method that is generally considered safe.

The PMHNP also encouraged Barbara to use her creative energy as another pathway for healing. Barbara was always creative in her painting and music, and she now decided to use piano and singing lessons to facilitate her healing process. The evidence supporting the use of music to reduce symptoms of depression is challenging to interpret due to the lack of specific information about the type of music therapy, design of studies, and small sample sizes (Chan, 2011). However, since there are minimal negative side effects associated with music therapy and music listening, and given Barbara's creative streak and fondness for music, the PMHNP encouraged and cultivated this creative endeavor as an important part of her path to recovery.

There are indications that spiritual activity is associated with reduction in depressive symptoms (Freinkel & Lake, 2007). Barbara had cultivated her spiritual life, which she reported as having an important positive effect on her mood and overall wellbeing. Numerous benefits of cultivating one's spiritual life have been reported in the literature, including increased religious activity, decreased incidence of mental disease, and improved overall health (Aukst-Margetic & Margetic, 2005; Jonas & Crawford, 2004; Koenig, 2004).

Spirituality through organized religious affiliation has also been associated with decreased risk of depressed mood in general (Freinkel & Lake, 2007). Yet it is interesting to note that there is literature suggesting that some religious practices may be more associated with positive outcomes (e.g., looking for new spiritual direction, providing spiritual support for others, using God as partner in problem solving, and actively giving God control of the situation) than others. Those who associated their religious practice with more negative outcomes reported feeling dissatisfied with relationships, attributing stressors to the Devil, passively waiting for God to change a situation, and identifying stressors as punishment from God as sources of negativity (Harris et al., 2008). For Barbara, it was important to be aware of some of these factors while continuing to practice her spiritual beliefs as she saw fit. By doing a careful spiritual assessment and exploring these issues with her therapist, Barbara was able to successfully continue on her spiritual path.

TIER 2 INTERVENTIONS

The positive effects of Omega 3 essential fatty acids (Omega 3) on mood have long been documented, with convincing epidemiological data associating its use with decreased levels of depression (Lake, 2007; Williams et al., 2006). There are indications that Omega 3 could have direct benefits on symptoms of depression like Barbara was experiencing (Appleton, 2010). A good starting dose for Barbara is EPA/DHA of 1000 mg (1 gram), which she could increase to 2000–3000 grams of combined EPA/DHA if needed, though this should be done in consultation with a medical provider (Emmons et al., 2012; Weil, 2011; Lake, 2007).

Epidemiological studies have demonstrated a correlation between low vitamin D levels and depression. Screening for vitamin D deficiency is especially important when there is minimal exposure to sunlight, and in the elderly (Sanders, 2011). There is some clinical validity for using vitamin D deficiency in persons with depressed mood, as well as positive effects on bone health and decrease in fall risks associated with adequate vitamin D levels (Sanders, 2011). Because Barbara's vitamin D level was 15, the PMHNP recommended a supplement in the form of Ergocalciferol 50,000 IUs once a week for two months, followed by supplementation with 4000 IUs of vitamin D_3 daily. Barbara planned to have her vitamin D levels checked in three months to ensure appropriate levels.

There is reliable evidence to suggest that adjunctive therapy of folate (folic acid) reduces symptoms of depression when selective serotonin reuptake inhibitors (SSRIs) are prescribed (Coppen, 2000). Since folate is a relatively safe, water-soluble vitamin, many experts recommend the use of this supplement (Hingle, 2007; Weil, 2011). In addition, some experts also recommend using vitamin B_{12} with folate, as folate can mask vitamin B_{12} deficiency (Hingle, 2007). Evidence suggests that vitamin B_6 may also play a role in the reduction of depressive symptoms in pre-menopausal women (Williams, 2005). This made it important for Barbara to take a high-quality multivitamin that includes a vitamin B complex. The PMHNP recommended that Barbara continue taking her daily multivitamin with B complex.

Barbara reported that she had always been interested in trying yoga, but "never got around to it." Yoga appears effective in decreasing symptoms of persons suffering from depression, although surprisingly few methodologically sound studies are reported in the literature (Gerbar & Brown, 2007). While the empirical evidence for using yoga to reduce depressive symptoms is not conclusive, the adverse effects of practicing yoga are few, as long as the same precautions are taken as with general exercise. Improved physical benefits and sense of wellbeing make this a viable option when paired with other evidence-informed approaches for persons suffering from mild to moderate depression (Gerbar & Brown, 2007). The PMHNP provided a list of yoga classes near Barbara's home, and she agreed to attend a class within the next month.

In recent years, there has been increasing evidence supporting the use of exercise to reduce mild to moderate depression. Numerous studies have demonstrated the importance of exercise in the treatment of depression (Rimer et al., 2012). Chapter 12 offers additional information about specific exercise regimens and referral information. Even moderate exercise three to five times a week appears to have considerable benefits (Rimer et al., 2012). A key factor when discussing the addition of exercise to Barbara's day was the PMHNP's non-shaming, non-judgmental approach. Barbara agreed to work with her therapist and primary care provider to find an appropriate exercise regime that might work for her over time in conjunction with interventions that helped her manage her eating disorder.

Mindfulness-based interventions (MBI) have been shown to reduce symptoms of depression and anxiety with people suffering from depression and anxiety (Baer, 2003; Hofman, 2010). MBI were found to alleviate various mental health symptoms, and despite the often considerable homework requirements, individuals seemed to adhere to the intervention throughout follow-up periods. The populations studied included people suffering from eating disorders, chronic pain, psoriasis, depression, fibromyalgia, anxiety, and cancer, as well as various healthy populations (Baer, 2003). Therefore, MBIs seemed to be applicable and feasible for Barbara's care.

Many different approaches fall into the MBI category, including mindfulness-based stress reduction and its related adaptations. In a 2010 review of the literature, MBI's preventative effects (including the prevention of depression) for healthy populations were indicated (Chiesa, 2010). When asked, Barbara chose to explore mindfulness-based exercises that were not overly lengthy, due to her reduced attention span. She used a brief mindful breathing exercise where she kept and redirected her attention on her breath for ten minutes, and each time she noticed that her mind wandered, she simply and non-judgmentally directed it back to her breath. Going forward, Barbara plans to use MBI in conjunction with her current spiritual practices, which include meditation.

TIER 3 INTERVENTIONS

The interventions belonging to this category require some collaboration with a professional to be safe and efficacious. Numerous forms of psychotherapy have been shown to be effective in the treatment of depression (Hilliard, 2001). Psychotherapy is typically recommended as first-line therapy in the treatment of mild to moderate depression and as adjunct to psychotropic treatment in severe depression and mild to moderate depression with psychosocial comorbidities (Sadock & Sadock, 2003). Clients should always be referred to a credentialed therapist for this intervention.

For Barbara, psychotherapy delivered by a qualified professional who specializes in the treatment of eating disorders is an important part of her treatment. Although the PMHNP is qualified to conduct psychotherapy, she recommended that Barbara continue with her psychologist because they have an established relationship to address past childhood issues and current issues related to her eating disorder.

TIER 5 INTERVENTIONS

Activities in tier 5 require full collaboration with professionals and are significantly intrusive. Considerable care should be taken when recommending these therapies, with particular attention paid to side effects, adverse effects, and interaction issues. Integrative mental health nursing includes conventional and non-conventional evidence-informed options as part of any treatment plan. The extent to which tier 5 interventions are used depends on individual preference, cost/risk/benefit analysis, presenting symptoms, and multiple individual factors. Unfortunately, once an individual sees a prescribing psychiatric professional, medications are usually the first, and sometimes the only, interventions included in the treatment.

The PMHNP discussed with Barbara the types of medications most appropriate in depression or when comorbid psychosocial issues exist. One of Barbara's concerns had been getting enough sleep. Because Barbara reported that a medication she was currently taking helped her manage her sleep, Barbara decided to continue quetiapine 25mg–50mg at bedtime until she developed other "quieting" strategies to help her initiate and maintain sleep (see Chapter 18).

Serotonin-selective reuptake inhibitors (SSRIs) are often considered a first-line treatment when prescribing to people who have never taken antidepressants before. Serotonin–norepinephrine reuptake inhibitors (SNRIs) and mirtazipine are also an option as a first-line treatment, but their side effects may be more problematic. Tricyclic antidepressants (TCAs) are an older type of antidepressant, and although they have efficacy that is comparable to that of the SNRIs and SSRIs, they have an higher risk in overdose and increased cardiovascular toxicity than those medication categories. Monoamine oxidase inhibitors (MAOIs) are a third basic class of antidepressants, but are often considered a last-line treatment due to their severe side effects from interactions with certain foods and other drugs. Other classes of antidepressants also exist, such as the norepinephrine-dopamine reuptake inhibitor (NDRI) bupropion, and the serotonin antagonist and reuptake inhibitors (SARIs) trazodone and nefazodone. SARIs are more frequently used in clinical practice as adjunct therapy and to manage some other drug side effects. For example, trazodone is widely used as a sleep agent but much less for its antidepressant effects.

Other psychotropic medications have reliable evidence as adjunct agents in the treatment of depression; these include select second-generation antipsychotics such as aripiprazole (Abilify) and quetiapine, as well as the mood stabilizer lithium. Due to their possible side effects, such as hyperglycemia, weight gain, hyper-lipidemia, and tardive dyskinesia, screening through laboratory tests and screening tools such the Abnormal Involuntary Movement Scale (AIMS) are an important part of Barbara's treatment plan, despite the relatively low dose of quetiapine she is currently taking (Sadock & Sadock, 2003, Chap. 13).

Although there is excellent clinical and scientific evidence supporting the benefits of various psychotropic medications to treat depressed moods, these medications do have limitations. Side effects of these medications and their interactions with other medications or food and herbal preparations are an ever-increasing concern. Cost is also often a significant issue, as well as the dependency on prescribing providers for medications. Some in the medical community have raised concerns over the creation of the field of "cosmetic psychopharmacology," where instead of using antidepressants to treat depressive disorders, we use them to feel "better than well" or rid ourselves of the normal, albeit uncomfortable, sensations and emotions that living life prompts in us. Others wonder if we are heading in this direction with the possible overprescribing of psychotropic medications (Elliott, 2010). Given these concerns, perhaps Principle 5 (i.e., trying less invasive/intensive therapies first) is a prudent course of action, alleviating depressed moods by sequentially using tiers 1–4 or using these therapies adjunctively with lower doses of antidepressants.

Outcome Evaluation

After a year of working together using an integrative approach that initially included medication, Barbara reported that she believes her vitamin D blood levels (near 80) helped her begin to manage her depressed mood and anxiety and engage in therapy and her music and painting. After another six months, Barbara self-discontinued the quetiapine with no problems. She reported feeling quite able to manage her sleep without medicine. Barbara also reported more confidence in managing depressed moods as they arose, while she continued to work on issues related to her eating patterns and work life with the support of her psychologist. Barbara and the PMHNP decided together to terminate their relationship.

During Barbara's early follow-up visits, evaluating the outcomes for Barbara by asking questions like "What would 'happy' look like to you?" remained important outcome indicators. An absence of symptoms and a feeling of general wellbeing are common goals in the treatment of depression, and traditional symptom outcome scales can be quite useful for a more objective description of depression symptoms. Other, less conventional approaches can also be used by qualified professionals to determine the change in the individual's health, including the flow of *qi*.

Summary

This chapter has provided a foundation for understanding depressed mood, a common type of mood disturbance, using an integrative mental health perspective. Nursing approaches are exemplified by a case study, Barbara S. Using an integrative mental health nursing approach, we must remember many integrative strategies for care lack adequate scientific evidence from a traditional biomedical view, but clinical evidence supports their use as adjunctive therapies in the treatment of moderate to mild depression. In addition, they serve as options for individuals who are not interested in a more biomedical approach to the treatment of mental health disorders. Nurses need to be open to what the person feels is important, what he or she wants to feel like, and what he or she needs to be able to do to feel content in their respective life.

SELECTED REFERENCES

American Psychiatric Association (2000). *Diagnostic and Statistical Manual of Mental Disorders, Fourth Edition-Text Revised* (DSM-IV-TR).Washington, DC: American Psychiatric Association.

American Psychiatric Association (2010). *Practice Guidelines for the Treatment of Patients with Major Depressive Disorder.* 3rd ed. Arlington, VA: American Psychiatric Association.

Baer, R. (2003). Mindfulness training as a clinical intervention: A conceptual and empirical review. *Clinical Psychology, Science & Practice, 10,* 125–143.

Chlan, M. F. (2011). The effectiveness of music listening in reducing depressive symptoms in adults: A systematic review. *Complementary Therapies in Medicine, 19*(6), 332. doi: 10.1016/j.ctim.2011.08.003

Elliott, C. (2010). *White Coat, Black Hat: Adventures on the Dark Side of Medicine.* Boston: Beacon Press.

Emmons, H., Bourgerie, S., Denton, C. & Kacher, S. (2012). *The Chemistry of Joy Workbook.* Oakland, CA: New Harbinger Publications.

Freinkle, A., & Lake, J. (2007). Religious beliefs, spirituality and intention. In J. Lake. and D. Siegel. (Eds.), *Complementary and Alternative Treatments in Mental Health Care* (pp. 365–380). Arlington, VA: American Psychiatric Publishing.

Harris, I. J., Erbes, C., Engdahl, B., Raymond, H. A. , Olson, A. M. W. & McMahill, J. (2008). Christian Religion Functioning and trauma outcomes. *Journal of Clinical Psychology, 64*(1), 17–29.

Jorm, A. F., Morgan, A. J., & Hetrick, S. E. (2008). Relaxation for depression. *Cochrane Database of Systematic Reviews, 4*, Article No.: CD007142.

Lake, J. (2009). *Integrative Mental Health Care: A Therapist's Handbook.* New York: W.W. Norton & Company.

Rimer, J., Dwan, K., Lawlor, D. A., Greig, C. A., McMurdo, M., Morley, W., et al. (2012). Exercise for depression. *Cochrane Database of Systematic Reviews.* Issue 7. Article No.: CD004366.

Sadock, J. S., & Sadock, V. A. (2003). *Synopsis of Psychiatry* (9th ed.). Philadelphia, PA: Lippincott, Williams & Wilkins.

21

Integrative Nursing Management of Fatigue

DIANA DRAKE

The Whole World is Tired

Fatigue is a complex and ubiquitous phenomenon. The prevalence of fatigue in healthcare settings and in the popular media suggests that the whole world is tired. In the clinical setting, the symptom of fatigue is beyond the occasional struggle with feeling overworked or too busy; it is a persistent state of weariness that can impact every level of health and wellbeing.

Fatigue can be either a symptom that is indicative of a serious underlying disease, or a simple signal that something is amiss in one's life. It is conceptually viewed within the triad framework of biochemical disease, psychological illness, and lifestyle factors. In the United States, it is estimated that a quarter of the population reports tiredness as a current health problem (Sabes-Figuera, McCrone, Hurley, King, Donaldson,, & Ridsdale, 2010). In a British study of primary care clinics, more than 10% of patients describe at least one month of feeling fatigue that was substantial (Nijrolder, van der Windt, & van der Horst, 2009).

Numerous references suggest fatigue is a disease of modern life, an accepted and self-managed consequence of the increased demands of productivity, multitasking, and information overload. Sleep specialist Naiman (2006) refers to the significance of the loss of true nighttime darkness (darkness) and the subsequent loss of reflection and dreaming as contributors to the heavy body feelings of persistent fatigue. Fatigue can also be viewed as a depletion of coping strategies. This phenomenon has been particularly studied among nurses who are exposed to repeated indirect trauma and suffering and acquire a resulting "compassion fatigue" (Yoder, 2008). The concept of fatigue as an inevitable or an expected part of living is prevalent, but this concept does not provide answers on how to mitigate what is happening and move towards optimal health.

THE CONCEPT OF FATIGUE AND THE PRACTICE GAP

From the patient's viewpoint, a lack of provider understanding, diagnosis, and treatment can translate into a lack of empathy or understanding of what an invisible complaint feels like (Elsass, Jensen, Morup, & Thogersen, 2007). The combination of the low yields from any particular diagnostic investigation and the lack of a physical cause in about one-fifth of fatigue cases creates a clinical perception by the patient that their complaint is not being taken seriously (Sabes-Figuera et al., 2010). As a subjective symptom, fatigue is more frequently reported by the patient than it is objectively assessed by a medical provider.

From the nursing viewpoint, the impact of fatigue on the patient's life may be underestimated, as few tools exist to measure fatigue in an otherwise healthy population. Fatigue related to chronic disease and cancer is better researched, and questionnaires exist to address these specific populations. Less is known about clinically healthy patients who are suffering from fatigue. Typically, survey tools aid in assessing both the intensity of fatigue-related symptoms and the impact of fatigue on specific types of functioning (Laranjeira, 2012). Some studies suggest that providers inquire more about the social and occupational consequences of fatigue in their patients' lives to improve fatigue clinical assessments and measure the impact of the condition (Sabes-Figuera et al., 2010).

The practice gap can perpetuate the toll of undiagnosed and untreated fatigue, resulting in an economic burden to the patient, their family, and the community. Decreased ability to function in the professional work setting, increased sick leave, work disability, and increased errors in judgment occur more regularly with a fatigue disorder (Laranjeira 2012). In a British study, 60% of the economic burden of fatigue was related to the patient's loss of income from the inability to work (Sabes-Figuera et al., 2010).

State of Science: Defining Fatigue

From the obvious to the extremely complex, the causes of fatigue can be as varied (can be as varied and intertwined) as the depleted individuals experiencing its effects. The symptom of fatigue is typically non-specific and often associated with a cluster of symptoms that have multiple causes. Fatigue is commonly found to be a symptom companion to sleep disorders, menopause transition, depression and anxiety, chronic health conditions, cancer, anemia, thyroid disorders, and grief. Fatigue persisting for at least one month is considered *prolonged* or *substantial fatigue*. Fatigue persisting for at least six consecutive months is considered *chronic fatigue*, and it is estimated that one in ten patients with fatigue have *chronic fatigue* (Sabes-Figuera et al., 2010). Laranjeira (2012) sums up the difference between the normal phenomenon of acute fatigue and the prolonged fatigue seen more often in the clinical setting, as follows:

> Prolonged fatigue is assumed to be a cumulative process and can occur if an individual is continuously exposed to one or more stressors during which there is no or inadequate opportunity to recover. Prolonged fatigue is not task specific, and compensation mechanisms are ineffective at reversing it within a short time. (p. 213)

Fatigue related to a disease diagnosis or a medical treatment is more prevalent. Cancer-related fatigue is often described as persistent and distressing, a subjective sense of physical, emotional, and/or cognitive tiredness or exhaustion related to cancer or cancer-related treatment that is not proportional to recent activity and interferes with the patient's usual functioning (Can, 2013). Regardless of the cause, the common ground in the fatigue experience is that it interferes with normal functioning for the patient.

In addition to the complexity of the fatigue phenomenon, its epidemiology is not well understood: it is rarely fatal and is challenging to assess and measure (Laranjeira, 2012). From the logic-based perspective of allopathic biomedicine, fatigue symptoms can appear shifting, vague, and fluctuating (Elsass et al., 2007).

Historical Picture of Fatigue: An Understandable Refuge

In addition to psychogenic pain, fatigue is the other great somatoform illness of the end of the twentieth century (Shorter, 1992). A symptom not fully explained by a medical condition, fatigue was first characterized in the 1700s as an illness that resulted in a lowness of spirits, heaviness, and abnormal delicacy (Elsass et al., 2007). Historically, gender differences labeled the female patient with fatigue as weak, prone to fainting spells, fits, and hysteria. Doctors in the 1880s advised long periods of rest for brain exhaustion and neurasthenia. In the mid–twentieth century, the archetype of the exhausted businessman and the nervous sub-invalid housewife was prevalent. Fatigue has historically been an understandable refuge where lesser demands are imposed on individual performance and clarity of thinking (Elsass et al., 2007).

In the twenty-first century, the search for accurate descriptions of fatigue continues. Integrative cardiologist Guarneri (2007) titles the chapters in her book on heart disease, The Fog of Stress, Echoes of Anger, Persistence of Grief, and The Landscape of Depression. This descriptive language deepens the understanding of the contributory factors in heart disease from the patients' perspective that were previously overlooked. Similarly, patients give words to fatigue imagery that can deepen the understanding of what it feels like to be inside the fatigue experience, locked doors, powerlessness, chaos and lack of clarity. From the patient perspective "It can be difficult to convince the system that your body is worn out when you don't understand why yourself" (Elsass et al., 2007, p. 86). Finding the accurate language to describe the experience broadens understanding for the patient and the integrative nurse.

The Fatigue Differential

Fatigue is the devoted companion of most types of physical and psychological disease; however, a physical cause of fatigue is only identified in a small percentage of the patients presenting with fatigue (Nijrolder et al., 2009). This makes it all the more difficult to differentiate fatigue as a distinct and uniquely individual patient experience that may exist with or without a physiological diagnosis. When fatigue is the result of an illness, the cure or treatment for the disease is likely to also resolve the fatigue. Examples of this are readily seen in thyroid-regulation medication, iron supplementation for anemia, and antidepressants that treat the deep fatigue of depression. Physical and mental health assessments, laboratory testing, and other diagnostic tools assist in most cause-and-effect conditions. Less clear to diagnose, but consistently intertwined with fatigue complaints, are fibromyalgia, chronic fatigue syndrome, adrenal insufficiency, Lyme disease, post-traumatic stress disorder, anxiety, and other chronic physical disorders.

Altered sleep is a frequently stated cause of fatigue by patients. Either an inadequate amount of sleep or poor-quality sleep can result in sleepiness with subsequent feelings of loss of attention and sensory connection to the world. Naiman (2006) suggests fatigue is distinct from sleepiness, and, although the two overlap, sleepiness and fatigue are different conditions that call for separate therapies. Fatigue is defined as a diminished capacity to respond or express one's self in the world, and healing requires deep rest and restorative therapies. Sleepiness can typically be relieved by a restorative sleep pattern, good nutrition, and reduced stress. Fatigue that is deeply rooted requires further healthcare assessment and a longer recovery.

The cycle of fatigue can be perpetuated by the same medical system that is trying to solve it. The patient struggling to be heard and have his or her condition diagnosed can be made more fatigued by the work of obtaining a diagnosis and treatment. Assigning the patient multiple treatments may induce more patient weariness in efforts to fix the problem. Integrative nursing principles encourage an approach that requires a high degree of sensitivity and awareness of the individuality of the patient in relationship to their disease. Carefully paced integrative interventions allow time for the patients to activate their innate healing ability (Maizes & Caspi, 1999).

The Integrative Nursing Perspective and Fatigue

The integrative nursing perspective offers another view of the complex and common condition of fatigue. Initial efforts in assessing the patient start with a foundation of person-centered, relationship-based care (Principle 4). Due to the poor specificity of the condition, deeply listening to the patient's story and understanding his or her history is essential to laying the foundation of integrative care. Integrative physicians Maizes and Low Dog suggest that broader questions in the patient interview will later create a framework for a broader choice of treatment modalities (2010).

Fatigue is redefined as a state of imbalance within the paradigm of integrative health. It is a multifactorial discord that has roots in the physical, psychological, spiritual, energetic, and/or environmental dimensions of the patient's life. The lack of a clear allopathic diagnosis does not diminish the presence or impact of fatigue for the patient. Without an allopathic diagnosis, the integrative nurse continues to consider the reality of the patient's experience and seeks to assist the patient in moving towards optimal health (Principle 1). The complex discord and imbalance of a fatigue diagnosis requires consideration of an interdisciplinary intervention approach with a full complement of evidence-based therapeutic modalities (Principle 5). The integrative nurse facilitates the shift from fatigue to optimal health, maintains the relationship of patient-centered care legitimizing the patient's experience of fatigue, and, as needed, increases the number of treatment strategies, moving from least intensive to more complex (Koithan, Verhoef, Bell, White, Mulkins, & Ritenbaugh, 2007).

Rebecca's Story: Case Scenario

Rebecca is 50-year-old female who has been referred to an integrative health clinic by an internal medicine physician for complaints of fatigue lasting more than four months. She had a complete physical assessment and laboratory testing with one abnormal finding of a low vitamin D level. Increasing supplementation brought her vitamin D level to normal; however, a "plateau of fatigue" still exists, and the patient is requesting an integrative approach to her fatigue diagnosis. She identifies the precipitating event as the November start of the busy holiday work season, during which "everything fell apart and I didn't have the energy to get up." Prior to that time, she does not recall feeling the "fatigue heaviness" she has identified over the past months.

- Work: Rebecca is a successful chef and owns a company supplying restaurants. Works 10–12 hours days supervising 25 people on a tight delivery schedule.
- Relationship: Lives with husband and two young adult children, describes marriage and family as "great, very happy" and supportive. Describes work relationships as friendly.
- Sleep: Sleeps seven hours without disturbance and wakes at 6:00 am. The most physically demanding part of her workday is between 6:00 am and 12:00 noon.
- Nutrition: Does not eat until 1:00 pm each day and feels exhausted afterwards. Drinks two glasses of wine or port at night with dinner at 8:00 or 9:00 pm. Diet assessment: fewer than five servings of fruits and vegetables per day, low fiber, minimal protein, states preference for pasta and white rice. Eats two meals a day, 8–10 hours apart, without snacks. (BMI is normal.)
- Supplements: vitamin D, 50,000 units per week.
- Restorative practices: No regular exercise, mind–body, or spiritual-based practice.
- Environment: Reports home (bed and couch) as a refuge from demands of work. Describes work environment as "exciting and demanding." Does not spend any time outdoors.

The integrative approach to Rebecca's case is based in integrative nursing principles that assist the healing process, regardless of the diagnosis. Understanding patient beliefs and values and the context of their lives shapes the integrative treatment plan. The healer credits consistency and coherence in the patient's illness perception to legitimize and validate the experience of his or her condition (Elsass et al., 2007). The dyadic dance of healing between the integrative nurse and the patient recognizes the complexities of the human–environmental system and understands that the patient cannot simply be reduced to a diagnosis (Principle 1).

Legitimizing the patient story creates a shift that triggers the patient's innate capacity for health and wellbeing (Maizes & Caspi, 1999) (Principle 2). Understanding that the patient once felt healthy and vital allows the integrative nurse to see the fatigue experience as an unfolding process that cannot be reduced to a diagnosis (Principle 1). The nurse's sense of healing intention, self-awareness, and nonjudgmental presence can itself promote a healing opportunity for the patient (Deary, Roche, Plotkin, & Zahourek, 2011). The integrative model of care stresses the belief within the caregiver that they are in themselves an important instrument of healing beyond the immediate modalities of medications and surgery (Jackson, 2004) (Principle 6). Healing intentionality on the nurse's part creates motivation and then action; this movement can shift the disease dynamic out of dysfunction and *stuckness*, towards a sense of healing and clarity (Koithan et al., 2007).

Assessing Fatigue

Assessing the symptoms from an integrative perspective starts with creating an opening for patients to feel comfortable enough to tell the story of their fatigue, the depth of their symptoms, and the impact on their functionality. The integrative nurse practices intentionality, bringing a conscious awareness to the assessment of the patient's body, mind, and spirit (Deary, Roche, et al., 2011). Unhurried, quiet, and comfortable environments can generate a more intimate response from the patient, reduce stress, and provide an opportunity for the nurse to listen deeply (Geimer-Flanders, 2009).

Assessment includes exploring with the patient what is behind the fatigue and the fullness of his or her experience. The integrative nursing perspective encompasses an understanding of patients living in a persistent state of flight-or-fight response, chronic stress and anxiety disorders, lifestyles that are frenetic and compartmentalized, poor nutrition, lack of restorative practices, loss of a spiritual connection, and the loss of compensatory strategies. Of equal importance to assessing the patient's illness experiences, integrative nursing seeks an understanding of what the patient felt like when they were healthy, what gave them joy and vitality. Assessing what the turning point or tipping point was for the patient in the fatigue progression can further illuminate the assessment. Patients often point to a specific incident or time when it started that may not appear relevant or connected to the provider (Elsass et al., 2007). Determining the key life intersections when the patient felt a fatigue imbalance can provide insight into his or her belief system about the disorder.

Relevant and evidence-based assessment tools to measure fatigue provide additional data for assessment. Currently, no gold standard that measures fatigue exists, and guidelines are ambiguous. Objective measurements focus on physiological processes or performance, such as errors or a change in reaction time. Subjective measures include the assessment interview, patient diaries, and questionnaires. When it is difficult for patients to describe their condition in words, visual images—either drawn by the patient or shown to them—can help define the impact of fatigue on the different aspects of self. Utilizing art expression in the assessment process can in itself be a healing practice (Jackson, 2004).

There are numerous clinical questionnaires to assess fatigue, including the Fatigue Severity Scale (Krupp, LaRocca, Muir-Nash, & Steinberg, 1989), the Fatigue Assessment Inventory (National Palliative Care Research Center, 2012), and the Piper Fatigue Scale (Piper, Dibble, Dodd, Weiss, Slaughter and Paul, 1998). The Fatigue Assessment Inventory is brief, commonly used, and available in several languages (Laranjeira, 2012). Developed in 1989, it is a 7-point rating scale of nine items. The complexity of the fatigue disorder often requires a more comprehensive assessment, which can be done through the added value of multiple tools. Examples of further assessment tools include, but are not limited to, the following: Sleep Quality Index (Buysse, Reynolds, Monk, Berman, & Kupfer (1989), PHQ 9 Depression Assessment (Kroenke, Spitzer, &Williams, 2001), Depression, Anxiety, Stress Scales (Lovibond & Lovibond, 1995), and the Functional Assessment of Chronic Illness Therapy–Spiritual WellBeing scale (FACIT-Sp) (Bredle, Salsman, Debb, Arnold, & Cella, 2011).

Fatigue is not always measurable by conventional methods, even with the best assessment tools. Integrative nursing considers that a patient may also benefit from approaches outside of the traditional biomedical system. Therefore, fatigue can be viewed and assessed from the perspectives of alternative healing systems; examples of this can be found in the traditional Chinese medicine (TCM) perspective, the Ayurvedic system, and through energy medicine principles. TCM may approach fatigue as the loss or blockage of *qi*, the vital energy moving through the body (Brown, R., 2008). The Ayurvedic system views fatigue through the three key constitutions, or mind–body types (Pitta, Vata, Kapha). An individual's balance within their mind-body type corresponds to the essential components of mind, body, and spirit being in balance. When the digestive fire (*agni*) of the body underperforms, fatigue and apathy can result (Gopal, 2008).

The chronic condition of fatigue may be also viewed as the result of a spiritual imbalance. Integrative psychiatrist Henry Emmons aptly describes spiritual imbalance as "a loss of an animating or creative force in his or her life, bringing on a state of apathy or darkness, like living in a cloud" (Emmons, 2006, p. 129).

Integrative nursing considers that the patient's positive coping strategies inherent in maintaining spiritual wellbeing and life satisfaction are impacted by chronic illness. Understanding the role that spirituality plays in illness and loss informs cross-cultural treatment interventions and aids in linking belief systems to intervention (Bredle et al., 2011). Spiritual support can come in many forms, based on the patient's beliefs, values, culture, and religion. Some examples of spiritual support may include: the compassionate presence of the caregiver, counseling from a spiritual or religious advisor, ritual and prayer, the intimacy and support of loved ones, and meditative reflection.

Understanding that integrative principles provide an alternate context in which to view and treat the patient's disease enriches the integrative nursing assessment process. Seeing the fatigue disorder as an imbalance of the body, mind, and spirit triad or as a blockage of vital energy flow allows the nurse to use a broader toolkit of integrative therapies (Jackson, 2004). As described in Principle 5, the nurse considers many forms of knowledge and multiple forms of evidence when choosing treatment interventions.

A comprehensive integrative assessment of the fatigued patient includes a careful history to determine the individual's fatigue pattern and to identify and understand the individual patient experience. Table 21.1 summarizes aspects to be considered in this assessment, and Rebecca's story serves as an example of its implementation.

Table 21.1: Integrative Nursing Assessment of Fatigue

Integrative Nursing	*Patient's Story of Fatigue Experience*
BODY Observe body language, posture, and movement. Be attentive to all aspects of the physical manifestation of fatigue.	• Symptoms, duration, and severity • Treatments and alleviating factors • Current medications • Sleep and/or rest patterns, immobility • Nutrition intake and any appetite or weight changes. Eating patterns • Anemia, pain, dehydration, nutritional deficiency, endocrine disorders • Complete physical evaluation
MIND Listen for the emotional impact of fatigue, the individual experience, contributing factors and a triggering event.	• Evaluation for depression, anxiety • Stress assessment • Financial resources • Impact on work and professional life • Relationship stress • Abuse: physical, sexual, emotional, financial
SPIRIT Be attentive to key imagery and language used to describe the fatigue experience. Be attentive to interwoven core beliefs.	• Core values and beliefs about fatigue • Restorative practices • Effects of fatigue on activities of daily living and lifestyle • Current or past trauma experiences • Past experiences of health, vitality, and joy

Clinical Decision-Making and Priority-Setting

Integrative nursing works to optimize health regardless of the symptom, meeting the patient where he or she is on the health–illness continuum. Consideration is given for age relevancy, life circumstances, patient goals, and willingness to change, while being attentive to physiological disorders, signs of depression, or psychological conditions.

The key goals of the integrative nursing interventions are to legitimize the story and the storyteller in their experience, and assist the patient in exploring a change in the story to move from imbalance and discord towards balance and vitality (Elsass et al., 2007; Koithan et al., 2007). The interventions focus on increasing resiliency and decreasing any maladaptive behaviors.

Prioritizing a broad integrative assessment sets the foundation for the choice and sequencing of interventions. The integrative nurse considers where the fatigue has had the greatest impact on the patient, the patient's beliefs and values about the disorder, and the adaptive behaviors the fatigue has necessitated in the patient's life. The integrative nurse recognizes the imbalance and discord found in the patient's work schedule, in her diet and meal timing, and in the lack of restorative practices. In Rebecca's case, the top three priorities to address in her fatigue disorder would be: (a) the immobilizing fatigue with a significant impact on work functionality; (b) the disproportionate ratio of rest or restorative therapies in relation to high-intensity productivity; and (c) her nutritional disregulation and deficit.

Integrative Fatigue Interventions

Clear and simple interventions that are non-taxing to the patient inform fatigue treatment interventions. Strong consideration is given to the amount of available energy the patient is working with and her own innate sense of how to move towards greater wellbeing. The patient guides the interventions and the timing of progress through treatments.

Rebecca is at an age of midlife transition, and health factors related to age have significant relevancy in intervention management (Greenblum, Rowe, Felber, & Greenblum, 2012). Based on Rebecca's assessment, interventions are targeted to address the area where her fatigue is having the greatest impact, her professional life. Assessment is an ongoing process; as new interventions are introduced, the patient is reassessed before increasing the intensity of additional treatment. In Table 21.2, the five tiers of integrative nursing interventions move from least to greatest intensity and provide evidence-based interventions grounded in integrative principles.

The Fatigue Intervention Table is useful to the integrative nurse in organizing an individual plan for the patient, which moves from simple treatment to more intensive interventions. In a meta-analytic review of non-pharmacological therapies for treating fatigue in cancer patients, the following three categories of treatment have the strongest

Table 21.2: Fatigue Interventions

Level of Intensity	Integrative Therapy Approach
Tier 1 Interventions	**Mind–Body Therapies** • Progressive Muscle Relaxation Technique • Guided Imagery **Nutritional Therapies** • Reestablish consistent eating patterns and increase nutritional value **Natural Products** • Aromatherapy: Lavender **Natural Products/Supplements** • Vitamin and nutrient supplements **Basic Foundation Integrative Nursing Therapies** • Energy Management
Tier 2 Interventions	**Movement Therapies** • Yoga class **Nutritional Therapies** • Nutritional evaluation **Natural Products/Herbs** • Ginseng
Tier 3 Interventions	**Mind–Body Therapies** • Mindfulness-Based Stress Reduction (MBSR) **Energy Therapies** • Reiki **Health Coaching** • Consistent guidance and support for healthy lifestyle
Tier 4 Interventions	**Whole Systems** • Ayurvedic • Traditional Chinese medicine
Tier 5 Interventions	**Pharmacological therapies** **Psychotherapy/behavioral therapy**

evidence base for managing fatigue: restorative approaches, supportive-expressive interventions, and cognitive-behavioral psychosocial interventions (Kangas, Bovbjerg, & Montgomery, 2008; Berger et al., 2008). Understanding this, the integrative nurse utilizes current evidence to guide the choice of interventions.

With a fatigue diagnosis, it is essential to consider the pacing and demands of the treatments offered. Whether choosing treatments from Tier 1 or Tier 5, all possible side effects need to be considered and potential relapses in progress adjusted for. Patients may move up or down among the tiers of interventions as necessitated by their response. The patient's innate healing ability plays a significant role in a dynamic progress towards wellbeing. Being attentive to the transformative shift in the patient response following a treatment choice can be key in integrative care evaluation (Koithan et al., 2007).

Tier 1 is the foundation that sets the stage for energy management, and this includes prioritizing and balancing work and rest cycles and cultivating the individual's awareness of restorative needs (Can, 2013). The restorative therapies of guided imagery and relaxation techniques are fundamental to mind–body medicine and have been shown to reduce stress response and anxiety (Rakel & Faass, 2006). They assist in down-regulating the autonomic nervous system, regulating respiration, and facilitating rest (Dayapoglu & Tan, 2012; Can, 2013). An example of this is found in the progressive muscle relaxation technique (PMRT), which is an integral intervention in dealing with a chronic disease. PMRT serves to assist the patient in voluntary stretching and relaxation of large-muscle groups through progressive exercises and respiration control. Guided imagery and/or music are added to enhance the relaxation response. The benefits of PMRT include facilitating sleep, reducing anxiety and the effects of stress, and reducing sensitivity to fatigue. A study utilizing PMRT to treat fatigue in multiple sclerosis patients found that a 5–20-minute PMRT session can effectively enhance sleep quality and preserve individuals' physical energy (Dayapoglu & Tan, 2012).

Tier 1 interventions also include addressing deficits in nutritional intake and disregulation of eating patterns that contribute to loss of energy. Evidence indicates that eating early in the day supports optimum functioning, and a consistent meal pattern with core nutrients supports energy needs throughout the day (Brown, J., 2008). Evaluation for a lack of essential nutrients that support immune functioning (such as Vitamin D, antioxidants, and probiotics) are considered in integrative care.

The last Tier 1 intervention is lavender aromatherapy, which has been widely used to modify mood and sleep. In a study on its use in midlife women with fatigue, 20-minute inhalation periods twice weekly were found to decrease heart rate variability and improve sleep quality during the 12-week study period (Chien, Cheng, & Liu, 2011). The benefits of aromatherapy include that it is relatively inexpensive and can be self-administered.

The second-tier interventions increase to more active forms of mind–body techniques. In a meta-analysis determining relevant effects on fatigue, yoga had a moderate confidence effect (Boehm, Ostermann, Milazzo, & Bussing, 2012). There have been few randomized controlled trials, but smaller studies indicate improvement in fatigue symptoms with cancer patients (Can, 2013). The physical exercise benefits of yoga can aid in attenuating anxiety, depression, stress, and fatigue. Studies show evidence for improving energy and reducing depression through a combination of yoga, exercise, and resonant breathing for 20 minutes twice a day (Brown, R., 2008).

In addition, Tier 2 interventions include further nutritional evaluation, which may include an elimination or anti-inflammatory diet to restore optimal absorption and gastrointestinal health (Teitelbaum, 2005). A nutritionist may be utilized for this intervention, or the integrative nurse can initiate basic dietary changes that include sound nutritional principles.

"Herbal adaptogens" are treatments that appear to increase the body's ability to adapt to stress and changing situations (Barton, Liu, Dakhil, et al., 2012). An herbal adaptogen is nontoxic to the user, generates a nonspecific response, and benefits the body as a whole. The adaptogen must also help create a state of balance in the patient and restore homeostasis. They are more commonly recommended by naturopaths, TCM, and Ayurvedic practitioners, but the integrative nurse who is knowledgeable in their use and potential side effects may choose to introduce them in the intervention recommendations. Ginseng is an example of an adaptogen used to treat fatigue. In a study done on fatigue related to cancer, the use of American ginseng at 2000 mg daily for eight weeks showed a reduction in general and physical fatigue without side effects (Barton et al., 2012). Ginseng, like many adaptogens, is Category C for level of evidence in fatigue treatment (Ulbricht, 2010), which indicates further studies are needed.

The Tier 3 interventions include the use of mindfulness-based stress reduction (MBSR), Reiki, and health coaching. MBSR is a cognitive therapy that is usually taught in group sessions over eight weeks. Fatigue and improved sleep patterns have shown statistically significant improvement in several studies, although larger randomized controlled trails are still pending (Can, 2013). There is a psychosocial component to group sessions that could indicate added value for spiritual wellbeing and supportive-expressive experiences (Kangas et al., 2008). Inherent in MBSR is learning self-management skills for stress and balance that are patient-centered and adaptable to any setting.

Reiki, a form of energy medicine, can provide restorative relief of stress and tension and promote self-healing in the patient (Lee, Pittler, & Ernst, 2008). Although large, randomized controlled studies of Reiki are lacking, smaller studies have shown Reiki to decrease fatigue and significantly improve quality of life when compared to a resting control group (Lee et al., 2008). Some of the biological responses to Reiki have included decreased levels of stress hormones, improved blood pressure and heart rate, decreased cortisol levels, and an improved sense of wellbeing (Coakley & Barron, 2012). "It is possible that the deep relaxation associated with Reiki, Healing Touch and Therapeutic Touch treatments, documented both qualitatively and through improved bio-physical markers, allows the body's self-regulated mechanisms to recalibrate...." (p. 62).

Tier 3 also includes the use of a trained health coach. A personal health coach can support the patient's self-discovery process and provide individualized supportive approaches over time (Wolever, Caldwell, Wakefield, et al., 2011). Strategies for prioritizing work–life balance and healthy lifestyle management are within the domain of health coaching and can complement and help sustain the integrative nursing interventions.

Tier 4 interventions involve assessment and ongoing treatment through alternate whole systems such as Ayurveda or traditional Chinese medicine. Ayurveda is a comprehensive system of natural health that originated in India over 5,000 years ago and is part of the yoga philosophy. Pilot studies in Ayurvedic treatments addressing depression, anxiety, and sleep disorders, which are all contributory factors in fatigue, showed significant relief (Sharma, Chandola, Singh, & Basisht, 2007). Further clinical trials are needed to translate the effects of Ayurveda therapies into biomedicine terms. TCM also offers another whole-system approach to fatigue. Research has been published on the benefit of TCM for pain treatment, but fewer studies are available on the use of TCM for fatigue. In a randomized controlled study on fatigue in breast cancer patients, significant improvement in mental and physical fatigue, as well as quality of life were noted (Molassiotis, Bardy, Finnegan-John, et al., 2012). In reviewing the evidence for interventions, the integrative nurse realizes the benefits of qualitative and quantitative research and appreciates that complex systems utilizing innovative approaches are not adequately captured by one method of measurement (Verhoef, Lewith, Ritenbaugh, Boon, Fleishman, & Leis, 2005).

Tier 5 interventions encompass pharmacological therapies such as antidepressants, anti-anxiety medications, and psychotherapy. The integrative nurse can continue to provide guidance and support for integrative therapies as the patient moves to more intensive interventions. The interventions started in Tier 1 continue to provide value at low cost, with few, if any, side effects. Patients' ability to self-manage and prevent recurrences of fatigue is promoted and maintained by the integrative nurse.

REBECCA'S INTERVENTIONS IN ACTION

Rebecca's intervention plan was based on her choices to make small nutritional changes for improving her energy throughout her work day, increase her rest and reflective activities, and try energy-based therapy.

- Increase from two to three meals with protein, and between-meal snacks.
- Eat first meal prior to starting morning work.
- Decrease alcohol intake.
- Referral to clinic Reiki therapist for one-hour sessions.
- Commit to a minimum of 20 minutes twice a day of restorative therapy of choice. Example: breath and relaxation techniques, listening to guided imagery tape, spending quiet time outside.
- Return to clinic in two months for ongoing support and reassessment.

Outcome Evaluation

Integrative nursing principles are grounded in relationship-based care, and treatment plans involve continuing follow-up and re-assessment for the patient recovering from a fatigue disorder. Many integrative therapies are based in a methodical change process that requires ongoing treatments and patient involvement. After allowing the patient to implement the first interventions, a secondary evaluation is done, utilizing fatigue questionnaires and the assessment process outlined earlier in this chapter. Assessing the top three concerns of the patient at the initial visit is a starting point for evaluating the effectiveness of the interventions.

Measuring the use and impact of integrative therapies can be improved by using a consistent questionnaire encompassing non-allopathic treatments throughout the assessment process (Quandt, Verhoef, Acury, et al., 2009). Alternatively, integrative nurses often assess for qualitative movements or shifts in the patient condition, recognizing that healing may not follow a clearly linear path as anticipated in allopathic treatments (Koithan et al., 2007).

Of importance in the evaluative process is the understanding that integrative nursing philosophy of care may be of value equal to or greater than the specific interventions applied. A Swedish study found significantly greater patient satisfaction and positive changes in health habits when an integrative health approach was used, as compared to a conventional care program in a similar population (Arman, Hammarqvist, & Kullbreg, 2011). Integrative care encompasses the individual dynamic balance of health and wellness and the essential role of the nurse as a healing facilitator, mediating and modifying the patient's journey along with the patient. Regardless of the diagnosis, the integrative nurse assists the patient in achieving optimal wellbeing within the context of their lives throughout their lifespan.

Summary

Fatigue without a physical cause remains clinically under-assessed and under-treated, regardless of its prevalence. Approaching the patient's fatigue experience from an integrative perspective allows the nurse to see the patient's story more fully and offer a broader range of treatment modalities. Validating the patient's experience of a chronic condition and its impact on his or her life is an essential component in assessing and treating fatigue. Current evidence-based studies show promising results for energy therapies, yoga, MBSR and PMRT, aromatherapy, nutritional support, and cultivating a restorative practice. Adaptogens, TCM, and Ayurveda are currently less researched by Western science but continue to provide a safe, alternate perspective on the fatigue experience and healing therapies.

Even as integrative nursing embraces the complex systems approach to healing, the nurse understands that she/he is a potent healing force in her right, with her own particular curative "manna." The presence and compassion of the nurse healer is a crucial synergistic adjunct to fatigue therapy. The key goals of the integrative nursing interventions are to legitimize the story and the storyteller in their experience and to assist patients in exploring a change in their story, a shift from imbalance and discord towards balance and vitality.

SELECTED REFERENCES

Barton, D., Liu, H., Dakhil, S., Linquist, B., Sloan, J., Nichols, C., et al. (2012). Phase III evaluation of American ginseng to improve cancer related fatigue: NCCTG trial NO7C2. *Journal of Clinical Oncology, 30*(Supplement abstract: 9001).

Berger, A., Kuhn, B., Farr, L., Lynch, J., Agrawal, J., & Von Essen, S. (2008). Behavioral treatment intervention trial to improve sleep quality and cancer-related fatigue. *Psycho-Oncology, 18*(6), 634–646.

Deary, L., Roche, J., Plotkin, K., & Zahourek, R. (2011). Intentionality and hatha yoga. *Holistic Nursing Practice, 25*(5), 246–253.

Elsass, P., Jensen, B., Morup, R., & Thogerson, M. (2007). The recognition of fatigue: A qualitative study of life stories from rehabilitation clients. *International Journal of Psychosocial Rehabilitation 11*(2), 75–87.

Kangas, M., Bovberg, D., & Montgomery, G. (2008). Cancer-related fatigue: A systematic meta-analytic review of non-pharmacological therapies for cancer patients. *American Psychological Association, Psychological Bulletin 134*(5), 700–741.

Koithan, M., Verhoff, M., Bell, I., White, M., Mulkins, A., & Ritenbaugh, C. (2007). The process of whole person healing: Unstuckness and beyond. *Journal of Alternative & Complementary Medicine, 13*(6), 659–668.

Laranjeira, C. (2012). Translation and adaption of the fatigue severity scale for use in Portugal. *Applied Nursing Research, 25*(3), 212–217.

Naiman, R. (2006). *Healing Night.* Minneapolis, MN: Syren Book Company.

Rakel, D., & Faass, N. (2006). *Complementary Medicine in Clinical Practice.* Boston, MA: Jones and Bartlett Publishers.

Sabes-Figuera, R., McCrone, P., Hurley, M., King, M., Donalson, A., & Ridsdale, L. (2010). The hidden cost of chronic fatigue to patients and their families. *BMC Health Services Research, 10*, 56.

22

Integrative Nursing Management of Pain

JUDY L. WAGNER AND SUSAN THOMPSON

The Burden of Pain

Pain affects everyone universally, regardless of age, gender, or ethnicity, and is one of the most common reasons patients seek medical care. Pain represents a significant institutional challenge as clinicians attempt to provide relief and reduce suffering. Both acute and chronic pain impose tremendous burdens for the United States in terms of healthcare costs, lost worker productivity, and emotional burdens to patients and families (Institute of Medicine of The National Academies [IOM], 2011). Approximately 100 million adults are affected by common chronic pain conditions—more than the number affected by heart disease, diabetes, and cancer combined—costing approximately $600 billion annually in direct medical treatment costs and lost productivity (IOM, 2011).

Despite the availability of effective therapies, studies continue to suggest that pain is undertreated (Wells, Pasero, & McCaffery, 2008). This unrelieved pain results in longer hospital stays, increased readmission rates, increased outpatient visits, and inability of patients to function fully (IOM, 2011). Pain experiences vary widely from person to person in terms of severity, duration, and response to treatment and can have profound emotional and psychological effects (IOM, 2011).

"PAIN" DEFINED

Pain is a highly individualized and subjective experience with no clear, objective measurement tool available for use when caring for patients. "Pain is whatever the experiencing person says it is, existing whenever he/she says it does" (McCaffery, 1968, p. 95). Acute pain typically lasts fewer days (less than seven) and occurs as a result of a single and treatable event such as traumatic injury, surgical procedure, or medical disorder, and is often associated with autonomic nervous system responses such as tachycardia, hypertension, and diaphoresis, which decrease with time (American College of Emergency Physicians [ACEP], 2009). Pain may also be caused by pathological and potentially life-threatening conditions, including cancer (ACEP, 2009).

Chronic pain is persistent pain that lasts longer than the expected time of healing and is continuous or recurs at intervals for months or years, and may occur without a known etiology (ACEP, 2009). Common examples of persistent pain include back and neck pain, arthritis, and diabetic neuropathy.

An Integrative Nursing Approach to Pain

The evolution of pain management over the last two decades has resulted in many technologically sophisticated diagnostic and therapeutic approaches (Audette & Bailey, 2008). This advancement has been accompanied by an array of pharmacological options to treat pain, including over-the-counter and prescription medications. Despite the growth in options to treat pain, it is not uncommon to find patients who continue to experience pain in spite of many therapeutic procedures and countless medications.

Inherent in this classic model of pain management is the viewpoint that the role of the healthcare professional is to *do* something or *fix* the pain, rather than work collaboratively with the patient to resolve the root cause of the pain or improve the functional consequences of the pain condition (Audette & Bailey, 2008). Alternatively, an integrative approach to pain management takes into consideration the whole person—physical, mental, emotional, spiritual, and social dimensions—and utilizes a full range of appropriate therapies to promote optimal healing. This includes focusing on a patient's lifestyle, beliefs, values, and sense of who they are, in addition to symptoms and test results. This integrative, relational approach emphasizes the body's innate capacity for healing and offers options that support healing. Consider the following scenario.

Case Scenario

Mr. S. was going for an amputation and was very agitated, picking at the air, pulling his curtain, hypersensitive to touch. Everything was painful to him. He was on call for the operating room and was waiting for the notification that they were ready for him.

Integrative Nursing Care

The integrative nurse approached Mr. S., took his hand, and offered to do acupressure, hand massage, and imagery. He nodded, agreeing to try it. She started with the hand massage and imagery, and when finished she asked again, "Are you ok with trying acupressure?" He agreed to that, and the nurse proceeded to apply pressure to points on his head/neck and shoulders. During the acupressure, a tear rolled down his cheek. The nurse asked, "Should I stop? Does it hurt too much?" Mr. S. answered, "No, but can I get one last foot massage before my foot is amputated?" She stopped applying acupressure and instead moved to the bottom of the gurney, uncovered his foot, and tenderly, lightly began to massage. Almost immediately, Mr. S. fell asleep and slept peacefully until the OR transport came to pick him up.

While the nurse brings his or her clinical experience and different "ways of knowing" to better understand what a patient may need for pain, no amount of wisdom and experience can match the innate ability of patients to know their own bodies, their discomfort, and what is needed to help them heal. In this case, the nurse "listens" with intuition; she "hears" the psychic, spiritual pain of Mr. S., and she reaches out to comfort him (Principle 4). Rather than ask Mr. S. about his pain and discomfort, quantifying its level of intensity and defining qualities and quickly offering an immediate intervention, she offers herself (Principle 2). This idea of the nurse "being the medicine" (personal communication, Quinn, 2012) goes beyond deep listening and incorporates different "ways of knowing," including intuition. One of the most important roles a nurse can play in pain management is "listening beyond the words"; the nurse becomes an effective instrument for pain management through the use of authentic compassion and intention (Quinlan-Colwell, 2009) (Principle 5).

Recognizing that she cannot remove the physical pain, the integrative nurse offers comfort through touch and massage. Research demonstrates that human-to-human touch is a significant element in promoting a patient's wellbeing (Field, 2011), and touch communicates the nurse's caring and concern (Principle 4). Furthermore, touch elicits the relaxation response, offering refuge from the psycho-spiritual pain of Mr. S.'s impending surgery (Principles 1 and 5). The nurse checks frequently with Mr. S. to assure his comfort with the various interventions and, when asked, willingly provides the requested foot massage. She knows that by honoring his physical body, she also supports the healing of his spirit (Principle 2).

Assessing Pain

Nurses play a critical role in the assessment and treatment of pain because of their frequent contact and relationships with patients in a variety of settings, assuming responsibility for safe, high-quality pain management based on their scientific knowledge and technical expertise. The unique position of the nurse requires an understanding of pain mechanisms, variables that influence pain perception and pain response, valid and reliable methods to assess pain, and a range of available methods to relieve it.

The complexity of the pain experience requires comprehensive nursing assessment that characterizes the pain, appraises the impact of the pain, and evaluates coexisting psychosocial factors. Comprehensive assessment includes completing a history to identify location of the pain, intensity, quality, chronology and pattern, precipitating factors, alleviating factors, and associated symptoms. Observing behaviors of the patient provides important nonverbal information, especially for patients who cannot provide a description of the pain.

Failure to assess pain is a major cause of inadequate pain management, and studies show that moderate to severe pain is often underestimated when clinicians do not obtain pain ratings from patients (McCaffery & Pasero, 1999). Pain is measured by self-report whenever possible. If self-report is not possible, other strategies must be used to assess pain, including nonverbal behaviors or by proxy reporting. Family members or others who know the patient well can provide credible information and actively participate in this assessment (Herr et al., 2006).

Two of the more widely used tools for assessing the extent to which the patient suffers with pain include the Initial Pain Assessment Tool and the Brief Pain Inventory, most often used with chronic pain conditions. The short-form McGill Pain Questionnaire is another general pain assessment tool often used in clinical practice and research. Pain rating scales (e.g., Visual Analog [VAS], Numeric Rating [NRS], and Faces) are often used in daily clinical practice to measure the intensity of pain. In order to provide adequate treatment and facilitate communication among healthcare professionals, pain should be routinely assessed and documented before and after treatments (McCaffery & Pasero, 1999).

Yet, listening to the patient's story is paramount when assessing pain. It has become an unfamiliar role for the nurse to approach patients with the intention of listening deeply. Rather, nurses more frequently ask patients about their symptoms, quantifying intensity and defining qualities, and quickly offer an immediate intervention. One of the most important roles a nurse can play in pain management is hearing authentically what the patient is saying about their pain, its characteristics, its history, and its effects on their mind, body, and spirit.

Patients often relate their satisfaction with pain management to their direct experiences with their healthcare providers, the quality of the patient–provider relationship, and the provider's ability to understand fully their experiences of pain (Beck et al., 2010). Creating a space where the patient feels heard without judgment is imperative when developing a solid nurse–patient relationship that puts the needs of the patient first. Developing a deep relationship with a patient can only occur when the nurse is fully present with the patient and uses self as a tool for healing. "For that moment, they are joined with the other who is patient...and so become part of the something larger than either alone. In this transpersonal healing process, they are each changed" (Quinn, 2009, p. 94).

Integrative Pain Interventions: The Right Therapy for the Right Situation

Not all therapies are appropriate or indicated for every patient condition. Integrative nurses choose from a full complement of evidence-based therapies. For decades, analgesics have been at the forefront in the management of acute and chronic pain. While this approach can be very effective, it is not without adverse physical and psychosocial consequences that can dramatically affect a patient's quality of life, especially with chronic use. Pharmacotherapy is considered one of the most invasive options in the treatment of pain, along with other interventions such as nerve blocks and surgical procedures. While there is certainly a place for these options, it is best practice to try the least invasive treatment option first if possible.

This is also true when considering the use of prn analgesics. Although narcotics are frequently used quickly in the treatment of pain, milder medications, such as NSAIDs and acetaminophen, can be used effectively, especially when used in conjunction with other non-pharmacological interventions. It is essential to acknowledge that patients have an innate ability to heal and can adapt to their physical conditions if provided with the tools that promote self-healing. By introducing therapies that potentially decrease, or in some cases eliminate, the need for high doses of pain medication, patients can take control of and better manage their pain. A key benefit from the use of these therapies is the cultivation of a sense of empowerment and control over a patient's ability to manage pain. Table 22.1 displays leading pain management techniques organized in order of least to most intensive.

MIND–BODY STRATEGIES

Our bodies follow our thoughts, and it is through this unbreakable connection that patients can take control of their pain and improve their quality of life. Reed, Montgomery, and DuHamel (2001) found mind–body methods (e.g., relaxation, imagery, mindfulness) "hold the greatest promise for benefit to the patient" (p. 821).

The *Relaxation Response* demonstrates how changes in thoughts can have profound effects on the body and its responses to internal and external stimuli (Benson & Stuart, 1993). The Relaxation Response utilizes the repetition of a word, phrase, prayer, sound, or muscular activity, which helps focus and calm the mind. Through stimulation of the parasympathetic nervous system, the Relaxation Response decreases blood pressure, heart and respiratory rates, muscle tension, and neurohormone output, all of which aggravate pain. This technique can be helpful with chronic pain, but it can also be used during acute pain episodes. The nurse can offer patients education and training by helping them identify words, phrases, or prayers that hold special meaning to them and simply guiding them through the steps of the Relaxation Response (Box 22.1).

Table 22.1: Integrative Approaches to Pain Management

Level of Intensity	Integrative Therapy Approach
Tier 1 Interventions	**Mind–Body Therapies** • Relaxation response • Guided imagery • Music • Distraction • Prayer **Basic Foundational Integrative Nursing Therapies** • Touch • Therapeutic listening, presence, therapeutic use of self **Hot/Cold Therapy**
Tier 2 Interventions	**Mind–Body Therapies** • Progressive muscle relaxation **Movement Therapies** • Yoga • Qi Gong • Tai Chi **Natural Products** • Aromatherapy **Hydrotherapy**
Tier 3 Interventions	**Mind–Body Therapies** • Hypnosis • Cognitive Behavioral [pain management] Therapy • MBSR meditation • Biofeedback **Energy Therapies** • Reiki • Healing/therapeutic touch • Acupuncture • Acupressure **Manipulative Therapies** • Massage • Reflexology **Over-the-counter analgesics (NSAIDs, acetaminophen)**
Tier 4 Interventions	**Whole Systems** • TCM (acupuncture) • Homeopathy **Manipulative Therapies** • Chiropractic **Prescription Analgesics** • NSAIDs • Non-narcotic analgesics **Transcutaneous Electrical Nerve Stimulation (TENS)**
Tier 5 Interventions	**Pharmacological Therapies** **Surgical Procedures** **Nerve Blocks**

Patients should practice this technique once or twice daily, regardless of pain level, to strengthen their ability to quickly fall into a relaxed state when needed, but it should also be done whenever pain levels become burdensome. Good times to practice are before breakfast and before dinner.

Box 22.1 Techniques to Elicit the Relaxation Response

The following is the generic technique taught at the Benson-Henry Institute.

1. Pick a focus word, short phrase, or prayer that is firmly rooted in your belief system, such as "one," "peace," "The Lord is my shepherd," "Hail, Mary, full of grace," or "shalom."
2. Sit quietly in a comfortable position.
3. Close your eyes.
4. Relax your muscles, progressing from your feet to your calves, thighs, abdomen, shoulders, head, and neck.
5. Breathe slowly and naturally, and as you do, say your focus word, sound, phrase, or prayer silently to yourself as you exhale.
6. Assume a passive attitude. Don't worry about how well you're doing. When other thoughts come to mind, simply say to yourself, "Oh well," and gently return to your repetition.
7. Continue for ten to twenty minutes.
8. Do not stand immediately. Continue sitting quietly for a minute or so, allowing other thoughts to return. Then open your eyes and sit for another minute before rising.

Practice the technique once or twice daily. Good times to do so are before breakfast and before dinner.

Meditation is a practice that has been used for thousands of years to ease suffering and calm the mind and body. It is a common misconception that meditation is used solely for relaxation, when actually relaxation and stress reduction are only two of its many benefits. Meditation does not let the mind rest, but rather trains it to have greater focus and clarity by calming the mind and reducing distractions (Davidson & Lutz, 2008). Since meditation is really about paying attention, it is likely that many people are already performing some form of meditation or mindfulness-based practice without knowing it (Kabat-Zinn, 1990). Common types of meditation are sedentary, done while sitting or kneeling with little or no movement; silent, which allows for movement and activities, but without any verbal communication and may include refraining from reading or writing; and movement or repetitive meditation, which incorporates some type of repetitive rhythmic movements (Kreitzer, 2005). Prayer is a familiar example of meditation.

Individuals who practice mindfulness-based techniques have been shown to have significant improvements in arthritic, back, and neck pain, as well as quality of life and psychological symptoms (Rosenzweig, Greeson, Reibel, Green, Jasser, & Beasley, 2010). One program that introduces individuals to these techniques is mindfulness-based stress reduction (MBSR), an eight-week training program that has been shown to be an effective method for easing the burden of chronic pain and improving quality of life (Teixeira, 2008). Whether meditation is learned during an MBSR program or another form of mindfulness-based training, it can be a useful tool when living with chronic pain, but is not frequently used in acute pain.

Guided imagery is another simple yet powerful and effective low-cost tool used to promote relaxation. In essence, the technique employs the use of one's imagination to regulate pain through sensory images; thus, the intensity of pain is decreased or becomes more acceptable (Mobily, Herr, & Kelley, 1993). Imagery, a fundamental aspect of holistic nursing practice, can be used to "reframe the experience or perception, facilitate problem solving, and ultimately increase one's sense of control over one's inner and outer life" (Brown-Saltzman, 1997). Imagery as a technique acts on the entire physiology by interacting with the image-making function of the brain (Schaub & Dossey, 2009).

Guided imagery as a clinical intervention has received significant attention in the literature as a strategy to relieve postoperative pain, pain related to cancer, and chronic pain (Antall & Kresevic, 2004; Schwab et al., 2007; Tusek, Church, & Fazio, 1997). A study on chronic headache pain revealed that patients who used guided imagery experienced decreased headache frequency, severity, and disability, and improved quality of life (Mannix et al., 1999). A 2011 systematic review showed that eight of nine randomized controlled trials suggested that guided imagery leads to a significant reduction of musculoskeletal pain (Posadzki & Ernst, 2011). Two studies explored the effectiveness of guided imagery with progressive muscle-relaxation in osteoarthritis, finding the intervention reduced pain and mobility difficulties while improving quality of life (Baird & Sands, 2004; 2006).

Theory suggests that guided imagery reduces sympathetic arousal by eliciting the relaxation response and enhancing immune function by increasing the pain sufferer's sense of self-efficacy and changing the meaning of pain (Lewandowski, Jacobson, Palmieri, Alexander, & Zeller, 2011). The mechanisms underlying the effectiveness of guided imagery are based on three operating principles described by Naparstek (1994), including (1) our bodies are not able to discriminate between sensory images and reality; (2) the experience of guided imagery produces an altered state that prepares us for more rapid and intense healing, growth, learning, and change; and (3) guided imagery generates a sense of mastery and control over what is happening to us; thus we feel better.

In preparing to use guided imagery, the environment must be conducive to relaxation by ensuring the patient is comfortable by either sitting comfortably or reclining, has privacy, and the space is free of distractions. The patient is then directed to close their eyes or focus on one spot in the room, and the imagery session begins. The following script is an example of guided imagery that may be used to elicit the relaxation response to alleviate both pain and anxiety (Box 22.2).

Box 22.2 Guided Imagery Script

Once you are seated or lying still, close your eyes and begin by taking three slow, deep breaths through your nose, filling up your belly, releasing slowly. Take another breath, seeing if you can send the warm energy of your breath to any place in your body that feels tense or sore....invite your body to release tension it doesn't need with the exhale....some parts release quickly, others take more time....notice a response....allow unwinding to happen....see if you can feel your breath going to all the places needing attention, beginning with the top of your head and slowly working down to the soles of your feet where your muscles are tense....allow your breath to loosen and soften....as you do this, you begin to feel safe, comfortable, and relaxed...any unwelcome or distracting thoughts that come to mind can be released with the exhale....so for a moment, your mind can be a clear space in stillness....and your body settled into a position of complete relaxation....now create in your mind an image of a beautiful place....this is a special place where you feel safe and you can find refuge from your cares....you might choose a place you've already been....or one you've always wanted to visit.... or one you just imagine as being peaceful and restorative.... look around and notice what you see with your eyes.... the colors and shapes.... the details of the scenery.... both to your right and left, above and below your head.... notice what is there.... listen to the sounds of this special place.... allow your ears to become familiar with what you hear, whether it's sounds of nature or beautiful music.... notice what you feel against your skin.... whether it's a soft breeze or balmy stillness, warm or cool, allow yourself to absorb the feeling.... breathe in the fragrance of this safe and relaxing place....spend as much time as you need in this place.... rest and be at peace.... allow all your senses to take it all in, with feelings of gratitude.... know that you can come back to this place any time you wish for respite and relaxation.... that each journey to this place acknowledges and engages the wisdom of your body.... bathing each cell with healing love, supporting the restorative work it was designed to do.... when you are ready.... look for a path that leads away from the spot where you have been resting, preparing yourself to return to the outer world.... take a moment to review your experience.... notice if there is something to bring back with you.... to remind you to use your mind and body this way.... when you are ready, you may return more relaxed and refreshed, with a sense of peace and confidence about all that lies ahead for you.

Guided imagery can be used for most people experiencing both acute and chronic pain; however, many studies have excluded patients who were diagnosed with a significant mental illness to avoid the potential for triggering an undesirable outcome. Although it may be ideal for the nurse to guide an imagery session, it is often most practical to use a CD or MP3 recording, which are available through libraries, stores, and online.

ENERGY THERAPIES

Energy healing embraces a mixture of ancient and modern practices that are thought to tap into a universal energy source to which everyone has access (DiNucci, 2005). Different cultures have names for this subtle energy source, including *chi, qi, mana,* and *prana* (DiNucci, 2005). The underlying assumption behind energy healing is that illness, disease, pain, or weakness may result from a disruption of a body's energy paths (Fazzino & McNulty, 2010). The term *energy healing* is used to describe an intentional process of using an external energy field to alter one's own or another's field to initiate physical, mental, emotional, or spiritual healing, using either direct contact or no-contact touch (Fazzino & McNulty, 2010; Slater, 2009).

Some of the most popular energy healing modalities include Reiki, Healing Touch (HT), and Therapeutic Touch (TT). *Reiki,* a Japanese term that means "universal life energy," was rediscovered in the early 1900s by Mikao Usui from the root system of ancient Tibetan healing arts (Birocco et al., 2012). It is performed by placing your hands either on or above different areas of the body to channel universal life energy to the patient, with a goal of encouraging the healing process. Practitioners of Reiki do not need to be prepared as healthcare providers; however, nurses may enjoy greater access and acceptability within a healthcare system and are in a unique position to incorporate this modality into direct care (Ringdahl, 2010). Although there are no uniform standards in Reiki education, three levels of training are available to those who desire to practice Reiki (Ringdahl, 2010).

Healing Touch was developed by Janet Mentgen in the 1980s and uses the hands to mediate energy through touch on the body and non-contact touch above the body to encourage relaxation and healing. The healing touch techniques are used to clear energy and bring energetic balance to the body (Fazzino & McNulty, 2010). Healing Touch is taught throughout the world in six course levels that lead to certification, which is based upon completion of the training as well as clinical practice (DiNucci, 2005).

Therapeutic Touch, developed by Delores Krieger and Dora Kunz in the 1970s, is based on the premise that a complex, dynamic energy field is formed by the body, mind, emotions, and intuition (Fazzino & McNulty, 2010). The technique involves several steps, including assessing a patient's energy field for imbalances, clearing the energy field, and directing the energy to areas that need attention (DiNucci, 2005). Training consists of two twelve-hour workshops, followed by certification after completing a one-year mentorship program that includes clinical practice (Therapeutic Touch International Association, 2012).

Although the nursing literature provides numerous examples of research on energy healing modalities, there is limited research linking these therapies to pain relief. After reviewing twenty years of research, Fazzino and McNulty (2010) reported that energy healing (i.e., Reiki, HT, or TT) either decreased use of pain medication or increased the time span between dosages when used as an adjunct to standard treatment. Perhaps the greatest strength of energy therapy modalities is that they pose few, if any, risks to patients. It has been noted, however, that there is potential for the release of emotions, and practitioners must be prepared to handle such a response (DiNucci, 2005).

MASSAGE

Massage soothes a patient's aching body, encourages circulation of blood and lymph to and from tissues, and promotes relaxation; evidence supports the impact of human-to-human touch as a significant element that promotes wellbeing (Field, 2011). Historically a part of nursing practice, this modality has been utilized less over time, given the presence of advanced technology, biomedical monitoring, complex medication management, and documentation demands. Massage has become a "complementary therapy" in nursing practice rather than a fundamental skill (Ruffin, 2011).

Massage has been shown to be effective in decreasing chronic pain and its associated symptoms of anxiety and nausea in cancer patients (Wilkinson, Barnes, & Storey, 2008), but it can also be useful in other forms of pain such as with the short-term management of acute neck pain (Sherman, Cherkin, Hawkes, et al., 2009). A simple five-minute massage on each foot can have a significant effect on pain, nausea, and relaxation in cancer pain patients (Grealish, Lomasney, & Whiteman, 2000) and is easily implemented into daily nursing practice with immediate effects.

While gentle massage is considered safe and effective, there are some precautions. Each patient's condition and needs should be assessed individually, but generally massage should be avoided in the presence of infection and fever, hemophilia, undiagnosed severe headaches, phlebitis, hypertension, hemorrhage, organ failure, inflammatory arthritis, neuralgias, deep vein thrombosis, and metastatic cancer (Abrams & Weil, 2009; Rosen & Faass, 2006). Nursing judgment, as well as discussions with the patient's provider, should always guide the use of gentle tissue massage in any patient. Unless the nurse has advanced training, light or medium pressure can be used in areas such as the neck and back, shoulders, hands, and feet. No leg massages should be performed on inpatients unless approved by the provider. Touching patients in a caring, therapeutic manner promotes wellbeing and healing in both the giver and receiver of this intervention (Ruffin, 2011).

AROMATHERAPY

Aromatherapy is the use of essential oils for the purposes of healing. Essential oils, the distilled extracts from plants, have been used for many years to relieve pain, promote healing, kill bacteria, and maintain health (Price & Price, 2007). Dating back as far as 5,000 years, ancient Chinese, Indians, Egyptians, Greeks, and Romans used essential oils in cosmetics, perfumes, and drugs, and for spiritual, therapeutic, hygienic, and ritualistic purposes (Battaglia, 2003). Although accepted as part of nursing in Switzerland, Germany, Australia, Canada, the United Kingdom, and France, aromatherapy has only recently become a part of nursing care in the United States (Halcón, 2010), and it is one of the fastest growing therapies among nurses (Buckle, 2009).

Essential oils are found in the secretory structures in plants and obtained by a process of distillation or expression (Price, 2007). Complex compounds, plant molecules are categorized based on the relationship between their chemical function and properties (e.g., antiviral, antibacterial, antifungal, analgesic, anti-inflammatory) (Price, 2007).

Clinical aromatherapy is defined as "the use of essential oils for specific, measurable outcomes" that are thought to work at psychological, physiological, and cellular levels (Buckle, 2009). Essential oils are most often used topically or by inhalation, including aromatherapy massage (Shi, Lee, Seo, Park, & Nguyen, 2012). Because it combines the therapeutic use of smell and touch, aromatherapy massage is an appropriate fit for nursing (Halcón, 2010).

Although there are many studies examining the use of aromatherapy for symptom relief, there is limited research specifically targeting pain relief. A blend of essential oils topically applied to the abdomen was found to reduce menstrual pain (Han, Hur, Buckel, Choi, & Lee, 2006); aromatherapy massage was found to provide relief for outpatients with dysmenorrhea and reduced the duration of menstrual pain (Ou, Hsu, Lai, Lin, & Lin, 2012).

Specific instructions about the use of essential oils are beyond the scope of this chapter, as there are several important safety aspects to this modality. While it is generally considered safe to use, clinical training is strongly encouraged for nurses before using aromatherapy in the clinical setting.

ACUPRESSURE

Acupressure is an ancient healing art founded in traditional Chinese medicine, utilizing the fingertips to apply gentle pressure to healing points on the body. These points, similar to the ones used in acupuncture, stimulate the body's innate healing properties by activating the movement of *qi* or energy through channels, or meridians, while releasing muscle tension and improving blood circulation (Reed-Gach, 1990). These pressure points can alleviate pain or tension in distant areas of the body and are considered an adjunct therapy to conventional treatments for generalized, non-inflammatory low back pain (American Society of Anesthesiologists, 2010).

There are several points on the body that can be used to relieve specific pain symptoms through direct, light to moderate fingertip pressure. The pressure point *Sanyinjiao* (SP6), located above the inner anklebone, has been shown to significantly reduce the pain from dysmenorrhea (Wong, Lai, & Tse, 2010) and decrease the pain of labor as well as length to delivery time (Lee, Chang, & Kang, 2005). Acupressure points on the lower back and sacral area have also been found beneficial in decreasing low back pain and improving functional status following one month of treatment (Hsieh et al., 2006). Auricular acupressure (pressure points on the ear) has been shown to be helpful in the management of cancer pain (Alimi et al., 2003). As with other modalities, further research is indicated (Lee & Fraizer, 2011).

Nurses can use acupressure easily and effectively in the clinical setting with patients experiencing chronic pain. In acute pain, pressure should be applied on *distant* healing points, never directly *on* the painful site itself. The amount of pressure also depends on the "robustness" of the individual. Patients who are elderly and/or frailer should have lighter pressure, while the young and/or healthier patients can tolerate a more moderate pressure. It should be noted that more intensive pressure is not necessarily needed to achieve positive results.

MOVEMENT THERAPIES

While movement therapies may not always be appropriate in acute care settings, nurses often recommend therapies that patients can use on their own at home to manage their chronic pain. Tai chi is a centuries-old system of movements from ancient Chinese traditions combining slow movements and postures with deep breathing and mental focus. Small studies have shown tai chi to be effective in reducing the symptoms of osteoarthritis (Song, Lee, Lam, & Bae, 2003), especially in osteoarthritis of the knee (Lee, Pittler, & Ernst, 2008). Patients with fibromyalgia have also shown improvement in functional symptoms after participating in tai chi sessions two times per week over twelve weeks (Wang et al., 2010), with the positive effects continuing at 24 weeks post-intervention.

Another form of movement therapy is yoga, which combines postures, movements, and breathing to bring the body and mind into balance. Yoga has been shown in small studies to have positive impacts on low back pain (Tekur, Singphow, Nagendra, & Raghuram, 2008; Williams et al., 2005) and knee and hand pain from osteoarthritis (Kolasinski et al., 2005; Garfinkel, Schumacher, Husain, Levy, & Reshetar, 1994).

SELECTED REFERENCES

American Society of Anesthesiologists. (2010). Practice guidelines for chronic pain management. *Anesthesiology, 112*(4), 810–833.

American College of Emergency Physicians. (2009). Optimizing the treatment of pain in patients with acute presentations. Retrieved from http://www.acep.org/content.aspx?id=48089.

Audette, J., & Bailey, A. (Eds.). (2008). *Integrative Pain Medicine: The Science and Practice of Complementary and Alternative Practice in Pain Management,* Totowa, New Jersey: Humana Press.

Benson, H., & Stuart, E. (1993). *The Wellness Book: The Comprehensive Guide to Maintaining Health and Treating Stress Illness.* New York: Fireside.

Birocco, N., Guillame, C., Storto, S., Ritorto, G., Catino, C., Gir, N., et al. (2012). The effects of reiki therapy on pain and anxiety in patients attending a day oncology and infusion services unit. *The American Journal of Hospice and Palliative Medicine, 29*(4), 290–294.

Institute of Medicine of The National Academies. (2011). Relieving pain in America: A blueprint for transforming prevention, care, education and research. Retrieved from http://books.nap.edu/openbook.php?record_id=13172&page=19

McCaffery, M., & Pasero, C. (1999). *Pain: Clinical Manual.* St. Louis, MO: Mosby, Inc.

Posadzki, P., & Ernst, E. (2011). Guided imagery for musculoskeletal pain: A systematic review. *Clinical Journal of Pain, 27*(7), 648–653.

Reed, W., Montgomery, G., & DuHamel, K. (2001). Behavior intervention for cancer treatment side effects. *Journal of the National Cancer Institute, 93*(11), 810–823.

Rosen, S., & Faass, N. (2006). Referring patients to clinical massage. In Raken, D., & Faass, N. (Eds.), *Complementary Medicine in Clinical Practice* (pp. 235–240). Sudbury, MA: Jones and Bartlett.

23

Integrative Nursing Management of Cognitive Impairment

REBECCA L. ROSS AND IRIS R. BELL

More than 16 million people in the United States currently experience cognitive impairment (Ward et al., 2012). Cognitive impairment (CI) is often an acquired disturbance of cognitive function affecting the ability to think, concentrate, divide attention, form memories, make decisions (executive function), use language, and/or perform perceptual-motor activities. CI is a feature of many different clinical and subclinical conditions with various etiologies, and ranges from mild to severe. These conditions include neurodegeneration, cerebrovascular disease, head trauma, infections, chronic inflammation, and nutritional disorders (DSM-V, 2013). Although age is a factor in mild cognitive impairment (MCI), Alzheimer's disease, vascular dementia, and cognitive difficulties can develop at any age (DSM-V, 2013). Loss or diminution of cognitive capacity is one of the most disabling problems that can degrade quality of life for the affected individual as well as their family support system (Kidd, 2008).

Conventional healthcare can contribute increasingly sophisticated diagnostic tests and medications that treat some types of CI and common concomitants, such as depression and anxiety. However, cognitively impaired individuals are often highly sensitive to the side effects of pharmacological agents, a mainstay of biomedical treatment of cognitive dysfunction and comorbid conditions. Consequently, an integrative approach to CI that employs various complementary strategies and minimizes use of drugs and polypharmacy is clinically essential. In this chapter, we focus on three leading categories of cognitive impairment and the care of persons affected by these conditions: (a) attention/concentration disturbances, (b) mild cognitive impairment, and (c) traumatic brain injury (TBI).

Types of Cognitive Impairment

ATTENTION AND CONCENTRATION DISTURBANCES

Attention and concentration disturbances may range from mild, intermittent symptoms of inattention, defined as an inability to direct one's consciousness to a person, thing, perception, or thought (Venes & Taber, 2013), to more severe disorders such as attention deficit/hyperactivity disorder–combined presentation, predominantly inattentive presentation, or predominantly hyperactivity/impulsive presentation (DSM-V, 2013). The average worldwide prevalence of attention/concentration disorders is 5.3% (Polanczyk, de Lima et al., 2007).

Attention-deficit/hyperactivity disorder (ADHD) is the most common neurodevelopmental disorder in children (Polanczyk et al., 2007), often persisting into adulthood (Polanczyk et al., 2007). ADHD is a chronic disorder that involves inappropriate and disruptive levels of inattention and/or hyperactivity and impulsivity, which often creates a significant negative impact on academic, social and vocational performance (DSM-V, 2013; Polanczyk & Rohde, 2007). While stimulant and non-stimulant medications have been the most well-known treatment for ADHD for several decades due to their high effectiveness, good safety profiles, and relatively minor adverse effects (Huang & Tsai, 2011), an increased interest in non-pharmacological interventions has gained strength in the last decade (Sadiq, 2007).

MILD COGNITIVE IMPAIRMENT

Mild cognitive impairment is often defined as an intermediate stage between the expected cognitive decline of normal aging and the more serious decline of dementia (Ward et al., 2012). However, Petersen and colleagues' (1999) original definition required a subjective memory complaint, impaired performance on objective memory tests, intact cognitive function, intact functional abilities, and a non-demented status. MCI is estimated to occur in approximately 3.5% of people age 60 and older and 15% for age 75 and older (Panza et al., 2005).

Affected individuals have self-reported and/or observer-reported memory problems, but otherwise normal cognitive skills and ability to perform activities of daily living. MCI may or may not progress to Alzheimer's disease, which is the most common form of dementia in the elderly. Major or Mild Neurocognitive Disorders Major or mild neurocognitive disorder due to Alzheimer's disease (AD) is a progressive, insidious neurodegenerative dementia involving memory loss, behavior changes, and gradual functional impairment in both instrumental (e.g., shopping, preparing meals, using the telephone, balancing a checkbook) and basic activities of daily living (e.g., feeding, dressing, toileting). Eventually, verbal capabilities also deteriorate. Temporoparietal function is greatly impaired, though other brain areas are also involved. Many AD patients exhibit a circadian rhythm of "sundowning," in which they become more agitated and confused later in the day and night. Wandering behaviors can develop. The gradual downhill course can take an average of 7.5 years before the diagnosis of dementia, with an accelerated cognitive decline thereafter (Wilson et al., 2012). A key pathophysiological feature of AD is beta amyloid deposition (plaques and neurofibrillary tangles), with phosphorylated tau-protein deposits associated with neuronal degeneration. In some racial/ethnic groups, apolipoprotein E is a biomarker for increased AD risk (Galasko, 2013).

Major or mild vascular neurocognitive disorder, commonly known as vascular dementia, is a memory disorder related to damage to cerebral blood vessels that can develop more suddenly than AD and progress in a stepwise fashion, as major and smaller silent strokes occur. Cognitive deficits in vascular dementia depend on the location of the strokes and blood vessel damage. If prefrontal or frontal brain regions are involved, vascular dementia can impair executive function and judgment, sometimes more than memory (Galasko, 2013). Approximately 10% of people with dementia have a mixed picture of both AD and vascular dementia. Individuals with any type of dementia are more prone to developing delirium during acute infections or from other intercurrent medical problems or medications (Lin et al., 2010).

MAJOR OR MILD NEUROCOGNITIVE DISORDER DUE TO TRAUMATIC BRAIN INJURY (TBI)

Traumatic brain injury (TBI) is defined as an injury to the brain occurring after birth that is not hereditary, congenital, degenerative, or induced by birth trauma. TBI commonly results in a change in neuronal activity, which affects the brain's physical integrity, the metabolic activity, or the functional ability (Faul et al., 2010). Every year, at least 1.7 million TBIs occur in the United States either as an isolated injury or along with other injuries. Causes of TBI include falls (35.2%), motor vehicle and traffic accidents (17.3%), occupational accidents (10%), recreational accidents (10%), and assaults (10%) (Faul et al., 2010).

There is a temporally related onset of symptoms with TBI, including headache, nausea, vomiting, dizziness and balance problems, fatigue, sleep disturbances, daytime sleepiness, sensitivity to light and/or noise, blurry vision, and memory and concentration problems. TBI often leads to impairments in multiple cognitive functions, including attention and concentration, working memory, memory, reaction time, processing speed, and executive function. A subset of affected individuals gradually recovers function over a period of weeks to months, but another subset experiences persistent cognitive impairments beyond the three-month point after injury. The chronic condition is sometimes labeled "post-concussive syndrome" (PCS). Quality of life, capacity for job performance, and relationships can all suffer from the aftermath of TBI and/or PCS (Draper et al., 2007).

Table 23.1 summarizes possible causative and contributing factors to these various cognitive impairments.

Table 23.1: Causes and Contributing Factors for Cognitive Impairment

Attention/Concentration Disturbances	Mild Cognitive Impairment	Traumatic Brain Injury
Age	Age	Age
Gender: Male = Female	Gender: Female > Male	Gender: Male > Female
• Males > % impulsiveness and hyperactivity	Family History	Brain injury from a:
• Females > % inattention	Genetic Factors	• motor vehicle accident
Family History	• Alzheimer's disease APOE-e4	• fall
Genetic Factors	mutations affected amyloid	• sports injury
Food Intolerance/Allergies	precursor protein, presenilin-1,	• explosive blast
Dietary Intake	and/or presenilin-2 proteins	Mechanisms may
• High sugar/ high carbohydrate, low protein diet	Head Trauma History	include injury-related
	Vascular Disease Risk	release of excessive
	Factors (hypertension, heart	excitatory amino acids
• High intake of processed foods	disease, stroke, diabetes, high	such as glutamate and/
	cholesterol)	or increased neuronal
• High intake of foods containing additives and preservatives	Oxidative Stress	oxidative stress.
	Inflammation	
	Chronic Stress	

An Integrative Nursing Approach to Cognitive Impairment

When caring for a person with cognitive impairment (CI), an integrative nurse considers the entire context of care with caregiving occurring at both the individual and family level of care. While all chronic conditions place stress on family caregivers, the caregiver burden with cognitive impairment is particularly overwhelming (Tomiyama et al., 2012). Further, CI often occurs in households where two elders reside, both with multiple health-related issues, one often caring for the other. Consider the following case where an integrative approach to care is particularly helpful.

The integrative nurse caring for Mrs. H would realize that, in order to successfully care for this woman, he or she must be actively engaged in managing the physiological and psychological sequelae of CI while simultaneously attending to the larger healing context (Principle 1). A more in-depth assessment is needed; ideally the nurse and nurse practitioner would work together with the patient, the family/ support system, and other pertinent people and agencies to gain a more comprehensive understanding of the onset and trajectory of Mrs. H's CI in a whole person, whole system context (Principle 4). Further assessment of the bodymindspirit domains of movement, exercise and rest, nutrition, personal and professional development, physical environment, relationships and communication, and spirituality will offer a comprehensive view of Mrs. H, the problems that she has been having, and their effect on her wellbeing and safety (Principles 1 & 2). Furthermore, a home assessment would be completed, paying particular attention to the effects of Mrs. H's forgetfulness on her husband's wellbeing (Principles 1 & 4).

Case Scenario

A 70-year-old woman, Mrs. H, presents to her primary care provider for a routine examination, the results of which indicate that her previously diagnosed and stable chronic disease conditions (non–insulin dependent diabetes mellitus and high blood pressure) are worsening as evidenced by a fasting blood glucose of 156 and a blood pressure reading of 158/92. The nurse knows that Mrs. H is the sole caregiver for her 75-year-old husband, who experienced a cerebral vascular accident (CVA) two years ago that resulted in moderate right-sided weakness, mild swallowing difficulties, and a moderately decreased ability to bathe or dress himself. After scheduling a follow-up appointment, the patient pulls aside the nurse and voices the following concern.

"I didn't want to bring this up with the nurse practitioner because I don't know whether it's anything to be concerned about or not," she confides. "But I'm worried about my memory. I seem to be forgetting where I've been putting things lately—my keys and important paperwork, like my bank statements. I usually have no trouble with everyday activities, but sometimes I just feel like I'm in a fog, especially when Mr. H has been restless all night and I haven't been able to get much sleep. I'm terrified that this could be the beginning of Alzheimer's disease. I am so worried that I won't be able to care for my husband and he will be taken out of our home that I am getting more and more anxious every day. Should I be concerned? Is there anything I can do to prevent it from getting worse?"

In light of her past medical history of diabetes and Mr. H's CVA history and current difficulty swallowing at times, it is important to assess this family's nutritional status, including food acquisition, food preparation, food intake, and other problems that may exist. Recognizing that caregiver burden, fatigue, and stress can contribute to CI but may also manifest as lapses in memory, the integrative nurse contemplates a referral to the dietician to learn about time-saving ways to prepare a diabetic meal with more fresh vegetables and low-fat protein sources that is easily adaptable for Mr. H. Her hope is that relieving her caregiver burden might boost Mrs. H's energy and improve her memory (Principles 2, 5, & 6).

Mrs. H. has also mentioned that her memory seems worse when Mr. H is restless the night before; it is important for the nurse to ask how much sleep and rest Mrs. H. is getting. In the same vein, it is also important to inquire if she is getting enough physical activity and social interaction to maintain her health and wellbeing (Principles 2 & 6). Depending on what deficits or needs Mrs. H and the nurse identify, it may also be appropriate to request services from friends, family members, and community agencies.

Such assistance might include requesting visits from members of her preferred spiritual community, formal in-home healthcare assistance for Mr. H, and respite care for Mr. H so Mrs. H has time to get out of the house and engage in personal development and recreational activities and nurture other relationships (Principles 3 & 6).

Assessing Cognitive Impairment

An integrative nursing assessment considers each patient's overall needs, regardless of the reason for the encounter. An integrative nurse views the patient as a whole human embedded within a complex biopsychosocial system and dynamic environment with which they are continuously interacting. Specific areas to assess are nutrition, physical environment, physical activity (movement, exercise, and play), sleep, relationships/ social environments and support systems, and spirituality/growth (Lake, 2005). It is equally important to assess the patient's perception of illness and to determine what priorities they have for the healing journey.

Several standardized measures are used to formally assess cognitive impairment, all of which can be used at baseline and for follow-up evaluation. Specific to attention/concentration disorders is the Conners-3 Scale for children (Conners, 2009) and the Adult Attention Deficit Disorder Scale for adults (Kessler et al., 2005; Rosler et al., 2006).

Specific to gross cognitive impairment, one measure commonly used to screen and assess moderate to severe CI (Alzheimer's disease, vascular dementia, and TBI) is the Mini-Mental Status Exam (Folstein et al., 1975; Rovner & Folstein, 1987). More refined tools used with mild to moderate CI include the Brief Cognitive Rating Scale (Vernooij-Dassen et al., 1996); Kendrick Cognitive Tests for the Elderly (Girardi et al., 2011); and the Montreal Cognitive Assessment (Freitas, Simoes, Alves, et al., 2012; Freitas, Simoes, Maroco, Alves, et al., 2012). Another widely used scale to assess status and progression of Alzheimer's disease is the Alzheimer's Disease Assessment Scale (Rosen et al., 1984; Verhey et al., 2004).

Recent literature indicates that greater cardiovascular disease and stroke risk are associated with increased cognitive decline in later life. Therefore, recommendations now include modifiable risk screening using the Framingham General Cardiovascular Disease and Stroke Risk scores as primary prevention measures that assess risk of cognitive decline in middle to later life (Kaffashian et al., 2013). In addition, the Cardiovascular Risk Factors, Aging and Dementia (CADIE) risk score is predictive of cognitive decline. These findings reinforce the importance of population-based early screening assessments as integral to supporting the innate healing capacity of the person. Early identification of risk provides a means to target modifiable risk factors such as high blood pressure, elevated blood glucose, and other vascular risk factors, thereby improving long-term health outcomes in high-risk populations (Kaffashian et al., 2013).

Specific to TBI, more intense neuropsychological testing by specialists should be done when medically necessary (National Institute of Neurological Disorders and

Stroke, 2012). For people with TBI and their caregivers, a workbook is available to facilitate self-assessment as well as coping and self-care at home (Mason, 2004).

Integrative Interventions for Cognitive Impairment

Interventions for cognitive disorders depend on the etiology or type of cognitive disorder that is being treated.

ATTENTION AND CONCENTRATION DISTURBANCES

Attention and concentration difficulties can affect a person across the lifespan and manifest differently, dependent on age and causative mechanisms. For instance, the challenges faced by a grade-school student are vastly different from those experienced by a chief financial officer of a multinational corporation. Yet intervention options may be similar. First-line approaches to mild attention and concentration difficulties are often integrative in nature. As depicted in Table 23.2, these can include restorative therapies, nutritional therapies, whole-systems therapies, and, when necessary, pharmacological therapies. Integrative approaches are often appealing to families, and studies show that a large percentage of children with ADHD are treated in this manner (Bader & Adesman, 2012).

Healthy eating has generally been found to have positive benefits, not only for problems of inattention and lack of concentration, but for physical, cognitive, and emotional health (Kuipers et al., 2012; Slavin & Lloyd, 2012). While some diet changes can be quite extreme, there are some that are much more common-sense, easy, safe, and beneficial to apply. Nutritional plans to reduce symptoms associated with ADHD include sugar-restricted diets, meals that incorporate a balanced protein–carbohydrate–fat ratio, omega-3 fatty acid, and other vitamin and mineral supplements (Bader & Adesman, 2012; Howard et al., 2011). One report links the ADHD-associated "Western-style" diet, high in fat and refined sugars, with increased ADHD symptoms, and the "ADHD-free" diet, (rich in fiber, folate, omega-3 fatty acids) to fewer ADHD symptoms (Howard et al., 2011).

The oligoantigenic (hypoallergenic/elimination) diet, which gained popularity in the 1980s and then waned, requires elimination of synthetic dyes, food additives, and preservatives (Harley et al., 2011; Kanarek, 2011). It requires significant diet restrictions, including elimination of cow's milk, cheese, wheat cereals, eggs, chocolate, nuts, and citrus fruits. While findings have shown a subset of children who have improved symptoms with this diet, it is time-consuming and disruptive to the family system (Millichap & Yee, 2012). However, it seems to be worthwhile for those motivated to try and where other therapies have failed (Pelsser et al., 2011).

Table 23.2: Interventions for Attention/Concentration Disturbances

Tier 1 Interventions	• **Mind–Body Therapies** Breath and relaxation Guided imagery • **Exercise and Movement** Walking, swimming • **Environmental Therapy: Nature, Silence** • **Dietary Interventions** Higher protein/lower carbohydrate diet Calorie-restricted diet for those who are overweight or obese
Tier 2 Interventions	• **Mind–Body Therapies** Meditation Establish contemplative, reflective periods in long workdays; physical activity/play periods for children • **Movement Therapies** Aerobic exercise Yoga Tai Chi Physical activity periods for children • **Nutritional Therapies** Nutritional evaluation using an elimination diet Ant-inflammatory diet, increasing phytonutrients, probiotics, decreasing intake of processed foods • **Natural Products** Herbal: ginko biloba Vitamins and supplements: omega-3 fatty acids, vitamin B complex with folate, vitamin C, vitamin E (mixed tocotrienes/tocopherols), SAMe
Tier 3 Interventions	• **Mind–Body Therapies** Mindfulness-based stress reduction course Cognitive therapy • **Energy Therapies:** Reiki Qi Gong Healing Touch • **Health Coaching:** Consistent guidance and planning for healthy lifestyle ADHD Life Coach
Tier 4 Interventions	• **Whole Systems Therapies:** Traditional Chinese medicine Homeopathic medicine, particularly successful with children
Tier 5 Interventions	• **Psychotherapy/Behavioral Therapy:** Cognitive Behavior Therapy adapted for ADHD Psychoeducation: ADD-friendly ways to organize life and overcome common barriers • **Pharmacological Therapies:** Non-stimulant medications Stimulant medications Anti-depressant medications

Moderately strong evidence indicates that omega-3 (found in fish and vegetables) helps with some inattention symptoms, though the research is still preliminary (Richardson & Montgomery, 2005). Still, omega-3s are used frequently, as the side effects are low and there are additional health benefits (Kotwal et al., 2012). Other dietary measures that have shown some initial promise include treatment of iron and zinc deficiencies (Konikowska et al., 2012).

Physical exercise, especially aerobic activities, has been shown to improve attention and concentration in children and adolescents (Field, 2012). In addition, mindfulness meditation has shown promise in adolescents and adults (Zylowska et al., 2008).

MAJOR OR MILD NEUROCOGNITIVE DISORDERS

For the most common causes of dementia, multi-modal integrative interventions that alleviate risk factors for AD and vascular dementia (Table 23.3) are pragmatic considerations (Kidd, 2008). Age, an obvious risk factor for dementia, is not a modifiable factor per se, although it may be possible to attenuate biological aging effects by reducing stress to lengthen telomere length, or using antioxidants to prevent cumulative cellular damage from oxidative stress and metabolic activity (Tomiyama et al., 2012). However, one cross-sectional epidemiological study suggests that multivitamin use is associated with relatively longer telomere length (a biological correlate of longevity) in women (Xu, Q. et al., 2009). Therefore, a stress reduction program with biofeedback, journaling, and/or progressive relaxation training with a good multivitamin supplement in their daily regimen may be a practical intervention for individuals with mild CI or early AD.

Therapy goals include improving blood vessel integrity, lowering high blood pressure and cholesterol, treating type 2 diabetes and dyslipidemia, reducing inflammation, improving mitochrondrial functioning, and protecting neurons against oxidative stress (Roberts, 2013), as well as adding cognitive stimulation and physical exercise (Cheng et al., 2013). For a younger person, reducing stress itself could lessen the long-term adverse impact of chronic excess cortisol levels, which are implicated as a permissive factor in hippocampal damage that leads to memory loss (Schwabe & Wolf, 2012). For prevention, journaling, meditation, guided imagery, and/or yoga could all lessen reactivity of the hypothalamic-pituitary-adrenal axis to stress (Shiralkar et al., 2013; Yadav et al., 2012). Research also supports using cognitive training, rehabilitation, and stimulation therapy to improve memory performance (Takeda et al., 2012).

Additional treatments (e.g., dietary changes and supplementation with omega-3 fatty acids, antioxidants, and specific herbal derivatives) are also supported by preliminary research (Parletta et al., 2013; Xu, Y. et al., 2006). While each therapeutic strategy identified in Table 23.3 has some supporting research evidence from animal and/or human studies, no single treatment has shown promise as an outstanding sole option

Table 23.3: Interventions for Mild Cognitive Impairment

Tier 1 Interventions	• **Mind–Body Therapies** Breath and relaxation Guided imagery • **Exercise and Movement** • **Environmental Therapy: Nature, Silence** • **Dietary Interventions** Mediterranean diet Anti-inflammatory diet • **Natural Products** Vitamin and nutrient supplements
Tier 2 Interventions	• **Movement Therapies** Yoga Tai Chi • **Mind–Body Therapies** Meditation group practice • **Nutritional Therapies** Anti-inflammatory diet: increasing phytonutrients, probiotics • **Natural Products** Herbal: ginko biloba, ginseng, green tea Vitamins and Supplements: vitamin B complex, vitamin C, D, E, Magnesium maleate, alpha lipoic acid, omega-3 fatty acids, co-enzyme Q 10
Tier 3 Interventions	• **Mind–Body Therapies** Music therapy • **Energy Therapies** Reiki Qi Gong Healing Touch • **Health Coaching** Planning and consistent guidance for a brain-healthy lifestyle (exercise, healthy diet, mental stimulation, quality sleep, stress management, active social life)
Tier 4 Interventions	• **Whole Systems of Care** Traditional Chinese medicine Holistic medicine Aromatherapy: lavender
Tier 5 Interventions	• **Psychotherapy/Behavioral Therapy** Reminiscence therapy, journaling to reduce stress • **Pharmacologic Therapies** Cholinesterase inhibitors (Aricept, Exelon, Razadyne, Cognex) and mentadine (Namenda) Anti-depressant medication

that can totally reverse memory loss (Ha et al., 2011; May et al., 2012; Witkin & Li, 2013). Yet, many of these interventions are relatively low risk and have multiple possible health benefits (Shah, 2013). Therefore, a clear and concise summary of the relative benefits and risks of a given intervention should be provided to the patient and family as the integrative nurse partners with them in decision-making.

Since dementia is a complex condition, it is likely that the most helpful program will involve a package of individually chosen options. As Csermely and colleagues (2005) have pointed out, using agents with partial but multiple actions may be preferable over the more usual strategy of single-action conventional therapy. With most conventional pharmacological treatments, the goal is to obtain focused effects on only one target cell type or receptor. However, people are complex adaptive systems or networks. As a result, forcing only one system out of many to change can cause imbalances and side effects from "unintended" downstream changes. Therefore, integrative nurses should consider most interventions as multi-focal rather than trying to find a single effective strategy (Csermely et al., 2005; Frautschy & Cole, 2010).

One of the most efficient ways to treat the person with memory problems as a complex system is to use nutritional and/or herbal interventions that inherently support more than one aspect of health. For example, many antioxidants have multiple anti-inflammatory potentials across multiple cells and tissues beyond the neurovascular/neurological system. At the same time, no one antioxidant necessarily works "best" for all types of oxidative stress in all cell systems (Fu & Li, 2011). Thus, combining a coordinated set of specific antioxidants, each at reasonable doses, may produce more benefit than any single item (Liebovitch, 2007).

Of course, many nutritional supplements, including antioxidants and herbs, can cause certain adverse effects and/or interact with conventional medications that older patients might also be taking. For example, high doses of vitamin E, gingko biloba, and other agents can cause increased anticoagulant effects, a notable concern for patients already taking warfarin or other anticoagulant drugs. Working with a knowledgeable pharmacist on possible drug–supplement interactions can be very helpful. Another useful resource is the National Institutes of Health Office of Dietary Supplements website (http://ods.od.nih.gov/) for fact sheets on specific substances. Finally, teaching patients about identifying reliable supplement manufacturers is essential.

Once dementia has developed, integrative interventions include a range of strategies to modify wandering and dangerous behaviors, especially agitation and aggression, and minimize reliance on drugs, whose side effects can cause additional confusion and falls (Hulme et al., 2010). Non-drug approaches for people with dementia may include light therapy (for restoring better circadian cycles for persons with sundowning), music therapy (Hulme et al., 2010; Padilla, 2011), and animal-assisted therapy (Takeda et al., 2012). In early stages of memory loss, meditation may also be helpful in reducing anxiety and stress reactivity (Innes et al., 2012). Aromatherapy with lavender may be beneficial in some cases (Hritcu et al., 2012), but the data are not consistently favorable, with suggested worsening of symptoms in patients who have a comorbidity of depression or anxiety disorders (Hawken et al., 2012; Padilla, 2011).

With respect to Mrs. H's concerns about her memory, we recognize that her caregiver burden is responsible for increasing the stress response, and that long-term stress can affect physiological systems (indicated by her rising blood sugar and blood pressure) as well as changes in mental status and memory. A combination approach might be most helpful as an integrative care strategy, evaluating Mr. H's restlessness and nutritional status while increasing Mrs. H's participation in stress-reduction therapies (walking, getting out in nature, visiting with friends) and supplementing her diet with omega-3–rich foods and antioxidants.

TRAUMATIC BRAIN INJURY

Many experts in the field of TBI believe that, in addition to any direct, focal physical damage to brain regions, the primary source of neuronal loss and dysfunction stems from oxidative stress in response to closed-head concussive effects in the sudden acceleration and deceleration of the brain within the confines of the bony skull. That is, the injury in concussion results largely in the excessive generation of reactive oxygen species that can damage or impair neuronal function and cerebrovascular function (Aiguo et al., 2010; Marcano et al., 2012). Frontal, temporal, and parietal lobes are particularly vulnerable to these types of injuries, with diffuse axonal injury involvement. As a result, integrative packages of care may revolve around supporting improvements in quality of life by blending multiple biological and lifestyle adjustment interventions (Table 23.4).

The primary biologically oriented intervention strategies reduce oxidative stress in the TBI brain and include a variety of antioxidant nutrients and selected herbal substances (Weber et al., 2012; Wu et al., 2006). Exploratory studies are also examining improved encapsulation and delivery vehicles, e.g., nanoparticles, for nutriceuticals and herbs that otherwise have poor gastrointestinal absorption and limited bioavailability (Bitner et al., 2012; Mathew et al., 2012; Nair et al., 2010; Ray et al., 2011), but otherwise potentially helpful antioxidant effects (Hsu et al., 2012; Marcano et al., 2012; Sonkaew et al., 2012).

Another promising, though controversial, therapy that demonstrated positive benefits in a double-blind placebo-controlled trial in people with TBI is classical homeopathy (Chapman et al., 1999). In addition, qualitative studies (Bell et al., 2004; Koithan, Bell, & Campesino, 2005; Koithan et al., 2007) as well as clinical case studies (Chapman, 2002) describe patient outcomes including improved function, quality of life, and behavioral symptoms associated with classical homeopathic treatment for TBI. Homeopathy is an over 200-year-old whole system of medicine that attempts to match the complete and unique bodymindspirit symptom pattern of the individual to a single homeopathically prepared medicine. Current thinking about mechanisms of action include evidence that these medicines are low-dose nanoparticle forms of their natural plant, mineral, or animal source material (Chikramane et al., 2010; Upadhyay & Nayak, 2011) that mobilize adaptive responses throughout the person as a complex adaptive system (Bell & Koithan, 2012).

As in dementia-spectrum memory disorders, certain types of psychosocial support (e.g., peer mentoring, and structured cognitive training) programs can also

Table 23.4: Interventions for Traumatic Brain Injury

Tier 1 Interventions	• **Movement Therapies:** Exercise and physical recreational activities • **Mind–Body Therapies:** Breath and relaxation • **Nature and Environment** Nature, silence • **Diet/Nutritional Therapies** Anti-inflammatory diet • **Natural Products** Vitamin and nutrient supplements
Tier 2 Interventions	• **Movement Therapies** Yoga Tai Chi • **Diet/Nutritional Therapies** Herbal: ginko biloba Vitamins and supplements: alpha lipoic acid, n-acetyl-cysteine, acetyl-l-carnitine, huperzine A, vinpocetine, vitamin E, oxyresveratrol
Tier 3 Interventions	• **Mind–Body Therapies** Music therapy • **Counseling and Supportive Therapies** Peer mentoring Internet-based rehabilitation support
Tier 4 Interventions	• **Diet/Nutrition Therapies** Multi-nutrient cocktail Vitamins and supplements: vitamin E, oxyresveratrol • **Whole Systems Care** Traditional Chinese medicine Homeopathy • **Mind–Body Therapies** EEG biofeedback Animal therapy
Tier 5 Interventions	• **Pharmacological Therapies** Non-stimulant medications Stimulant medications Norepinephine and dopamine reuptake inhibitor medication • **Psychotherapy, Behavioral Therapy** Cognitive Behavior Therapy adapted for TBI Psychoeducation regarding specific deficits incurred due to TBI

help alleviate the adverse impact of TBI on quality of life (Serino et al., 2007). Electroencephalographic (EEG) biofeedback (neurotherapy) may also facilitate rehabilitation improvements in core cognitive dysfunctions of people with TBI (Duff, 2004). For individuals with limited geographical access or other barriers to rehabilitation programs, Internet-based training (e.g., online calendar reminders, online problem-solving) is being explored (Egan et al., 2005; McDonald et al., 2011; Wade et al., 2010). In addition to conventional treatment options for the anxiety and depressive mood disorders that often accompany TBI, interventions such as tai chi may offer additional benefits, including improved sleep, improved balance, improved cognitive function, and reduced fall risk (Yeh et al., 2008).

Conclusion

Cognitive impairment is but one aspect of a whole human experience embedded within a whole system. Therefore, a thorough assessment for a patient with CI is best accomplished using an integrative nursing approach, one that honors the complexity of the situation and the unique expression of that condition within the context of family and caregiver systems. It is also important for nurses to remain mindful of the burden caregivers may be experiencing and assist in caring for them as well as the identified patient with CI. The development of a comprehensive integrative nursing care plan that takes into account a patient and caregiver(s) immersed in their unique, complex, biopsychosocial system and dynamic environment with which they are continuously interacting will best serve the patient and their health and wellbeing needs.

SELECTED REFERENCES

APA. (2013). *Diagnostic and Statistical Manual of Mental Disorders, Fifth Edition* (DSM-V). Washington, DC: American Psychiatric Association.

Bader, A., & Adesman, A. (2012). Complementary and alternative therapies for children and adolescents with ADHD. *Current Opinion in Pediatrics, 24*(6), 760–769.

Cheng, S. T., Chow, P. K., Song, Y. Q., Yu, E. C., Chan, A. C., Lee, T. M., et al. (2013). Mental and physical activities delay cognitive decline in older persons with dementia. *American Journal of Geriatric Psychiatry, 21*(2). doi:pii:S1064-7481(13)00065-1. 10.1016/j.jagp.2013.01.060.

Faul, M., Xu, L., Wald, M. M., Coronado, V., & Dellinger, A. M. (2010). Traumatic brain injury in the United States: National estimates of prevalence and incidence, 2002–2006. *Injury Prevention, 16*, A268–A268.

Galasko, D. (2013). The diagnostic evaluation of a patient with dementia. *Continuum (Minneapolis, Minn.), 19*(2 Dementia), 397–410.

Lake, J. (2005). *Integrative Assessment and Treatment of Cognitive Impairment.* U.S. Psychiatric Congress Session Reports. Accessed on March 13, 2013, at www.progressivepsychiatry.com/powerpoint/USPsychCongo5_Cognitive.pdf.

Padilla, R. (2011). Effectiveness of environment-based interventions for people with Alzheimer's disease and related dementias. *American Journal of Occupational Therapy, 65*(5), 514–522.

Polanczyk, G., & Rohde, L. A. (2007). Epidemiology of attention-deficit/hyperactivity disorder across the lifespan. *Current Opinion in Psychiatry, 20*(4), 386–392.

Slavin, J. L., & Lloyd, B. (2012). Health benefits of fruits and vegetables. *Advances in Nutritional Research, 3*(4), 506–516.

Takeda, M., Tanaka, T., Okochi, M., & Kazui, H. (2012). Non-pharmacological intervention for dementia patients. *Psychiatry & Clinical Neurosciences, 66*(1), 1–7.

24

Integrative Nursing Care of the Human Spirit

JANET F. QUINN

The spiritual issues are already there. All one needs to do is to ask one's patients whether they would like to talk about them.

—*Daniel Sulmasy*

With these words, physician and Franciscan friar Daniel Sulmasy elegantly and with great parsimony sums up the focus for this chapter (Sulmasy, 2006, p. 167). As whole human beings, we are spiritual beings. As spiritual beings, we are inclined to ask the *big questions,* particularly when we are ill or frightened or in other ways out of right relationship (Box 24.1). "For many of us, it is only illness or the approach of death that turns us toward the questions we were born to ask" (Bartlow, 2000, p. 4).

These big questions, the search for our true selves, meaning, the sacred, and the transcendent underlie all spiritual issues in healthcare, and whether we are conscious of it or not, the issues are already there. Thus, while the symptom of "spiritual distress" can arise in the healthcare context, it is important to identify it as a subset of a much larger concern for integrative nurses; namely, tending the human spirit. This chapter will explore an integrative nursing approach to spirituality: how the integrative nurse tends the human spirit and addresses the symptom of spiritual distress.

What Is Spirituality?

While there is broad general recognition that religion is the outer expression of beliefs contained in the teachings and sacred texts of particular traditions, including its rituals, practices, observances, and related lifestyles, there is no authoritative definition of "spirituality" in the general healthcare or the nursing literature (Narayanasamy, 1999, 2001; Chiu et. al., 2004; McSherry & Jamieson, 2011). In a passage from her book *Suggestions for Thought* (1860/1994), quoted in Macrae (2001, p. 21), Florence Nightingale wrote:

What do we mean by spirituality?...Feelings called forth by the consciousness of a presence of higher nature than human, unconnected with the material,

Box 24.1 *Some of Life's Big Questions*

Who am I?
Why am I here?
What is ultimately Real?
Is there a God? What kind of God?
Why do I have to suffer with this?
What is this about?
Am I being punished?
Who am I now that this has happened?
What matters most, especially now?
Does my life have meaning?
What happens when we die?
How do I live knowing I will die?
How can I connect with my Source
What is my true nature?
Who or what is my highest self?
Does something of me survive death?

these we call spiritual influences; and this we are conscious is the highest capability of our nature.

In modern nursing literature, concepts like meaning, purpose, connectedness, mystery, transcendence, and energy have been used to define spirituality (Chiu et al., 2004; McCarroll et al., 2005). The most frequently cited definition of spirituality in the nursing literature, according to McSherry and Jamieson (2011), is the one offered in 1989 by Murray and Zentner, "who suggest spirituality is a universal phenomenon that is deeply personal, sensitive, and often a hidden area of human life that applies to all people, those with a religious belief and those with no religious belief" (p. 1758). An interdisciplinary consensus conference on spirituality in palliative care defined spirituality as "the aspect of humanity that refers to the way individuals seek and express meaning and purpose and the way they experience their connectedness to the moment, to self, to others, to nature, and to the significant or sacred" (Puchalski et al., 2009, p. 887).

Some authors have suggested that the more inclusive definitions of spirituality make the spiritual dimension indistinguishable from positive psychology, and for this reason they, like Nightingale, reserve the term *spirituality* for its association with the transcendent (Koenig, 2007; Pargament, 1999). One of these authors, Sulmasy (2006), defines spirituality as the characteristics and qualities of one's relationship with the transcendent, explaining that everyone thus may be said to have a spirituality. "Some call the transcendent God, others do not personalize it, and still others reject it, as with atheists, which is still a relationship, albeit one which will necessitate a personal search for meaning and value in light of the rejection of the transcendent" (p. 14).

Thus, "it would appear that nurses and health care professionals are still uncertain about the meaning of spirituality and the delivery of 'spiritual and religious care'" (McSherry & Jamieson, 2011, p. 1759).

How, then, should we proceed? First, each nurse should find her or his own working definition of spirituality, as this will have a direct effect on the capacity to provide spiritual care. Second, the integrative nurse should recognize that, since there are about 7 billion people on the planet, there are 7 billion different *experiences* of spirituality, and potentially, that many definitions (Zinnbauer, 1997). While there are many useful reference tools that outline the beliefs and practices of the world's major religions, they cannot predict any unique individual's spiritual beliefs or needs. Furthermore, some of the latest surveys suggest that people, especially the younger generation, are increasingly describing themselves as "spiritual but not religious"; that is, not affiliated with a particular faith tradition (Pew, 2012). In the final analysis, for the purposes of tending the human spirit and meeting the spiritual needs of patients (clients, families, communities), we might say that *spirituality* and *spiritual distress*, like pain, *is what the patient says it is* (Malinski, 2002).

This non-definitive way of approaching spirituality in clinical practice may at the outset create anxiety or concern in the integrative nurse, who is trying to address these issues in a caring, compassionate, competent way. But, if you take a moment to sit with this definition—that *spirituality is what the patient says it is*—you might find that it is profoundly liberating. It does not require you to know at the outset what will unfold in the interaction, or to have answers, solutions, or even comprehension of the patient's beliefs. It actually requires other ways of knowing (Carper, 1978; Munhall, 1993).

The spiritual is an integral pattern of being-knowing-doing that is fundamentally ineffable; it is a mystery that opens itself to the listening heart, speaking in a language of its own. Nursing's ways of knowing, including the intuitive and the aesthetic, provide vehicles to meet the spirit of another and to tend it with care, gentleness, and reverence. In particular, Munhall (1993) suggests "unknowing," which is a position of full openness, the ideal attitude to assume when engaging a conversation about a patient's spirituality.

> Openness to a range of spiritual perspectives (or lack thereof) is part of ethical nursing practice. Nurses need not feel they must be knowledgeable in particular spiritual traditions, but they are required to be open to inviting or allowing reflection by the individual on the spiritual dimension of his or her experience of illness and suffering. Also, nurses may deem self-reflection on their own spiritual beliefs to be beneficial to their practice. (CNA, 2010, p. 3)

RATIONALE FOR ADDRESSING SPIRITUALITY
IN NURSING PRACTICE

The Moral Imperative

The most important reason to address the spiritual dimension in healthcare is that *not* to do so is to provide incomplete care, which is both negligent and immoral. If the human is by definition more than a body, as nursing philosophy, history, theory, and scholarship agree, and if health and healing are not limited to the absence of disease but are the emergence of wholeness of bodymindspirit, then the spirit must be cared for. "Spirituality is *intrinsic* to the practice of health care," writes Sulmasy (2006).

> The purgation of spirituality from Western health care practice that began slowly during the Renaissance and accelerated sharply during the last half of the twentieth century has been a historical anomaly and a moral mistake. Spirituality is integral to health care practice.... *Attention to spiritual needs is a moral imperative. It is not simply a moral option—something that ought to be permitted or tolerated.* (2006, p. 169, emphasis added)

The Human Imperative

America continues to be a country in which the vast majority of people are religious and/or spiritual, and they want their spirituality included in their healthcare. Estimates of the percentage of patients who are open to being asked about their spirituality vary from approximately 4% to 80%, depending on the situation (Ehman, Ott, Short, Ciampa, & Hansen-Flaschen, 1999; King & Bushwick, 1994; Maugans & Wadland, 1991). A poll reported in *USA Weekend* indicated that 60% of those aged 18 to 34 years and 67% of those aged 55 to 64 years would like to be asked about their spirituality (McNichol, 2002). McCord et al. (2004) reported that, in a survey of 921 adults, 83% of respondents wanted physicians to ask about spiritual beliefs in at least some circumstances.

In 2006, a Gallup poll reported that 49% of Americans identify as religious, 40% identify as "spiritual but not religious," 7% identify as both spiritual and religious, and 3% identify as neither. The spiritual but not religious (SBNR) group is the newest national demographic, and it is growing, particularly amongst younger people. Data from Pew (2012) indicate that "one-fifth of the U.S. public—and a third of adults under 30—are religiously unaffiliated today, the highest percentages ever in Pew Research Center polling" (p. 9). Some members of this unaffiliated group are engaging in other emerging models of spiritual expression, including Interfaith and InterSpiritual orientations (Teasdale, 1999; see http://www.interfaithcongregations.org/). We live in a time when there is unprecedented access to the sacred literature and practices of every culture on the planet. Increasingly, people are taking advantage of this to craft deeply personal and sometimes very eclectic paths on the spiritual journey (Mabry, 2006).

If these data are close to normative, then we can assume that roughly the same percentages apply to healthcare professionals and the people we care for. These data constitute an important rationale for including spirituality in healthcare.

The Legal and Ethical Imperative

The Joint Commission on Accreditation of Healthcare Facilities requires that all institutions have a plan for addressing spiritual needs, but leaves the "how to" up to individual healthcare facilities (2008). Thus, each nurse needs to be aware of the policies and procedures related to spiritual care in her/his facility. The American Nurses Association (ANA) Code of Ethics includes the need for nurses' respect for each person's spiritual wellbeing and beliefs, while their guidelines for nursing assessment include the spiritual needs of patients (ANA, 2012). McSherry and Jamieson (2011) observe that there are numerous international organizations that have endorsed the position that nurses and healthcare professionals should be attending to the spiritual dimensions of care.

The Evidence Imperative

In recent decades, research into the potential health benefits of religion and spirituality has skyrocketed. There are now over 3,000 quantitative original data-based studies on religion/spirituality and health, the vast majority of which show positive associations (Koenig, 2011). Entire texts have been written summarizing these data (Matthews & Clark, 1998; Koenig, 1999; Koenig, King, & Carson, 2012; Koenig, McCullough, & Larson, 2001; Levin, 2001).

While these data are compelling, we need to be extremely careful that we do not allow it to turn spirituality into a utilitarian means to an end, rather than a noble and essential end in itself. Larry Dossey wrote in the foreword of Levin's 2001 book:

> Perhaps the major challenge we face is how to avoid trivializing religious and spiritual practices. When laypersons and professionals discover the impact of these measures on health, they may begin to regard them as the latest item in the medical tool kit. Seen in this way, prayer becomes merely the latest aspirin, the newest penicillin. Prayer and spiritual practices have far greater benefits, I believe, than aiding physical health. They are our bridge to the Absolute, however named—God, Goddess, Allah, Universe, Tao. In my view, this benefit of religion dwarfs any physical advantage it may convey. (Levin, 2001, p. ix)

Sulmasy (2006) concurred: "Regardless of outcomes, spiritual issues are an intrinsic part of health care. The spiritual transcends outcomes" (p. 167).

An Integrative Nursing Approach to Tending the Human Spirit

How do we reintegrate spirituality and care for the human spirit into nursing practice? While care of the whole person, including the spirit, has always been part of nursing's focus, it has been severely marginalized in current nursing practice by the dominant biomedical model. To reintegrate spirituality into clinical practice, nursing, unlike medicine, does not need to change its fundamental paradigm. Rather, nurses need to reaffirm its presence in their practice, learn more deeply about it, and ground their being-knowing-doing in it. Box 24.2 lists the essential elements of an integrative nursing approach to tending the human spirit.

Every encounter is a bodymindspirit meeting (Principle 1). There is no time or place when nursing care does *not* involve the spiritual dimension, regardless of the nurse's or patient's awareness of it. Providing spiritual nursing care requires a process of becoming aware of what is already present and then attending to it with increased intentionality and focus. "Spiritual nursing care is an intuitive, interpersonal, altruistic and integrative expression that is contingent on the nurse's awareness of the transcendent dimension of life but reflects the patient's reality" (Sawatzky and Pesut, 2005, p. 23).

The opportunity to tend the spirit is present in every nursing encounter as we support comprehensive health and healing (Principle 2). It is accomplished through nurses' being-knowing-doing as they hold a space for spiritual wellbeing and/or healing with

---

Box 24.2 An Integrative Nursing Approach to Tending the Human Spirit

In tending the human spirit, the integrative nurse:

1. Encounters every person as bodymindspirit meeting bodymindspirit, thus integrating awareness of and attention to the spiritual dimension of self and other in our being-knowing-doing.
2. Identifies patients' spiritual and/or religious beliefs, preferences, and practices to support them as part of a comprehensive, integrative approach to health and healing.
3. Recognizes when there is either a need or desire for additional spiritual wellbeing, support, and/or guidance, or actual spiritual distress.
4. Formulates and implements a plan with the patient to address these needs, including assisting patients with increasing their spiritual self-care, and/or
5. Makes appropriate referrals if the extent or nature of the patient's needs or distress is beyond one's personal or professional scope of practice.

authentic presence, tone of voice, eye contact, touch, energy, consciousness, love, and compassion (Quinn, 1992, 2002; Watson, 2005; Koerner, 2011).

Spiritual care unfolds through the ongoing caring/healing relationship enacted in every nurse–patient encounter (Principle 4). While helpful in making sure that the spiritual needs of patients are not overlooked (and required in some instances), formal spiritual assessment is not necessary to provide spiritual nursing care, and when it has been used, is not sufficient to ensure adequate care of the spirit. Spiritual care is not done when the form has been completed and referrals made, but is an ongoing part of the person-centered, caring and healing relationship.

There are rich and deep paradoxes in the spiritual life, which have been written about in the literature of every religious tradition. For example, on the spiritual journey, pain is not necessarily bad; discomfort is not necessarily to be quickly resolved; distress is not always a sign that something is wrong; and suffering may be a door to liberation or enlightenment, something to open to, surrender to, and embrace. Another example: the "dark night of the soul," described by the mystic St. John of the Cross, might be seen as a form of "spiritual distress," mimicking in some ways (but not in others) depression or even despair. Yet it is not a problem to be solved, or a process that any outsider should attempt to help someone complete or "resolve" on a timeline. To do so can do more spiritual harm than good, like trying to help a butterfly free itself from its cocoon. "A prescriptive nursing process approach implies influencing, and in some cases reframing, the spirituality of patients and thereby extends beyond general notions of spiritual support...this approach extends the nursing role beyond appropriate professional boundaries, making it ethically problematic" (Pesut and Sawatzky, 2006, p. 127).

Specific nursing interventions must reflect spirituality and spiritual needs as validated by the patient and must be offered rather than prescribed, leaving the patient free to accept or decline, completely free from any coercion, including suggestions that they "should" do these things to get a better health outcome (Principle 5). These principles and elements provide the foundation for clinical decision-making about integrative spiritual care interventions, from least invasive to more intensive. Sawatzky and Pesut (2005) summarize the process perfectly: "Spiritual nursing care begins from a perspective of being with the patient in love and dialogue but may emerge into therapeutically oriented interventions that take direction from the patient's religious or spiritual reality" (p. 23).

Integrative Spiritual Assessment

Tending the human spirit is accomplished through the being-knowing-doing of the integrative nurse, who provides a "container," a sacred space, for the processes of spiritual assessment and, when appropriate, intervention. Spiritual assessment and spiritual intervention are not separate, linear steps. Rather, they are inherently interconnected and interdependent dimensions of a whole-person/whole-system approach to spiritual caring, like the concept of *yin* and *yang* in traditional Chinese medicine.

For example, the moment we bring our wholeness of being-doing-knowing as part of the assessment, we have opened a space for patients to share this very personal dimension of their life. Just this invitation is a potentially powerful intervention, which can be very helpful to those who are facing the big questions that often arise in the face of a health challenge. Simultaneously, in that intervention, the nurse listening with the whole self may hear a faint voice of inner spiritual strength that can be supported, or identify spiritual distress and the need for intervention.

Each aspect of integrative nursing practice is inherently influenced by and influences the others. Therefore, the core competencies for providing spiritual care arise from and flow between the dimensions of being-knowing-doing, depicted as a spiral surrounding and holding the space for the process of spiritual nursing in Figure 24.1.

SPIRITUAL ASSESSMENT TOOLS

Integrative nurses may choose (or be required to use) one of the multiple tools available for conducting a spiritual history/screening/ assessment. Koenig (2007) suggests that even a single question (e.g., "Do you have any spiritual needs or concerns related

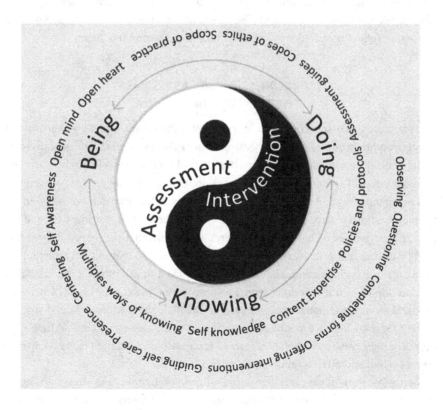

FIGURE 24.1 Core Competencies for Spiritual Nursing Care

to your health?") can be enough to open the conversation and let the patient know that this is an area of interest to the healthcare professional (p. 44). Koenig also offers guidelines for choosing an instrument for clinical use. The questions should be: brief, taking only a few minutes to administer; easy to remember; effective in gathering the most essential information; patient-centered, focused on patient's beliefs and the role they play in health and illness; and valid and credible.

One of the frequently used tools that meets these criteria is the FICA guide, developed by Puchalski and Romer (2000). Using the easily remembered income-tax term "FICA" as an acronym, the letters serve to remind the interviewer of four general directions for questions related to Faith, Importance of faith, Church (or spiritual Community), and Action steps needed. Other easy-to-remember and brief intake tools have been developed, including the SPIRIT tool (Maugans, 1996) and the FACT tool (LaRocca-Pitts, 2008).

There are several instruments for spiritual assessment that have been developed in nursing, for example, the T.R.U.S.T. Model for Inclusive Spiritual Care (Scott-Barss, 2012) and the Spiritual Assessment Tool (Dossey, Keegan, & Guzzetta, 2000, p. 106). While not brief, they can help the nurse think about how to start or deepen a spiritual assessment dialogue. Reviewing the plethora of questions can relieve anxiety about what to ask in an initial assessment. The questions can also remain in the background as possible follow-up questions when a spiritual conversation has begun.

INTEGRATIVE SPIRITUAL ASSESSMENT/
INTERVENTION IN ACTION

As previously discussed, coming to know (assess) the spirituality of another is not a linear or additive process, nor is it checking off boxes or disinterestedly/disconnectedly filling in blanks on standardized forms. It is more like a dance or a flow where any and all dimensions of the nurse and the patient are simultaneously present, influencing and being influenced. As the integrative nurse takes in the information shared in dialogue, questions to expand understanding of what she or he is hearing arise, and the conversation deepens. One might discover, for example, that the person feels deeply held by God in this as in every time in his or her life and so requires only the support to maintain that connection. Or, one might be moved to ask more questions, based on intuition or in response to observed pain or words that convey spiritual struggle. Answers prompt additional questions, and so the dialogue continues. Sacred space is created for shared silence, taking deep breaths, allowing the story to unfold in its own time. The integrative nurse holds that sacred space within which right relationship may emerge in self and other (Quinn, 1992).

Being-knowing-doing cannot be separated from each other in the integrated nurse or in the integrative process of spiritual assessment and intervention. Consider each of the actions that follow as a nurse might conduct a spiritual assessment, and imagine

Case Scenario

Before engaging with the patient, a 48-year-old man hospitalized to rule out colon cancer, you center yourself in the present moment, letting go of other thoughts, concerns, and agendas. You make an intention to be open and unknowing; you enter into intersubjective space with this other person, the sacred space of your shared energy field, with gentleness and respect for the mystery of this other who sits unknown before you with inherent dignity and value and his own spiritual story. You notice a pair of prayer beads around his neck and a spiritual book on his nightstand. You remember the policies and procedures of your system that guide spiritual assessment, and you have questions from the formal tools you can use in your awareness.

Integrative Nursing Care

You feel a comfort in yourself and an openness in the patient, so you ask about the beads—"I see you are wearing what looks like prayer beads around your neck; can you share something about them with me? What is their meaning for you?" You sit down so that you are at the same level and you meet his gaze with openness; you re-center, remembering that you wish to be a sacred space, to receive this unfolding mystery. And so your spiritual dance with this other has begun. Through this very gentle flow, you have opened the door; you have invited the soul to step forward, and you have accomplished what is perhaps the most important part of "spiritual care": you have let this other know that you see him as a whole person, and that his spirituality is not only accepted, but important to you, as deserving of time and space as the care of his body or mind.

During your conversation, the patient shares that his Sufi prayer practices are very important to him, but it has been difficult to maintain them because it seems that every time he begins, he is interrupted by one or another of the staff. Knowing that you know nothing about Sufism, you take a moment with this information to listen within for what is most important about what the patient has shared. You respond by asking if it would be helpful to have a Do Not Disturb sign that he could put on his door when he wants to do his practices. He smiles broadly and then tells you that he will include you in his prayers of gratitude. You ask if he would be willing to share what Sufism is about for him, and the dialogue continues as you listen both to what is said and to how your own being is responding. You follow up by asking if there are any other spiritual needs or concerns that he would like addressed. You complete the conversation and chart appropriately, alerting other staff. Finally, you obtain the sign and place it at the bedside where the patient can access it.

yourself in this scenario. See if you can feel the integrality of being, knowing, and doing in the following case study.

Integrative Interventions for Tending the Human Spirit

There are three broad categories of interventions that integrative nurses use to tend the human spirit.

BEING AN INSTRUMENT FOR HEALING THROUGH BEING-KNOWING-DOING

The caring and integrated nurse-self is perhaps the most potent instrument for tending the spirit of another human being. Core competencies for this sacred work include:

- *Spiritual self-knowledge*: Engaging in ongoing inquiry and self-discovery concerning "the big questions" of life so that we are comfortable engaging those questions with others.
- *Spiritual self-care*: Exploring and participating in multiple ways of tending our own spirits so that we remain vital and spiritually alive, and so that we can help others use these modalities for spiritual self-care.
- *Ability to center oneself*: To become still in mind, heart, and body so that we may become the healing environment, a sacred space for those we seek to serve.
- *Authentic presence*: Bringing the fullness of who we are into the present moment, letting go of attachments, agendas, hopes and fears, anything that distracts from the simplicity of being fully in the moment, attentive and available to the other.
- *Listening deeply*: Listening not only with the physical senses but with the "ears of the heart" and/or intuition, for the still, small voice of the spirit of both self and other.
- *Compassion*: Allowing oneself to be touched by the vulnerability of the other, responding with an authentic, heartfelt outflow of loving energy and the deep wish for their happiness, peace, and wellbeing.
- *Self-awareness/reflection*: The capacity to notice what is happening in our own bodymindspirit as we sit in presence with another, and the skill to manage it and reflect on it as necessary to maintain our inner freedom.
- *Commitment to personal wholeness*, including spiritual wellbeing: The gift we have to offer is who we are, so it becomes imperative, if we wish to be of service, to continually cultivate our health and wholeness at every level.

The integrative nurse models a healthy physical, emotional, spiritual life for others.

- *Openmindedness and openheartedness*: We recognize that people may have very different spiritual orientations than we do, but we keep our minds and hearts open to the truth, goodness, and beauty that reside in the depths of every human being. We do the inner work that it takes to become truly non-judgmental of others who are different from us.
- *Capacity for unknowing and dwelling in mystery*: In the domain of the human spirit, we cannot know anything for sure, but we can cultivate the ability to be with our own and others' spiritual experience without the need to fix it or to leave if it is uncomfortable.

OFFERING SPIRITUAL CARE MODALITIES

The integrative process of spiritual nursing will yield the necessary data for clinical decision-making related to spiritual care. Depending on what emerges, nursing care planning may involve the use of integrative and/or spiritual modalities to provide explicit spiritual care within the boundaries of the principles discussed and scope of practice.

People are spiritually unique; there is no one-size-fits-all spiritual care or spiritual practice. Some people are more extroverted (exterior) by nature, while others are natural contemplatives (interior). Some find the best way to connect with spirit is through the body or being in nature, while others prefer the quiet solitude of a hermitage, and still others, prayer groups or organized worship. Nurses offering spiritual care modalities must also be culturally sensitive, recognizing that, for example, "individually focused, inner spiritual pursuits may have little relevance for those who come from societies that emphasize a communal spirituality" (Pesut et al., 2008, p. 2807).

Regardless of the starting point (see Table 24.1) for spiritual care modalities, the whole person, bodymindspirit, is impacted by any modality, wherever it originates. For example, we can identify meditation as an interior, individual activity. But when people are meditating, there are also changes in their bodies; their brains are very different, their heart rate and blood pressure decrease, and their skin conductance changes. Meditation may also help us be calmer and less reactive in our relationships and more likely to try to create healing spaces where we work.

Some of the approaches in Table 24.1 move back and forth between the inner (subjective) and outer (objective or physical) experience. Some of these are modalities that nurses provide directly through the use of self-as-instrument (e.g., being fully present, deep listening, supporting, holding space, and providing time and space). These might be thought of as "least intensive" interventions on the continuum of least intensive/invasive to most (Principle 5). Others enhance capacity for self-care (e.g., teaching,

Table 24.1: Modalities for Tending the Human Spirit in Health and Healing

Approaches to tending the spirit through the individual, inner experience	Approaches to tending the spirit through the body

• Spiritual practices from one's religion or as given by spiritual guides
• Meditation consistent with patient beliefs, experiences and desires, for example:
  • Simple breath meditation
  • Zen
  • Vipassana
• Contemplative practices, such as Centering Prayer
• Spiritual reading and/or spiritual study
• Integral Inquiry practice with "Big Questions"
• Cultivating deeper self-awareness
• Forgiveness practices
• Prayer of all varieties, both active and listening
• Reflective journaling
• Imagery and visualization
• Writing/reading poetry
Any inner activities that bring people closer to their spiritual ideal, by whatever name/language
	• Performing ritual practices of one's religious tradition or spiritual path
	• Mindful eating
	• Mindful exercise/movement work
	• Fasting
	• Yoga
	• Pranayama breathing
	• Walking meditation, including the Labyrinth
	• Sacred dance, including Dances of Universal Peace
	• Listening to or making music
	• Singing/chanting/repeating mantras
	• Emotional Freedom Technique
	• Tai Chi
	• Qi Gong
	• Mindful cooking for self and loved ones
	• Viewing and/or making Art
	Any physical activities that bring people closer to their spiritual ideal, by whatever name/language

Approaches to tending the spirit through the shared inner experience between/among people	Approaches to tending the spirit through natural, social, cultural, and institutional environments
• Sitting in Sacred Space with nurse and allowing the questions to arise and be met • Spiritual direction • Group spiritual direction • Pastoral care/counseling • Spiritually oriented therapy • Centering Prayer group • Being with loving family/friends • Support groups • Ministry of availability—being willing to be fully present to others who are struggling • Seeking healing in broken relationships • Loving-kindness meditation practice *Any shared inner activities that bring people closer to their spiritual ideal, by whatever name/language*	• Seeking/using appropriate referrals • Being in nature • Being with animals and pets • Organized religious/spiritual services/celebrations • Working for social change • Participating in group service activities and causes that feed the soul/spirit • Gardening • Creating/utilizing sacred space • Caring for the environment in meaningful ways • Loving-kindness practice in work and other outer, system settings *"Anything you do every day can open into the deepest spiritual place, which is freedom." —Rumi*

providing reading and study materials, guiding spiritual practices, suggesting websites, or making referrals). These are somewhat more "intensive" on the continuum.

MAKING APPROPRIATE REFERRALS

While integrative nurses can address spiritual concerns and spiritual distress through a multitude of ways of being-knowing-doing as discussed, there are times when a referral to a spiritual care professional is an important intervention, sometimes representing the far end of the least-to-most intensive interventions for spiritual care. Depending on preferences and needs of the client, and on policies and available resources within the institution and community, referrals for spiritual care can be made to chaplains, spiritual directors, and/or pastoral staff of the patient's religious congregation. These referrals do not replace the tending of the human spirit that is part of ongoing integrative nursing care, but add to and support it. Some common reasons for making a referral to spiritual care professionals include: (a) a patient or family request; (b) expressions of spiritual guilt, anger, shame, resentment, hopelessness, ethical dilemmas, or other indications of spiritual distress that are beyond the skills of the nurse; and (c) institutional protocol.

Outcome Evaluation

Naming a specific outcome for spiritual nursing care may not be appropriate or even possible. Spiritual states of ease or distress are what the person/patient says they are, and there may not be "resolution" of spiritual distress by the time the nurse–client encounter terminates. The integrative nurse continues to provide spiritual nursing care by holding the space for the unfolding, moment-by-moment spiritual narrative of the client, and to provide ongoing encouragement and support, and referral, as indicated. If objective, scored assessment tools have been used, then post-intervention scores can be assessed as outcomes.

Perhaps the most appropriate outcome evaluation is process-based, rather than outcome-specific. Documentation should reflect that spiritual assessment has taken place and that spiritual needs have been identified, with appropriate interventions made. Follow-up to make sure that referrals have been made and that the patient has been seen is part of outcome evaluation. In addition, patients should be reassessed to determine if, from their point of view, their spirituality has been adequately addressed or if there is more that the nurse can do.

SELECTED REFERENCES

Burkhardt, M. A., & Nagai-Jacobson, M. G. (2002). *Spirituality: Living Our Connectedness*. Albany, NY: Delmar.

Koenig, H. G. (2007). *Spirituality in Patient Care*. West Conshohocken, PA: Templeton Press.

Koenig, H. G. (2011). *Spirituality and Health Research: Methods, Measurements, Statistics, and Resources*. West Conshohocken, PA: Templeton Press.

Murray, R. B., & Zentner, J. P. (1989). *Nursing Concepts for Health Promotion*. London: Prentice Hall.

Narayanasamy, A. (1999). A review of spirituality as applied to nursing. *International Journal of Nursing Studies, 36*, 117–125.

Pesut, B., Fowler, M., Taylor, E. J., Reimer-Kirkham, S., & Sawatzky, R. (2008). Conceptualising spirituality and religion for healthcare. *Journal of Clinical Nursing, 17,* 2803–2810.

Puchalski, C., Ferrell, B., Virani, R., et al. (2009). Improving the quality of spiritual care as a dimension of palliative care: The report of the consensus conference. *Journal of Palliative Medicine, 12*(10), 885–903.

Quinn, J. F. (1992). Holding sacred space: The nurse as healing environment. *Holistic Nursing Practice, 6*(4), 26–36.

Sawatzky, R., & Pesut, B. J. (2005). Attributes of spiritual care in nursing practice. *Holistic Nursing Practice, 23*(1), 19–33.

Sulmasy, D. P. (2006). *The Rebirth of the Clinic.* Washington, D.C.: Georgetown University Press.

IV

Integrative Nursing Applications

25

Integrative Nursing in Acute Care Settings

LORI KNUTSON AND VALERIE LINCOLN

With the increasing need to explore cost-effective healthcare delivery options, the use of complementary and alternative medicine (CAM) has steadily expanded (Ananth, 2011; Gannotta et al., 2009; Dusek, Finch, Plotnikoff, & Knutson 2010; Knutson, 2006; Lincoln, 2003). This increase has prompted various agencies and organizations to survey hospitals about the integration of CAM in their acute healthcare settings in the United States and other countries. The progression and integration of CAM into the acute healthcare environment follows the increase in consumer use over the past several decades (Barrett, 2003) and is driving force for the incorporation of integrative healthcare in the acute healthcare setting (Clement, Chen, Burke, Clement, & Zazzali, 2006; Mann et al., 2004). The expansion of clinical focus to include integrative healthcare is evident in the disciplines of both medicine and nursing and is often included in medical curricula, including residencies and fellowships, and in all levels of nursing education, including doctorate studies in nursing practice programs (Lincoln, 2000).

The phenomenon of hospital-based integrative services is seen across all regions of the country and in all cross-sections of the acute care hospital industry, including community-based and academic institutions, and for profit and not-for-profit organizations. Ananth (2011) completed a survey of over 714 institutional respondents of hospitals to assess the degree of CAM therapy used in the hospital setting as well as the motivators of the integration of these therapies in the acute care hospital environment. The report found that the top inpatient modalities included pet therapy, massage, music or art therapy, guided imagery, relaxation, and Reiki. The survey further revealed a wide range of reasons hospitals offered CAM therapies, the highest motivator being patient demand at 85%. Hospitals that offer integrative services do so for various reasons, such as consumer preference, market factors and differentiation strategies, a growing emphasis on patient satisfaction as a legitimate outcome of care, organizational mission, resource availability, and other service-expansion approaches. Mann et al. (2004) has identified seven models of integrative care, two of which focus on inpatient acute care models: hospital-based integration and integrative medicine in academic medical centers. The following rationales characterize some reasons for this progressive development: improving patient and family experiences of healthcare in an inpatient setting; honoring a commitment to provide integrated care; expanding patient care options; improving communication and relationships between patients and caregivers; reducing dependency on pharmaceutical and technological interventions; providing greater attention to wellness; disease prevention and self-care; enhancing the reputation of the hospital; and other potential benefits such as nursing and service staff retention. At this point in time, however, most acute care hospitals do not offer multiple integrative services.

Woodwinds Health Campus: An Exemplar of a Community-Based Hospital

Woodwinds Health Campus (WHC) is an example of a community-based hospital that emerged in 2000 in response to the community's desire to have a local community hospital in Woodbury, Minnesota. The hospital represents an organization embracing an innovative and integrative approach to healthcare. Woodwinds is a collaboration between HealthEast Care System and Children's Hospitals and Clinics. Upon opening, Woodwinds was a 70-bed inpatient hospital with a vigorous outpatient center, emergency care center, primary and specialty clinics, and the host of a Natural Care Center within the hospital itself. The Natural Care Center is one of several outpatient holistic centers of Northwestern Health Sciences University (NWHSU). This multidisciplinary clinic offers care from the chiropractic, naturopathic, massage, traditional Chinese medicine, and Healing Touch traditions, as well as a host of retail products.

The success of the integrative model at Woodwinds is evidenced by the need to add two additional eight-bed units to accommodate the volume of inpatients and the expansion of this model to other acute care hospitals within the HealthEast Care System, an impressive accomplishment in these challenging fiscal times for the healthcare industry. Factors contributing to success of the Woodwinds model include: the vision and guiding principles, the optimal healing environment, the holistic nursing model, the Holistic Practice Council, the delivery of select healing arts therapies and integrative services such as acupuncture and certified massage therapy, and the efforts of the holistic leadership to emulate the healing healthcare model (HHM) of servant leadership and compassionate service. In short, it is all about the overarching culture of healing person, place, and community at Woodwinds. There is resonance with each of the fundamental principles for integrative nursing practice. In particular, Woodwinds provides access to nature in the healing gardens, a labyrinth, and nature-based artwork and images. Additionally, the Woodwinds patient and employee customers appreciate the seamless access to select healing arts therapies in conjunction with their traditional care. Distinctively, the healing healthcare model has a strong focus on self-care and healing for the staff as a primary contribution to the overall healing environment.

VISION AND GUIDING PRINCIPLES

The vision of Woodwinds is to be an innovative, unique, and preferred resource for health. The healing healthcare model promotes health and healing of body, mind, and spirit through relationships, choices, and learning. The values and guiding principles of Woodwinds describe an organization that is committed to integrative, innovative, collaborative, responsive, and compassionate service to the community (Lincoln & Johnson, 2009).

WOODWINDS' GUIDING PRINCIPLES AND VISION

The core values and standards of the Woodwinds Health Campus' organizational mission are foundationally supported by the integration of the practice of holistic nursing. Both the organizational philosophy of servant leadership and the integration of a holistic nursing model are considered innovations within the healthcare system.

Woodwinds Guiding Principles

Deliver *patient- and family-centered service* that encourages and supports active involvement in one's own health care.

Promote a *"seamless" system* that truly supports an environment of customer service—maximizing the collaborative nature of the campus.

Use *all resources responsibly*—remembering the impact on the overall financial health of the organization.

Challenge the status quo and apply *innovative thinking* by continuously embracing and implementing change.

Create and sustain a *healing environment* that promotes health and quality of life in harmony with nature and spiritual awareness.

Foster choice by providing a spectrum of care with integration of select complementary approaches to health and wellbeing.

Improve the health of the community by actively partnering to identify and address their priority needs.

Create a *culture supporting* individual *wellbeing*, fostering equal and respectful *relationships* and responding to the *challenges* of the future.

Serve as a *learning laboratory* for the sponsor organizations—integrating new systems and processes when it is the right thing to do and utilizing existing systems where appropriate.

Apply the efficiencies of ambulatory/outpatient services to the systems and processes across the entire campus.

Woodwinds Purpose

Promote health and healing of body, mind, and spirit for all through relationships, choices, and learning.

Woodwinds Vision

To be the innovative, unique, and preferred resource for health by fundamentally creating the healthcare experience in a way that has not been done before.

Woodwinds Values

Compassionate service: Placing the needs of those we serve above our own; treating individuals with dignity, respect, and empathy.

Ethical practice: Demonstrating the highest standards of integrity, honesty, and loyalty.

Meaningful collaboration: Working together with patients, families, co-workers, and outside partners to strengthen mutually beneficial collaborative relationships.

Human potential: Growing through personal development, fulfilling work, and continual teaming while encouraging growth in others.

OPTIMAL HEALING ENVIRONMENT

Although Woodwinds was created and operational before the concept of an optimal healing environment (OHE) was published by the Samueli Institute, the efforts of Woodwinds are synergistically supported by the seamless integration of the overall healing environment as described by Jonas and Chez (2004). This seminal work provides a comprehensive review of the factors affecting the inner environment of the persons in a healing relationship (developing healing and intention, experiencing personal wholeness, and cultivating healing relationships), as well as the outer environmental factors (applying collaborative medicine, creating healing organizations, and building healing spaces). The bridge between the two realms of the inner and outer environments are represented by practicing healthy lifestyles, both an inner and outer process.

Recognizing the unique opportunity to create a healing environment from the bottom up, Woodwinds took a multidisciplinary approach to the principles and pillars of this model (Lincoln, 2000). The overarching Woodwinds culture recognized and focused upon these "six P's" of the Woodwind's model: people, philosophy, place, process, policies, and practice (Figure 25.1).

The design is comprehensive and integrated. The culture of compassionate service and servant leadership is evident in the staff and the community volunteers. The designed environment enhances this culture in many ways. For example, the interior halls are curved to eliminate a straight rectilinear, institutional feel. Every patient room is private and large enough to accommodate support persons and caregiver needs. All rooms look out onto a large campus imbued with nature. The healing power of nature is supported by outdoor spaces, a healing garden, and a large labyrinth that is also visible from within the hospital. Two gazebos are available for both patient and staff

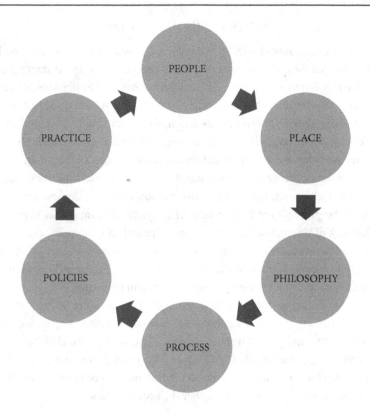

FIGURE 25.1 Woodwind's Model: People, Philosophy, Place, Process, Policies, and Practice

renewal. The vast majority of the extensive artwork is inspired by nature. In addition, the chapel embraces the visual support of earth, wind, fire, and water to embody the desire for a spiritually inclusive environment. Local Ojibwa elders assisted in the blessings of the healing space and healing gardens. Classical elements are also emphasized throughout the campus; some departments have aquariums to invoke the water of the land, and multiple fireplaces provide warmth and light in most patient and family sitting areas. The overall design calls forth the iconic north woods cabins of Minnesota.

The healing environment is also supported by having no overhead paging; interpersonal communication is supported by less invasive technologies. There are no specified visiting hours. Many meetings are "called" by the use of brass or crystal bowls and a moment of heart-centered awareness before the business of the day begins.

The staff and volunteers are carefully selected, not only for their clinical competence, but for their willingness to embrace the opportunity to practice from a place of respect, compassion, and healing. Woodwinds continues to attract and retain these kinds of employees and volunteers, which is reflected in staff satisfaction and engagement, patient satisfaction, and very successful clinical outcomes.

HOLISTIC NURSING MODEL

The holistic nursing model (HNM) (Lincoln & Johnson, 2009) was adopted by the Woodwinds nursing division to guide patient-centered care in all nursing departments. The philosophy, core beliefs, and standards developed by the American Holistic Nurses Association (AHNA) are essential parts of the orientation classes for new nursing division employees. These classes are required of all nursing division personnel and also offered to all Woodwinds staff. The concepts embodied in the standards incorporate a sensitive balance between art and science, intuitive and analytical skills, and the use of the healing capacity of the body, mind, and spirit. Leadership and management personnel as well as staff nurses and other employees personally and professionally commit to the principles of holistic care. The holistic nursing model is founded on both the work of Koerner on "healing presence" (2012) and the *caritas* core principles of Watson's "Caring Science" (2008). This nursing framework assists staff in aligning the principles of holistic nursing with the passion of the caregivers through the access of our compassionate *caritas* consciousness and healing presence.

We recognize that each clinical shift brings challenges to the delivery of compassionate, holistic care. Like all fast-paced acute care nursing divisions, we, too, live with increased acuity, quick patient turnover, high patient volume, and challenging clinical circumstances. Approaching these challenges with healing presence and *caritas* consciousness facilitates a healing moment, sets the intention to be of service to others and our co-workers, and allows us to remember the present moment.

THE HOLISTIC PRACTICE COUNCIL

A major vehicle for change-agency and leadership of the holistic nursing model is the Holistic Practice Council. The leadership is shared by the Clinical Lead for Integrative Services and a staff member. The membership includes nursing personnel from each unit, nursing leadership, patient care associates, and representatives from other disciplines and departments. The Council supports the application of the holistic nursing model by facilitating education, evidence-based practice, and research. The Council has partnered to develop: holistic nursing educational and practice competencies, procedures related to select Healing Arts Therapies (HAT), educational programming such as annual education and competency validation, the annual Woodwinds Health Campus Healing Healthcare Conference, and larger house-wide initiatives such as the Prayer Shawl Ministry and the Pause for Prayer process. The Prayer Shawl Ministry is facilitated by the Council leader and hosts both volunteer staff and volunteer community members who donate their time and prayers to create prayer shawls. These shawls provide comfort for both patients and families who face life-challenging circumstances but are also available for employees who face the same struggles. The Pause for Prayer initiative serves patients, staff, or family members who request the spiritual support of others' healing intention. A few seconds of healing flute music is played overhead to call the spirit of healing to the others' consciousness. This is done for both patients and staff who are facing deep challenges. Like in many organizations, a few moments of a lullaby are played overhead to announce the birth of a child into our larger community.

To aid leaders in facilitating accountability for all employees and their use of the holistic nursing model, the Council developed annual competency checklists. Annually, each staff member submits a "reflective practice" story that influenced his or her awareness or learning about the nature of healing. They are also asked to submit a holistic personal goal and a holistic professional goal, in addition to ensuring that a minimum of three contact hours per year are focused on holistic topics of their choosing.

HEALING ARTS THERAPIES AND INTEGRATIVE SERVICES

The integrated use of select HAT allows the caregivers to offer many choices to improve the patient experience and also empowers the patients and their families to participate in the healing process. The current roster of HAT offered by caregivers includes essential oils; guided imagery; healing music; energy-based healing such as Healing Touch, Reiki, and therapeutic touch; acupressure; and hand and foot massage. The RN staff practice in alignment with the Minnesota State Board of Nursing Statement of Accountability, which directs nursing practice when delivering complementary or alternative therapies (see http://mn.gov/health-licensing-boards/nursing/licensees/practice/integrative-therapies.jsp).

Within the first year of operation, the Healing Arts Therapy Volunteer program (HATV) was established to lead and supervise the delivery of select therapies that augment the care of the direct caregivers (Lincoln, Nowak, Briggs, Schommer, Fehrer, & Wax, in press). The volunteers offer Healing Touch, Reiki, massage, guided imagery, use of essential oils, and healing music. Integrative services offered by specialty-certified or licensed professionals such as certified music practitioners (CMP), certified massage therapists (CMT), or acupuncture practitioners (LAC) are also robustly offered with a goal of making them available "for every patient's consideration, every shift."

The overwhelmingly successful postgraduate fellowship program in acupuncture created and offered in partnership with NWHSU quickly became a productive hospital-based employee acupuncturist model, uniquely and uniformly supported by our medical and nursing staff. Acupuncture is offered free of charge in all of the inpatient units, from medical-surgical to maternity care, and in outpatient units such as the emergency department and the new integrative cancer care clinic. CMT is offered as a fee-for-service therapy. Most patients receive essential oils, healing music, or guided imagery, while 25% to 35% of patients receive energy-based healing or acupuncture treatments during their hospital stay.

HOLISTIC LEADERSHIP

The Integrative Service department (IS) at Woodwinds is highly valued in the care model. The budget for Integrative Services is integrated into the operations budget for programs currently without philanthropic support. The department is led by a clinical leader to champion these grassroots initiatives, including education, practice, clinical research, and clinical outcome evaluation of these services. The clinical lead's responsibilities include serving as the primary investigator of the Institutional Review Board (IRB)-approved Healing Arts Therapy Research Registry, which currently hosts approximately 20,000 study patients. This registry is a partnership endeavor with the Medical Director, the Physician Leadership group, the Holistic Practice Council, and the Woodwinds Leadership Team.

Personal and organizational evolution towards deeper healing and consciousness is essential to the overall culture at WHC. These expectations are mirrored by the CEO as well as staff and volunteers. Other departmental leaders are responsible for many expansion initiatives, such as offering *oshibori* with essential oils in breast care services along with a selection of natural teas, offering integrative services in the outpatient cancer care clinic, and offering acupuncture for patients undergoing bone marrow biopsies. Each monthly leader meeting covers an agenda topic that supports the leader's personal or leadership holistic knowledge, in addition to classical management topics. The entire leadership team co-participates in the evolution of holistic care, including completing annual holistic leadership goals and holistic personal goals that enhance personal and departmental wellness.

Allina Health/Abbott Northwestern Hospital/Penny George™ Institute for Health and Healing: An Exemplar of a Tertiary Care Center

Allina Health, a not-for-profit healthcare system, provides care for Minnesota and western Wisconsin. With over ninety clinics, eleven hospitals, fifteen pharmacies, hospice, home care, medical equipment, and emergency medical transportation, it is the largest healthcare system in the upper Midwest. It has over 24,000 employees, 5,000 associated and employed physicians, and 2,500 volunteers.

Abbott Northwestern Hospital (ANH) is part of Allina Health and is the largest not-for-profit hospital in the Twin Cities area, with 633 available beds. Each year, the hospital provides comprehensive healthcare for more than 200,000 patients and their families from the Twin Cities area (Minneapolis–St. Paul) and throughout the upper Midwest. More than 5,000 employees, 1,600 physicians, and 550 volunteers work as a team for the benefit of each patient served. For more than 125 years, Abbott Northwestern has had a reputation for quality services. The hospital is well known for its centers of excellence: cardiovascular services in partnership with the Minneapolis

Heart Institute®, mental health services, medical/surgical services, Neuroscience Institute, Orthopedic Institute, physical rehabilitation through the Sister Kenny Rehabilitation Institute, Spine Institute, Virginia Piper Cancer Institute™, perinatology, obstetrics and gynecology through Womencare, and the Penny George™ Institute (PGI) for Health and Healing

Founded in 2003 through the support of the George Family Foundation and the Ted and Dr. Roberta Mann Foundation, the Penny George Institute for Health and Healing has created a national model of patient care built on the foundation of integrative health. Through its range of inpatient services, Outpatient Clinic, LiveWell Fitness Center, Integrative Health Research Center, and community and professional educational programs, the Penny George Institute is the nation's largest hospital-based integrative health program.

VISION AND MISSION

The Penny George Institute (PGI) seeks to transform healthcare by blending the art of healing and the science of curing to optimize the health of the whole person—mind, body, and spirit.

The Penny George Institute's vision is to transform healthcare locally through the provision of outstanding integrative care to patients and employees in all settings across Abbott Northwestern and its related institutions. It is anticipated that the PGI will transform healthcare nationally through the development and dissemination of integrative care practices that demonstrably enhance quality, ensure safety, and reduce costs.

Since 2003, the PGI's inpatient care team has provided more than 60,000 consults to hospitalized patients at Abbott Northwestern. The inpatient team consists of twenty-two highly skilled integrative healthcare professionals—eight licensed acupuncturists, six massage therapists, six holistic nurses, a music therapist, and a reflexologist. Consults for services are primarily requested for pain management and anxiety; however, other indications include gastrointestinal issues, musculoskeletal conditions, mental health, sleep disturbances, and general wellbeing. Each weekday morning, the PGI practitioner team meets to assign an average of 25 to 30 new patient referrals. On a typical day, 60 to 75 patients will receive an integrative medicine consult or service. The PGI's inpatient professionals are fully integrated into the hospital. They receive formal referrals, make rounds with physicians, consult with nurses, provide bedside therapies, and document their care in the electronic health record system (EPIC).

All of the PGI's practitioners are cross-trained in a multitude of complementary therapies. Patients receive individualized care developed in partnership with the care team to enhance their experience and outcomes. Patients may be seen before surgery or immediately after surgery, and some practitioners have accompanied patients during a procedure or surgery. Patients may receive one or more of these therapies: acupuncture/acupressure; aromatherapy; energy healing including Reiki and Healing Touch;

healing art; Korean hand therapy; mind/body therapies including relaxation response, guided imagery, and biofeedback; music therapy; reflexology; or massage therapy.

PRE-HOSPITAL PROGRAM

The Pre-Hospital Program helps people prepare for an upcoming surgery or procedure at Abbott Northwestern Hospital. It is designed for patients who are anxious about their visit, worried about pain, need help developing a self-care plan, or want to learn skills to enhance recovery. Through mind–body skills training, participants discover tools, skills, and information that will help make their hospitalization and recovery a positive, healing experience. A mind–body coach helps participants learn to use skills like meditation, breath work, relaxation techniques, guided imagery, biofeedback, and self-care practices. The participants learn to apply their new skills toward reducing pain to a tolerable level, shifting feelings of anxiety to feelings of calm and confidence, planning for and experiencing a positive outcome after surgery, taming the stress response, and eliciting the relaxation response.

THE ART OF HEALING

At Abbott Northwestern Hospital, creative arts are used to support healing, and research is being conducted to measure the impact of the arts in patient care. The Art of Healing program offers positive, creative, and constructive arts programming for patients, visitors, employees, and volunteers. Patients can explore art as a healing tool during their hospitalization. Music therapy is used to reduce anxiety, stress, and pain. Exhibits, concerts, classes, and other events explore the healing aspects of art. The Caring for the Caregiver program offers a series of classes designed to support Abbott employees and volunteers in the art of self-care, including visual journaling, movement, and the meditative aspects of painting. The PGI is a member of the Society for Arts in Healthcare. This national organization demonstrates the valuable role the arts can play in the healing process and encourages and supports research into the benefits of arts in healthcare.

TRANSFORMATIVE NURSE TRAINING PROGRAM

The Transformative Nurse Training (TNT) program is one example of Abbott Northwestern's commitment to excellence in nursing. The program brings nurses back to the essence of nursing practice and teaches the foundations and principles of holistic nursing. Over the course of six day-long sessions, nurses acquire practical skills to promote and enhance self-care and care for patients, including massage, guided imagery, physiological relaxation response, meditation, Oriental medicine, nutrition, and more. An important and unique component of the program is mentorship. After completing the course, participants have the opportunity to work with an integrative health nurse clinician to integrate what they have learned into their own lives and use it to enhance patient care. This has led to increased nurse engagement and patient satisfaction and has improved patient outcomes. Researchers are evaluating the changes in nurses' attitudes and their knowledge and application of therapies that are addressed in the TNT program. Since it was established in 2006, more than 250 nurses from ANH have participated in the 48-hour training program. In 2011, a TNT Train-the-Trainer program was developed, enabling TNT's expansion to all eleven hospitals within Allina Health. Beyond its local expansion, TNT is now providing training to nurses at two Department of Veterans Affairs hospitals in California as part of a scientific study.

INNOVATIVE RESEARCH CONDUCTED BY THE INTEGRATIVE HEALTH RESEARCH CENTER

The Integrative Health Research Center (IHRC) establishes measurable patient outcomes and identifies best practices through data analysis and clinical trials. The IHRC maintains a balance of basic science, randomized controlled trials, and observational studies in support of Allina Health's research goals. Led by Jeffery Dusek, Ph.D., the IHRC collaborates with Harvard Medical School teaching hospitals (Massachusetts General Hospital) in using innovative gene expression to detect genomic mechanisms of how integrative therapies affect the body and mind. In randomized controlled trials, the IHRC uses psychological and biological measurement to understand how integrative therapies influence clinical outcomes. IHRC research involves patients across ANH's centers of excellence. With a large inpatient integrative service and documentation in an electronic health record system, the PGI maintains the largest integrative medicine dataset of its kind in the country. Using this dataset, the IIRC is unique in its ability to conduct observational studies assessing the best practices and effectiveness of integrative services in the "real world" setting of an acute care hospital. Through rigorous research, the PGI is testing new models of care and is sharing this knowledge through training and publishing and by replicating its programs and services at other Allina Health facilities and beyond.

In 2011, the IHRC received a $2.4 million National Institutes of Health grant for research in an observational study of a model for the delivery of CAM therapies and an evaluation of the effectiveness of CAM therapies for pain management in an acute care inpatient hospital. The aims of the study are:

Aim 1: Quantitatively describe a model for delivering CAM therapies to understand selection of patients and CAM therapies for pain management.
Aim 2: Examine the effects of selected CAM therapies on immediate change in pain.
Aim 3: Examine the effects of selected CAM therapies on duration of pain change.

Allina Health, through the efforts of the PGI, is committed to transforming healthcare through a whole-person approach. Integrative nursing is key to the success of this goal.

Furthering the advancement of nursing in the delivery of whole-person care serves the patient, the nurse, and the field of nursing as a whole.

The Evolution of the Innovation of Integrative Medicine and Integrative Nursing in Acute Care Hospitals

Many hospitals and hospital systems are adopting components of integrative nursing by utilizing HAT, offering the practice of holistic nursing, being grounded in holistic nursing theory, and emphasizing care for the caregivers, in addition to using select specialty-licensed or certified integrative therapies such as acupuncture, certified massage therapy, music therapy, biofeedback, and so on. Often these components are integrated into a singular unit or clinical service line at a time.

Hospitals such as Winter Haven Hospital in Winter Haven, Florida, have strongly emphasized Caring Science as the foundation of their nursing practice. Other Caritas Charter Healthcare organizations include two hospitals of the John C. Lincoln system of Phoenix, Arizona; Baptist Hospital of Miami, Florida; the Gundersen Lutheran hospital of La Crosse, Wisconsin; Mountain States Health Alliance of Johnson City, Tennessee; Albert Einstein Healthcare Network of Philadelphia, Pennsylvania; the Bon Secours Health System of Marriottsville, Minnesota; and the Chesapeake Regional Medical Center of Chesapeake, Virginia.

Many academic and tertiary care centers are also integrating a holistic model of care. The University of California–Los Angeles Health System has made efforts at both the Westwood and Santa Monica campuses to offer comprehensive programming and staff education related to many therapeutic interventions under the programmatic rubric of "Urban Zen" to meet their specific patient care needs. These include: yoga, Reiki, use of essential oils, and mindfulness awareness techniques. Other institutions, such as the Mayo Clinic, have several hospitals offering various healing arts therapies for specific patient populations. The same is true for Gundersen Lutheran Hospital in LaCrosse, Wisconsin, and the hospitals of ProHealth Care of the Waukesha, Wisconsin, region.

In the Twin Cities, most hospitals have added components to enhance the healing environment and offer integrative therapies, including the University of Minnesota Medical Center, Fairview, and the University of Minnesota Amplatz Children's Hospital. Additionally, many smaller community hospitals such as Transylvania Regional Hospital in Brevard, North Carolina, and the North Hawaii Community Hospital in Kamuela not only focus on healing arts therapies but emphasize and focus on transcultural care. This assessment of the evolution of integrative nursing in the acute care setting is a dynamic, ever-evolving representation of the diffusion of integrative care in this country and others. This represents an innovation in optimizing the healing environment in the acute care hospital experience.

The Future

With the advent of the Affordable Care Act (see http://www.healthcare.gov/law/index. html), which passed into law in 2010, hospitals are rewarded via Medicare payment for quality of care and maintenance of high levels of patient satisfaction. Two key components of the patient-satisfaction measure (Hospital Consumer Assessment of Healthcare Providers and Systems—http://www.hcahpsonline.org/home.aspx) include:

1. "How responsive hospital staff are to patients" and
2. "How well caregivers [referring to hospital personnel] manage the patients' pain."

Integrative nursing practice, as defined by the principles of *person-centered and relationship-based care, informed by evidence and using the full range of therapeutic modalities from least intensive/invasive to more*, is an opportunity for hospitals to fully realize their quality and patient satisfaction outcomes, leading to optimal reimbursement. Additionally, it is believed that hospitals will see improved nurse retention and the associated financial gains when nurses are trained in integrative principles and interventions.

SELECTED REFERENCES

Ananth, S. (2011). Complementary and alternative medicine survey of hospitals. http://www. SamueliInstitute.org.

Barrett, B. (2003). Alternative, complementary, and conventional medicine: Is integration upon us? *The Journal of Alternative & Complementary Medicine, 9*(3), 417–427.

Clement, J. P., Chen, H. F., Burke, D., Clement, D. G., & Zazzali, J. L. (2006). Are consumers reshaping hospitals? Complementary and alternative medicine in U.S. hospitals, 1999–2003. *Health Care Management Review*, April–June, *31*(2), 109–118.

Dusek, J. A., Finch, M., Plotnikoff, G., & Knutson, L. (2010). The impact of integrative medicine on pain management in a tertiary care hospital. *Journal of Patient Safety, 6*(1), 48–51.

Gannotta, R. J., Zoller, J., Brantley, J., & White, A. (2009). *Perceptions of Medical Directors and Hospital Executives Regarding the Value of Inpatient Integrative Medicine Programs.* Columbia, South Carolina: Medical University of South Carolina.

Jonas, W., & Chez, R. (2004). Toward optimal healing environments in health care. *Journal of Alternative and Complementary Medicine, 10*(Suppl 1), S1–S6.

Koerner, J. G. (2012). *Healing Presence: The Essence of Nursing.* New York: Springer Publishing Company.

Lincoln, V., & Johnson, M. (2009). Staff Nurse Perceptions of a Healing Environment. *Holistic Nursing Practice*, May–June, 183–190.

Lincoln, V. (2000). Nontraditional healthcare: Emerging into integrative healthcare. In Condon, M. C., (Ed.), *Women's Health: An Integrated Approach to Wellness and Illness.*, pp. 180–194. Upper Saddle River, NJ: Prentice-Hall Health.

Watson, J. (2008). *The Philosophy and Science of Caring.* Denver, CO: University Press of Colorado.

26

Integrative Nursing in the Community

JUDITH FOULADBAKHSH AND SUSAN G. SZCZESNY

Communities have been defined in many different ways, but what remains consistent is the nature and importance of relationships. This includes, but is not limited to, relationships with (a) other individuals and families, whether close or far away; (b) diverse populations; (c) the physical, emotional, and spiritual environment; and (d) the services and systems available, including those that promote health and provide care. Thus, nurses have viewed communities as their client (Hanchett, 1979), partner, and those they serve. In this chapter, we aim to provide an integrative view of nursing in the community that encompasses this broad view of communities. This will include discussion about how integrative nursing is positioned in the community, the role of integrative nurses and their view of community as a system, and the types of therapeutic interventions and healthcare delivery models that support integrative care. In this way, the physical, psychosocial, and spiritual needs of individuals, families, communities, and their environment can be addressed in a holistic and comprehensive manner. This, we believe, is necessary to fully promote health and healing, prevent disease, assure comfort when ill, and ease the transition at end of life. Recognizing the interconnectedness of individuals, their communities, and the environment is essential to the development of nurse–client partnerships that support health of the body, mind and spirit.

Defining the Community

"Community as client" takes into account the philosophical premise of systems theory and related concepts such as boundaries, geographical and non-geographical, that expand and contract in response to stress and strain to promote adaptation. Hence, a community may be a physical area or a non-physical entity, such as a community of high-risk pregnant adolescents who are not confined within a geographic location. Viewing the community as the client allows the nurse to provide care for the larger group, with ultimate benefits for the individual members as well. In a reciprocal manner, the comprehensive care of individuals benefits communities, society, and the surrounding environment. Consistent with a system's view, change in a part affects the whole, wherein parts are inseparable, coexisting, and interdependent. Thus, community nursing focuses on all levels of relationships and recognizes the interconnectedness of individuals, families, groups, and society, all of which influence health promotion and wellness. So no matter how small or large the change enacted by nursing care, one must always consider the ripple effects extending out from and inward to the individual, and the influence exerted on communities along the way.

Conceptual Framework: Integrative Community Care

COMMUNITY/PUBLIC HEALTH NURSING PRACTICE

As global boundaries disappear, nurses working in the community encounter increasing population diversity and rapid exposure to different systems of healthcare from around the world, most with differing philosophical views and beliefs. Within our Midwestern community, for example, there are thousands of different cultural and subcultural groups, most with diverse health beliefs, practices, and traditions that affect their health. Also important are the ongoing changes within conventional Western medicine, which is increasingly recognizing potential benefits of diverse global systems of healthcare and related therapies as evidence emerges. So how do these factors affect nursing practice in the community and the models we currently use as a guide? And what is the nurse's role in promoting an integrative care model that incorporates the key principles discussed in earlier chapters?

"Public health nursing," also referred to as "community health nursing," remains grounded in a population-based perspective using a multidisciplinary team approach to interprofessional practice. These caring/healing relationships aim to create healthy communities that support healthy people. Practice models incorporate assessment of population health status, identification of health indicators, consideration of all levels of prevention (primary, secondary, and tertiary), and individual, family, community, and systems-focused nursing interventions. Inherent in public/community health are the creation and maintenance of healthy environments and socioeconomic conditions that foster and support health (American Public Health Association, 1999). Given the above-described scope of practice, as "new" paradigms of care emerge, with differing philosophical beliefs, therapies, and practitioners, changes are imminent and highlight the need for new integrative models of care.

Integrative Care in Communities

Use of an integrative approach in the care of communities requires understanding of the complexity of human nature and the healing process, and how adaptation occurs in individuals and community systems (as previously discussed in Chapter 1). This approach aims to create a balance between an *individual* (personal system) and *collective* (community system) focus (Goddard, 2006), which is vitally important to community nursing care. Of great importance is our understanding of whole systems, and that a change in a part affects the whole. Complex systems, such as communities, go through periods of stress and strain, always seeking to adapt and achieve homeokinesis (dynamic stability). Community health nurses understand these principles and know that promoting health-behavior change on an individual level will ultimately affect change at the family and community level. Understanding the subjective and objective aspects of health and illness from an individual and collective perspective also allows us to see where gaps in care occur (Kreisberg, 2008) and to plan appropriate and creative healing interventions.

An integrative approach can also help us "simultaneously address the health and wellbeing of nurses, the healthcare team, the patients, families and significant others, the healthcare system/structure, and the world" (Dossey, 2008, p. 23). As highlighted in the sixth Principle presented in Chapter 1, integrative nursing focuses on the health and wellbeing of caregivers, who are integral to community and its members.

PROMOTING HEALTHY ENVIRONMENTS: ROLE OF COMMUNITY HEALTH NURSES

Also critical to the promotion of health and healing and the prevention of illness are the development and maintenance of healthy environments. While nurses have focused on the healing properties of nature and the environment since the Nightingale era, the need to create optimal healing environments in the community continues to be of critical importance. An optimal healing environment is one in which "the social, psychological, spiritual, physical, and behavioral components of health care are oriented toward support and stimulation of healing and the achievement of wholeness" (Jonas & Chez, 2005, p. S1). Community health nurses recognize that humans are inseparable from their environments (Principle 1) and play a vital role in fostering optimal healing environments using integrative care strategies. Community health nurses are consistently vigilant in assessing environmental safety, always on the alert to detect potential health hazards, whether physical, biological, social, or psychological. The principle of *biophilia*, which emphasizes the significant role of nature in the healing process, has been fundamental to community health practice since its early days, reinforcing the significance of healthy environments in health and wellness.

Incorporating the principles of integrative care, nurses caring for communities and the individuals within continue to be strong advocates for environmental protection and positive change. Creating and sustaining environments that are nurturing, supportive, and safe is indeed an ethical mandate for nurses caring for communities and may involve grassroots initiatives, political action, and policy development. Integrative community care also promotes ecologically sound environments that support the bodymindspirit, with opportunities for healthcare that include conventional, complementary, and traditional healing therapies that are culturally appropriate. Community health nurses remain a vital force in maintaining healthy, "green environments" as they witness firsthand the impact of unhealthy environments on all levels of health. Thus, community health nurses who incorporate integrative and holistic principles continue to lead the way with an eco-nursing perspective as they advocate for ethical and moral standards that protect our environment and our world, while being a vital force in maintaining "green environments and communities."

The ecological commitment of community health nurses is evident in their initiating and voicing support for "green spaces" in communities, such as parks within crowded, tenement-filled inner-city areas, where children play while adults relax and connect with neighbors, further strengthening relationships. They continue to advocate clean air, free from pollutants and pesticides, in urban and rural areas, while also promoting recycling and education about environmental safety. Community health nurses have always integrated the principles of caring for the mind and the spirit, for individuals and the community at large, recognizing the profound negative effects of overcrowding, poverty, violence, and despair on health and wellbeing. All levels of prevention have promoted an awareness of the importance of supporting the environment while maintaining health among the interconnected systems.

Integrative Community Health Nursing Model

Models—pictorial representations of concepts and relationships—help illustrate a process, providing insight and direction. For our work in the community, which we define as integrative nursing practice, we follow a model that reflects the reciprocal flow of energy between the individual, community, and global levels (Figure 26.1). Energy (as depicted by arrows) includes relationships, information, communication, exchange of matter, networks, and connections, which can be physical, psychological, social, and/or energetic in nature.

In this model, communities and societies are nestled in between the global and individual levels and provide an interface through which communication flows, is enhanced, and/or is restricted. The global community, we believe, has had an increasingly profound influence on individuals, families, societies, and local communities, largely due to our growing awareness of international events and crises, overwhelming expressions of need and compassionate offers of assistance, and mounting concerns about prevalent global problems. In response, as individuals and communities, we express concern as well as stress and fear. As these global networks become more evident, we begin to see how change in one part of our world affects us all. This has been evident in how we have responded to natural disasters; for example, after the devastating tsunami in Japan, the world watched with fear and concern about the global effects of nuclear

Integrative Community Health Nursing Model

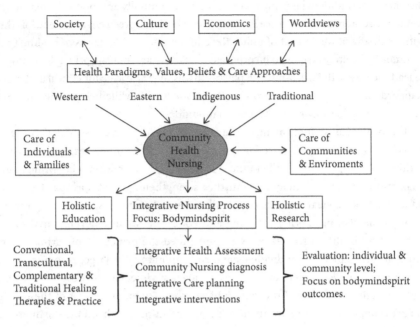

FIGURE 26.1 Integrative Community Health Nursing Model

radiation. The rallying of community resources was profound, reflecting worldwide commitment to the physical, emotional, and energetic needs that were manifested, and the development of partnerships to provide community care.

Also reflected in our model is the increasing interest in culturally diverse traditional and alternative whole systems of healthcare that exist across the world. This interest has been facilitated by technological advances in the rapid spread of information as well as the individual desire for more holistically based healing amidst dissatisfaction with mechanistic conventional medical care. At present, complementary, alternative, and traditional therapies are being used by the vast majority (almost 80%) of individuals in North America (Balneaves et al., 2012; Fouladbakhsh, 2010), highlighting the increased opportunity to holistically support the health of individual, communities, and environments with integrative care practices.

Our model also illustrates the integrative nursing process, which includes assessment of complex community systems and their members, creative care planning, and intervention, all of which demonstrate respect for individual, family, and community values and beliefs. While not different from our regular methodology of practice, this approach recognizes the importance of an *integrative nursing assessment* and *integrative care planning and intervention*. These phases of the nursing process are viewed as more comprehensive and sensitive to understanding: (a) the interplay of the bodymindspirit in relationship to health; (b) the influence of cultural and spiritual beliefs and traditions on health and healing; and (c) the use of healing practices and therapies that support whole-system healing. This is critically important to understanding our patients and their environments, which reflect traditions, customs, and use of conventional and alternative care providers. An integrative assessment provides the basis for the community healthcare plan and subsequent comprehensive, holistic care. Our model also stresses the need for integrative interventions that promote health (primary prevention) and support the body, mind, and spirit of individuals and communities through the healing process (secondary prevention). Integrative community nursing often focuses on less invasive methods and caring relationships that support multilevel healing. End-of-life care, often guided by community-based hospice nurses, is reflective of tertiary prevention, promoting comfort while maintaining dignity at this time of transition (individual and family system change). Also inherent within this model is the expansion of provider boundaries to promote multidisciplinary relationships and interprofessional practice. This level of integrative community practice would include the voices of alternative healthcare practitioners as well as conventional care providers, all of whom effectively collaborative with equality and mutual respect.

Integrative Approaches for Community Health Problems

Historically, public health efforts focused almost exclusively on the control of communicable diseases, with a major shift occurring as antibiotics and immunizations became widely available. Primary, secondary, and tertiary levels of prevention remain our framework for practice, with initiatives focused on risk-reduction to promote physical and psychological wellbeing (primary prevention) and to care for those with chronic illness (secondary prevention) and end-of-life concerns (tertiary prevention). Often the focus is on the increasing prevalence and burden of chronic illness, which has resulted in lack of access to and availability of health services, increased cost of care and financial burden, and decreased productivity. Individuals with chronic illness have been increasingly seeking comfort and healing using complementary and integrative therapies, especially among those with cancer (Fouladbakhsh, 2008; 2010; Mann, Gaylord, & Norton, 2004; Schiff, Attias, Hen, Kriendler, Arnon, Sroka, & Ben-Arye, 2012).

Prevalent chronic illnesses that are now considered to be public health problems because of their effect on the community, society at large, and the environment include osteoarthritis, obesity, post-traumatic stress disorder (PTSD), chronic low back pain, HIV/AIDs, diabetes, autism, and cardiovascular disease. Environmental community health problems of high significance include homelessness, school and workplace violence, substance abuse, and environmental degradation. A discussion on integrative nursing care as related to selected public health problems follows.

Osteoarthritis (OA) currently affects 27 million American adults and is expected to increase over the next two decades, affecting 25% of the population (Lawrence, 2008; Murphy & Helmick, 2012). This condition has devastating effects on mobility, physical functioning, and quality of life (QOL), with profound implications for productivity and cost of care (Yelin, Cisternas, Pasta, Trupin, Murphy, & Helmick, 2003). Non-traditional therapies that have been used to manage OA include yoga, tai chi, acupuncture, and natural supplements, which have varying degrees of effectiveness and have been studied predominantly in individuals with knee involvement (Fouladbakhsh, 2012). Data indicate improvement in gait and balance, reduction of back pain, and increased strength, flexibility, and balance with yoga practice (Ulger & Yagli, 2011; Raub, 2002; Bukowski, Conway, Glentz, Kurland, & Galantino, 2006). Similarly, tai chi has been found to increase knee extension and decrease pain and fear of falling among elders with OA (Song, Roberts, Lee, Lam, & Bae, 2010; Shen, James, Chyu, Bixby, Brismee, Zumwalt, & Poklikuha, 2008). Although further data are needed, the integration of therapies that focus on healing the bodymindspirit may improve balance and independence, prevent falls, and improve wellbeing. Nutraceutical supplements, specifically glucosamine and chondroitin, are also widely used to manage OA progression and symptoms. Thus, it is highly probable that a community health nurse will encounter individuals using these readily available non-prescription supplements and must use an integrative assessment to determine their appropriateness and safety.

Obesity, which is often grouped with other eating disorders, also continues to rapidly escalate in the United States as well as worldwide, with higher prevalence in ethnic minorities (Benavides & Caballero, 2009; Flegal, Caroll, Ogden, & Curtin, 2010; Forrest & Leeds, 2007; Ogden, Carroll, Kit, & Flegal, 2012). This presents a dire picture, given the increased prevalence and earlier onset of diabetes, cardiovascular disease, and other highly burdensome chronic conditions that are related to being overweight or obese (Gregg, Cheng, Cadwell, Imperator, Williams, Flegal, & Williamson, 2005). Although most attention has focused on the use and misuse of dietary supplements and weight-loss products such as ephedra, studies of other complementary and traditional therapies are beginning to emerge in the literature. Although further research is needed, preliminary data support the use of yoga to decrease stress and inflammatory responses (Kiecolt-Glaser, Christian, Preston, Houts, Malarkey, Emery, & Glaser, 2010) and improve sleep and mood (Fouladbakhsh, 2011; Fouladbakhsh, Davis, & Yarandi, 2012; Harinath, Malhotram Pal, Prasad, Kumar, Kain, et al., 2004), all of which are related to obesity, binge eating, and other nutritional disorders (Guarracino, Savino, & Edelstein, 2006; Sojcher, 2011; Carei, Fyfe-Johnson, Breuner, & Brown, 2010; McIver, O'Halloran, & McGartland, 2009). Yoga practice also resulted in decreased fatigue, improved QOL, and reduced waist circumference among obese breast cancer survivors (Littman, Bertram, Ceballos, Ulrich, Ramaprasad, et al., 2012). Similarly, tai chi improved body mass index (BMI), was safe and effective, and reduced inflammatory biomarkers of oxidative stress (C-reactive protein) among obese individuals with diabetes (Chen, Ueng, Lee, Sun, & Lee, 2010), potentially strengthening their constitution and enhancing wellbeing at many levels.

Positive outcomes of bodymindspirit practices, such as yoga and mindfulness-based stress reduction, on prevalent community problems such as autism, mental health, and PTSD have been demonstrated, although further study is indicated (Bohlmeijer, Prenger, Taal, & Cuijpers, 2010; Rosenblatt, Gorantla, Torres, Yarmush, Rao, Park et al., 2011; Strauss, Coeytaux, McDuffie, Nagi, & Williams, 2011). In addition, these therapies are now being viewed as having potential preventive benefits with regard to school, community, workplace, and prison violence, due to their stress-reducing effects.

Role of Nursing and Nursing Leadership

The integration of non-conventional evidence-based healing therapies into nursing practice in the community has profound implications. Community health nurses are in a prime position, whether in official public health agencies, schools, faith-based organizations (parish nurses), homeless shelters, or home/hospice care, to practice within an integrative framework. This will allow nurses to more comprehensively assess needs of community members and provide, refer, and recommend beneficial healing interventions. The nurse should also be a strong community and patient advocate and educator, which includes political activism and legislative involvement to eradicate known health hazards and support an ecologically balanced environment. Community health nurses are also skilled at establishing community partnerships, which are important in a number of ways, such as assessing and planning healthier communities, decreasing morbidity and mortality, and improving the community and its environment. Because nurses are the most numerous of healthcare providers, they are also uniquely situated to provide leadership in the transition to integrated healthcare in the community.

It is our belief that integrative nursing care happens in communities in two ways: spontaneously and planned. Having a holistic, integrative view of nursing can arise as a natural part of a nurse's philosophy of life, health and healing, and personal experience. Integrative care may also occur spontaneously as a natural part of a community's life, affecting the individuals in it and the environment that surrounds them. Nurses working with ethnic communities, for example, Chinese and Native Americans, must consider their different worldviews and perspectives on life, health and illness, and healing approaches. This experience also provides a different way of viewing human–environment caring relationships and their influence on health and wellbeing, thereby promoting integrative care.

Integrative nursing care can also be *planned* at the individual and community levels using the principles identified in Chapter 1. Needed is a comprehensive worldview that shifts away from a disease-oriented model to one emphasizing whole-person/

whole-system healing. Collaboration with peers may also promote integrative nursing practice and stimulate interest in self-care and wellbeing of the caregiver. Nursing leaders can also support education and clinical practice that incorporates the principles of integrative nursing care.

Exemplars of Integrative Community Care Programs

INTEGRATIVE COMMUNITY HEALTH CLINICAL PRACTICE

Fenway Community Health Center (FCH), Boston, Massachusetts: This community center originated in 1971 as a grassroots initiative in response to the AIDS epidemic, and it continues to provide integrative services to the lesbian, gay, bisexual, and transgender (LGBT) community. The FCH model of integrated community-based care is comprehensive and culturally sensitive, addressing the physical, psychosocial, and spiritual needs of this vulnerable community. A comprehensive range of health services is provided, and nurse practitioners participate in interprofessional teams that provide compassionate care to promote healing. Complementary and traditional therapies such as yoga, massage, and acupuncture have been integrated into the care model for over two decades to promote comfort while managing pain, musculoskeletal problems, anxiety, fertility issues, detoxification, and more (Mayer, Mimiaga, VanDerwarker, Goldhammer, & Bradford, 2007; Mayer, Applebaum, Rogers, Wilson, Bradford, & Boswell, 2001).

Veterans Affairs Integrative Health Clinic and Program (IHCP), Salt Lake City, Utah: This program provides "nonpharmacological biopsychosocial management of chronic nonmalignant pain and stress-related depression, anxiety and symptoms of PTSD" (Smeeding, Bradshaw, Kumpfer, Trevithick, Stoddard, et al., 2010, p. 823) and actively incorporates integrative nursing participation for a highly vulnerable and increasingly prevalent at-risk community population. This program was initiated by a nurse with support from the nursing director (personal communication, S. Smeeding, July 6, 2012). A board-certified family nurse practitioner is involved in integrative assessments, establishment of treatment plans that include healing interventions, follow-up, and referrals for care. Nurses are also actively involved in the provision of complementary therapies, including acupuncture and medical hypnosis (RN licensed acupuncturist and advanced practice nurses, respectively). In addition, the "Choose to Heal Stress" and "Quit Smart" multi-modal programs include therapies to support whole-system healing. Longitudinal study reveals improved QOL for veterans, high patient and provider acceptability, and low cost of care (Smeeding et al., 2010).

Welcome Inn Integrative Health Team, Royal Oak, Michigan: The Welcome Inn, a program sponsored by the South Oakland County Citizens for the Homeless, provides daytime services for homeless adults during the cold winter months, including shelter, nutritious meals, social work services, and integrative health care. The development of this nonprofit organization was prompted by community outrage over the freezing death of a homeless individual in the local neighborhood. The integrative health team includes nurses, students, and other individuals who provide integrative care that focuses on supporting the healing process on a whole-person level. Caring relationships are established to determine physical and psychosocial needs and provide referrals for conventional care services. The healing team also provides an array of complementary and non-traditional therapies to maximize wellness, reduce stress, and assist individuals with the physical and emotional healing process. Community partnerships have been established with conventional healthcare providers and alternative practitioners who provide care without cost for the uninsured.

The team also offers education on many health topics such as nutrition, and a full range of therapeutic modalities reflecting Principle 5 of integrative nursing practice. These therapies, viewed as less invasive and having the potential for bodymindspirit healing, include massage sessions, yoga classes, Healing Touch, and reflexology treatments. The integrative approach of the health team has served to promote health and healing through early detection of physical and emotional problems and provide comfort and improved QOL while reaffirming the dignity of individuals faced with homelessness.

COMMUNITY EDUCATION

CAMEO Program, Vancouver, British Columbia, Canada: This program, funded by the Lotte and John Hecht Memorial Foundation and the Canadian Institute of Health Research, was developed based on the needs of cancer patients in British Columbia with regard to knowledge and decision-making about complementary medicine (CM). A lack of information and provider communication was identified, as well as insufficient support in making CM decisions, addressing an important gap in cancer care (Balneaves, Truant, Verhoef, Ross, Porcino, Wong, & Braxier, 2012). The *CAMEO* (Complementary Medicine Education and Outcomes) program (see www.bccancer. bc.ca/cameo) provides CM information and resources to patients across the cancer trajectory, along with an array of education and decision-support interventions, promoting open communication and facilitating integrated care. The *CAMEO* team is led by a nurse researcher and includes nurse clinicians who provide CM education in the cancer community.

The Community Cancer Connections Project at the College of Nursing at the University of Arizona is also an exemplary program focused on integrative community health. The mission of this project is to offer community-based, integrative oncology resources and education using a distributive resource and learning platform (see www. linkin.nursing.arizona.edu). The project focuses on the health and wellbeing of the cancer community (survivors, family, friends, and providers), with a future plan to offer coaching and advocacy for the cancer community.

INTEGRATIVE COMMUNITY HEALTH RESEARCH

Nurses have led the way in holistic research for over four decades, with studies examining specific therapeutic modalities and their effects on various outcomes. Understanding the effects of a whole-systems approach to health and healing within communities, however, requires investigation. Research that is guided by an integrative nursing framework is needed to clearly identify how this approach will benefit individuals, communities, and the environment in which they live.

While our research has not yet focused on a whole system of care per se, it offers a glimpse into the potential benefits of approaching the care of lung cancer patients in a more holistic and integrative manner. By offering a system of yoga focused on breathing ease and stress reduction, we have been able to examine effects of the practice on overall QOL for an under-served population with a complex and daunting illness. The study team, using a holistic philosophy that aims to compassionately accept individuals wherever they are in their life journey, worked closely with participants over a nine-month period. Yoga allowed us to teach patients about the power of the breath and meditation as a healing practice, which became integrated into the daily lives of the participants and researchers. The effect of this holistic research on the study team was also profound, strengthening their interest in therapeutic healing practices and fueling the spirit of research within (Fouladbakhsh, Szczesny, Kowalewski, & Blair, 2013).

In sum, these community-based programs and initiatives provide insights into the importance of integrative care and its effects on whole person and community health. It is imperative that future endeavors focus on the innate healing capacity of individuals and the adaptability of community systems, building in approaches that strengthen caring community connections, partnerships, and healthy environments.

Aspirational Vision

The epidemic of chronic illness and environmental degradation is expected to continue, with dire consequences for individuals, families, communities, and the planet. Although this has been acknowledged and attempts at management are in process, an integrative perspective has been lacking. New solutions are clearly needed, with significant potential existing within integrative care at all levels of practice. Healing of individuals, communities, and the earth is possible if everyone becomes accountable in the process. It has never been more important that nurses at all levels of care become an active part of the solution. Whether caring for a community of hospitalized patients, staff nurses, high-risk individuals, or community neighborhoods, the philosophy of holistic bodymindspirit care and integrative practice apply.

SELECTED REFERENCES

Dossey, B. (2008). Theory of integral nursing. *Advances in Nursing Science*, *31*(1), E52–E73.

Esbjorn-Hargens (2009). *Integral Ecology: Uniting Multiple Perspectives on the Natural World*. New York: Random House/Integral Books.

Fouladbakhsh, J. M., Szczesny, S., Kowalewski, K., & Blair, D. (2013). Honoring the spirit of research within: The Yoga and More (CAM) Research Interest Group. *Journal of Nursing Education & Practice*, *3*(2), 132–140.

Gaboury, I., Boon, H., Verhoef, M., Bujold, M., Lapierre, L. M., & Moher, D. (2010). Practitioners' validation of framework of team-oriented practice models in integrative health care: A mixed methods study. *BMC Health Services Research*, *10*, 289.

Mann, D., Gaylord, S., & Norton, S. (2004). Moving toward integrative care: Rationales, models, and steps for conventional-care providers. *Complementary Health Practice Review*, *9*, 155–172.

Smeeding, S. J., Bradshaw, D. H., Kumpfer, K., Trevithick, S., & Stoddard, G. J. (2010). Outcome evaluation of the Veterans Affairs Salt Lake City Integrative Health Clinic for chronic pain and stress-related depression, anxiety, and post-traumatic stress disorder. *Journal of Alternative & Complementary Medicine*, *16*(8), 823–835.

Song, R., Roberts, B. L., Lee, E. O., Lam, P., & Bae, S. C. (2010). A randomized study of the effects of T'ai Chi on muscle strength, bone mineral density, and fear of falling in women with osteoarthritis. *Journal of Alternative & Complementary Medicine*, *16*(3), 227–233.

Strauss, J. L., Coeytaux, R., McDuffie, J., Nagi, A., & Williams, J. W. Jr. (2011). *Efficacy of Complementary and Alternative Medicine Therapies for Post-Traumatic Stress Disorder*. Washington, DC: Department of Veterans Affairs, Health Services Research & Development Service.

Ulger, O., & Yagli, N. V. (2011). Effects of yoga on balance and gait properties in women with musculoskeletal problems: A pilot study. *Complementary Therapies in Clinical Practice*, *17*(1), 13–15.

Yelin, E., Cisternas, M. G., Pasta, D. J., Trupin, L., Murphy, L., & Helmick, C. G. (2007). Medical expenditures and earnings losses among persons with arthritis and other rheumatic conditions in 2003 and comparisons with 1997. *Arthritis & Rheumatism*, *56*(5), 1397–1407.

27

Integrative Nursing in Mental Health: Models of Team-Oriented Approaches

MERRIE J. KAAS, BARBARA PETERSON, AND GISLI KRISTOFERSSON

Models for Team-Oriented Approaches to Integrative Mental Health Care

NEED FOR INTEGRATED, INTEGRATIVE MENTAL HEALTH CARE

Mental illness and substance use disorders are the newest epidemics of this century (Kessler & Ustun, 2008). Mental illness is a major cause of disability in the United States and globally, and the economic burden of mental illness is growing (Greenberg et al., 2003; Mark et al., 2011). Mental health problems such as depression, schizophrenia, post-traumatic stress disorder, and dementia are included in the list of highest-cost chronic health problems, along with arthritis, cancer, chronic pain, diabetes, and vision and hearing loss. Care of patients with coexisting multiple chronic conditions costs seven times as much as those with one chronic condition. The cost to the person with mental illness includes early mortality; people with serious mental illness die, on average, 25 years earlier than the general population, largely due to treatable medical conditions such as cardiovascular, pulmonary, and infectious diseases (National Association of State Mental Health Program Directors, 2006).

The American mental health care system is costly, yet not all those who need treatment receive it (Greenberg et al., 2003). Early diagnosis and treatment of mental health disorders could reduce the lifetime burden of chronic diseases. Because mental health and physical health concerns are so closely related, adults and children with mental illness, more than any other patient population, need interprofessional, coordinated approaches to address their myriad physical and mental health needs. Collaboration among healthcare providers is needed to provide safe, high quality, holistic care for patients with mental illness. Integrated, team-oriented mental health care models are needed.

INTEGRATED MENTAL HEALTH CARE

The Patient Protection and Affordable Healthcare Act (HR 3590, "Obamacare") passed by our Congress in 2010 provides new opportunities for improved healthcare based on principles of preventative healthcare and healthcare teams. As U.S. healthcare reforms continue to evolve, it is clear that new *integrated* healthcare system models are being developed to address mental health care disparities by combining primary care services with mental health care to provide coordinated care for persons with mental illness and substance use disorders. These *integrated* healthcare system models are meant to improve access to mental health care, manage the economic burden and suffering by people with mental illness who do not have adequate health care, and manage costs associated with increasing disability attributed to coexisting medical and mental illnesses (Parks et al., 2006). However, too often healthcare systems that treat patients with serious mental illness have a fragmented model of care in which mental health professionals work in "silos" with little or no team collaboration between each other or with medical care practitioners.

The Substance Abuse Mental Health Services Administration (SAMHSA)—Center for Integrated Health Solutions (www.integration.samhsa.gov) disseminated its *Standard Framework for Levels of Integrated Healthcare* to advance the discourse about the integrated nature of these healthcare system models. This framework describes a continuum from the simplest to the most complex levels, starting from coordinated care, then to co-located care, and finally to integrated care. Each level is described in terms of communication among team members, clinical delivery of health and mental health screening, the patient experience, coordination of information sharing among team members and across systems, the organizational support for integrated services, and the allocation of financial resources across services and teams. A summary table describing these levels in more detail is found at www.integration.samhsa.gov. This table provides an organizing schema for integrated healthcare systems, whether providing mental health care services in primary care settings, or primary care services in mental health care settings. These new healthcare models attempt to decrease the mind–body service gap in our mental health care system today. What is missing from this discussion is how to create new integrated mental health care models that embody the bodymindspirit health paradigm, not just close the "mind–body" gap between physical and mental health care system services.

INTEGRATIVE MENTAL HEALTH CARE

These limitations of current models of mental health care, with the emphasis on biological determinants of mental illness, subsequent pharmacological interventions, and the separation of mental health care from medical care have led mental health care practitioners to consider a new paradigm in mental health care—*integrative* mental health.

Integrative mental health considers a whole person approach to understanding mental illness by addressing bodymindspirit determinants that affect the person's health and wellness. Integrative mental health addresses prevention and treatment of mental illness through combinations of the best conventional and non-conventional personalized approaches to mental health care determined through a shared decision-making process between the patient and practitioner (Lake, Helgason, & Sarris, 2012).

People suffering from the emotional pain of mental illness seek help from many avenues to address the cause of their suffering and obtain relief. However, because of dissatisfaction with conventional approaches to mental health care, more are choosing non-conventional, complementary and alternative medicine (CAM) therapies to replace or augment conventional therapies (Sirois, 2008). Studies have revealed that persons diagnosed with multiple chronic conditions, including mental illness, use CAM therapies significantly more than the general population does, including relaxation techniques, spiritual or energy treatments, vitamins, herbs, or other natural substances (Lake, Helgason, & Sarris, 2012). The majority of patients seeking complementary and alternative mental health practitioners self-refer; only a small percentage of people are referred by their medical care provider, and often these CAM services are limited because of cost. While these mental health conditions are best managed by a collaborative team of practitioners, communication or coordination of care is rare (Simon, Cherkin, Sherman, Eisenberg, Deyo, & Davis, 2008).

The passage of the Patient Protection and Affordable Healthcare Act provides a rare opportunity for the development of new mental health care teams that include CAM practitioners. This healthcare legislation mandates non-discrimination among licensed practitioners for insurers who provide group and individual healthcare coverage (Weeks, 2012). Licensed integrative practitioners have an opportunity to participate more fully in mental health care teams with other traditional mental health providers to support the patients' health and wellness and alleviate the symptoms of mental illness (Weeks, 2012).

Increasing numbers and diversity of team members within and across systems of mental health care add complexity to healthcare delivery and require additional teamwork to be effective. How new mental health care teams can deliver effective care is still unknown. However, it can be useful to examine current integrative mental health care programs to identify team approaches of integrated care. Using a conceptual framework of team orientation, the authors describe the level of teamwork and propose components for future integrated, integrative mental health programs.

Exemplars of Integrative Mental Health Teams

The three examples below incorporate some level of a team approach to integrative mental health care.

THE WHOLENESS CENTER

Located in Fort Collins, Colorado, the Wholeness Center (www.wholeness.com) exemplifies holistic, integrative approaches to mental health services. Founded and developed in 2010 by Dr. Scott Shannon, the clinic offers conventional and integrative modalities to provide holistic mental health care to patients. Each patient seeking treatment at the Wholeness Center undergoes an initial assessment to get a comprehensive picture of the mind, body, and spirit issues. Included in the assessment are physical assessment and laboratory studies of mental, emotional, and social concerns, as well as a naturopathic assessment of nutrition, diet, and lifestyle issues. Patients are seen for chronic mental health issues such as autism, ADHD, and mood disorders. Many children with developmental issues such as autism or ADHD also have significant dietary and gut issues, allergies, ear infections, a history of frequent antibiotic treatments, poor diets, or nutritional malabsorption.

The multidisciplinary treatment team at the Wholeness Center includes: adult and child psychiatrists, family therapists, naturopathic doctors, counselors, psychologists, acupuncturists, a clinical social worker, a nutrition specialist, a psychiatric nurse practitioner, and a massage and cranio-sacral therapist. The Wholeness Center staff offer a wide range of evidence-based integrative therapies such as acupuncture, massage and cranio-sacral therapy, Reiki, neurofeedback, nutritional and supplement education and recommendations, biofeedback, medications and medication education groups, hyperbaric oxygen therapy, biomedical therapies, dialectic behavior training skills classes, mind–body therapies, meditation and stress reduction classes, family therapy, and group therapy. At the Wholeness Center, child/adolescent psychiatrists and psychiatric nurse specialists, who are trained in integrative mental health, collaborate with patients and families to maximize the combined benefits of medication management and complementary and alternative therapies. The Wholeness Center employs a psychiatric nurse practitioner as one of four prescribers. This psychiatric nurse practitioner also has expertise in diet and nutritional problems and metabolic issues, and provides patient education. The treatment team also includes the patient and family, who jointly share ideas and expertise to develop a comprehensive treatment plan. Dr. Shannon notes (personal communication, April 18, 2013) "that a major problem with traditional mental health providers is they don't address the physical aspects of the patient and only try to work from the neck up. For example, they don't look at nutrition deficits, somatic concerns, metabolic problems, mitochondrial aspects, all important contributors to mental health issues, especially those with chronic conditions." Shannon goes on to say providers need to look at all spheres of the patient's life—including family dynamics and relationships, parenting, metabolic issues, and genetic issues—to understand mental health issues from a bodymind-spirit, integrative perspective.

Patients seeking mental health services from the Wholeness Center do so for several reasons, such as: the clinic philosophy fits with their own, traditional care hasn't been effective, or they have been referred by a friend who has been helped at the Wholeness Center. Primarily serving the local Fort Collins area, the clinic is also nationally recognized for its unique contribution to mental health, and about 20% of patients travel from out of state to be seen by a Wholeness Center practitioner. Dr. Shannon says,

> I started the Wholeness Center to demonstrate the practical value of Integrative Mental Health. I teach health care professionals around the globe and I had seen the value of this type of care in my small practice but had no specific clinical model to share. Now, I have a workable model that is both cost effective and quite popular. My deepest hope is that the type of care that we practice at Wholeness Center will become an inspiration to help heal the current mental health care system in this country, which mirrors the chaos, isolation and fragmentation that our patients experience. (Personal communication, April 20, 2013)

RESILIENCE TRAINING PROGRAM AT ABBOTT NORTHWESTERN

The Resilience Training Program (http://www.wellness.allinaheath.org) located at the Penny George Institute for Health and Healing at Abbott Northwestern Hospital in Minneapolis, Minnesota, was founded and developed by Henry Emmons, M.D. It is an outpatient program that focuses on an integrative approach to mental health problems. Dr. Emmons is widely known in the field of integrative mental health and is the author of two books on the subject, *The Chemistry of Joy* and *The Chemistry of Calm*, as well as a workbook called *The Chemistry of Joy Workbook*, with Susan Bourgerie, MA, LP; Carolyn Denton, MA, LN; and Sandra Kacher, MSW, LICSW. Together, they form a group called Partners in Resilience and co-manage the Resilience Training Program as well as other projects.

The Resilience Training Program is an eight-week, skills-building, group-based program meant to increase a person's innate resilience for healing and thus increase his or her wellbeing and resistance to internal and external stressors (Dusek, 2009). Described as "an integrated approach for those experiencing depression, anxiety and other stress-related conditions" (Allina Health, 2013), the program is based on Dr. Emmons's book *The Chemistry of Calm* (2006). One of the key goals of the program is to decrease symptoms of mental illness and future relapses for participants. The Resilience Training Program is especially designed to address the needs of people who want to reduce their reliance on psychotropic medication, including those with a history of not tolerating these well (Allina Health, 2013).

The program begins with an initial integrative assessment by a psychiatrist who specializes in integrative approaches to identify presenting symptoms and determine potential causes of distress, and the goals of the patient for seeking treatment. Dietary and nutritional assessments, including laboratory tests, are completed by a clinical nutritionist using a functional nutritional approach to explore the potential impact of the patient's diet and nutrition status on symptoms. An exercise assessment is completed by an exercise physiologist to determine current functional status. An eight-week group mindfulness program aimed to increase the mindfulness skills of participants is also an integral part of the program. Potential nutritional approaches and supplementation may be used to restore balanced brain chemistry. Upon referral, additional integrative therapies are provided nearby at the Penny George and Roberta Mann Institute for Health and Healing.

Through self-report measures, initial program outcome data suggest that the Resilience Training Program is effective in mitigating psychiatric symptoms. Outcomes of the Resilience Training Program were measured using the Perceived Stress scale, the Center for Epidemiological Studies–Depression, Spielberger's State-Trait Anxiety Inventory, and single-item questions related to sleep and fatigue (Dusek, 2009). Among the 47 participants who had concluded the Resilience Training Program, there was a significant reduction in symptoms in numerous areas, including state and trait anxiety and perceived stress (Dusek, 2009).

The Resilience Training Program team includes a psychiatrist, a clinical nutritionist, and an exercise physiologist, along with many other healthcare professionals, depending on patient need. The nurses on the team collect initial participant information from the intake calls and coordinate the initial assessment with the new program participants. The process is team-based with a holistic, individualized approach to mental health care through interdisciplinary collaboration (Henry Emmons, personal communication, April 15, 2013).

TOUCHSTONE MENTAL HEALTH CARE HEALTH AND HEALING CENTER

Touchstone Mental Health (www.Touchstonemh.org) is a nonprofit mental health center located in Minneapolis that provides a range of community-based programs for people with mental illness. Touchstone's mission is to "Inspire Hope, Healing and WellBeing" through person-centered care to support a healthy mind, body, and spirit by encouraging each person to define their life goals—physical, mental, emotional, spiritual, social, vocational, and interpersonal. Touchstone services include intensive residential treatment, assisted living, intentional communities, intensive community rehabilitation and targeted case-management, home and community based services, and behavioral healthcare coordination. Touchstone has developed a first-in-the-country Community Health and Wellness Center designed for people with mental illness and physical health concerns. This Community Health and Wellness Center is situated in a new assisted-living complex with forty customized apartments, which was designed and built using current evidence-based healing environmental design and located in an area impacted by poverty. The goal of this Center is to be a non-stigmatizing place that brings all the physical and mental health experts together who have an interest in working with people with mental illness. Center participants are Minneapolis and other metropolitan residents who have a mental illness.

Integrative health services provided by Touchstone's Community Health and Wellness Center include: education for health, wellness, and lifestyle management; physical health care education in areas of sleep hygiene, medication management, dental care, nutrition classes and weight management; gardening for healthy diet; diabetes and cardiovascular management skills; physical fitness groups; bodymind-spirit groups such as mindfulness and acupuncture; healing arts; life skills groups; and family support. "The program goal is to provide integrative health approaches within an integrated environment," notes Martha Lantz, LICSW, MBA, Executive Director. The Path to Wellness Journey includes a comprehensive, holistic assessment done within the Center by an integrative psychiatric nurse practitioner. The integrative mental health care team meets with the individual to develop an individualized, whole health plan. The individual will then choose the Center offerings that best fit his/her needs and comfort level. Health and Wellness Center staff teams work with community partners, peers, and families to support the individual's journey toward improved wellness. The integrative health team includes psychiatric nurses, social workers, nutritionists, psychiatrists, personal training experts, dieticians, and primary care and specialty practitioners.

Conceptual Framework for Team-Oriented Models of Care

Boon, Verhoef, O'Hara, and Findlay (2004) conceptualized a framework for team-oriented healthcare practices that is similar to SAMHSA's levels of system collaboration. This framework describes seven types of team-oriented approaches to integrated healthcare, from less to more coordinated. Their model is adapted here to compare current models of integrative mental health care. Using the Boon et al. framework, these models are differentiated by philosophy, structure, process, and outcomes. The levels of team approaches for integrative mental health care are described in Table 27.1.

COMPARISONS ACROSS LEVELS

In moving from parallel models to unified models of team-oriented mental health care, diversity of thought and philosophy increases because of the fostered engagement of

Table 27.1: Team Approaches to Integrative Mental Health Care

Model	Description
Parallel	Independent mental health care practitioner working in a common setting performs his/her job within his/her formally defined scope of practice and documents patient information in a separate record; there is little communication among practitioners, and when it occurs, it is about a specific problem.
Consultative	Expert advice is requested and given from an integrative mental health professional to another professional via direct personal communication, including an electronic or hard copy formal letter or referral note; separate patient records exist, but documentation can be shared if there is a written authorization by the patient.
Collaborative	Integrative mental health practitioners, who normally practice . independently from each other (e.g., acupuncturists, massage therapists), share information concerning a particular patient who has been (is being) treated by each of them. Sharing among practitioners and the patient/family could come through common treatment plans, consultation documentation, phone calls, person-to-person discussions with and without the patient present; probably each provider continues to keep his/her own patient records.
Coordinated	Formalized administrative structure requires communication and the sharing of patient records among integrative mental health practitioners who are members of a mental health care team intentionally gathered to provide treatment for a particular mental health care problem (e.g., psychiatric crisis), rehabilitation issue (e.g., housing), or to deliver a specific therapy (e.g., medication management). A case coordinator (or case manager) is responsible for ensuring that information is transferred to and from relevant practitioners and the patient; there is generally one common patient record kept by the case coordinator/manager.
Multidisciplinary	Based on a treatment plan, one or two integrative mental health care team members direct the services of a range of ancillary members who may or may not meet face-to-face; each individual team member continues to make his/her own treatment decisions and recommendations, which may then be integrated by the team leader and communicated through face-to-face team meetings or electronically; the mental health care team may not include all mental health care professions; each team member documents in a common patient record.
Interdisciplinary	Integrative mental health practitioners teams make group decisions about patient care (usually based on a consensus model); development of treatment plans for all patients is facilitated by regular, face-to-face team meetings; each integrative mental health team member understands and respects the disciplinary role of the others to implement the treatment plan; team members record progress with the implementation of the treatment plan using a collaborative document.
Unified	Integrative mental health practitioners provide a seamless continuum of decision-making and patient-centered care and support through continual communication, both face-to-face and electronically; mental health care team members employ an interprofessional team approach guided by consensus building, mutual respect, and a shared vision of wellness that permits each practitioner and the patient to contribute his/her particular knowledge and skills within the context of shared decision-making; team documentation is shared in a common patient record and reviewed by individual team members for progress toward meeting patient goals.

team members from different disciplines, including the patient. Future team members could now include qualified practitioners of acupuncture, yoga, and mindfulness; music and art therapists; in addition to psychotherapists and medication prescribers. Each mental health care team member adds his or her individual and discipline-specific philosophical frameworks which guide his/her clinical practice. As mental health practices evolve from parallel to unified, these disciplinary distinctions become less critical as the team of practitioners focuses on holistic, interprofessional approaches to mental health treatment guided by the individual's social and cultural determinants of health.

The structure of team-oriented practice models increases in complexity from parallel to unified because of the increased number and diversity of team members who communicate shared treatment decisions. As unified mental health care teams evolve, the team structure changes from one with a clearly defined hierarchy of roles to less formal structures of service to best fit a shared decision-making philosophy. At this level, many team members provide similar services such as patient education, mindfulness, and acupressure. While this seems simplistic and natural, engaging all team members and the patient in decision-making with equal votes can prove transformational.

The increasing complexity of structure from parallel to unified necessitates communication among team members and the patient that is respectful, direct, and ongoing. It appears that communication among team members is easier and less restricted with electronic health records. However, consensus-building and developing a shared vision for the patient's whole health cannot always be developed and described electronically. Other communication venues need to ensure that the mental health team "talks" to all the members of the team, including the patient.

Patient/person-centered outcomes mandated by the Patient Protection and Affordable Healthcare Act are developed by healthcare teams that might include physicians, integrative practitioners, nurses with different scopes of practice, and the patient. As parallel healthcare teams develop more into unified teams, person-centered outcomes become more holistic, yet complex because of all team members' thoughts about the patient's treatment outcomes, the patient's vision of his/her own health outcomes, and expected outcomes of the disease or illness process. As more unified mental health care teams evolve, common screening tools used by both practitioners and patients are developed with defined outcome measures to monitor patient progress. Because unified teams are more diverse, integrative mental health team members will communicate more efficiently with each other and the patient to ensure that the appropriate health and mental health outcomes are identified and monitored.

Comparison of the Exemplar Models

Each of the integrative mental health care models is an also exemplar of integrated care. All three programs are community-based, focused on the needs of people with mental health concerns. All three programs offer both mental and physical health on-site services with the goal of maximizing the individual's mental health and physical wellness, starting with a comprehensive, holistic assessment, which then becomes the basis of an individualized wellness and treatment plan. Each program has its own integrative mental health team composed of different integrative mental health practitioners who provide both conventional and non-conventional forms of treatment. Person-centered care and individualized treatment or wellness plans are an important aspect of all these programs.

Each of these programs functions at a different level of integrated complexity. The Resilience Training Program team functions at the interdisciplinary level of team development. The Resilience Training Program is smaller, with fewer team members, who each have a specific role and integrative mental health specialty, providing diversity among team members. Team members know each other well, and many have worked together for a long time. The integrative team members make group decisions with the patient about treatment options, meet in face-to-face meetings, and document their work in a common patient record.

The integrative mental health teams at the Wholeness Center and Touchstone's Health and Wellness Center appear to function at the multidisciplinary level of development. Both have many integrative mental health practitioners, some who are more a part of a team than others because of the needs of the client. Teams are developed based on the individual's mental health or physical health care needs. Some of the integrative mental health practitioners retain their own client records onsite, but there is a common treatment plan to which the practitioners contribute. The selection of the integrative mental health team leader is unknown for each of these two programs.

The role of the integrative mental health nurse is clearly identified as an advanced practice nurse at the Wholeness Center and Touchstone's Health and Wellness Center. The psychiatric nurse practitioners complete initial holistic assessments, including diagnostic evaluations, and prescribe medications. It is unknown whether they also conduct psychotherapy or provide additional psychoeducation. The Resilience Training Program nurse coordinates the plans for new participant initial assessments and is a team member but does not provide any specific integrative mental health practices.

The Future of Integrated, Integrative Mental Health Care

It is likely that with changes brought about by the Patient Protection and Affordable Healthcare Act, the inclusion of integrative practitioners as a part of the mental health care team will be an important development in mental health care. As new *integrative* mental health programs develop to provide *integrated* physical and mental health services to improve the health and wellbeing of clients, it will be necessary to develop new and effective team structures and processes to ensure that all team members, including the patient, can communicate with each other via different modalities (e.g., online, hard copy, and face-to-face) for consensual decision-making. Integrative mental health care teams will need to find common documentation systems that can capture the holistic health and mental health needs of the patient. Common interdisciplinary screening tools will need to be used for the assessment of physical and mental health concerns, and decisions will need to be made about the specific team member responsible for following up with assessment findings and monitoring any evidence-based outcomes. Interprofessional education related to disciplinary roles and scope of practices will be important as more integrative practitioners join the team. Cross-discipline practices will need to be defined so that the patient receives seamless care.

It is an exciting time for integrative mental health nursing because our holistic, person-centered, integrated approaches to patient care and our skills as team leaders provide us with the opportunities to lead the development of these new models of integrated, integrative mental health care.

SELECTED REFERENCES

Boon, H., Verhoef, M., O'Hara, D., & Findley, B. (2004). From parallel practice to integrative health care: A conceptual framework. *BioMedH Services Research, 4*(15). doi: 10.11186/1472-6963-4-15. Retrieved from http://www.biomedcentral.com/1472-6963/4/15

Dusek, J. A. (2009). Evaluation of an 8-week resilience training program in moderate to severely depressed patients. *Explore, 5*(3), 160. doi: 10.1016/j.explore.2009.03.046

Emmons, H. (2006). *The Chemistry of Joy: A Three-Step Program for Overcoming Depression Through Western Science and Eastern Wisdom*. New York: Simon & Schuster.

Greenberg, P.E., Kessler, R.C., Birnbaum, H.G., Leong, S.A., Lowe, S.W., Bergland, P.A., Corey-Lisle, P.K. (2003). The economic burden of depression in the United States: How did it change between 1990 and 2000? *Journal of Clinical Psychiatry, 64*(12), 1465–1475.

Kessler, R. C., & Ustun, T. B. (Eds.). (2008). The WHO World Mental Health Surveys. *Global Perspectives on the Epidemiology of Mental Disorders*. Cambridge, UK: Cambridge University Press.

Lake, J., & Spiegel, D. (2006). *Complementary and Alternative Treatments in Mental Health Care*. Arlington, VA: American Psychiatric Publishing.

Lake, J., Helgason, C., & Sarris, J. (2012). Integrative mental health (IMH): Paradigm, research, and clinical practice. *Explore, 8*(1), 50–57.

Mark, T. L., Levit, K. R., Vandivort-Warren, R., Buck, J. A., & Coffey, R. M. (2011). Changes in U.S. spending on mental health and substance abuse treatment, 1986–2005, and implications for policy. *Health Affairs, 30*(2), 284–292. doi: 10.1377/hlthaff.2010.0765

Parks, J., Svendsen, D., Singer, P., & Foti, M. E. (Eds.) (2006). *Morbidity and Mortality in People with Serious Mental Illness*. Alexandria, VA: National Association of State Mental Health Program Directors (NASMHP) Medical Directors Council.

Simon G. E., Cherkin, D. C., Sherman, K. J., Eisenberg, D. M., Deyo, R. A., & Davis, R. B. (2008). Mental health visits to complementary and alternative providers. *General Hospital Psychiatry, 26*(3), 171–177.

Sirois, F. M. (2008). Motivations for consulting complementary and alternative medicine practitioners: A comparison of consumers from 1997–2005. *BMC Complementary and Alternative Medicine, 8*, 16.

Weeks, J. (2012). Health care legislation includes gains and shortfalls for integrative medicine.... plus more. *Integrative Medicine, 9*(2), 18–20.

28

Integrative Nursing of Older Adults Across the Continuum

LINDA L. HALCÓN, CONSTANCE SCHEIN, AND CORJENA CHEUNG

Overview and Background

Although the status of elders in communities varies by group and subculture, for many in the United States this stage of life is not well defined or understood. Indeed, media characters and common stereotypes often seem limited to comic, shallow, or tragic images of old age. Integrative nurses can play an important role in helping older adults experience optimal aging by incorporating into their practice the six Integrative Nursing Principles described in Chapter 1. Emphasizing the breadth of integrative nursing, Pugnaire Gros of McGill University in Montreal described integrative nursing as "the science of health promoting interactions" (Pugnaire, 1981). As defined earlier in this text, *integrative nursing care* is "informed by evidence, uses a full range of therapeutic modalities, and is delivered within a caring-healing relationship by someone who is actively engaged in their own healing journey." Engagement in one's own healing on all levels is particularly salient in the care of the elderly because nurses who have not come to terms with mortality and aging in their own healing journey will find it difficult to be truly present in caring-healing relationships with older adults. Appreciation of the developmental tasks of elderhood is a keystone for nurses' self-knowledge and the care of older adults.

DEFINITION OF OLDER ADULTHOOD

Defining older adulthood may seem as straightforward as choosing a cutoff point on a numerical scale. Such an approach is limited in that it does not individualize elderhood or take into account the external and internal experience of being an older adult. *Older adults* or *seniors* sometimes have been defined as those as young as 50 to 55 years of age. For example, many people clearly remember receiving an invitation to join a national seniors' organization prior to their fiftieth birthday. Often this invitation occasions reflection about what it means to have "senior" status, since many people do not feel "old" at 50, or even at 65. Indeed, average lifespans and working lives are considerably longer than they were for previous generations, and 65 years no longer seems like a generalizable marker of the transition to elderhood. In looking for cutoff points, 70 years may be a more reasonable age to mark the legal transition to senior status. For demographic purposes, advanced elderhood is often said to begin at 85 years. In the spirit of person-centered integrative nursing (Principle 4), it makes sense to encourage elders to self-define their life stage, except where there are legal implications.

DEVELOPMENTAL TASKS OF OLDER ADULTS

Whereas health professionals are often quite familiar with the developmental stages and tasks of childhood, less attention has been paid to the tasks of older adulthood. An understanding of human development in the senior years can help nurses better appreciate the innate body/mind/spirit capacities for health and wellbeing of individuals in this population (Principle 2). These capacities at times may be hard to recognize because the focus on deficits and problems inherent in Western biomedical approaches may inhibit recognition of older adults' strengths.

Although functional differences between early and late elderhood are generally recognized by developmental theorists, the developmental tasks of the two groups of elders often are not differentiated. Because the focus of older elders becomes progressively more internal than external, this lack of differentiation may reflect the relative invisibility of tasks that are more focused on "being" in a "doing" culture like the United States. Erik Erikson characterized the developmental task of all ages of older adults as "integrity vs. despair," defining integrity as acceptance of one's life and death, and despair as failure to find meaning in one's life, often expressed by anger or bitterness (Harder, 2012). Another theorist, Robert Peck, identified three main tasks leading to ego integrity for older adults, but he also did not differentiate between older and younger seniors. The tasks, according to Peck, are to: (1) find satisfaction in who they are as people, separate from family and work roles; (2) adapt to physical aging through body transcendence rather than becoming self-absorbed in one's limitations; and (3) reflect positively on the meaning of one's life and accomplishments while transcending the ego, rather than becoming preoccupied with death (Berk, 2010, Chapter 18). Going deeper into the meaning of older adulthood, Bill Plotkin describes two distinct phases of elderhood and their developmental tasks in *Nature and the Human Soul: Cultivating Wholeness and Community in a Fragmented World* (2008). Early elderhood, according to Plotkin, is embodied by the accomplished adult who moves away from striving to achieve, and toward his/her inner life, even though he or she may remain very active in the world. The focus of early elderhood is mentoring and "caring for the web of life" (p. 391) through deep appreciation of the interdependence of all life forms. The challenge of this age, according to Plotkin, is to focus on "surrender[ing] to the ways in which life...wants to manifest through the individuated self" (p. 391), rather than focusing on the ego's agenda. This early phase of older adulthood is often marked by deep appreciation of the earth and humanity, along with a desire to creatively support community in its many forms. Plotkin characterizes the shadow side of early aging as "pasture and playtime" (p. 408). This shadow stage often results in the despair described by Erikson when physical and mental decline no longer allow participation in recreational activities and travel.

Ideally, according to Plotkin, a younger elder will enter late elderhood with gratitude for the world and her place in it and a psychospiritual shift into surrender and non-attachment. The only real "task" of this age is to make final peace through forgiveness of oneself and others in preparation for leaving one's life. Plotkin's description of the developmental stage of older elderhood corresponds to the psychosocial stage of *gerotranscendence* described by Joan Erikson, widow of Eric Erikson (Berk, 2010). Gerotranscendence can be seen as "a cosmic and transcendent perspective directed forward and outward, beyond the self" (p. 475). Such elders continue to be involved socially in the world and yet spend more time in inner reflection, displaying "heightened inner calm and contentment" (p. 475). Understanding these stages and tasks of older adulthood gives integrative nurses increased ability to identify the subtler capacities and evidence for health and wellbeing that can give new meaning and purpose to the lives of older adults (Principle 2).

Older Adults and Integrative Therapies

Integrative nursing includes not only a mindset and philosophy of care, but knowledge of the evidence for using integrative modalities and the skills to apply that knowledge when appropriate. Nurses may be asked to provide expert advice to patients, families, or other caregivers, or to provide integrative modalities directly if they are qualified. Whether in care settings or in the community, there is increasing recognition of the benefits of including integrative therapies in the range of therapeutic modalities available to support the health and healing of older adults (Principle 5).

Integrative nurses can increase their competency in integrative therapies by reading the current research and knowing what types of integrative therapies are commonly used by older adults so that they can accurately advise and offer information on their benefits and sometimes risks. Due to natural aging processes, older people are especially prone to a broad range of chronic health conditions that can require long-term healthcare management. Pharmacotherapy poses considerable risks and challenges to this population. Age-related changes in drug metabolism arise from decreased renal and hepatic function, higher fat–lean muscle mass ratio, and decreased serum protein levels. As a result, drug-related adverse effects may occur in older adults more frequently and at doses much lower than would be observed in younger individuals (Bruckenthal, Reid, & Reisner, 2009). In addition, drug interactions and treatment non-compliance may make stable blood levels of pharmaceuticals and predictable pharmacokinetics more difficult to attain. Because of these factors, non-pharmacological treatment options such as integrative therapies are especially attractive for older adults. The range of possibilities includes lifestyle/nutrition programs that have normalized blood sugar in those with type 2 diabetes and some forms of heart disease, to using imagery or aromatherapy to assist with anxiety or insomnia.

Indeed, evidence over time suggests that many older adults do use integrative or complementary and alternative therapies (CAT) to address their health needs. Data from the 1999 National Health Interview Survey (NHIS) suggested that more than one in four adults over 55 years had used at least one of twelve complementary or alternative modalities in the previous year, very similar to 25 to 34 year olds and only slightly less frequently than 35 to 54 year olds (Ni, Simile, & Hardy, 2002). The Alternative Health/Complementary and Alternative Medicine supplement to the 2002 National Health Interview Survey reinforced these and other large cross-sectional study results suggesting that a significant portion (35%–37 %) of older adults used CAT (Eisenberg et al., 1998; Tindle, Davis, Phillips, & Eisenberg, 2005). More recently, results of the 2007 NHIS indicated that complementary and alternative medicine (CAM) usage remained high within all subgroups of older adults: 41% of 60–69 year olds, 32% of those 70–84, and 24% of those 85 and over (Barnes, Bloom, & Nahin, 2008). Of the five major categories of CAM, older adults were most likely to use biologically based therapies, mind–body therapies, and manipulative and body-based therapies, in that order. Similarly, Cheung, Wyman, and Halcón (2007) found that the top five CAM modalities used by community-dwelling older adults were nutritional supplements, spiritual healing or prayer, megavitamins, herbal supplements, and chiropractic care.

The National Center for Complementary and Alternative Medicine (NCCAM) and the National Institute of Health (NIH) Senior Health provide evidence-based resources on integrative therapies for older adults for healthcare providers and consumers. The Natural Standard and Cochrane Reviews also provide information about a range of therapies with a conservative view of the evidence. In addition to the information provided on NIH websites (Table 28.1), integrative nurses can obtain journal articles on a broader range of therapies and evidence through online databases such as PubMed, Medline, Cinahl, and The Allied and Complementary Medicine Database (AMED).

According to a survey conducted by the American Association of Retired Persons (AARP) and National Center for Complementary and Alternative Medicine (NCCAM) (2007), among people aged 50 or older, 69% of those who use integrative therapies do not talk to their physicians about it. They may be afraid that their physicians will disapprove or react negatively. This lack of communication between older patients and their medical care providers is a concern because of the increased risk of drug–herb and drug–supplement interactions in this population. We hope that future research will capitalize on these synergies and antagonisms, investigating the potential for reducing the use of pharmaceuticals by combining or replacing

Table 28.1: NIH Examples of Integrative Therapies for Common Conditions in Older Adults

Condition	Integrative Therapies	Health Outcomes
Cardiovascular Disease	Garlic Ginkgo Biloba Meditation Tai Chi	Prevent blood clots Lower risk of developing peripheral artery disease Lower pulse and blood pressure Lower blood pressure
Cancer	Acupuncture Chinese Herbal Medicine Hypnosis Massage Yoga	Reduce chemo-induced nausea and vomiting Increase survival rate in colorectal cancer Reduce hot flashes Reduce pain and improve mood Improve fatigue
Osteoarthritis	Acupuncture Glucosamine Chondroitin Massage Tai Chi Yoga	Relieve moderate to severe pain Reduce pain and improve function Reduce low back pain Control pain Reduce low back pain

Source: NCCAM, 2012; NIH Senior Health, 2012.

them with safer botanical medicines. Nurses should elicit and document information on integrative therapies used and appropriately advise older adult patients, both to ensure safe care and to advance knowledge about potentially harmful interactions. After reviewing the scientific evidence, a nurse can advocate for patients who express a desire to continue supplements or herbs during medical treatments, brokering arrangements that are acceptable to all parties. Consideration should be given to both evidence-based practice and practice-based evidence in assessing appropriate modalities.

The following case example illustrates how an integrative nurse might review the evidence and guide an older patient with osteoarthritis. DG is a 72-year-old widow who has been living with arthritis for over 25 years. Arthritis is among the most prevalent chronic health conditions and the leading cause of disability in older adults. DG does not like the side effects of medications; therefore, she lives with pain and stiffness in her joints every day. She takes glucosamine chondroitin supplements to help manage her arthritis symptoms and is interested in trying other natural remedies.

Prevalence studies show that arthritis is one of the most common health conditions for which older adults utilize integrative therapies (Carrington et al., 2008; Cheung, Wyman, & Halcón, 2007). Caspi, Koithan, and Criddle (2004) attribute such high use to the disease's prevalence, its poorly understood etiology, the lack of definitive cures, a variable disease course, the severity of pain and discomfort, and the disease's adverse impact on functional status. Acupuncture, herbal remedies, and supplements including chondroitin, glucosamine, and S-adenosyl-methionine (SAMe) have been found effective in relieving the pain of osteoarthritis (Soeken, 2004). Sale, Gignac, and Hawker (2006) also found that, despite reports of pain, only 21% of older adults with osteoarthritis take their prescribed pain medications, and 95% reported using at least one herbal remedy for their arthritis.

Applying Principle 5 (*Integrative nursing practice is informed by evidence and uses the full range of therapeutic modalities to support/augment the healing process, moving from least intensive/invasive to more, depending on need and context*) to the case of DG, an integrative nurse might initiate dialogue with her about her condition and her openness to other integrative therapies, listening deeply for meaning and also providing up-to-date information on safety and efficacy. In this discussion, an herbal product or acupuncture might be discussed if she wishes to expand her therapy repertoire, taking into account the evidence summarized above. Less invasive approaches to pain relief, such as imagery, acupressure, aromatherapy, and energy healing, also could be explored.

Senior Living and Care Options

Older adults are inseparable from their environments (Principle 1), and because many older adults are no longer members of the formal workforce, their living situation is a major environmental factor that can enhance or impede movement toward health. Every older adult's environment and perception of his or her environment is unique; however, senior living choices are influenced by societal trends. Over the past century, senior living and senior care models have shifted from home to institution and back to home. A hundred years ago, older people lived and died at home or in the homes of family members. As more seniors began to live longer, and with the advent of Medicare and Medicaid, greater numbers of older adults entered hospitals for lengthy stays when they became too ill to care for themselves. In response to the rising cost of hospital care, nursing homes were popularized as less acute environments than hospitals, projected to lessen the financial burden on families and the healthcare system overall. As increasing numbers of older adults with chronic diseases began to live longer, however, the cost and volume of nursing home care also became a concern. Assisted-living models emerged as another, less costly option to meet the needs of older adults who do not need skilled nursing services but want or need more support than often would be present in an independent-living setting. Now other new options for "aging in place" are emerging to help older adults stay in their homes and communities as long as possible. Aging in place is a concept that involves adaptations to support independent living by bringing needed services to the home and mobilizing community support. This model often results in cost savings because the residence itself is not part of the care package. In addition, improved quality of life may be associated with staying in an accustomed and

The Eden Alternative

The Eden Alternative was one of the first major initiatives for aging in place. Founded over twenty years ago to counter loneliness, helplessness, and boredom among older adults, Eden Alternative is an international nonprofit organization that promotes a philosophy and principles to effect culture change in all senior living environments. A network of thousands of associates, mentors, educators, and registered aged homes currently endorses the philosophy, and the organization addresses all settings where elders live, including home and community. The Eden Alternative Principles are consistent with integrative nursing, as illustrated by their Principle 2: "An Elder-centered community commits to creating a human habitat where life revolves around close and continuing contact with plants, animals, and children," and Principle 7: "Medical treatment should be the servant of genuine human caring, never its master" (Eden Alternative, 2013).

maximally independent environment. Although care settings have gone full circle from home to home, it is critical to recognize that "home" is not the same as it used to be. For the most part, the family is no longer there. Some families have been able and willing to accommodate their elders, but most rely on more formal healthcare and social services options.

Public discourse is needed to find a new balance of personal, family, and public responsibility for elders, and there is a great need for creativity to ensure the conditions for optimal wellbeing of older adults who need temporary or long-term assistance. "One size fits all" will not work for seniors or families, or for our society as a whole. Kreitzer's WellBeing Model (2011; Figure 28.1) provides a framework for designing and evaluating senior living options for optimal wellbeing. This model includes six dimensions of wellbeing: health, relationships, security, purpose, community, and environment. An individualized wellbeing approach that addresses each of these dimensions supports older adults in attaining their maximal connectedness and contentment at this stage of life, regardless of the setting.

Building design can be used to manifest creative thinking aimed at enhancing wellbeing in all its dimensions, not only *environment* and *security*. In some European and Asian countries, senior living facilities may include smaller personal spaces dispersed around larger public spaces (Lee & Loomis, 2007). This type of living encourages socialization and mutual assistance (relationships, community, and purpose). Older American adults often desire large private spaces, however, reflective of the American dream of the large single-family home. Alternative approaches to space allocation may need considerable marketing in the United States, but they may also reduce isolation and enhance social wellbeing. At the farther end of the care continuum,

Wellbeing

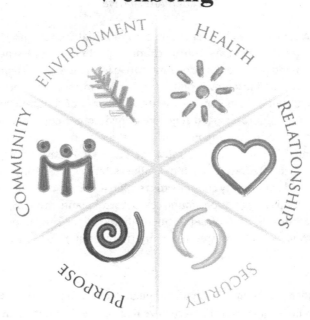

Mary Jo Kreitzer, RN, PhD, FAAN
Director, Center for Spirituality & Healing

UNIVERSITY OF MINNESOTA
Center for Spirituality & Healing

FIGURE 28.1 Kreitzer's WellBeing Model

a Dutch nursing home for dementia patients was designed like a small village, with streets, shops, restaurants, a movie theater, a hairdresser, and staff members dressed as shopkeepers. The aim of this facility is to feel like normal community living, rather than an institution, to reduce the stress of residents (Moise, 2012).

Some senior living complexes, especially faith-based facilities, are designed to provide spiritually rich environments consistent with residents' faiths and cultures. In a broad sense, this may include philosophies that recognize the strengths that elders bring to the world and their need for continued learning and purpose no matter what their physical or mental condition. Some of these designs may challenge the current cultural myths of aging and dementia care. For example, the vision of AgeSong in the San Francisco Bay area is to "create a more accepting, loving and caring human being based on the idea of developing the virtues of the elder within all of us" (AgeSong, 2013).

Exposure to the natural world is important in order to enhance seniors' living environments. Integrative nursing recognizes the healing and restorative power of nature for body, mind, and spirit (Principle 3). Nature-based therapies are included in

The Goodman Group

The mission of The Goodman Group, based in Minnesota, is to "create and manage living environments that emphasize quality of life and enable residents and staff to achieve an optimum level of wellbeing" (www.thegoodmangroup.com, accessed November 5, 2012). This company has incorporated a focus on mind, body, and spirit in its senior living facilities for over ten years. Their interest encompasses exploring new and meaningful building designs that foster wellness and community and incorporate nature, as well as experimentation with integrative health and healing modalities. On-site intergenerational learning centers bring together seniors and preschool children. Key initiatives aim to enhance the environment, engage residents and staff, empower the spirit, extend function, and energize the psyche. The Goodman Group evaluates the impact of their wellbeing model on health, satisfaction, and longevity using metrics that include: balance/core strength, mobility/gait, pain, quality of life, spiritual wellbeing, connectedness, mental health, anxiety, and cognition (Katie Westberg, CTRS, CDP, National Director of Life Enrichment, The Goodman Group).

many senior living settings, and older adults living in the community typically arrange their own nature therapy by having a pet or walking in the park. In care settings, nature-based therapies include building designs to maximize sunlight and views of nature, indoor plants and birds, and opportunities for gardening and being with animals. Integrative nurses recognize the importance of exposure to nature in all of its forms, and they can be instrumental in arranging or providing opportunities to be in and part of the natural world.

Although some innovations in elder care involve housing or institutional design, others offer services that encourage healthier lifestyles and thus reduce the risk of disability and chronic diseases. The range of lifestyle amenities varies, but may include beautiful natural settings, proximity to arts and cultural centers, libraries, fitness centers, schools or daycare facilities, banks, restaurants, religious facilities, and barber/beauty shops. Lifestyle enhancements, such as personal training or onsite fitness centers, are becoming more prevalent in senior residences and care settings. Also, plant-based whole foods menus are more common with increased recognition that food really is medicine. The irrefutable evidence on the health effects of lifestyle factors has the potential to revolutionize the standard of care for older adults, and integrative nurses play an important role. There are many examples of very comfortable and thoughtfully designed, full-spectrum senior living complexes (Appendix A). Ownership models range from private for profit to not for profit, and some include a portion of subsidized units that are more affordable.

Nursing Roles, Leadership, and Practice Model

It is inevitable that nurses will provide care to older adults who are either using integrative therapies or are open to trying different integrative therapies for managing their health conditions. Knowledge about older adults' use of integrative therapies is especially helpful for nurses who are front-line healthcare providers. Most healthcare professionals, however, underestimate their patients' use of integrative therapies and are not prepared to discuss it (Brems et al., 2006). Integrative nurses must be the exception.

Nursing is poised to lead a broader discussion of health and healthcare with and for the aging population. Integrative nursing principles provide the foundation and contribute to viewing older adults' health in terms of relationships, wellbeing, and transitions. A nurse's ability to understand what is both supportive of health and desired by the elder and how these two can fit together is essential (Principle 4). Professional relationships are shaped by the interactions and the degree of engagement achieved between elders and caregivers.

Schein (Figure 28.2) proposes a practice model that shows how different types of engagement can assist older adults to move through any type of transition to new states of stability and wellbeing. Engagement refers to the nurse's ability to respond to the elder's current situation, including his or her needs, desires, and hopes for health and wellbeing. Situation-responsive nursing (Gottlieb & Rowat, 1987) facilitates the engagement process, which can then lead to learning and stability regardless of the situation. The challenge on an individual basis is to adapt approaches to accommodate seniors' goals and expectations.

As people age, they move through multiple transitions that can influence their overall wellbeing in the areas described by Kreitzer (2012; Figure 28.1). *Health* is a frequent area of need or a transition state for older adults; however, *relationships, security, purpose, community,* and the *environment* can affect their health and are equally important in determining their overall wellbeing. Integrative nursing attends to all of these. Not only are there different types of transitions, but there are different ways of entering into transitions. Transitions may be self-imposed or externally imposed by health or circumstances.

Using Schein's model, potential nursing roles may include creating environments where people desire stability. The role of nursing is not to engineer stability but to engage in personal advocacy to create readiness and a desire for stability. Advocacy involves understanding when a transition has taken place and offering services and supports directly, or passing along information to those who can study the situation more in depth. Integrative nurses may also participate in institutional or community advocacy for older adults with transitional needs. Engagement, in Schein's model, may be self-initiated or imposed. *Voluntary engagement* between a nurse and older adult may occur where there is no known change in health status but there is a general

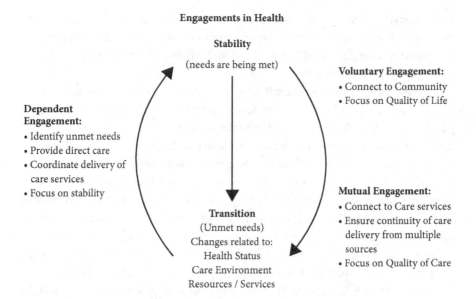

Engagements in Health

Stability

(needs are being met)

Dependent Engagement:
• Identify unmet needs
• Provide direct care
• Coordinate delivery of care services
• Focus on stability

Voluntary Engagement:
• Connect to Community
• Focus on Quality of Life

Transition
(Unmet needs)
Changes related to:
Health Status
Care Environment
Resources / Services

Mutual Engagement:
• Connect to Care services
• Ensure continuity of care delivery from multiple sources
• Focus on Quality of Care

FIGURE 28.2 Schein's Model

motivation to make connections and improve health. For example, a 78-year-old woman who lives alone but has noticed increasing isolation, weight gain, and difficulty with home upkeep might seek advice. In this situation, an integrative nurse might first listen deeply to her concerns and goals, bringing to her attention possible lifestyle modifications (exercise, nutrition), supports (housing changes to minimize upkeep and enhance socialization), and integrative therapies (mindfulness, massage, aromatherapy, nutritional supplements) that could be part of an individualized program to reach her optimal wellbeing. *Mutual engagement*, however, may be initiated as a result of negative changes in health or another wellbeing factor that led an older adult to engage in positive actions to prevent predictable declines in health or other factor. Mutual engagement requires more formal interactions that can facilitate the desired goal of improved health—for example, an elderly man with a newly diagnosed heart condition requiring frequent contact with healthcare providers to minimize or reverse the changes in his health status. An integrative nurse in this situation might provide support to the patient as well as his family. In addition to nutrition and exercise changes, he and his family members may want to include stress-reduction techniques, reflective and nature-based practices, or energy healing, if informed of the potential benefits. Through mutual engagement, he might be motivated to seek a new level of stability with improved health. Finally, there are the transitions that eliminate any opportunity for stability without significant interventions and dependency on systems, relationships, and community. *Dependent engagement* occurs as a means of survival and is often seen as a crisis both by the individual and the caregivers, formal and otherwise, with whom they develop relationships to manage the transition. Rather than focusing on what is known medically to be the expected outcome, nurses can make a greater difference by letting go of their agenda and looking more honestly at the needs and desires of clients (Principle 4).

Looking for readiness to engage in change is a significant part of the healing relationship with seniors. Younger, active seniors who have not experienced significant physical or mental decline may seek information about health from friends, family, and the Internet when less dramatic transitions occur. These elders can greatly benefit from credible and holistic sources of health promotion information coming from a wellbeing perspective. Nurses in all settings can help older adults improve their integrative health literacy, leading to a healthy and reflective population of older adults who achieve the developmental milestones of elderhood and help shape the options available for senior living when they reach the point of needing care. Voluntary engagement can greatly reduce the time of needing care, and expanding life years while reducing care years will reduce costs and increase the quality of life for all seniors.

Older adults are thirsty for health knowledge and want to be as healthy as possible. They, possibly more than younger adults, can see the effects of lifestyle on themselves and others. They may also understand the limits of treatment approaches compared to prevention. As many older adults move through the care continuum, from independent living, to assisted living, to nursing homes, integrative therapies and healing practices can be helpful in reestablishing stability (Figure 28.2) (Kolanowski et al., 2010). For example, adaptive yoga and tai chi may be used in any setting to maintain and improve balance and mobility. Likewise, mindfulness, imagery, massage, energy techniques, aromatherapy, or acupressure can help with insomnia, anxiety, or restlessness. Integrative nurses may provide therapies themselves or refer to or arrange for appropriate services.

Challenges and Opportunities

SYSTEMS CHANGE

Rapid shifts in consumer awareness are driving changes in the healthcare system. Whereas challenges remain for integrative nursing of older adults, increasingly there are opportunities as well. One challenge is that integrative services and non-biomedical approaches and modalities often are not covered by Medicare currently, nor are preventive and health promotion services. The Affordable Care Act with its emphasis on Accountable Care Organizations and health outcomes is likely to encourage new models that emphasize wellness and health promotion. Already there is new national recognition of the need to consider non-invasive and non-pharmacological approaches first when engagement with the healthcare system occurs. For example, the Medicare Minimum Data Set (MDS 3.0) for pain management now requires documentation of non-pharmacological strategies to address pain, and the Center for Medicare and Medicaid Services expects the use of non-pharmacological approaches prior to using antipsychotic or other psychoactive medications for off-label uses such as dementia or Alzheimer's disease (DHHS, 2012). Recognizing the power of relational and nature-based care, the Center for Medicare and Medicaid Services recommends the following behavioral interventions to help prevent use of pharmaceuticals: (a) consistent assignments of staff in care settings, (b) regular one-on-one interactions, (c) getting outside at least once a day, and (d) use of complementary and alternative approaches (American Medical Directors Association, 2012).

PAYMENT AND CARE MODELS

Current care and payment models focus almost exclusively on deficits; however, there is now widespread recognition that the real goal is to keep people as healthy as possible for as long as possible. New payment and reimbursement models that focus on positive health outcomes and include prevention and community-focused integrative nursing should be explored. One example of this is the homecare organization Buurtzorg Nederland in the Netherlands, which has achieved large cost savings and at the same time demonstrated excellent patient health outcomes and satisfaction using a nurse-led model and a very flat organizational structure (Nandram, 2012). This model is exciting because it incorporates a focus on the health and wellbeing of the nurses as well as on those they serve (Integrative Nursing Principle 6). In the United States, more thinking is needed about the family and community component of the new care continuum models. Especially for older seniors (85 and older) and those who are extremely frail, how will communities and families be part of the support system? Smaller, more dispersed housing and care models that maximize self-care and informal supports may allow more seniors to remain in their communities.

Aspirational Vision

Integrative nurses will help shape the future health and healthcare of older adults. One of nursing's professional roles is to be a change agent for health systems, society, and our own profession. In order to shift the culture, integrative nurse leaders need the openness to interpret new findings and carry out disruptive innovations when this is called for. Higher education must give nurses the skills to challenge rules and systems effectively. In practice settings with older adults, we desperately need nurses and leaders willing to risk conflict in order to do what is right and get results.

In the United States, we must change our view of aging as a necessary evil to a time of hope and wellness. The human form is not destined to depart this world in a state of passive acceptance of decline, loss, and hopelessness, but rather with emphasis on capability, wellness, and health. Kreitzer's Wellbeing Model (Figure 28.1) and Schein's Model (Figure 28.2) provide a framework for viewing the lives and health of older adults and providing care. Health is not seen as the absence of illness, but rather a mindset that is focused on creating an optimal approach to realizing the full capacity of health and wellness. The integrative nursing principles provide guidance to nurses as they educate and empower seniors to take charge of their health and demand the system change so that it will truly support healthy aging.

SELECTED REFERENCES

AARP & NCCAM. (2007). Complementary and alternative medicine: What people 50 and older are using and discussing with their physicians. Retrieved from http://assets.aarp.org/rgcenter/health/cam_2007.pdf.

Berk, L. (2010). Emotional and social development in late adulthood. In *Development Through the Lifespan* (5th ed.). Upper Saddle River, NJ: Pearson Higher Education Publishing. Retrieved from http://www.pearsonhighered.com/showcase/berkexploring2e/assets/Berk_ch18.pdf.

Carper, B. (1978). Fundamental patterns of knowing in nursing. *Advances in Nursing Science*, *1*(1), 13–24.

Carrington, R., Papaleontiou, M., Ong, A., Breckman, R., Wetington, E., & Pillemer, K. (2008). Self-management strategies to reduce pain and improve function among older adults in community settings: A review of the evidence. *Pain Medicine*, 9(4), 409–424.

Cheung, C., Wyman, J., & Halcón, L. (2007). Use of complementary and alternative therapies in community-dwelling older adults. *Journal of Alternative & Complementary Medicine*, 13(9), 997–1006. doi:10.1089/acm.2007.0527

Gottlieb, L., & Rowat, K. (1987). The McGill model of nursing: A practice-derived model. *Advances in Nursing Science*, 9(4), 51–61.

Kreitzer, M. J. (2012). Spirituality and Well-Being: Focusing on what matters. *Western Journal of Nursing Research*, 34(6), 707. doi:10.1177/0193945912448315

Nandram, S. (2012) In search for the spiritual innovation at the Dutch elderly home care organization Buurtzorg Nederland. *Amity Case Research Journal*, February, 1–6.

Plotkin, B. (2008). *Nature and the Human Soul: Cultivating Wholeness and Community in a Fragmented World*. Novato, CA: New World Library.

Tindle, H., Davis, R., Phillips, R., & Eisenberg, D. (2005). Trends in use of complementary and alternative medicine by U.S. adults: 1997–2002. *Alternative Therapies*, 11(1), 42–49.

29

Integrative Nursing: Palliative Care and End-of-Life

JULIE KATSERES AND KATHLEEN A. NELSON

The most visible creators are those artists whose medium is life itself.
The ones who express the inexpressible—without brush, hammer, clay, or
* guitar.*
They neither paint nor sculpt.
Their medium is simply being.
Whatever their presence touches has increased life.
They see, but don't have to draw. . .
Because they are the artists of being alive.

—Donna J. Stone
(Reprinted with permission from Stonegate Press)

Death during the 1800s (Civil War) generally occurred at home shortly after the onset of illness, with the emphasis of care on easing symptoms (American Association of Colleges of Nursing (AACN), 2010). The United States comprised mainly self-reliant, agricultural families for whom death from infections and injuries was a constant in daily life; even children were exposed to the normalcy of death at an early age (Keegan & Drick, 2011; Wyatt, 2011). The old and sick were cared for by family members, and death was viewed as a natural part of life (Keegan & Drick, 2011; IOM, 1997). The growth of science and industry in the early twentieth century brought improvements in sanitation, living, and working conditions, resulting in an increase in length of life (AACN, 2010). Additional life-saving and life-prolonging breakthroughs such as antibiotics, pain medications, chemotherapy, and radiation positively influenced length of life, and the focus of health care shifted from easing suffering to curing disease, with death itself being equated to medical failure (Keegan & Drick, 2011; AACN, 2010).

Since the 1950s, care of the dying has transitioned from being provided by loved ones in the home to being delivered by healthcare professionals in institutions, despite 61%–80% of people stating they want to die at home surrounded by family and loved ones (Benson, 1999). Unfortunately, healthcare professionals do not feel equipped to provide this care (Duke & Northam, 2009; Ferrell et al., 2006; Robinson et al., 2004; Rothman et al., 1998). With more than 80% of people dying in hospitals and nursing homes, what was embraced as a natural part of life has shifted to something arouseing fear, and feelings of hopelessness and failure (Treece et al., 2006).

In an attempt to intervene, the first U.S. hospice was established in New Haven, Connecticut, in 1978, based on a British model established in 1967, with Congress passing the Medicare Hospice Benefit in 1982, which created guidelines for enrollment (Horowitz, 2009; Keegan & Drick, 2011). While the palliative care movement began in the late 1980s, a controlled trial funded by Robert Woods Johnson Foundation in 1992 demonstrated continued poor patient–physician communication, aggressive and futile treatments at end of life, and poor symptom management in seriously ill hospitalized patients (Teno et al., 1997). Efforts to improve the knowledge and skill in healthcare students and providers are evident in such programs as the End-of-Life Nursing Education Consortium series, palliative care fellowships, and hospice and palliative care certifications.

The purpose of this chapter is to disarm the fear and awkwardness around death by exploring integrative nursing principles that guide palliative and end-of-life care, review settings where nursing provides care to the dying, and examine integrative modalities helpful in the transition of living to dying, where death is something that happens to us, while dying is something we do (McSherry, 2011).

Principals Guiding Care Practices

Nursing has long embraced a holistic approach to providing care. Since Florence Nightingale's time, nurses have viewed our practice as including mind, body, and spirit; as well as being both a science and an art (Ferrell et al., 2010; Sheldon, 2000). Conversely, our current healthcare system fosters an environment advocating efficiency and multitasking, creating impersonal task-oriented interventions geared toward physical management (doing), with little to no attention paid to psychosocial and spiritual domains (being) (Sheldon, 2000).Unfortunately, it is all too common to hear nurses make comments such as, "I've given him all the medications available; I don't know what more to do for him."

Palliative care involves alleviating the effects of disease without curing. It encompasses a team-oriented approach, attending to aggressive symptom management, and affords emotional and spiritual support personalized to the patient's and family's needs and wishes (National Hospice & Palliative Care Organization (NHPCO), 2011). Therefore, palliative care utilizes a model of quality, compassionate care for people facing life-limiting illness or injury that embraces the whole. As a result, palliative care has true synergy with integrative nursing—nursing care that is system-focused on the whole person/whole systems, grounded in relationships, and delivered by interprofessional teams that include both conventional (allopathic) and integrative care modalities. The principles of integrative nursing are directly applicable to palliative care.

HUMAN BEINGS ARE INSEPARABLE FROM THEIR ENVIRONMENTS

Palliative care is a model that helps to create an environment for peaceful transitions. Standards of Practice for Hospice Programs (NHPCO, 2010) not only design inpatient facilities to provide homelike environments, but incorporate mindbodyspirit interventions to assist patients with meeting preferences in a changing environment or life circumstances. These standards include environmental safety and security as well as provide uninterrupted services despite changes in patient care settings. Keegan and Drick (2011) advocate for a specially designed room referred to as "the Golden Room" for hospitals and care facilities as a way of providing a healing space for patients and families as they shift from aggressive, cure-focused care to assertive symptom management and assistance in dying with dignity.

HUMAN BEINGS HAVE AN INNATE CAPACITY FOR HEALTH AND WELLBEING

Palliative care supports people as they evolve along their life journey. While the focus changes from curing illness to healing of the mindbodyspirit, palliative care helps patients and their caregivers find peace and authenticity through this process and at the end of life. It is not unusual to bear witness to statements such as, "This illness/cancer has been a blessing in disguise in finding true meaning and happiness in my life," and "I never realized what I truly have and am now so grateful."

NATURE HAS HEALING AND RESTORATIVE PROPERTIES THAT CONTRIBUTE TO HEALTH AND WELLBEING

Nature's restorative properties can help promote mindbodyspirit wellbeing in the end-of-life context, not only for patients but for families and caregivers, including professional care teams. Many hospice units utilize a variety of strategies to bring "the outside in." Incorporating natural surroundings in processing life transitions has been shown to be beneficial in finding meaning and value in one's life.

INTEGRATIVE NURSING IS PERSON-CENTERED AND RELATIONSHIP-BASED

Patient and family-centered care is the first criterion of ten guiding hospice standards (NHPCO, 2010). Interdisciplinary teams strive to collaborate and facilitate patient, family, and caregiver directed palliative care on admission and throughout the journey, recognizing shifts in need and process. Hope and dignity are concepts crucial in this journey.

Hope is our primary conscious and unconscious motivator; it is ever present—its form is what changes (Fanslow-Brunjes, 2008). Families as well as healthcare providers express fear and worry about "taking away hope" when charged with delivering bad news. However, conveying this information has not been shown to negatively impact hope (Gum & Snyder, 2002). Fanslow-Brunjes (2008) describes hope as a life force, the essence of self, which propels one forward, while Duggleby and Wright (2001) depict hope as an inner resource that one draws upon to endure suffering. Hope is fluid, and emotional states change as circumstances shift and unfold (Kersten et al., 2012; Fanslow-Brunjes, 2008; Gum & Snyder, 2002).

Fanslow-Brunjes (2008) describes four stages of hope: hope for cure, hope for treatment, hope for prolongation of life, and hope for a peaceful death; while others refer to the process of redefining goals in the setting of changing circumstances, thus keeping hope alive (Kersten et al., 2012; Gum & Snyder, 2002). Uncontrolled pain; worries about abandonment, isolation, becoming a burden on family members, and loss of dignity were found to negatively impact hope (Herth 1990). Nurses' perspectives on their role they play in preserving patients' hope centered on understanding the individual's hope, focusing on the patients' quality of life, and building trust with patients (Reinke et al., 2010).

Dignity is frequently mentioned in nursing literature, described as a human attribute or right in life as a quality of being worthy, honored, or esteemed (Milton, 2008). Haddock (1996) characterizes dignity as the shared humanity of patient and nurse, while recognizing the uniqueness of the individuals. In a cross-sectional cohort study of patients who were terminally ill with cancer and receiving care from a palliative care program, an increased risk of dignity impairment was correlated with increased perceived change in appearance, increased sense of being a burden to others, increased dependency on others, increased pain intensity, and being an inpatient (Chochinov et al., 2002). Thus, achieving good pain and symptom control, feeling supported, and having one's personal needs attended to minimizes the potential that one's dignity will be undermined (Chochinov, 2012). The Nursing Outcomes Classification (NOC) recognizes dignified life-closure as an outcome, defined as "personal actions to maintain control during approaching end of life" (Moorhead, 2004).

INTEGRATIVE NURSING PRACTICE IS INFORMED BY EVIDENCE AND USES THERAPEUTIC MODALITIES

A full range of therapeutic modalities is used within palliative care to support and augment the healing process, moving from least intensive/invasive to more, depending on the need and context. Specific modalities utilized in palliative care and at the end of life are addressed later in this chapter.

INTEGRATIVE NURSING ALSO FOCUSES ON HEALTH AND WELLBEING OF CAREGIVERS

According to Ferrell et al. (2010), nurses attending End of life nursing education consortium (ELNEC) training reconnect with why they became nurses and are reminded of the sacred work of palliative nursing the importance of illness as a human experience, and explore skills that foster the nurse–patient relationship. Self-care is a lifelong journey and involves more than diet and exercise. It also attends to caring relationships, peer support, healing environments, and self-reflection (McElligott, 2013). Use of self-reflection is an essential practice in providing palliative care, as the art of palliative care is getting comfortable with the discomfort of "gray" in a black-and-white milieu. "Holding space" for people to process information, internal, external, and existential, is hard work.

Settings

Rothman et al. (1998) illustrate medical students' perceptions of a "good death" as one that is anticipated and dignified, in which all involved acknowledge its imminence, and that may occur in a home or healthcare facility; whereas a bad death was deemed impersonal and violent, as witnessed in an emergency room setting.

THE INTENSIVE CARE UNIT AND THE EMERGENCY ROOM

The initial attempt to avoid putting a patient through a "bad death" is sometimes made on the patient's arrival in the emergency room. The conversation between the physician and the patient/family to acquire a patient's code status may be one of the most inconsistent, uncomfortable, and misunderstood processes for all parties involved (Downar & Hawryluck, 2010). The graphic description of the mechanics behind resuscitation seems to be directly proportional to the prognosis of the individual. The physician's intent may be to spare the patient from a less-than-optimal outcome, but does a patient hear much past, "If your heart stops or you stop breathing…?"

A proposed change in terminology is one way to reframe the issue of code status to a more patient-centered approach. Using the acronym "AND" for "Allow Natural Death" instead of "Do Not Resuscitate" is a gentler style that may be more reflective of the patient's wishes than a statement that implies many things will not be done (Meyer, 2012).

Education continues to be an effective change-agent. Physicians receiving additional training in conversations related to end-of-life communication successfully facilitated ethical and informative goals of care discussions (Dickens, 2009; Downer & Hawryluck 2010). The use of a critical care nurse liaison trained in palliative and end-of-life issues yielded reports of improved communication, and increased sensitivity to cultural and religious issues (Robley & Denton, 2006).

INPATIENT AND HOME HOSPICE CARE

The National Consensus Project (2009) endorses the need for specialized training for nurses providing palliative and hospice care. A 2002 study evaluating the effectiveness of hospice nurses in both the home and hospital setting found a positive impact from indicators in the areas of symptom control, family readiness, and comfort, despite lengths of stay averaging less than two weeks (Brokel & Hoffman, 2005).

PRISONS

Approximately 10% of the 1.6 million incarcerated individuals are serving life sentences in U.S. prisons (Belluck, 2012). Managing end-of-life care has become a necessity for our prison system. Similar issues of symptom control, maintaining dignity, and fear of dying alone, concern prison hospice programs (National Prison Hospice Association (NPHA), 2011). Inmates serving as volunteers bring a unique perspective to hospice care, which focuses on the impact of the "family member/caregiver" role. "Family" is redefined for many prisoners to be "other inmates" (NPHA, 2011). These individuals must be considered when developing a bereavement program. Many inmate hospice volunteers have professed both spiritual and emotional growth attained through experiencing a desire to care for another human life, sometimes for the first time (Tillman, 2000).

Modalities

Suffering is universal, necessary, and unavoidable. It is woven throughout nature and human existence. We experience "little deaths" of loss and grief every day. In our own life journey, we endure pain and suffering in our process of attaining growth and new skills.

Martins and Basto's (2011) study on nursing interventions to relieve suffering found the process of alleviating suffering at the end of life evolves between the nurse and the patient in two stages: "perceiving the patient's suffering" and "alleviating suffering," which are intercepted with "suffering with the patient." In suffering with the patient, the nurse identifies with his/her own mortality and becomes more capable of dealing with suffering and death.

Emotional interventions include listening intently, talking to support the patient, touching the patient, fostering the nurse–patient relationship by creating a bond of confidence, giving love and compassion, and focusing on the patient's experiences, thereby extending empathy. Spiritual interventions encourage the search for meaning; being present; facilitating a connection with nature, family, and friends; supporting the patient's beliefs and religious practices such as prayer; and providing therapies such as music, therapeutic touch, meditation, imagery, humor, and laughing.

Physical interventions provide comfort through maintaining hygiene, repositioning and massage to relieve pressure zones, and managing pain and symptoms (Martins & Basto, 2011).

Surveys of hospice's use of integrative therapies found 70%–86% of the participating hospice agencies had integrative therapies available for their patients (Horowitz, 2009; Running et al., 2008). Massage therapy (60%–87%), music therapy (48%–74%), energy healing (50%–65%), and guided imagery (45%–48%) were the most frequently used modalities offered; with aromatherapy (45%), acupuncture (11%–32%), pet therapy (32%), meditation (29%), art therapy (19%–22%), reflexology (15%–19%) and hypnotherapy (15%–16%) following (Horowitz, 2009; Running et al., 2008). The Hospice and Palliative Nurses Association has deemed that nurses play an important role in incorporating integrative therapies into practice (HPNA, 2003).

LIFE REVIEW

Life review, a form of reminiscent therapy, seeks to address the struggle of finding meaning in one's life for the person facing death. Using a structured format of questions, the patient shares and reflects upon events of importance, people of influence, and attributes for which s/he would like to be remembered. Sharing one's story diminishes psychological distress and provides peace of mind (Ando et al., 2010). Allen et al. (2008) developed a "legacy intervention" incorporating family members' responses relating to how the patient brought meaning to their lives, and memories that would be preserved long after the patient's parting. The exchange between patient and family in the creation of this legacy notebook proved to diminish the patient's depression, increased meaning-based coping, and strengthened overall wellbeing.

FORGIVENESS

Forgiveness is an active release of pain and expectation that is causing suffering (Grieco, 2008). It requires shifting one's energy from hatred, blame, and being right, toward healing, peace, and resolution, and may involve forgiveness of others, God/ Spiritual Source, or oneself (Grieco, 2008; Wyatt, 2011). Forgiveness is not done for someone else, but for oneself, as a personal, private act; an unseen decision of the human heart. It doesn't necessarily mean to forget, condone, or absolve; but rather is a process of extending love and compassion that often leads to transformation in taking responsibility for one's actions, tolerance toward others, reconciliation, and redemption (Burkhardt & Nagai-Jacobson, 2009; Wyatt, 2011).

There are many forgiveness processes published; most have common themes of beginning with the will or desire to forgive, followed by an internal exercise of letting go of the hurt, anger, and resentments. The process culminates with opening the heart to love and compassion in order to heal and become whole (Burkhardt & Nagai-Jacobson, 2009; Grieco, 2008; Wyatt, 2011).

MUSIC

Music has been shown to reduce physical symptoms such as pain and anxiety, increase tolerance for treatment, and ease emotional and spiritual distress, while improving quality of life and the relationship between patients and caregivers (Black & Penrose-Thompson, 2012; Horne-Thompson & Grocke, 2008; Schmid & Ostermann, 2010). Music can be active (person participates in creating music) or passive (listening to music played by someone else), with the personal preferences of the patient taken into consideration. While trained music therapists have the in-depth understanding and training to use music as a tool to attend to a variety of conditions, nurses may also utilize this modality as a means of comfort and care.

"Music thanatology" is a special type of music offered via live harp and vocals at the deathbed. The goal is to accompany the dying person through the transition from life to death using a prescriptive set of music addressing the complex physical and spiritual needs of the dying (Black & Penrose-Thompson, 2012). Limited research has been conducted in this relatively new field; however, the current literature indicates music vigils decrease agitation and wakefulness while evoking hope, calmness, and relaxation (Black & Penrose-Thompson, 2012).

LIGHT TOUCH/MASSAGE

Touching signifies caring and love. The use of bilateral hand massage for people at end of life can be comforting while noninvasive. It relies on caring touch that can be administered by professional and nonprofessional personnel, including family, and requires minimal effort from the recipient. There are at least two hand-massage protocols in the literature that were developed by nurses and are easily taught to staff to establish competency (Buckle, 2011; Kolcaba et al., 2004).

AROMATHERAPY

The use of aromatics has a long history of being associated with the spiritual transition into the next life, funeral preparations, and assisting in the bereavement process. When appropriately used, aromatherapy can facilitate significant healing on physical, emotional, and spiritual levels (Buckle, 2003; Whyte et al., 2007). Essential oils can be utilized in the management of many symptoms such as pain, nausea/vomiting, anorexia, fatigue, grief, anxiety, depression, anger, insomnia, and spiritual distress (Battaglia, 2003; Price & Price, 2007). The selection of oil(s) should be made by patient preference, with the nurse offering two to three choices aimed toward a specific goal/symptom. It may be beneficial to rotate oils or blend oils to minimize developing a negative response to a particular scent and symptom. Following are a few examples of essential oils helpful for specific indications. These may be inhaled directly or indirectly via a diffuser, or be combined with a carrier oil or lotion and lightly massaged to a targeted area.

Anger—*Rosa damascena* (rose otto)

Anxiety—*Cananga odorata* (ylang ylang), *Citrus aurantium* var. *amara* (neroli), *Citrus bergamia* (bergamot), *Jasminum grandiflorum* (jasmine), *Ocimum basilicum* (sweet basil), *Pelargonium graveolens* (geranium)

Depression—*Anthemis nobilis* (Roman chamomile), *Cananga odorata* (ylang ylang), *Citrus bergamia* (bergamot), *Jasminum grandiflorum* (jasmine)

Sadness/sorrow/grief—*Jasminum grandiflorum* (jasmine), *Rosa damascena* (rose otto)

Spiritual distress—*Citrus bergamia* (bergamot), *Lavandula angustifolia* (true lavender), *Ocimum basilicum* (sweet basil), and *Origanum majorana* (sweet marjoram)

RITUALS

In many institutions, additional tributes may be implemented, such as covering the deceased with a special quilt while transferring the body to the morgue, placing a memento or symbol outside the patient's room indicating that the patient has died. This evokes a moment of recognition not only by other staff, but by the family and other patients. Regular debriefing sessions within a nursing unit or interdisciplinary team may also allow time for reflection and healing. Post-mortem care is the last thing you will do for your patient before s/he leaves your care. Do it with pride, care, and respect.

Summary

Palliative care is *not* withdrawing care, but rather shifting the focus of care from curing disease and illness to a journey of living with disease/illness, focusing on the quality of life, while at the same time finding value and meaning in the transitions toward dying with dignity. The skill set required in providing palliative nursing care is congruent with integrative nursing. The principles that guide integrative nursing are woven throughout palliative care and are reflected in the mindbodyspirit approach. Continued efforts at facilitating the naturalness of death as a part of life provide opportunities for patients, families, and healthcare professionals to minimize fear, foster growth and healing, and bear witness to the sacredness of dying.

SELECTED REFERENCES

American Association of Colleges of Nursing (2010). End of life nursing education consortium (ELNEC). Available from www.aacn.nche.edu/elnec. Accessed February 22, 2012.

Chochinov, H. (2012). *Dignity Therapy: Final Words for Final Days.* New York: Oxford University Press.

Downar, J., & Hawryluck, L. (2010). What should we say when discussing "code status" and life support with a patient? A Delphi analysis. *Journal of Palliative Medicine, 13*(2), 185–195.

Ferrell, B., Virani, R., Jacobs, H. Malloy, P., & Kelly, K. (2010). Arts and humanities in palliative nursing education. *Journal of Pain & Symptom Management, 39*(5), 941–945.

Keegan, L., & Drick, C. (2011). *End of Life: Nursing Solutions for Death with Dignity.* New York: Springer Publishing Company.

Kersten, C., Cameron, M., & Oldenburg, J. (2012). Truth in hope and hope in truth. *Journal of Palliative Medicine, 15*(1), 128–129.

McSherry, C. (2011). The inner life at the end of life. *Journal of Hospice & Palliative Nursing, 13*(2), 112–120.

Meyer, C. (2012). Allow Natural Death—an alternative to DNR? Available from http://www. hospicepatients.org/and.html. Accessed April 3, 2012.

National Hospice & Palliative Care Organization (2010). NHPCO Standards of Practice. Available from http://www.nhpco.org/nhpco-standards-practice. Accessed March 30, 2013.

National Hospice & Palliative Care Organization, NHPCO. (2011). What is hospice and palliative care? Available from http://www.nhpco.org/i4a/pages/index.cfm?pageid=4648. Accessed April 14, 2012.

30

Integrative Nursing and the Environment

SUSAN LUCK

No amount of medical knowledge will lessen the accountability for nurses to do what nurses do; that is, manage the environment to promote positive life processes.

—Florence Nightingale, 1859, Notes on Nursing

At the heart and spirit of Florence Nightingale's legacy is the knowledge that our external environment is inextricably interconnected to the health and wellbeing of all species and ecosystems, a concept that is reflected in the first principle of integrative nursing—human beings are inseparable from their environments.

In this time of increasing concerns about the impact of the environment on the health of individuals and communities, identifying and reducing health risks associated with environmental exposures and potential hazards in the workplace, community, and home is becoming part of our nursing practice. In continuing Nightingale's voice as an environmentalist, nurses are organizing and leading initiatives in healthcare and are increasingly becoming environmental advocates for their patients, families, and communities. By assessing the environments in which people live, work, and play, nurses are integrating environmental awareness, education, and strategies and thus improving health outcomes, from local to global levels. Nurses with environmental health knowledge are closing the information gap by educating consumers, colleagues, hospital administrators, school personnel, parents, and communities.

The International Council of Nurses (ICN) in a position statement titled *Reducing Environmental and Lifestyle Related Health Risks* (2012) expresses concern regarding the enormous human suffering caused by the growing burden of environmental and lifestyle-related, preventable, noncommunicable diseases. They ask that nurses and national nurses associations play a strategic role in helping reduce environmental and lifestyle health risks related to noncommunicable diseases. ICN (2012) views nursing as a steward of the environment; human health is dependent on the health of our lands, oceans, and air, elements of a person's environment.

The American Nurses Association (ANA) in their landmark document *ANA's Principles of Environmental Health for Nursing Practice with Implementation Strategies* (2007) put forth a call to action, encouraging nurses to gain a working understanding of the relationships between human health and environmental exposures and to integrate this knowledge into their practice. These principles are applicable in all settings where registered nurses practice, and are intended to protect nurses themselves, patients and their families, other healthcare workers, and the community and to recognize our role as environmental health leaders. As part of this integrative nursing worldview, the ANA has provided a foundation for the development of principles of environmental health for nursing practice that includes the belief that human health is linked to the quality of the environment, and that air, water, soil, food, and products should be free of potentially harmful chemicals. The ANA document states that a healthy environment is a universal need and fundamental human right, and that environmental and social justice is a right of all populations; disparities in health are not acceptable.

Dossey (2010) describes Nightingale as one of the early proponents of the precautionary principle; she understood that nurses have an ethical and moral responsibility to take anticipatory actions to prevent harm. The precautionary principle avers that precautionary measure should be taken when activities cause a threat to human or environmental health, even when the effects of those actions are not fully undestood (Raffensperger, 1998). The precautionary principle supports taking action in the face of uncertainty, shifting burdens of proof to those who create risks, analyzing alternatives to potentially harmful products and practices, and utilizing participatory decision-making methods. It also advocates taking the life cycle of chemicals, products, or technologies into account and adding a proactive phase of requiring pre-market analysis for potential environmental harm.

A 2013 Institute of Medicine (IOM) report describes a patient's "environment" as comprising three sectors—home, community, and workplace—wherein chemical and physical hazards may be encountered via various media such as contaminated soil, water, and air. For nurses working in all healthcare sectors, a review of the patient's home, community, and work life must be included in an integrative and comprehensive health assessment to gain a more complete picture that can identify potential risk factors. For example, the report includes "fish consumption" under the heading of "home" environment and "source of drinking water" under "community." Specifics of work duties and agents handled, including cleaning products and solvents, as well as personal-care products and a review of ingredients, allow a nurse to tailor guidelines and recommendations. For women of childbearing age, this assessment can optimize their health and that of their future pregnancies, as research is increasingly focused on preconception environmental exposures. Routine intake questions about hobbies, habits, and home and work environments might identify exposures associated with adverse reproductive consequences that can be minimized during the pre-conception period. Elements of the environmental history elicited during the pre-conception visit may identify key determinants of a future healthy pregnancy. The workplace is usually the principal source of exposure to toxins with unambiguous reproductive and developmental effects. These toxins are often found in industry sectors, including healthcare, in which many women work. Numerous studies have shown that nurses are particularly vulnerable to workplace exposures.

Nurses and other healthcare providers have wide-ranging roles in addressing environmental factors in policy, public health, and clinical practice. Public health initiatives include risk recognition, assessment, exposure reduction, remediation, monitoring, and avoidance. The complex web of disease and environmental contributors is amenable to some straightforward clinical approaches, along with health advocacy and educating healthcare providers and communities to assess, identify, and address multiple toxins in the home, workplace, and community. Addressing environmental contributors to chronic disease has broad implications for society, with large potential benefits including improved health and productivity.

Living in the Modern World

Today, roughly a quarter of all human disease and death in the world can be attributed to what the World Health Organization (WHO) in its *World Cancer Report* (2003) broadly defines as "environmental factors"; the organization predicts that cancer will increase by 50% by 2020 if measures are not put into place. Environmental health factors play a significantly larger role in developing countries, where contaminated water and sanitation, along with indoor and outdoor air pollution, make major contributions to mortality.

In the past few decades, production of synthetic chemicals has increased a thousand-fold in the United States alone, with estimates of more than 80,000 "largely unregulated" chemicals on the market today. Each year, an estimated 2,000 new chemicals are introduced for use in such everyday items as foods and personal-care products, according to the National Toxicology Program, Department of Health and Human Services (2012). Bioaccumulation of these compounds is fueling metabolic and systemic dysfunction, often working synergistically to create new chemical compounds. Research studies on systems most affected by these compounds include the immune, neurological, and endocrine systems. This toxic "body burden" can trigger autoimmune disease, asthma, allergies, cognitive deficits, mood changes, reproductive problems, glucose dysregulation, and obesity. Biological responses to multiple stressors can exacerbate potential epigenetic changes that can lead to obesity, metabolic syndrome, cardiovascular disease, type 2 diabetes, and Alzheimer's and Parkinson's, all diseases that may be associated with contributory environmental factors, including air pollution, heavy metals, and various endocrine-disrupting chemical exposures (Luck, 2012).

The links between exposure to everyday chemicals and cancer risk has been "grossly underestimated," according to the National Cancer Institute (NCI) *Report on Reducing Cancer Risk* (2009), which urges the Obama Administration to identify and eliminate environmental carcinogens from workplaces, schools, and homes. In 2012, Health and Human Services Secretary Kathleen Sebelius, along with other federal agencies, released the "Environmental Justice Strategy and Implementation Plan," outlining steps that will be taken to protect communities facing greater health and environmental risks. This report, in collaboration with the National Breast Cancer Fund (2013), concludes that preventing exposure to environmental risk factors is the most promising path to decreasing the incidence of breast cancer and is the "key to reducing the burden" on individuals, families, and society. Exposure to a multitude of pesticides in our air, water, and food is a growing concern globally. Pesticides pervade the environment and are making children sicker than they were a generation ago, according to the research released by the Pesticide Action Network (October, 2012). More than 1 billion pounds of pesticides are used annually nationwide and have contributed to an array of health problems in youths, including autism, cancer, birth defects, early puberty, obesity, diabetes. and asthma. The authors' conclusions were based on dozens of recent scientific studies that have tied chemicals to children's health, and their report sought to bring collective meaning to those findings. "Children are just much more vulnerable to pesticide exposure," noted co-author Kristin Schafer, senior policy strategist at the Pesticide Action Network. This research raises the question of whether many of the health problems seen in children could be prevented with new environmental regulations. The May 2011 issue of the *Journal of Health Affairs* describes the staggering economic impact of toxic chemicals and pollutants in the environment. One of the reports cites $76.6 billion annually in the United States alone as the cost of pediatric healthcare for children with reduced cognitive abilities due to preventable childhood lead exposure and environmentally caused attention-deficit hyperactivity disorders resulting from toxic chemicals. Childhood asthma, exacerbated by particulate-matter air pollutants, childhood obesity and its comorbidities due to endocrine-disrupting chemicals found in certain foods and products, and health consequences of mercury from contaminants in fish, were all implicated in the research (Trasande & Liu, 2011).

Dr. Phillip Landrigan, a pediatrician and epidemiologist at Mount Sinai School of Medicine in New York and director of the Children's Environmental Center, has extensively advocated new federal regulations for pesticides entering our food supply (Landrigan, 2011), and he cites peer-reviewed studies on children exposed to organophosphates in the womb showing lower-than-average intelligence and impaired cognitive function. A review of the research indicates that the risk of lymphoma and leukemia increased significantly in children when their mother had been exposed to pesticides during the prenatal period (Vinson, 2011). The importance of sowing the seeds of health early in life prompted Leiss and Kotch (2010) to issue a "wake-up call" about the importance of environmental health for mothers and children, advocating that it is time to tackle intensive and extensive exposures that impair development in a multitude of ways. They call for improved environmental regulation and control, better public education to combat avoidable exposures that are routinely occurring as a result of ignorance, more research, environmental justice, and coverage of environmental health in the training of healthcare professionals. As a result of known adverse reproductive and developmental effects linked to environmental exposures, in addition to the current routine queries about a patient's alcohol and smoking history, key environmental determinants of a future pregnancy outcome should also be elicited during the preconception visit. These determinants include: mercury intake via fish consumption; nitrate exposure from well-water sources; and exposure to chemical, physical, or biological hazards in the workplace and home. Eliciting a detailed environmental history permits tailored recommendations to optimize a woman's health and that of her future pregnancy (Table 30.1).

Table 30.1: Integrative Health and Wellness Assessment Tool (Copyright symbol needed) International Nurse Coach Association, 2012

Environmental Assessment	Always	Almost Always	Once in a While	Almost Never	Never
1. I have a healthy, non-toxic home environment.	☐	☐	☐	☐	☐
2. I have a healthy, non-toxic work environment.	☐	☐	☐	☐	☐
3. I am aware of how my external environment affects my health and wellbeing.	☐	☐	☐	☐	☐
4. I share environmental awareness with others in my workplace and community.	☐	☐	☐	☐	☐
5. I try to make healthy environmental choices when I can.	☐	☐	☐	☐	☐
6. I notice allergies or other symptoms when I am in my home.	☐	☐	☐	☐	☐
7. I notice allergies or other symptoms when I am in my workplace.	☐	☐	☐	☐	☐
8. I check my home for mold.	☐	☐	☐	☐	☐
9. I change my air filters (air conditioning) regularly.	☐	☐	☐	☐	☐

(continued)

Table 30.1: (Continued)

Environmental Assessment	Always	Almost Always	Once in a While	Almost Never	Never
10. I use gas heat in my home with good ventilation	☐	☐	☐	☐	☐
11. I keep my car in a garage under my bedroom.	☐	☐	☐	☐	☐
12. I use a water filter in my home.	☐	☐	☐	☐	☐
13. I check my basement for radon.	☐	☐	☐	☐	☐
14. I have hobbies that involve using chemicals (painting, stained glass, woodwork, etc.)	☐	☐	☐	☐	☐
15. I spray pesticides in my home, garden, or lawn.	☐	☐	☐	☐	☐
16. I use a flea collar or other topical chemical treatments on my pets.	☐	☐	☐	☐	☐
17. I am exposed to secondhand smoke.	☐	☐	☐	☐	☐
18. I am aware that what I apply to my skin is absorbed into my body.	☐	☐	☐	☐	☐
19. I wear commercial perfume.	☐	☐	☐	☐	☐
20. I read labels and check ingredients for parabens, pthalates, etc., and try to choose non-toxic personal care products (shampoo, skin lotion, makeup, hair spray, etc.).	☐	☐	☐	☐	☐
21. I avoid food colorings, flavoring, and additives in my foods.	☐	☐	☐	☐	☐
22. I use commercial household cleaners, disinfectants (chlorines), and solvents (degreasers) in my home or workplace.	☐	☐	☐	☐	☐
23. I dry-clean clothes and remove the plastic before I hang them in my closet	☐	☐	☐	☐	☐
24. I use air fresheners or burn incense or scented candles in my home or office.	☐	☐	☐	☐	☐
25. I use a microwave oven to prepare food.	☐	☐	☐	☐	☐
26. I microwave my food in paper or glass and avoid plastic.	☐	☐	☐	☐	☐
27. I use a cell phone and hold it away from my ear.	☐	☐	☐	☐	☐
28. After purchasing new products (shower curtain, carpeting, mattress, furniture, car, etc.), I ventilate the area or leave the product outside until the "off gas" smell disappears.	☐	☐	☐	☐	☐

©2011. International Nurse Coach Certificate Program (INCCP) (www.intergrativenursecoach.com). Adapted from Barbara Dossey & Lynn Keegan. (2008), Self-care assessment tool. In Dossey and Keegan. *Holistic Nursing: A Handbook for Practice*; Sudbury, MA: Jones & Bartlett Publishers.
The format is designed for the survey software of Healthcare Environment (www.hcenvironment.com).

Endocrine Disruptors

Hormone- and endocrine-disrupting chemicals (EDCs) are substances that interfere with the release, transport, metabolism, binding, action, or elimination of the body's natural hormones. According to the National Institute of Environmental Health Sciences (NIEHS), part of the National Institutes of Health, this category of chemicals known to interact with our hormones is of growing concern across the health spectrum. EDCs appear to interfere with the body's endocrine system and produce adverse developmental, reproductive, neurological, and immune effects in both humans and wildlife. A wide range of substances, both natural and manmade, are thought to cause endocrine disruption, including pharmaceuticals, dioxin and dioxin-like compounds, polychlorinated biphenyls, DDT and many other pesticides, and plasticizers such as bisphenol A. EDCs may be found in many everyday products, including plastic bottles, metal food cans, detergents, flame retardants, food, toys, and personal-care products such as cosmetics. The NIEHS supports studies to determine whether exposure to EDCs may result in human health effects, including lowered fertility and an increased incidence of endometriosis and some cancers. Endocrine disruptors appear to pose the greatest risk during prenatal and early postnatal development when organ and neural systems are forming. Environmental chemicals that show estrogenic effects have been well studied. Although environmental exposures affect us throughout our lives, there are certain times in our lives, known as "critical windows," when some exposures or issues are of greater concern. Just as toxins in the environment may last a long time and may interact synergistically, toxins in our bodies can accumulate and become a lifetime part of our "body burden."

Epidemiological evidence increasingly suggests that environmental exposures early in development play a role in our susceptibility to disease in later life. While the environmental links to breast cancer are still being researched, recent studies strongly suggest that exposure during fetal life to the xenoestrogenic, hormone-disrupting compound bisphenol A (BPA) may be implicated in breast cancer decades later (Ayyanan et al., 2011; Sengupta et al., 2013; Yang et al., 2013). BPA is used in the manufacturing of various plastics and resins for food packaging and consumer products and mainly enters the human body as a result of leaching from the packaging into food and drink. In 2013, nearly 100 researchers studying the health effects of BPA gathered at NIEHS to provide an update on their findings. They presented research that BPA exposure during fetal mammary gland development, even at low doses, has resulted in significant alterations in the gland's morphology that varied from subtle ones observed during the exposure period to precancerous and cancerous lesions manifesting in adulthood. "Exposure *in utero* is extremely important because that's the time organs are being formed," observed Dr. Ana Soto, a professor at Tufts University School of Medicine in Boston and one of a team of scientists who worked on the new research. "The risk of breast cancer starts in the womb," and it thus could be a critical factor in understanding why so many women without known risks are developing breast cancer. In an important new study that builds on previous research findings (Muna, Nahar, Chunyang, Kurunthachalam, & Dolinoy, 2013), BPA was evaluated in first- and second-trimester human fetal liver samples to evaluate gene expression specific for BPA metabolism. This research provides new evidence that, when there is considerable exposure to BPA during human pregnancy, the capacity for BPA metabolism and biotransformation is altered in various enzymatic pathways in the human fetal liver. This research continues to examine potential health risks of *in utero* BPA exposure on future breast cancer risk.

While the chemical industry continues to argue that BPA is not harmful to humans, on February 12th, 2013, the congressionally mandated Interagency Breast Cancer and Environmental Research Coordinating Committee (IBCERCC) report made seven clear recommendations to enhance research on breast cancer prevention by building the evidence base for environmental exposures that can trigger the onset of disease. The report includes the largest-to-date analysis of peer-reviewed science on breast cancer and the environment, including many animal and human studies that provide plausible evidence that chemical exposures increase breast cancer risk. Many gaps in research and policies were identified, and the agency researchers are calling for a national, comprehensive, cross-governmental breast cancer prevention strategy.

BPA is now also considered an environmental "obesogen" as research reveals that compounds in the environment appear to increase an individual's risk of obesity. The obesogen hypothesis "proposes that perturbations in metabolic signaling, resulting from exposure to dietary and environmental chemicals, may further exacerbate the effects of imbalances in diet and exercise, resulting in an increased susceptibility to obesity and obesity-related disorders" (Grun & Blumberg, 2009). Experimental data in animals show that brief exposure early in development to chemicals with estrogenic activity can increase weight gain later on. At two months of age, mice treated at birth with the estrogenic drug diethylstilbestrol (DES) weigh the same as untreated mice. However, by the time they were six months old, the treated mice had considerably greater fat mass than the untreated controls.

Scientists have long been concerned about chemicals in the environment that mimic estrogens found in the body. Researchers have found links between these "xenoestrogens" and such problems as decreased sperm viability, ovarian dysfunction, neurodevelopmental deficits, and obesity. But experimental limitations have prevented them from exploring one of the most serious questions posed by exposure to xenoestrogens: what happens when—as in the real world—an individual is exposed to multiple estrogen-mimicking chemicals at the same time, including pesticides, plastics, and personal-care products? Researchers at the University of Texas have used new techniques to study exposure to low doses of multiple xenoestrogens. Cheryl Watson, senior author of a paper on the study in the journal *Environmental Health* (2013), reported, "These compounds work at very low concentrations—at the parts per trillion or parts per quadrillion levels—and when you mix them together they affect estrogenic signaling differently and more dramatically than they do individually. We need to pay attention to this, because estrogens influence so many things in both males and females—reproduction, the immune system, metabolism, bone growth." Studies have detected measurable levels of bisphenol A and bisphenol S. According to Watson, 90% of Americans are exposed to dozens of xenoestrogens more or less continually.

Nursing Legacy: Nursing Advocacy

As nurses, and as front-line healthcare providers, we have a unique role as advocates within our communities and our healthcare facilities, creating positive environmental change from the inside and changing healthcare policies and practices. The following are organizational mandates that can inspire us to move our nursing legacy forward.

NURSING LEGACY: NURSING ADVOCACY

In December 2008, 50 nursing leaders were selected to represent the nursing profession at a four-day invitational meeting to develop a strategic plan for environmental health nursing. They represented nursing sub-specialty organizations ranging from nurse midwives, school nurses, and nurse practitioners, to critical care, neonatal, and public health nurses, and state nursing associations. A national organization, the Alliance of Nurses for Healthy Environments, was formed, along with an organizational structure to engage national efforts in education, practice, research, policy, and advocacy. The "Global Green and Healthy Hospitals Agenda" is an effort to build on the good work happening around the world and engender an approach to sustainability and health that can be replicated by thousands of hospitals and health systems in a variety of countries and health settings. Together with global partners, "Health Care Without Harm" has brought nursing leadership to the healthcare sector through its mission to promote the health of all people and implement ecologically sound and healthy alternatives to workplace healthcare practices that pollute the environment and contribute to disease. For example, the incineration of medical waste is a leading source of dangerous air pollutants such as dioxin and mercury, and the use of hazardous chemicals indoors may contribute to the high rates of asthma among healthcare workers. In January of 2013 in Geneva, Switzerland, world governments finalized a global, legally binding treaty on mercury, the bio-accumulative heavy metal that is poisoning the world's fish supply, threatening public health and the environment. Among other measures, the treaty text mandates an end to the manufacture, import, and export of mercury thermometers and sphygmomanometers by 2020. This is a major victory for those working to "green" the health sector around the world.

As part of its efforts to create healthier work environments for nurses, the American Nurses Association (ANA) (2012) encourages hospitals to be more environmentally conscious in their day-to-day operations via the "Healthier Hospitals Initiative," a three-year plan to improve the health and safety of patients, hospital employees, and communities (http://www.nursingworld.org/MainMenuCategories/WorkplaceSafety/ Healthy-Nurse/ANAsPrinciplesofEnvironmentalHealthforNursingPractice.pd). Nurses across Canada have been active in "greening" the Canadian health system through initiatives that support energy conservation, waste reduction, and the use of environmentally preferable products. Beyond their contributions to greening their workplaces, Canadian nurses are also engaged through their professional associations in developing health policy that supports sustainable development within the health system, as part of "green teams" focusing on promoting energy efficiency, product longevity, non-toxicity, and creating healing environments.

The Agency for Toxic Substances and Disease Registry (ATSDR) (2010) began its "Environmental Health Nursing Initiative," a collaborative effort to increase and sustain environmental health knowledge and skills in nurses and other health professionals. The goal of the initiative is to make environmental health an integral component of nursing practice, education, and research, knowledge, skills, and awareness among nurses who serve individuals and communities. The mandate states that nurses are important to environmental health because they play key roles in protecting the health of all people; are in direct contact with patients, families, and communities from many cultural and socioeconomic backgrounds; and have the credibility and access that enable them to provide scientifically sound information about environmental issues and toxic exposures.

Summary

Florence Nightingale and subsequent nurse scholars have written about the impact of the environment on human health and the nurse's role in optimizing environments for healing. Since Nightingale's time, numerous scholars have documented that environmental conditions play a major role in the health of individuals and populations. As nurses become more informed about the environment as a determinant of human health, they will be able to advocate more effectively and continue to uphold Nightingale's legacy and impact the health and wellbeing of all, local to global.

SELECTED REFERENCES

Agency for Toxic Substances and Disease Registry (ATSDR). (2012). Environmental Nursing Initiative. Available at: http://www.atsdr.cdc.gov/EHN/.

American Nurses Association (ANA). (2007). Principles of Environmental Health for Nursing Practice with Implementation Strategies.

Andra, S. S., & Makris, K. C. (2012). Thyroid disrupting chemicals in plastic additives and thyroid health. *Environmental Science Health Center Environmental Carcinogen Ecotoxicology Review*, *30*(2), 107–51.

Healthcare Without Harm. A comprehensive environmental health agenda for hospitals and health systems around the world. Available at: www.noharm.org http://www.hcwh.org www.greenhospitals.net.

Healthier Hospitals Initiatives, Clean Med, and Healthcare Without Harm. Available at: http://healthierhospitals.org and at http://www.cleanmed.org/.

Institute of Medicine (IOM). (2013). Environmental decisions in the face of uncertainty. Consensus Report, February 8, 2013. Board of Population Health and Public Health Practice. Available at: http://www.instituteofmedicine.org/.

Luck, S. (2012). Environmental health. In Dossey, B. M., & Keegan, L. (Eds.), *Holistic Nursing: A Handbook for Practice* (6th ed.; pp. 633–677). Burlington, MA: Jones & Bartlett.

Nahar, M., Sathyanarayana, S., Focareta, J., Dailey, T., & Buchanan, S. (2012). Environmental exposures: How to counsel preconception and prenatal patients in the clinical setting. *American Journal of Obstetrics & Gynecology*, *207*(6), 463–70.

National Cancer Institute. (2009). Reducing environmental cancer risk: What we can do now. Available at: http://www.cancer.gov/cancertopics/understandingcancer/environment/

Pesticide Action Network. (2012). Annual report: A Generation in Jeopardy: How Pesticides Are Undermining Our Children's Health and Intelligence. Available at: http://www.panna.org/publication/generation-in-jeopardy.

V

Integrative Nursing: Models of Education

31

Pre-Licensure Nursing Education for Integrative Nursing

TEDDIE POTTER, LINDA L. HALCÓN, AND MARY M. ROWAN

A Brief Historical Context

The concepts of integrative nursing are not new in pre-licensure nursing education. Many nurse educators and theorists assert that nursing by definition is "integrative and holistic" because patients are viewed as whole "bodymindspirit" beings belonging to multiple systems, including nature, that affect healing and health. With increasing emphasis on high-technology care and empirical evidence in the later part of the twentieth century, this holistic aspect of nursing was largely ignored by the biomedical healthcare system; however, it was not forgotten by nursing educators. Pre-licensure nursing education continued to emphasize interventions such as presence, therapeutic listening, stress relief, touch, spiritual care, and attention to patients' culture as critical elements of nursing care. Undergraduate nursing students were and are still encouraged to attend to their own journey of wellbeing in order to fully develop as nurses. These strategies were not called "holistic" or "integrative," but they often were considered parts of independent nursing care (Snyder & Lindquist, 2001; Chlan & Halcón, 2003).

Although many aspects of integrative nursing are not new, public interest in complementary and alternative therapies (CAT) has led to renewed affirmation and clarification of integrative nursing within pre-licensure nursing education. Nurse educators recognize that many of these interventions could aid nurses in actualizing concepts of integrative nursing and therefore have begun to consider which CAT skills and knowledge should be included in pre-licensure nursing education and which are more appropriately left to continuing education or advanced training.

In addition, nurse historians examined past nursing interventions, suggesting that the use of some traditional herbal remedies be reinstated in nursing practice (Libster, 2012). The importance of including cultural considerations was also stressed (Leonard, 2001). CAT modalities, as independent nursing interventions, were debated, with many state boards of nursing regulating their use (Sparber, 2001).

Currently, emphasis is placed on providing students a conceptual foundation of broad knowledge with some emphasis on CAT skill development. There is room for interpretation in the standards and guidelines, however, and each school has a unique internal environment; therefore, pre-licensure nursing programs vary in naming and adopting integrative nursing concepts and CAT applications.

ESSENTIAL INGREDIENTS OF A PARADIGM SHIFT

Undergraduate education is slowly shifting to greater recognition and acceptance of integrative nursing and therapies that are less invasive (e.g., acupressure, aromatherapy, touch, movement therapies) than some of the common biomedical interventions. Key institutional elements that facilitate this shift include: a culture of faculty innovation; a core group of committed faculty; strategic alliances within and outside of the institution; CAT research expertise; support from administration and alumni; and student interest. Although it is not necessary that all be present in order to more explicitly incorporate an integrative approach to nursing in pre-licensure nursing education, each of the elements, described below, can play an important role.

A *culture of faculty-driven innovation* sets the stage for change. This can take the form of faculty publications on new conceptual models or theories that support integrative health and healing. Faculty-authored texts or chapters on integrative health and healing topics can help establish an institutional reputation for innovation. Similarly, an institutional history that includes other, non-related types of innovations can also be drawn upon to establish historical precedent for cutting-edge changes in general.

A *core group of interested and committed faculty* is necessary. Without such a group, sustained attention to integrative health and healing within the governance and curricular development structure is not possible. It may be helpful to form a time-limited task force to examine opportunities and barriers to change with this group placed within an official school committee for legitimacy, consultation, and accountability. Additionally, faculty development opportunities should be provided for faculty members so that they may gain experience, knowledge, and perhaps an increased emphasis on self-care (Booth-LaForce et al., 2010; Halcón et al., 2001).

Strategic alliances within and outside of the institution can be critical in supporting proposed curricular changes. There is an interprofessional interest in growing public awareness of integrative care approaches. Therefore, institutional support may be found in other health professions where similar curricular changes are underway. Informal support for increased emphasis on broad conceptualizations of health and the importance of stress and environmental factors may be found at any level of administration or in areas such as ecology, nutrition, and student health and recreation services. External alliances can also facilitate change, including other schools of nursing and nursing professional organizations (e.g., American Holistic Nurses Association) or in research associations (e.g., the International Society for CAM Research).

With the focus on evidence-based practice in nursing education, *faculty research* and dissemination of the results in publications and at conferences can be critical. Not all faculty interested in integrative nursing have the resources for conducting research. However, many interested and knowledgeable faculty members can support curricular changes by critiquing the evidence and writing review articles for contributing publications that can be assigned as course readings. *Support from the administration* can be a catalyst for curricular change. Administrators can remove barriers and provide resources. *Alumni* can likewise have an influence on administration by providing a supportive voice for innovative changes. They can let administrators know that they are proud to be alumni of a cutting-edge school working to make nursing education more integrative and holistic.

Although students do not determine curricula, *student interest* can slow or speed paradigmatic changes in pre-licensure nursing. Student surveys can be used to determine attitudes and skills in integrative nursing. Surveys can provide data to both measure the effectiveness of curricular changes and provide direction for future educational programming. If findings suggest that students are looking for deeper learning in integrative nursing, this can support continued changes.

The American Association of Colleges of Nursing Essentials

More than 25 years ago, the American Association of Colleges of Nursing (AACN) directed a national panel of nurse leaders to define the knowledge, clinical skills, values, and other essential abilities for graduates of baccalaureate nursing programs in the United States. While there were prior attempts to develop competency guidelines for professional nursing education, the document published in 1987 by the AACN was the first national effort to "define the essential knowledge, practice, and values" of professional nursing (p. 54). Periodically AACN continues to update these essential abilities for graduates of baccalaureate nursing education programs, disseminating the reports to nursing schools and policymakers across the United States. The guidelines are revised in order to stay current with changing conditions in nursing and healthcare and best-practice evidence.

In the United States, language describing health and healing beyond biomedicine has shifted from *alternative*, to *complementary and alternative*, to *integrative health and healing practices*. AACN documents reveal a parallel history of the evolution of integrative healthcare in the United States, particularly as it pertains to nursing education. Despite the absence of specific terminology related to complementary and alternative therapies or integrative health and healing, elements congruent with integrative health and healing were found throughout the original published AACN (1987) document. For example, there were several references to the importance of culture as part of the nursing knowledge necessary to determine health needs, such as "cultural and spiritual beliefs and practices related to health, illness, birth and death and dying" (p. 59). Furthermore, the 1987 AACN *Essentials* stated that nursing knowledge should encompass "health practices and cultures, belief systems, and the environment" (p. 60).

The 1998 AACN *Essentials of Baccalaureate Education for Professional Nursing Practice* reflected the changing beliefs and values of the public, as well as nurse educators and leaders from across the country. Complementary and alternative modalities were expressly described as "essential nursing core knowledge." For example, the provider-of-care role required evaluation and assessment of the "usefulness in integrating traditional and complementary healthcare practices" (AACN, 1998, p. 16).

In the most recent revision of *The Essentials of Baccalaureate Education for Professional Nursing Practice* (AACN, 2008), sample content for curricula is provided for each of the core elements. Although the various elements are generally described in conceptual terms such as, "[d]eliver compassionate, patient-centered, evidence-based care that respects patient and family preferences" (p. 31), sample content does include complementary and alternative therapies (AACN 2008).

While the American Association of Colleges of Nursing represents baccalaureate and higher-degree nursing education, the National League for Nursing (NLN) represents vocational/technical and associate degree nursing programs in addition to baccalaureate nursing education. The NLN outcomes and competencies for graduates of nursing programs include similar recommendations related to preparing graduates for holistic, culturally competent, and patient-centered nursing care (National League for Nursing, 2011). Around the United States, nurse educators use the AACN and NLN competencies to guide curriculum development. The following is a case study illustrating the journey one school of nursing took to intentionally thread integrative healing content through the curriculum.

Case Study: University of Minnesota School of Nursing BSN Curriculum

The University of Minnesota (UMN) was an early leader in integrative nursing. Two nursing faculty members edited a widely used integrative nursing textbook, first published in 1985 and now in its sixth edition (Snyder, 1985; Snyder & Lindquist, 2011). Several faculty members served as chapter authors, and some had established programs of CAT research; thus a *core group of interested faculty* was easy to identify. In the late 1990s, a group of ten nursing faculty members in *strategic alliance* with the Center for Spirituality and Healing, an interdisciplinary center in the Academic Health Center, stepped up efforts to infuse integrative nursing throughout the curriculum. The goals of faculty were to increase student awareness of holistic nursing and complementary and alternative therapies (CAT), expose students to examples of relevant healing practices, apply the use of healing practices to cases, consider how regulatory policies guide the use of integrative therapies, and incorporate appropriate approaches and concepts into professional practice and self-care.

In 2000, an R-25 interdisciplinary grant from the National Center for Complementary and Alternative Medicine (NCCAM) was awarded to the Center for Spirituality and Healing to incorporate CAT into the curricula of the College of Pharmacy and Schools of Medicine and Nursing at the UMN, strengthening curricular change activities. Surveys were conducted of faculty, graduate students, and undergraduate students in nursing, medicine, and pharmacy (Kreitzer et al., 2002; Halcón et al., 2003). The nursing faculty data were used to design faculty development activities and to support faculty in adding more content to their courses. Dependence on a few faculty champions for content expertise was one of the early and ongoing weaknesses of this effort. Data from senior BSN students helped both in assessing the curriculum and in determining where additional content might be most useful. Findings indicated that general curricular content was congruent with integrative health and healing principles, such as moving from least to more intensive treatments, but there was very little specific content about modalities. For the most part, students reported that they did not have sufficient knowledge to personally provide integrative therapies in their practice. Later studies in other undergraduate nursing programs (Keimig & Braun, 2004) yielded similar findings.

The UMN survey results stimulated faculty discussion of whether the curricular goal was clinical competence to perform specific modalities, versus being competent to advise clients on issues related to CAT. Along with the student survey, curricular mapping and faculty interviews were conducted to identify integrative course content and teaching materials. In a few instances, duplicative content was identified and corrected through this process. Although there were isolated student objections to integrative nursing content, faculty continued to explore the scholarly literature and include more content about integrative nursing and CAT in their courses.

This curricular effort was strengthened by the availability of free evidence-based online modules designed for health professionals. These modules provided an excellent introduction to integrative therapies and made it easy to incorporate content into existing courses (see Center for Spirituality and Healing Online Modules: Integrative Healing Practices http://www.csh.umn.edu/modules/index.html). For example, an existing online module on botanical medicines was added to the pharmacology class, and the modules on culture and faith traditions and traditional Chinese medicine were assigned in a transcultural nursing and global health course.

Clinical courses began including readings of CAT literature; for example, specific therapies that might be helpful in gerontological nursing.

Comprehensive data collection, gap analysis, and strategic planning resulted in integrative nursing content's being threaded throughout the undergraduate nursing curriculum at the UMN. An introduction to integrative therapies is now a required component of the foundational course for first-year students. In addition to material explicitly designed for healthcare providers, students engage in online learning designed for use by consumers or potential consumers of healing practices. Many such resources are now available online (for example, see http://www.healthandhealingny.org/highlights.asp). In order to strengthen experiential learning, integrative therapy skills such as aromatherapy, massage, energy healing, and music therapy were added to the skills lab, garnering positive student feedback (Chlan et al., 2005). In 2012, all BSN students attended a day-long series of presentations and experiential sessions on CAT modalities within an integrative nursing framework.

Courses in the BSN curriculum include material on integrative approaches specific to particular patient populations. For example, the maternal–child course incorporates healing practices when teaching about pain (e.g., modifying pain sensations with massage), environmental modification (aromatherapy or music therapy), and culturally appropriate foods believed to promote healing In a similar fashion, a course focused on the acute care of adults and older adults includes an experiential workshop day during which students explore healing practices such as Reiki, mindfulness-based stress reduction (MBSR), botanical therapy, and hand massage. In an upper-division professional practice course, students explore the state policies related to nursing licensure and the use of integrative therapies.

Research funding and publications were important in establishing integrative nursing expertise at the UMN. In recent decades, faculty members have published articles on topics such as imagery in pediatrics (O'Connor-Von, 2000), aromatherapy in wound care (Halcón, Swiontkowski, Tsukayama, Thiel, & Lillehei, 2010), music therapy for ventilator-dependent patients (Chlan, Engeland, Anthony, & Guttormson, 2007), journaling (Snyder, 2009), Reiki in premature infants, American Indian health paradigms (Struthers, Eschiti, & Patchell, 2004; Struthers & Eschiti, 2005), and mindfulness meditation in transplant patients (Kreitzer, Gross, Ye, Russas, & Treesak, 2005).

Finally, the presence of a core faculty group with expertise in integrative health and healing as well as a nursing specialty (pediatrics, gerontology, or public health nursing) was one of the strengths of this approach. Broad involvement of diverse faculty facilitated the threading of integrative nursing content throughout the curriculum and prevented integrative nursing from being a silo in the curriculum.

Transforming Nursing Education and Practice

Our history is only an introduction to the conversation. Currently, there is a call from various sectors to rethink nursing education (Benner et al., 2010). The time is right for the integrative philosophy to become the unifying framework for nursing scholarship and practice.

The Institute of Medicine report *The Future of Nursing: Leading Change, Advancing Health* (2010) urges nurses to be full partners with other healthcare professionals in the redesign of healthcare in the United States. The report acknowledges nurses' unique ability to coordinate effective sustainable plans of care for clients. As the skills and knowledge of nurses gain recognition, nursing's inherently integrative approach should also be illuminated.

In *Educating Nurses: A Call for Radical Transformation,* Benner, Sutphen, Leonard, and Day (2010) concluded that nursing education in the United States lacks depth and breadth, especially related to situational knowledge. They wrote, "Educators in nursing need to improve the teaching of nursing science, natural and social sciences, leadership, and humanities" (p. 13). These two ground-breaking reports support the need for an alternative nursing education paradigm to guide nursing education and practice.

Yet, before attempting to create an alternative, it is important to understand the current situation. In Potter's (2010) examination of eight of the most popular nursing fundamental textbooks, we find a starting point. Five of the eight current fundamental textbooks included a sentence or two about holism or holistic nursing, but they did not describe integrative nursing. The textbooks also failed to use holism or integrative principles as a framework for nursing education. If complementary or integrative therapies were mentioned at all, they appeared in a special box or were added on at the end of a chapter. None of the texts proposed integrative nursing as a philosophical template for professional nursing.

Marginalization of the integrative nursing philosophy is most evident in the history of nursing content in the fundamental textbooks. Potter (2010) found the history of nursing content in the fundamental textbooks made scant mention of autonomous nursing roles. Most of the exemplars were representatives of the acute-care model or military nursing, and few examples of nursing's long history of community care were noted.

Potter (2010) also analyzed the autobiographies written by historic nurse exemplars. Common themes from these autobiographies included the interconnection of humans and nature, the importance of a global perspective, the use of multiple ways of knowing, the value of astute observation, and the necessity for medicine to be individualized. These historically unique characteristics of nursing epistemology align with many core elements of integrative nursing, including the role of environments, the healing power of nature, relationship-based individualized care, and the application of a full range of therapeutic modalities.

Nursing education research (Benner et al., 2010) and multidisciplinary research on the future of the nursing profession (Institute of Medicine, 2010) are calling nursing to step up to its full potential. Nursing history offers many autonomous and relationship-based nursing exemplars. It is time to bring the wisdom of the past into the future through implementation of an integrative nursing philosophy.

SHIFTING THE PARADIGM

Thomas Kuhn's groundbreaking work *The Structure of Scientific Revolutions* (1970) offers important guidance as we think about shifting the paradigm for nursing education. Kuhn posits that the evidence on which our actions are based does not accumulate at a predictable and organized fashion. Instead, knowledge creation is episodic, with significant evolution of ideas occurring when the old models fail to adequately address anomalies.

We are at this point in healthcare today. Our current system fails to address complexity and unexpected whole-system anomalies. The historical principles of integrative nursing may provide the paradigm to address these emerging anomalies and offer an alternative healthcare system.

Nurse educators and leaders can tip the balance towards a new paradigm by taking several intentional actions. Shifts that need to take place include changing the way integrative healing is taught in nursing curricula, challenging reductionist thinking that separates the whole into parts, shifting more of the responsibility for health and healing from the provider to the client, and shifting the way we think about nature.

Yet, nursing undergraduate education remains strongly linked to the current healthcare system with its requisite skills and knowledge, despite having the revised AACN 2008 *Essentials*. Nursing programs do a delicate dance, balancing content required for practice with the knowledge, skills, attitudes, and experiences that are required for systems change and adoption of a new order.

Nursing leaders need to shift the thinking of the profession so that integrative principles are considered core. The key way to accomplish this shift is through research and publications that provide evidence of the efficacy of an integrative approach to patient care. This textbook furthers the transition to a new paradigm by offering guidance for curriculum development. The following content areas are specific places where a curricular shift needs to occur.

Currently, social conditions, nature, and health are often thought of as independent from one another. This fragmented view fails to acknowledge complex relationships and hinders innovative thinking. Nursing students need to be taught how to "connect the dots" using the depth and breadth of global human knowledge to solve pressing health challenges. A transdisciplinary approach to nursing education will facilitate this competency in nursing students. "Transdisciplinarity compliments disciplinary approaches. It occasions the emergence of new data and new interactions from out of the encounter between disciplines" (De Freitas, Morin, & Nicolescu, 1994). Nurses need to know that knowledge from other fields of study can significantly expand their grasp of the relationship between social conditions, nature, and health. Likewise, nurses must gain confidence that nursing knowledge provides a unique contribution to interprofessional dialogues about complex healthcare challenges.

The old healthcare paradigm was built on the underlying assumption of patient/client passivity or the provider message, "I will tell you what you need to know when you need to know it." Integrative nursing calls nurses to have a different type of relationship with patients and clients. It encourages all people to actively participate in their own health and healthcare. Empowering active participation is a radical departure from the norm. Partnership with healthcare recipients is not an expected behavior in many Western cultures; therefore, nurse educators need to teach communication skills, model patient–nurse interactions, and encourage reflective practice.

Finally, nursing education needs to start to shift the relationship biomedicine has with nature. One look at common popular myths illuminates our lack of accurate information about nature. "Bacteria are always dangerous and need to be killed with antibiotics." "Severely immune-compromised patients should not be in the same environment with a plant." "Given adequate time and resources, science will be able to triumph over any disease or health problem that nature creates." Another commonly held attitude is that nature causes illness and challenges healing. These attitudes demonstrate how far we have strayed from Florence Nightingale, who wrote:

> It is often thought that medicine is the curative process. It is no such thing; medicine is the surgery of functions, as surgery proper is that of limbs and organ. Neither can do anything but remove obstructions; neither can cure; nature alone cures. Surgery removes the bullet out of the limb, which is an obstruction to cure, but nature heals the wound. So it is with medicine; the function of an organ becomes obstructed; medicine, so far as we know, assists nature to remove the obstruction, but does nothing more. And what nursing has to do in either case is to put the patient in the best condition for nature to act upon him. (Nightingale, 1860/1969, p. 133)

Conclusion

To summarize, the following steps can help nurse educators establish the integrative philosophy as the foundation for nursing scholarship and practice:

- Teach nursing history that illuminates models of integrative nursing.
- Make certain that integrative principles are woven through each and every course in the curriculum.

- Promote transdisciplinary thinking that supports a whole-systems approach to healing.
- Teach theory and practical skills that empower the client to be an active participant in his or her own health and healing.
- Throughout every course of the curriculum, provide students with evidence demonstrating the body's own reparative ability so nature is seen as an ally rather than a foe.

The next generation of nurses is being socialized through nursing education today. Will they be taught to base their career on current assumptions about the role of nature, a narrow range of acceptable modalities, a limited epistemology, and a belief that patients are meant to be passive? Nursing educators must make sure the answer to this question is "No." Fully embracing integrative nursing in the curriculum will guide future nurses to partner with individuals and communities, creating environments where nature can heal.

SELECTED REFERENCES

American Association of Colleges of Nursing. (2008). *The Essentials of Baccalaureate Education for Professional Nursing Practice*. Washington, DC: AACN.

Benner, P., Sutphen, M., Leonard, V., & Day, L. (2010). *Educating Nurses: A Call for Radical Transformation*. San Francisco: Jossey-Bass.

Booth-LaForce, C., Scott, C., Heitkemper, M., Cornman, B., Bond, E., & Swanson, K. (2010). Complementary and alternative medicine (CAM) attitudes and competencies of nursing students and faculty: Results of integrating CAM into the nursing curriculum. *Journal of Professional Nursing, 26*(5), 293–300.

Chlan, L., Halcón, L., Kreitzer, M. J., & Leonard, B. (2005). Influence of an experiential education session on nursing students' confidence levels in performing selected complementary therapies. *Complementary Health Practice Review, 10*(3), 189–201.

Halcón, L., Chlan, L., Kreitzer, M. J., & Leonard, B. (2003). Complementary therapies and healing practices: Faculty/student beliefs and attitudes and the implications for nursing education. *Journal of Professional Nursing, 19*(6), 387–397.

Halcón, L., Leonard, B., Snyder, M., Garwick, A., & Kreitzer, M. J. (2001). Incorporating alternative and complementary health practices within university-based nursing education. *Complementary Health Practice Review, 6*(2), 127–135.

Institute of Medicine. (2010). *The Future of Nursing: Leading Change, Advancing Health*. Washington, DC: National Academies Press.

Kreitzer, M. J., Mitten, D., Harris, I., & Shandeling, J. (2002). Attitudes toward CAM among medical, nursing, and pharmacy faculty and students: A comparative analysis. *Alternative Therapies, 8*(6), 44–53.

National League for Nursing. (2011). *NLN Competencies for Nursing Education*. Retrieved from http://www.nln.org/facultyprograms/competencies/index.htm.

Sparber, A. (2001). State boards of nursing and scope of practice of registered nurses performing complementary therapies. *The Online Journal of Issues in Nursing, 6*(3). Retrieved November

19, 2012, from http://www.nursingworld.org/MainMenuCategories/ANAMarketplace/ANAPeriodicals/OJIN/TableofContents/Volume62001/No3Sept01/ArticlePreviousTopic/CmplementaryTherapiesReport.html.

Snyder, M. (1985). *Independent Nursing Interventions*. (2nd ed.). New York: Wiley & Sons.

Snyder, M. & Lindquist, R. (Eds.). (2011). *Complementary and alternative therapies in Nursing*. (6th ed.). New York, Springer Publishing Company. (3rd edition 1998, 4th edition 2002, 5th edition 2006, 6th edition 2010).

32

Graduate Nursing Education for Integrative Nursing

MARY V. FENTON, LINDA L. HALCÓN, AND MARIE NAPOLITANO

Graduate nursing education has taken multiple paths to incorporate the concept of integrative nursing as a component or basis of nursing master's specialty programs and doctoral programs, including Doctor of Philosophy (PhD) and Doctor of Nursing Practice (DNP) programs. Schools of nursing seeking guidance on how to include integrative nursing may want to refer to the principles of this text and the standards for holistic nursing developed by the American Holistic Nurses Certification Corporation (AHNCC) to recognize and endorse the programs that integrate holistic nursing principles. Criteria have also been developed to recognize advanced holistic nursing practice through the AHNCC certification process.

But the process of introducing concepts of integrative nursing into graduate curricula has not been undertaken with the focused national consensus processes that the American Association of Colleges of Nursing (AACN) sponsored with the development of its *Essentials of Baccalaureate, Masters' and Doctoral Education for Advanced Nursing Practice* over the past fifteen to twenty years (AACN, 2012). The *Essentials* define the core curricular elements and framework and expected graduate outcomes for higher-education programs in nursing regardless of focus, major, or practice setting. Due to the lack of a similar consensus process, however, the concepts of integrative nursing in graduate education have not been included in the graduate *Essentials* documents, and, if present in curricula, they are usually added to current courses, presented as electives, or included as a minor component. Exceptions are the core programs that have made integrative and/or holistic nursing the basis for a graduate program, minor, or specialty (Fenton & Morris, 2003). This chapter will focus on the various ways concepts and principles of integrative nursing in several select programs have been incorporated into graduate nursing programs, with examples of educational models. Recommendations to increase and sustain the efforts are presented.

Integrative Nursing in Graduate Education

The term *integrative nursing* is defined as a way of being-knowing-doing that advances the health and wellbeing of patients, families, and communities through caring/healing relationships. *Integrative nurses* are defined as nurses who use evidence to inform traditional and emerging interventions that support whole-person/whole-systems healing. This definition reflects a broad view of health and healing not only at the individual whole-patient, family, and community levels, but also at the whole-systems level. The term "integrative nursing" encompasses many of the terms and concepts that nurses have historically used to describe various aspects of a whole-person/whole-systems approach to healthcare, including holistic nursing, alternative and complementary modalities, caring, and individual and whole-systems healing. In the late 1990s and early 2000s, there was an increasing interest in holistic and alternative and complementary modalities (CAM) from the public and health professionals alike. Many authors published recommendations that these concepts be included in nursing school curricula (Fasano-Ramos, 1999; Halcon et al., 2001; Melland & Clayburgh, 2000; Pepa & Russell, 2000; Rauchhorst, 1997; Richardson, 2003; Sok et al., 2004; Stuttard & Walker, 2000). Recommendations ranged from teaching students how to elicit information and evaluate the use of such therapies by patients, to reviewing the research evidence of such practices, to offering in-depth courses in specific modalities (Reed et al., 2000). The American Holistic Nurses Association (AHNA) set standards for holistic nursing practice and components of the holistic curriculum for baccalaureate programs. Several graduate advanced-practice masters' programs offer entire programs, minors, and electives that provide in-depth preparation in CAM and holistic care (Frisch, 2003; Sierpina, 2001; Sofhauser, 2002). Other authors have defined "holistic nursing" as a context or framework for alternative/complementary modalities and differentiated the philosophy of holistic care from the actual treatment techniques of applying CAM modalities (Frisch, 2001).

It is challenging to identify nursing graduate programs and courses incorporating integrative nursing principles when reviewing school and/or program websites, due to varying terminology, lack of clarity in course title and course descriptions, and integration of concepts throughout programs and courses. One online survey study of 125 accredited nursing schools found over 74 different titles of courses identified by faculty as consistent with tenets of integrative or holistic nursing (Fenton & Morris, 2003). A recent review of websites of a sample of schools of nursing identified from the earlier study revealed fewer programs that explicitly identify their programs as integrative/holistically focused. Of the 31 school of nursing websites reviewed, only five indicated integrative and/or holistic nursing as the basis for an entire graduate program, minor, or specialty, and five included integrative/holistic concepts as a graduate minor. Whether this finding reflects a true decline in the focus on integrative and holistic nursing in nursing education programs needs to be explored, but if so, it has implications for how nursing is being taught now and in the future.

Examples of Doctoral Nursing Programs

The University of Portland's Doctor of Nursing Practice program

The Doctor of Nursing Practice program (DNP) program at the University of Portland (Oregon) is an example of a doctoral program developed from an integrative health viewpoint. The program began in May 2008 and is offered to post-baccalaureate nurses prepared as family nurse practitioners, and to post-master's nurse practitioners (APRNs). The program includes an integrative health (IH) component consisting of five courses; program outcome measures and course competencies reinforce the integrative perspective. The National College of Natural Medicine and the Oregon College of Oriental Medicine, located in Portland, provided support for the program because APRNs see increasing numbers of their graduates' patients. With increasing use of integrative approaches to care, including therapies such as acupuncture or herbs, APRNs needed to understand these integrative principles and practices, recommend appropriate therapies, refer to practitioners, and be part of an interprofessional healthcare team.

School of Nursing (SON) faculty believe that integrative health honors the innate ability of the body to heal, values the relationship between patient and healthcare provider, and integrates complementary and alternative medicine when appropriate to facilitating healing (Frisch, 2001). An integrative philosophy runs deep at the SON, refocusing care on whole persons, bodymindspirit, and health and healing even when it is not possible to cure. Required IH courses include (1) Integrative Health: Concepts of Health and Healing; (2) Integrative Health: Approaches to Care; (3) Integrative Health: Mind–Body Connections; (4) Integrative Health: Botanical Therapy; and (5) Nutrition Therapy.

IH is interwoven throughout the DNP program. Program outcome measures require students to demonstrate knowledge and skill sets to practice from an integrative perspective. The establishment of increasing numbers of IH private and large institutional healthcare practices in Oregon provides clinical sites for FNP students and potential post-graduation positions (University of Portland 2012).

The University of Minnesota School of Nursing Doctor of Nursing Practice program

The University of Minnesota's SON incorporated integrative health and healing into its graduate-level curricula in the late 1990s and is another example of a nursing graduate program developed from an integrative perspective. The development process included faculty and administrators of the SON and the interdisciplinary Center for Spirituality and Healing of the Academic Health Center (Halcon et al., 2001) Student and faculty interest was high and was an important factor in removing barriers to change (Halcon et al., 2003; Kreitzer et al., 2002). Early strategies (e.g., experiential faculty programs, on-line modules on modalities, topics that could be incorporated into existing courses) leveraged the natural partnership between the School of Nursing and the Center for Spirituality and Healing and facilitated the assimilation of integrative health and healing in graduate nursing education (UMN, Center for Spirituality and Healing, 2012).

The healthcare environment in Minnesota also provided incentives for change. Practitioners of all types with skills in integrative health and wellness were in high demand in acute, long-term, and ambulatory care facilities. It became clear that all nursing graduate students needed a strong core of integrative health and healing, with options to specialize in this content area. There was and still is local and national demand for specialists prepared to lead the transformation of healthcare to an integrative model. A two-pronged approach was adopted as the M.S. degree program was phased out and the DNP developed. First, faculty agreed to incorporate substantive integrative health and healing content in all DNP specialties. Twelve of fourteen specialty areas require a mandatory three-credit overview of integrative therapies and include integrative content specific to their specialty populations. One of the two opted-out specialties, nurse anesthesia, later incorporated significant content in a way that better fit the needs of the specialty. Second, the Integrative Health and Healing (IHH) DNP specialty area was developed to prepare advanced practitioners of holistic and integrative nursing across all levels of care and individuals to systems (UMN, 2012).

The DNP Program admitted its first students in the fall of 2009 and graduated its first cohort in the spring of 2012. This program of study prepares graduates with skills necessary for working with individuals, families, communities, and health systems to develop integrative approaches to health promotion, disease prevention, and chronic disease management, with special emphasis on managing lifestyle changes and incorporating the use of complementary therapies. Graduates work in hospitals, outpatient settings, health plans, corporate and community organizations, and in private practice. Courses offer students the opportunity to strengthen their disciplinary and interdisciplinary expertise. The focus is on non-pharmacological interventions with emphasis on optimal healing environments, botanical medicines, clinical aromatherapy, mind/body healing, functional nutrition, energy healing, health coaching, self-care, advanced integrative health and healing skills and program planning, applied research, and policy development. Program faculty include experts from the School of Nursing and the Center for Spirituality and Healing, adding to the richness of teaching and mentoring.

To promote a feeling of community, two evening salons are held each semester and include a light dinner provided by faculty (Manthey, 2010). After an opening "centering" exercise, each person in the circle states what is on his or her mind about integrative nursing that evening. Usually a theme emerges, and there is a group discussion of that topic. At the close, each person again reflects on what is on his or her mind about integrative nursing. Initially the salons were limited to IHH DNP students, but other doctoral students expressed an interest in integrative practice, requesting to join in. This has provided a fertile ground for discussion of common interests and exploratory collaboration.

Future directions include finding creative ways to engage non-local students in this area of study. The DNP degree can be completed in an online distance format combined with several short on-site intensives each semester; however, it is challenging to find appropriate distance clinical sites that can provide students optimal experiences in settings with existing integrative programs.

Texas Tech University Health Science Center (TTUHSC) School of Nursing DNP program

Texas Tech School of Nursing offers post-master's DNP programs in Executive Leadership and Advanced Practice for nurse practitioners and nurse midwives. Students are introduced to the concept of reflective journaling and holism in healthcare and develop a holistic nursing conceptual framework in an introductory course to use as a base for their practice for the remainder of the program. One course in particular, Integrating Complementary and Alternative Modalities (CAM) into Healthcare Systems, is required for those in Advanced Practice. The course uses the field of integrative healthcare as a venue for developing the student's role to improve healthcare for rural and vulnerable populations with limited access to conventional health services. Students utilize research evidence and gain knowledge about and experience with various complementary and non-traditional therapies. Critical reviews of the application of evidenced-based research approaches to examine the effectiveness and safety of CAM in advanced nursing practice are synthesized within an analysis of healthcare systems (Texas Tech UHSC, 2012).

Examples of Integrative and Holistic Master's Degree Programs

Several masters' programs are endorsed by the American Holistic Nurses Credentialing Center, indicating a focus on holistic/integrative healing and nursing practice (AHNCC, 2012). The programs include advanced practice master's programs with holistic specialty components, concentrations or tracks in holistic nursing and advanced practice programs, and clinical nurse leader programs with holistic nursing concepts integrated through select courses. New York University, which has an advanced practice adult primary care/holistic nursing master's program, includes a three-course specialty component in advanced holistic nursing focused on contemporary practice roles of the holistic nurse practitioner, psychoneuroimmunology, nursing strategies in holistic primary care of adults, and common health problems across the lifespan (Dean, 2001; NYU, 2012).

Tennessee State University (2012) offers a Master of Science in Nursing in Holistic Nursing. The curriculum includes content and experience in advanced holistic assessment, psychoneuroimmunology, stress management, guided imagery and hypnosis, pharmacology, herbology, complementary healing modalities and ancient healing practices, and integrative medicine combining Western medicine with other healing approaches. Clinical hours lead toward certification in hypnosis, Chinese medicine, Reiki, Healing Touch, aromatherapy, herbology, guided imagery, acupressure, or other healing modalities.

Florida Atlantic University (FAU) offers a 15-credit Advanced Holistic Nursing Track as part of its advanced practice master's program (Purnell & Lange, 2011). Students may choose one of three focal areas: mind–body practices, manipulative and body-based practices, or energetic healing practices (FAU, 2012). Metropolitan State University's (2012) website notes a holistic philosophy and specific program objectives for both its nursing masters and developing DNP program. They offer tracks in Public Health Nursing Leadership and in Leadership and Management, in which a core course—Foundations of Integrative Care—is required and serves as an elective in the Nurse Educator Track.

Examples of schools endorsed by AHNCC that integrate holistic principles and concepts within the courses but also offer specific courses in holistic nursing are Xavier University (2012) in Cincinnati, Ohio; Dominican University of California (2006), which offers a Clinical Nurse Leader Program (Jossens & Ganley, 2006); and Capital University (2012), which offers concentrations in Administration, Nursing Education, Legal Studies, and Theological Studies. While these programs explicitly identify an integrative and/or holistic focus on their websites, there are probably other schools with a similar focus that was not readily apparent.

Teaching Integrative Nursing Practice in Graduate Education

There are varied approaches to nursing graduate education based on principles of integrative/holistic nursing practice in the literature and as proposed in this book.

Integrative/holistic nursing can be utilized as the major construct for the program, as described above, or as one of the major concepts or concentration areas reflected in the program and courses. Examples of teaching integrative nursing practice provided here are applicable to both master's and doctoral programs, but due to the recent rapid expansion of DNP programs, we have chosen to provide examples of ways faculty could teach and integrate principles of integrative/holistic care within the AACN *Essentials of Doctoral Education for Advanced Nursing Practice*, believing that will be the future. We have selected two AACN DNP *Essentials* as examples of how principles of integrative nursing can be incorporated into graduate programs using the University of Minnesota DNP program as an example for Essential II (Organization and Systems Leadership for Quality Improvement and Systems Thinking) and the University of Portland DNP program as an example for Essential VIII (Advanced Nursing Practice).

AACN DNP ESSENTIAL II: ORGANIZATIONAL AND SYSTEMS LEADERSHIP FOR QUALITY IMPROVEMENT AND SYSTEMS THINKING

It is clear that the transformation of systems and organizations requires new ways of thinking about organizations and leadership. There are leadership models that are consistent with integrative nursing principles and show promise of shifting the underlying assumptions of existing leaders, faculty, and students; these models can be incorporated into the leadership curricula of graduate nursing programs. A description of one of these models, Whole Systems Leadership, can be found at the University of Minnesota Center for Healing and Spirituality (UMN, CSp/H, 2012). Based on complex systems science, Whole Systems Leadership emphasizes the importance of connections and the importance of many small actions in creating new futures. The six core characteristics of the model are:

1. *Deep listening:* Conversations have the power to transform our understanding and generate innovative options for action. A key component of successful conversations is deep listening, which means listening to learn and temporarily suspending judgment.
2. *Awareness of systems:* Whole Systems Leadership understands communities, organizations, and groups as adaptive, changing systems. With an awareness of systems, you get a fuller perspective of the situation, which expands and refines your options for action.
3. *Awareness of self:* Developing self-awareness is the necessary beginning to developing skillful ways to respond to situations. If you are not aware of your motivations, feelings, and beliefs, you cannot make effective decisions about how to behave.

4. *Seeking diverse perspectives:* A whole-systems approach thrives on the respectful inclusion of all voices. From this viewpoint, conflicting opinions do not present a problem; rather, they present a potential resource that can sharpen thinking and lead to innovative options for action.

5. *Suspending certainty, embracing uncertainty:* Suspending certainty enables you to see beyond your habitual lenses to get a broader and potentially more accurate view of what is going on. It also creates room for diverse views so that new or different knowledge can come forth.

6. *Taking adaptive action:* Adaptive action means learning from everything you do. It means taking the time to recognize patterns and reflect on their meaning before jumping to a solution. It balances an inclusive, deep listening approach with a bias towards action.

Theory U, developed by Otto Scharmer (2012), is another relevant leadership model for graduate nursing education. Theory U is based on the concept of "presencing," described as a shift to an inner state that invites in future possibilities that want to emerge. Using deep listening, leaders and others undergo the following five-stage process of "discovering the future by doing:"

1. *Co-Initiating:* Build common intent—stop and listen to others and to what life calls you to do.

2. *Co-Sensing:* Observe, observe, observe. Go to the places of most potential and listen with your mind and heart wide open.

3. *Presencing:* Connect to the source of inspiration, and go to the place of silence and allow the inner knowing to emerge.

4. *Co-Creating:* Prototype the new in living examples to explore the future by doing.

5. *Co-Evolving:* Embody the new in ecosystems that facilitate seeing and acting from the whole.

In their last clinical course, IHH DNP students apply principles and practices of contemporary whole-systems leadership to help healthcare agencies or facilities, such as hospitals or long-term care organizations, create new integrative health and healing programs or services. Funded by a grant by the George Family Foundation, most students have been able to attend Otto Scharmer's Presencing Institute and other national or international conferences to further develop their expertise in whole-systems leadership.

Other leadership models are applicable to leadership in integrative nursing. Such models include an emphasis on systems thinking, deep listening and observation, and becoming willing to embrace uncertainty and go beyond old engagement and organizational patterns. These skills, along with knowledge of integrative therapies, are needed for the transformation of the current healthcare system.

AACN DNP ESSENTIAL VIII: ADVANCED NURSING PRACTICE

Essential VIII specifies the practice competencies that all DNP graduates are expected to demonstrate in an area of specialization within the larger domain of nursing. The example below demonstrates how the specialization of integrative health can be incorporated into a DNP program to meet the criteria for Essential VIII.

Integrative health is incorporated into multiple aspects of advanced nursing practice in the University of Portland's DNP program, including coursework, program competencies, NP management course outcomes and clinical assignments, and program-wide case presentations and opportunities for clinical placements in primary care practices using multiple types of practitioners. An advisory committee, composed of IH practitioners, reviews the curriculum and assists with identifying clinical sites.

Courses address different aspects of IH, reinforcing basic principles such as effective relationships, self-care, maintenance of health, and healing from whole-systems perspectives. "Integrative Health I" examines the concepts of integrative health and its place within conventional medicine and nursing. Philosophies of health and healing are explored from multiple disciplines through various therapeutic approaches. Self-care and motivational interviewing are introduced and threaded through all IH courses. Course outcomes are demonstrated through a theoretical analysis paper on health and healing and a reflective journal examining a self-care practice. "Integrative Health II" explores multiple whole-systems approaches such as Oriental medicine, Ayurveda, naturopathy, chiropractic, and homeopathy from the perspectives of these systems practitioners. IH practices are critically evaluated based on available evidence. A significant course outcome is the ability to build collegial relationships with these practitioners. Student learning activities include reflective journaling on self-care and experiential immersion clinical experience with IH practitioners. "Integrative Health III" explores psychoneuroimmunology, interpersonal neurobiology, and other scientific evidence linking mind and body in health and disease. Various mind–body therapies are examined for integration into NP practice. Student activities include undertaking the mindfulness-based stress reduction program with a reflective journal on the experience. "Integrative Health IV" explores the conceptual approaches to herbal therapy and botanical medicine. Competency is developed in accessing appropriate evidence, identifying clinical indications, knowing potential risks of herbs and dietary supplements, and communicating with patients about botanicals. Student activities include writing a position paper regarding the student's personal view of plants and an herbal paper addressing multiple aspects of a selected herb. "Integrative Health V" addresses aspects of nutrition as a health process from the pathophysiology of digestion to the evidence for specialty diets, the impact of industrial food products on health, vitamins, and clinical challenges in changing patient dietary behavior. Course outcomes are demonstrated through a paper addressing aspects of a specialty diet, an experience of recording personal food intake with analysis, and a position paper on one of the four foods discussed in Pollan's (2001) book, *Botany of Desire*.

NP management courses require students to use an IH approach with patients in clinical settings while developing skills in patient–clinician relationships, patient-centered communication, and use of appropriate level of health literacy. Management knowledge and skills include use of herbs and supplements, alternative practices such as cupping, and complementary practitioners such as acupuncturists, identifying cultural beliefs and practices such as *susto* being the etiology and the *curandero* as healer; addressing nutrition, sleep, activity, stress, and coping; and family as defined by the patient. Evaluations of course assignments include criteria that assess the quality of the IH approach. Students use Natural Standards as a complimentary practice database and to evaluate level of evidence for complimentary practices.

PROGRAMMATIC NEEDS

To be successful in developing and implementing such programs, there is a critical need for faculty with both education and experience in integrative health. For example, faculty who teach in the University of Portland program include an adult nurse practitioner with a doctorate in acupuncture and Oriental medicine who maintains an integrative practice as a nurse practitioner in internal medicine and has published studies examining use of integrative medicine in primary care; a family nurse practitioner with a certificate in integrative medicine from the University of Arizona who practices with an integrative family medicine group and has published and presented on complimentary practices and an integrative perspective in nursing; a clinical nurse specialist in mental health who integrates Reiki into her therapy practice and focuses on research with complementary therapies and cancer in both her graduate and post-graduate education; and the dean of the School of Nursing who implemented and evaluated a one-year faculty development for integrative health at the University of Portland and served on the Oregon College of Oriental Medicine research advisor group for their federal grant to infuse research into their programming. Faculty development is essential for all graduate faculty, not just those teaching integrative/holistic nursing and the integration of CAM modalities, in order for students to have the opportunity to take an integrative approach in all courses.

Recommendations to Increase and Sustain Graduate Integrative Nursing Programs

There appear to be fewer integrative/holistic nursing graduate specialty programs within schools of nursing in the United States today than ten years ago (Fenton & Morris, 2003). In some cases, programs were started by faculty champions but without the institutional support to sustain the effort over the long term. Competing administrative, financial, and environmental demands have undermined sustained efforts towards graduate nursing programs focused on integrative health and healing. Yet the need for integrative approaches to advanced nursing practice and research has not decreased, and the need for integrative transformation of healthcare has grown. Graduate nursing education programs must incorporate integrative concepts and skills in their curricula despite institutional or professional barriers. Concrete examples of actions that could be taken include:

- Faculty and administrators taking the lead in modeling self-care and incorporating reflective practices such as journaling into teaching and administrative roles encourages creative thinking. Faculty may include such practices as components of the curriculum throughout the program or as components of courses in evidence-based practice of integrative/holistic practices, including CAM.
- The engagement of nursing deans, directors, and faculty in learning about integrative/holistic practice and education is essential to both developing and sustaining a focus on integrative/holistic concepts. Bringing in experts to consult with faculty and administration and present CE programs is a useful strategy.
- The incorporation of innovative ways to interweave integrative principles and holistic practices such as deep listening into the day-to-day functions of schools of nursing creates productive and supportive environments. For example, at the University of Minnesota, the faculty chair and the dean instituted practices at faculty meetings and executive meetings to ensure that all voices would be heard. At Texas Tech, the DNP program was created at faculty retreats using a "talking stick" for faculty members to state their intent for the new program. This practice resulted in a norm of creativity and collaboration at these retreats.
- The AHNA can be helpful in promoting recognition of integrative nursing programs, as nurses interested in integrative health and healing read this organization's publications. Encouraging recognition of programs through the AHNA process and advanced certification in holistic nursing through AHNCC can help sustain an integrated/holistic approach in a school of nursing curriculum. Efforts are underway to bring this certification more in line with current advanced-practice nursing credentialing.
- The Consortium of Academic Health Centers for Integrative Medicine offers interdisciplinary opportunities for health professionals. The mission of the Consortium is to advance the principles and practices of integrative healthcare within academic institutions. The Consortium provides its institutional membership with a community of support for their academic missions and a collective voice for influencing change.

- Integrative nursing faculty and students should be integrated with other specialties. At the University of Minnesota, the IH nursing faculty host a salon twice every semester for students and faculty interested in integrative nursing networking. Attendees include DNP students from all specialties, graduates, PhD students conducting research on integrative topics, and interested faculty.
- Providing faculty exposure to integrative nursing with online resources in specialty areas and opportunities to attend conferences and meet with clinical experts in their areas provides ways to promote integrative/holistic nursing in courses. Several years ago, University of Minnesota faculty were provided with online resources, and now faculty include examples of integrative/holistic evidence-based programs or practices in their courses.

A Vision for the Future

Our vision for the future of graduate nursing programs is that there will be no need for separate integrative nursing programs and curricula because healthcare systems will be focused on integrative care. We envision that all graduate nursing specialties will include sufficient knowledge of integrative practice and modalities to produce graduates who serve as competent resources for the public, institutions, and policymakers. In this future, expert integrative nurses will bring health to their workplaces and educational institutions and will be sought out for their ability to provide foundations for transformation. We need leaders from all disciplines that have skills in integrative therapies and integrative leadership to help transform our health systems.

SELECTED REFERENCES

American Association of Colleges of Nursing. (2012). The Essentials of Doctoral Education for Advanced Nursing Practice, (2007). Available at: www.aacn.nche.edu/publications/position/DNPEssentials.pdf. Accessed June 30, 2012.

American Holistic Nurses Certification Corp/AHNCC. (2012). Available at: http://www.ahncc.org/home/endorsedschools.html. Accessed June 4, 2012.

Fenton, M. V., & Morris, D. L. (2003). The integration of holistic nursing practices and complementary and alternative modalities into curricula of schools of nursing. *Alternative Therapies in Health and Medicine, 9*(4), 62–67.

Frisch, N. (2003). Standards for holistic nursing practice: A way to think about our care that includes complementary and alternative modalities. *Online Journal Issues in Nursing, 6*(2); Available at: http://www.nursingworld.org/ojin/tocic15tpc15_4.htm. Accessed June 6, 2012.

Halcón L., Leonard, B., Snyder, M., Garwick, A., & Kreitzer, M. J. (2001). Incorporating alternative and complementary health practices with university-based nursing education. *Complementary Health Practice Review, 6*(2), 127–135.

Jossens, M. O., & Ganley, B. J. (2006). Integrated health practices: Development of a graduate nursing program. *Journal of Nursing Education, 45*(1), 16–24.

Manthey, M. (2010). A new model of healing for the profession of nursing. *Creative Nursing, 16*(1), 18–20.

Melland, H. I., & Clayburgh, T. L. (2000). Complementary therapies: Introduction into a nursing curriculum. *Nursing Educator, 25*(6), 247–250.

Purnell, M. J., & Lange, B. (2011). Creating a graduate holistic nursing program. *Holistic Nursing Practice,25*(3), 140–146.

Rauchhorst, L. (1997). Integration of complementary therapies in the nurse practitioner program. *Clinical Excellence for Nursing Practice, 1*(4), 257–265.

33

Continuing Professional Development for Integrative Nursing

MARY KOITHAN AND KATHY CHAPPELL

Then comes intellect. It wishes to satisfy the wants which intellect creates for it.

—*Florence Nightingale (Cassandra, 1860)*

en and women come into the profession of nursing because of their desire to nurture, to help, to make a difference in another person's life, to
offer comfort, to care. Nurses are called to this profession because of their
moral commitment to care for another human being in some of their most vulnerable
times, and to facilitate, support and assist them in their search for health and wellbeing
(Nightingale, 1859; Quinn, 2000; Watson, 2011). The knowledge and skills that nurses
master during their pre-licensure programs and the first years of their careers enable
them to provide safe, competent, and compassionate care in an ever-changing healthcare system. And yet, in a rapidly changing healthcare environment, they often find
themselves wondering how they lost the "care." They find themselves without the time
to talk quietly with the young teen undergoing tests for leukemia, to hold the hand
of the eighty-year-old woman whose husband has just been taken into surgery, or
to dry the tears of a young mother whose child has been rushed into the emergency
department.

Like our colleagues in medicine, some will leave the profession having lost the purpose of what they came to do (Remen, 2001). Others will seek formal graduate education. Still others will look to professional development (e.g., continuing education
courses, certificate programs, competency programs) to satisfy their desire for professional growth. An environmental scan indicates a plethora of professional development opportunities in integrative nursing with offerings across multiple learning
platforms (symposia and conferences, residential intensives, online asynchronous
sessions, asynchronous media-supported classes, and agency-supported in-service
sessions) and multiple venues. This chapter facilitates your search to find meaning in
our chosen field; to recapture nursing's soul.

Nursing's pioneer, Florence Nightingale, provided a basis for nursing professional development in 1859, stating that systems must be in place to *"satisfy the wants which intellect creates."* Nursing professional development satisfies the wants through continual engagement in lifelong learning wherein registered nurses develop and maintain the ability to practice as competent and fulfilled healthcare providers. Florence Nightingale demonstrated, through her actions and her written word, that nurses must always be engaged in scientific inquiry, use thoughtful analysis, and be open to learning experiences throughout their careers in order to provide high-quality, patient-centered care (Nightingale, 1859).

Overview of Professional Development in Nursing

Nursing professional development (NPD) has been defined as a career-long continuum of formal and informal educational activities that are informed by wide-ranging sources of evidence, including clinical or practice-based evidence as well as scientific and theoretical evidence (American Nurses Association/National Nursing Staff Development Organization, 2010). Formal, structured activities include such areas as academic coursework, continuing education programs, certification, and skills-based competency courses. Informal, self-directed learning activities include such areas as point-of-care learning or searching the literature for new evidence (Figure 33.1).

In the United States, NPD formally began in 1969 when the American Nurses Association convened a national conference to provide an opportunity for academic providers of continuing nursing education (CNE) to explore the educational needs of nurses in the practice setting, as distinct from the needs of those in the pre-licensure academic setting, recognizing that ongoing education was a necessary component of safe, effective professional practice. In 1972, the ANA established the Commission on Continuing Education, and, in 1974, it published *Standards for Continuing Education in Nursing*. A formal accreditation system for continuing nursing education was launched in 1975 following development of the standards. Guidelines for staff development were developed and published in 1976, as the importance of continuing professional development in the practice setting became evident. In 1991, the American Nurses Credentialing Center (ANCC) was created as a subsidiary of the ANA, and the work of credentialing NPD was transferred to the ANCC. The ANCC continues to develop and implement criteria for organizations that provide continuing nursing education through accreditation. ANCC also offers certification to individual registered nurses who work as nursing professional development specialists (American Nurses Association and National Nursing Professional Development Organization, 2010).

The National Council of State Boards of Nursing (NCSBN) and the individual state nursing boards support NPD through establishing standards for the

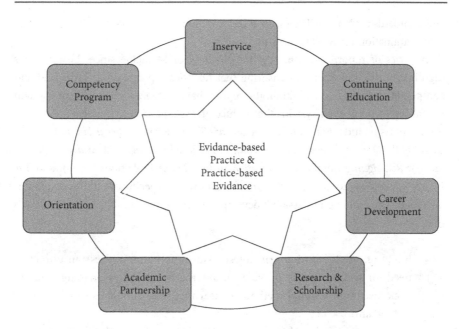

FIGURE 33.1 This figure depicts the scope of practice of nurses working in professional nursing development roles. Nursing Professional Development, as cited in American Nurses Association/National Nursing Staff Development Organization (2010), *Scope and Standards of Professional Nursing Development.* Washington DC: ANA Publishing. Reprinted with permission. All Rights Reserved.

entry-level examination (National Council Licensure Examination, or NCLEX) as well as requirements for re-licensure in each state such as continuing education. In addition, state boards of nursing develop the scope of practice standards for registered nurses practicing in each state; respond to complaints and determine disciplinary actions as needed; and collect and analyze nursing workforce data. The NCSBN advocates for nurses at the national level in areas such as workforce, education, and practice. Some state boards of nursing also develop standards for and approve providers of continuing nursing education (National Council of State Boards of Nursing, 2010).

There are several associations and organizations that support the work of nurse educators in the practice setting, including the Association for Nursing Professional Development (ANPD; formerly known as the National Nursing Staff Development Organization), the Professional Nurse Educators Group (PNEG) and the Alliance for Continuing Education in the Health Professions (ACEHP). The focus of these groups is to improve the ability of nurse educators to provide high-quality educational activities for registered nurses that have a positive impact on the practice of nursing and/or patient outcomes. The ANCC and ANPD have also collaborated to develop the Scope and Standards for Nursing Professional Development as well as an individual certification examination for NPD specialists.

A series of reports published by the Institute of Medicine since the 1970s has highlighted the importance of ensuring that healthcare providers are educated and competent to practice. In addition, the reports have criticized the healthcare system for failing to implement systems that reduce errors and increase patient safety. The IOM reports include: *Educating the Healthcare Team* (1972), *To Err is Human* (2000), *Crossing the Quality Chasm* (2001), *Health Professional Education: A Bridge to Quality* (2003), *Redesigning Continuing Education in the Health Professions* (2009), and *The Future of Nursing* (2010). The IOM's most recent report specifically addresses the importance of continuing professional development (CPD) for healthcare professionals that is:

- Based on adult learning principles: ensures activities address an unmet need for the healthcare provider, is interactive, employs ongoing feedback, uses multi-modal methods of learning, and simulates the clinical setting; and
- Built on a foundation of five core competencies, including the ability of the healthcare practitioner to: provide patient-centered care, work collaboratively in interprofessional teams, utilize evidence-based practice, understand and apply quality improvement tactics, and effectively utilize information technology (IOM, 2010).

Improving the health and wellbeing of patients, families, and communities through safe, patient-centered care is at the heart of integrative nursing. Therefore, opportunities to develop knowledge, skills, and abilities to deliver integrative nursing are paramount in our current healthcare environment. Yet, how do nurses judge the quality of programs available to them? How do nurses select among the various professional development opportunities in integrative nursing?

The Context of Professional Development in Nursing

Responsibility for ensuring that registered nurses have access to and are engaged in quality continuing professional development activities rests with the individual nurse, with organizations that employ registered nurses, and with the professional and regulatory agencies that are accountable for the delivery of safe, high-quality patient care. The infrastructure that supports continuing professional development activities includes accrediting, certifying, and licensing bodies.

ACCREDITING BODIES

Accreditation is defined as the process by which a voluntary, nongovernmental agency or organization appraises and grants accredited status to institutions, programs, or services that meet predetermined structure, process, and outcome criteria (U.S. Department of Education, 2013). Within nursing, the largest credentialing body for CNE is the American Nurses Credentialing Center's Accreditation Program. The ANCC Accreditation Program accredits two types of organizations: (a) "Accredited Providers," organizations that are granted accredited status to provide CNE activities; and (b) "Accredited Approvers," organizations that are granted accredited status to approve other organizations or individuals who provide CNE activities. Accredited organizations must meet strict standards related to planning, implementing, and evaluating CNE activities. These accreditation standards are congruent with those from other accrediting bodies in medicine (Accreditation Council for Continuing Medical Education, ACCME) and pharmacy (Accreditation Council for Pharmacy Education, ACPE), and are designed to ensure that CNE activities are developed using adult education design principles, planned independently from the influence of commercial interest organizations, and designed to improve the professional practice of nursing and/or patient outcomes.

The process of applying for accreditation requires that an organization submit an application and supporting documentation that demonstrate how it has met predetermined criteria for the specific credential. The application and supporting documentation are evaluated by qualified reviewers and validating interviews with the applicant organization. Additional evidence is requested if necessary, and a final summary report or evaluation is generated by the review team. A separate body, the Commission on Accreditation, makes the final determination of accreditation. Initial applicants may receive up to two years of accreditation, and re-accrediting applicants may receive up to four years of accreditation. Accreditation may not be awarded if the applicant fails to meet criteria requirements.

Courses that are provided by accredited organizations assure the professional nurse seeking integrative nursing CNE that the education is of high quality and appropriate for continuing professional development. For a list of ANCC-accredited organizations, visit www.nursecredentialing.org/Accreditation/AccreditedOrganizations.

The ANCC also credentials providers of interprofessional education collaboratively with ACCME and ACPE, and credentials skills-based competency courses designed to validate a nurse's skill or skill set in the clinical setting. The process of application and accreditation is similar to the accreditation process for a single professional unit; however, organizations providing interprofessional continuing education (IPE) must demonstrate that at least 25% of their educational activities use a "for the team, by the team approach" recommended by the IOM (2009) report on redesigning continuing education for the health professions. A team of reviewers from nursing, medicine, and pharmacy review applicant organizations, and accreditation is granted by the individual governing commission or board for each discipline. A list of organizations credentialed for interprofessional education can be found at www.nursecredentialing. org/Accreditation/AccreditedOrganizations. As integrative nursing embraces collaboration and patient-centered care, this credential is a growth opportunity for organizations interested in providing continuing education that supports integrative nursing professional development.

Organizations and individuals can seek approval for educational activities from ANCC Accredited Approvers. These educational activities must meet the same quality standards as courses offered by accredited organizations and are delivered with oversight from the accredited organization. For organizations and individuals who are providing recognized continuing education through an approver unit, visit the individual Accredited Approvers' websites. Additionally, some state boards of nursing and other professional associations approve a small number of continuing-education providers.

CERTIFYING BODIES

Certification is defined as a process by which a nongovernmental agency or association certifies that an individual has met certain predetermined standards specified by that profession for specialty practice. Its purpose is to assure various publics that an individual has mastered a body of knowledge and acquired skills in a particular specialty (American Board of Nursing Specialties, 2005). Nurses individually certified in NPD have met stringent education and practice eligibility requirements and have passed a rigorous examination demonstrating they possess a unique body of knowledge and skills related to the specialty area. In addition, certifying bodies require that individual nurses holding specialty certifications participate in regular professional development activities, including active practice in NPD (planning, implementing, and evaluating CNE; participating in educational activities; presenting, publishing, and conducting research; precepting new educators; and volunteering in professional nursing associations).

Participating in integrative nursing professional development activities offered by appropriately certified nurse educators provides further assurance that the education meets high quality standards. The National League for Nursing offers a certification exam for nurse educators practicing primarily in the academic setting, called the Certified Nurse Educator (CNE) credential. Alternatively, ANCC offers a certification exam for nurses specializing primarily in continuing education in the practice setting, called the Nursing Professional Development (NPD) credential (RN-BC). To determine if a nurse educator is certified, simply look for either credential to be listed with their name and title. Additional information can be obtained at www.nln.org/certification/index.htm and www.nursecredentialing.org/Certification/NurseSpecialties/NursingProfessionalDevelopment.

LICENSING BODIES

Licensing bodies establish criteria for both initial licensure and re-licensure, which assures the public that those practicing nursing have met minimal safety and professional standards. In the United States, licensure of registered nurses is under the purview of the state boards of nursing. For initial licensure, state boards of nursing utilize the NCLEX initial licensing examination, which was developed and is maintained by the National Council of State Boards of Nursing. Requirements for re-licensure are determined by the individual state boards of nursing and may include mandatory participation in continuing nursing education and/or specific types of mandatory education, as determined by each Board (National Council of State Boards of Nursing, 2010). Participating in continuing nursing education activities for integrative nursing satisfies these licensure requirements in states requiring continuing education, as the knowledge and skills acquired are directly applicable to practice and enhance the quality and safety of patient care.

Professional Development and Integrative Nursing: Opportunities and Systems

Several formal systems have emerged over the years that support professional development opportunities in integrative nursing. The American Holistic Nurses Association (AHNA) was founded in 1981 by Charlotte McGuire as an organization that provided ongoing opportunities for professional engagement for nurses who were suffering because of changes in staffing patterns and nurse shortages that dramatically changed the nature of nursing to a profession that was "becoming less patient and wellness focused" (AHNA, 2013). Since 1981, AHNA has been the leading professional organization committed to providing holistic and integrative nursing continuing education and professional development. AHNA's vision is a world in which nursing nurtures wholeness and inspires peace and healing that are fostered by activities that (a) ensure the incorporation of integrative healing modalities across nursing education; (b) educate the public and healthcare providers about complementary modalities of care; (c) participate in the political arena to ensure a focus on and access to wellness activities; and (d) participate in creating and disseminating evidence about the effectiveness of healing interventions (AHNA, 2013). AHNA is an ANCC-Accredited Provider and Approver of CNE, creating an extensive network of continuing development opportunities for nurses across the globe.

Several academic centers have developed courses and certificate (academic and non-academic credit) programs focused on integrative nursing, including the University of Minnesota's Center for Spirituality and Healing, the University of Arizona's Center for Integrative Medicine, the University of Arizona's College of Nursing, Rush University College of Nursing, and Boston University. Individual courses are offered throughout the United States at leading academic institutions, and increasingly, programs (conferences, courses, residential intensives) are available to nurses internationally. For example, the International Society for Complementary Medicine Research (www.iscmr.org/) sponsors annual conferences in locations around the world to disseminate the latest evidence and best practices in complementary healing strategies and integrative care.

Annual conferences are also beginning to emerge. The Integrative Healthcare Symposium, begun in 2004, annually gathers an interprofessional audience in New York City to discuss integrative care (www.ihsymposium.com/). Topics in the most recent meeting included nutrition, integrative women's health, world medicine, integrative nursing, bodymindspirit interventions, and integrative specialty tracks such as integrative pediatrics and oncology. The Society for Integrative Oncology (www.integrativeonc.org/) is an interdisciplinary organization founded in 2003, committed to the delivery of integrative, seamless care to improve the lives of people affected by cancer. They meet annually to discuss the latest evidence and novel approaches that promote health and wellbeing in oncology practice. The Consortium for Academic Health Centers for Integrative Medicine, active since 2004, sponsors several interprofessional conferences each year about a variety of topics, including education and training, innovative approaches to integrative healthcare, and advances in scientific evidence supporting integrative care (www.imconsortium.org/home.html). Scripps Center for Integrative Medicine in San Diego, California, also offers an annual interprofessional Integrative and Holistic Nursing conference (www.scripps.org/services/integrative-medicine). This conference, begun in 2009, focuses on developing competencies in nutrition, bodymindspirit care, and evidence-supported integrative healing strategies with interactive afternoon sessions about touch therapies, compassionate communication, mindfulness, and qi gong.

Finally, independent education companies, many of which are ANCC-Accredited or Approved Providers, offer opportunities that include courses and certificate programs. The Birchtree Center for Healthcare Transformation (www.birchtreecenter.com/), founded in 2000, offers education and consultation services focused on healing, transformation, and caring. Allegra Learning (www.allegralearning.com/) offers online continuing education and certificate programs in integrative nursing, integrative mental health care, and meditation. Several certificate programs (online, in-person, and media-supported asynchronous learning platforms) in holistic nurse coaching are available through providers such as the Bark Coaching Institute (www.barkcoaching.com/contact.php), the Integrative Nursing Institute (inursecoach.com/education/

inccp-curriculum/), and the Caritas Coach Education Program (www.watsoncaring-science.org/education-programs/caritas-coach-education-program-ccep/).

CREDENTIALED PROFESSIONAL DEVELOPMENT
OPPORTUNITIES IN INTEGRATIVE NURSING

There are several options available for integrative nurses seeking NPD courses or programs in integrative nursing provided by accredited organizations. AHNA has been continually accredited by ANCC since 1997. As both an Accredited Provider and Approver, AHNA provides a single access point to a large number of programs focused on holistic and integrative nursing. The AHNA, also recognized by the California State Board of Nursing as a provider of continuing education, offers courses ranging from a single contact hour to programs over several days appealing to a variety of learners, distributed via online media (webinars, asynchronous online courses), print materials (research and practice-focused journals, self-study modules), and live events. For a list of currently available courses, visit www.ahna.org/Education/EarnContactHours/tabid/1202/Default.aspx.

AHNA also approves individual CNE activities using a peer-review process that assures the learner that a program or course has been planned and implemented according the ANCC standards of professional education and that the content is consistent with the scope and standards of holistic nursing (AHNA, 2013). Applications are received from international organizations and individuals. A wide variety of courses is available, which range from individual integrative therapeutic modalities to integrative nursing processes of care (e.g., coaching, assessment, appreciative inquiry, compassionate communication, patient advocacy). To find a course approved by AHNA, you can search their database (www.ahna.org/Education/EarnContactHours/ApprovedPrograms/tabid/1206/Default.aspx) by topic or location.

Program Endorsement is awarded to certificate programs that are congruent with the mission, vision, and purpose of AHNA, and with the Scope and Standards of Holistic Nursing Practice and the state of the science and practice of holistic nursing. Endorsed programs complete a rigorous peer-review process with consent to endorse by the AHNA Leadership Council. Courses that earn an endorsement by AHNA are consistent with the principles of integrative nursing, relationship-based care, and nursing self-care. Integrative nurses can find these programs listed at www.ahna.org/Education/ProgramEndorsement/tabid/1207/Default.aspx.

The ANCC Nursing Skills Competency Program (NSCP) is a credential awarded to a course that is designed to validate a nurse's skill or skill set in the clinical setting. Skills or skill sets may be specific to a setting or specialty, skills recently included in academic nursing programs, skills needed to re-enter the nursing field, or new skills developed since the nurse's initial preparation as a registered nurse. The applicant must demonstrate that the course has been designed to measure knowledge, skills, and professional ability competency so that participants are prepared to safely administer the skill in a practice setting.

The Caritas Coach Education Program, accredited by the ANCC's NSCP in 2012, is a six-month program that is delivered using a mixed-methods approach that includes intensive residential weekends, independent study, and guided mentoring. This program prepares a knowledgeable, experienced, and reflective healthcare professional to practice using a heart-centered approach, translating an ethic based on the "Science of Human Caring" into the current healthcare system (Watson Caring Science Institute, 2013). Graduates of this program work with patients and families within acute care, long-term care, and ambulatory community-based agencies, as well as within the private-practice setting. Others teach students in academic institutions, disseminating the principles of caring science, *caritas* practice, and integrative nursing.

Exemplars of Integrative Nursing Professional Development Programs

We offer an in-depth description of three exemplar programs that support ongoing professional development in integrative nursing as a way of highlighting the breadth and depth of opportunities for lifelong learning.

THE BIRCHTREE CENTER

The BirchTree Center (2013) offers programs for individuals as well as organizations that support the "renewal of the patient–practitioner relationship based on values of caring, healing, wholeness, and human connection." Participants come to this program seeking new perspectives and caring methods, renewal of their commitment to be present with patients and facilitating healing in others, and learning about holistic and integrative intervention strategies. Programs on transformational leadership principles and best practices for a variety of integrative therapies are also offered.

Live events and retreats are typically held in the United States several times throughout the year. Topics include manifesting the healing environment, best practices in integrative therapies and modalities of care, enlightened healthcare focused on transforming the healthcare experience, and holistic nursing certification preparatory courses. Web-based learning is also offered through collaborative relationships. Online courses include end-of-life care, ending violence, and holistic nursing recertification preparation.

Envisioning and fostering healthcare system transformation, BirchTree also offers consultation and educational services to healthcare organizations that focus on creating healing environments that celebrate the human potential and personal connections.

The BirchTree team helps organizations redefine and repurpose their nursing services so that they deliver relationship-centered care in a framework that supports the renewal of both patient and providers. Nursing staff members learn and experience self-care and self-renewal skills as well as integrative interventions that can be woven into the fabric of the institutions' patient-care units. Knowledge and skills in the use of intentionality, innate wisdom, and creativity are cultivated to help create transformative healthcare environments (BirchTree, 2013).

THE UNIVERSITY OF ARIZONA'S CENTER FOR INTEGRATIVE MEDICINE

Dr. Andrew Weil founded the Arizona Center for Integrative Medicine (AzCIM) in 1994 to create, educate, and support a community that embodies the philosophy and practice of healing-oriented medicine, addressing mind, body, and spirit health and wellbeing (http://integrativemedicine.arizona.edu). AzCIM offers a broad range of educational opportunities for advanced-practice nurses (nurse practitioners, clinical nurse specialists, nurse midwives, and nurse anesthetists) including a rigorous, postgraduate two-year fellowship in integrative medicine, and continuing-education courses in a variety of topics approved by the AHNA (AzCIM, 2013).

The fellowship is designed to be a distance-learning program using a combination of online educational modules, interactive online discussions moderated by CIM faculty, and three-week-long residential intensives held in Tucson, Arizona. Curriculum segments include nutritional health, botanical and natural products, mind–body medicine, complementary/alternative therapeutics and alternative systems of medicine (e.g., traditional Chinese medicine, Ayurveda, manual medicine, homeopathy), and integrative approaches to a variety of healthcare specialty practices. Residential intensives typically include sessions with internationally renowned scholars and healthcare providers; one-to-one interaction and experiential sessions with healthcare providers credentialed in various modalities of care (e.g., Healing Touch, hypnosis, botanical medicines, massage, Reiki); and discussion groups with cohort fellows about practice ethics, business acumen, evaluation and quality improvement, and research.

Individual asynchronous online educational courses are also available for all nurses, although much of the content is directed toward advanced practice. Courses range by the numbers of CNE hours provided and include topics such as anti-inflammatory diets, nutrition and cardiovascular health, an integrative oncology series, integrative mental health, and environmental medicine. Courses are designed to be case-based and interactive and include video-supported educational modules.

The Center also supports an annual state-of-the-science Nutrition and Health Conference, now in its tenth year. An eclectic group of international researchers and scholars, clinicians, educators, and chefs gather to discuss the latest nutritional research and best practices focused on promoting health and healthful living through nutrition and food. Always a premiere event in the integrative healing community, this conference has a wide variety of learning opportunities for all types of nursing professionals.

THE UNIVERSITY OF MINNESOTA'S CENTER FOR SPIRITUALITY AND HEALING

Founded in 1997, the Center for Spirituality and Healing (CSp/H) is an interprofessional Center of Excellence at the Academic Health Center at the University of Minnesota. With an extensive list of collaborating organizations and over fifty faculty members, the center "enriches health and wellbeing by providing high-quality interdisciplinary education, conducting rigorous research, and delivering innovative programs that advance integrative health and healing" (www.csh.umn.edu/).

In addition to its academic courses and the Integrative Health and Healing, Doctor of Nursing Practice (DNP) Program that is offered through the School of Nursing, the CSp/H offers post-baccalaureate certificate programs in Integrative Therapies and Healing Practices, with focus areas in health coaching, clinical applications, leadership in optimal healing environments, and nature-based therapy. Twelve credit hours are required to complete this certificate, with the ability to transfer coursework to an accredited graduate-degree program. In addition, participants can select to enroll in the Health Coaching option for continuing education credits only, participating over a four-month period in a mixed-methods course delivery method that combines online learning with two four-day intensive weekends.

A myriad of innovative programs are also available. Participants in the Mindfulness-Based Stress Reduction Program learn how to manage their stress and take control of their lives. A combination of evening and morning programs and day-long retreats over an eight-week period facilitate growth in mindfulness meditation practices, yoga and gentle stretching, and other activities that encourage body mindspirit balance, rejuvenation, and wellbeing. In addition, the CSp/H offers this program in both web-based and telephonic delivery methods to increase access to this information. Continuing education is offered through the University of Minnesota College of Continuing Education.

The Purpose Project is a series of lectures and interactive sessions designed to facilitate a deeper understanding of personal and professional meaning. Working On Purpose™, Living On Purpose™, and Leading On Purpose™ programs help people discover the power of purpose at all stages and phases of life. Professional purpose sessions include the Thought Leadership Hub, where ongoing conversations focus on a particular aspect of purpose and the implications for health, science, learning, society, and the workplace. The Wellbeing Series offers healthcare professionals as well as the lay public opportunities to engage with faculty associates of the CSp/H about emerging science and evidence supporting optimal health and wellbeing. A combination of on-line resources, live events with internationally acclaimed speakers, books and print materials, blogs, and podcasts are available about topics such as positivity, nutrition and health, empathy, vulnerability, and emotion.

Travel study opportunities also exist to enhance students' knowledge and understanding of culturally based healing practices, natural products, and differing world-views of healthcare. In January each year, the CSp/H offers six courses on Hawaii's Big Island (Hawaii) exploring native Hawaiian healing practices, Reiki, aromatherapy, acupressure, and imagery. Courses can be taken for academic credit or for continuing education, with scheduling spaced to allow participants to take up to three courses over a ten-day period. Additional travel courses are available, including courses that focus on the role of plants in human affairs and indigenous Peruvian healing traditions.

Research and clinical practice are also part of the Center's portfolio with extensive community, national, and international partnerships supporting the achievement of their mission. By offering a wide variety of professional development opportunities in integrative nursing, the University of Minnesota is positioned as a leader in this emerging nursing specialty.

Looking Forward: Envisioning the Future of Professional Development in Nursing

It is widely recognized that today's healthcare environment is fast-paced, complex, and highly technical. Professional registered nurses must be engaged in lifelong learning in order to deliver safe, high-quality care that has a demonstrated positive impact on patient outcomes. As the delivery of healthcare evolves, so does the future of NPD.

SHIFT FROM DISCIPLINE-CENTRIC TO INTERPROFESSIONAL EDUCATION

The future of NPD will require a shift from discipline-centric education for individual members of the healthcare team to an interprofessional focus promoting team-based care. Mounting evidence demonstrates that the failure of healthcare providers to collaborate, communicate, and successfully function in teams has devastating outcomes for patients that can only be addressed by significant change in the way that we educate healthcare professionals (Institute of Medicine, 1972, 2001, 2009, 2010; Greiner, & Knebel, 2003; Health Professions Network Nursing and Midwifery Office, 2010; Kohn, Corrigan, & Donaldson, 2000; Interprofessional Education Collaborative Expert Panel, 2011).

The World Health Organization (WHO) defines *interprofessional education* (IPE) as occurring "when students from two or more professions learn with, from and about each other to collaborate and improve health outcomes" (WHO 2010). One purpose of interprofessional education is to improve interprofessional collaborative practice (IPCP), which occurs "when multiple health workers from different professional backgrounds work together with patients, families, carers, and communities to deliver the highest quality of care" (WHO 2010). Creating a supportive environment for interprofessional education and interprofessional collaborative practice that includes developing faculty, tools, and resources to support interprofessional learning will be critical work for the future.

EMPOWERING AND INCLUDING THE PATIENT IN PROFESSIONAL DEVELOPMENT

The patient is rapidly becoming an integral member of the healthcare team, and NPD will need to ensure that the patient is included in designing and delivering professional development activities. While nurses have long been the "voice of the patient" in the healthcare setting, patients should now become a member of the planning team for an educational activity, sharing first-hand experiences of a disease process or treatment interventions to ensure these perspectives are included in the activity. In addition, future CPD will see healthcare providers and patients learning together to facilitate communication and to improve health literacy and informed choices. Programs such as the Promise Project and the Wellbeing Series offer a glimpse into the future of NPD in integrative healthcare.

PROFESSIONAL DEVELOPMENT BASED ON AN IDENTIFIED GAP

Participating in professional development activities should result in improved knowledge, skills, and abilities to provide safe, high-quality patient care; to teach or mentor others to provide safe, high-quality care; and to provide leadership for the nursing profession. It is essential, then, that professional development activities be designed to address gaps that may exist between a nurse's current state of practice and the desired state or outcome of practice, regardless of the practice setting. Rather than planning generic programs that meet the broad needs of a large audience, CPD may be more uniquely focused on specific goals and objectives that individual nurses require to provide safe, high-quality care. Therefore, mechanisms that encourage and facilitate the development of individualized CPD programs of study must be developed. For the integrative nurse who is seeking to satisfy his or her professional development needs, that would mean thinking creatively about carving a professional path forward.

FINDING VALUE IN SELF-REFLECTION AS A METHOD OF PROFESSIONAL DEVELOPMENT

Historically, professional development activities have been focused on knowledge or skills acquisition. While it is important to ensure that nurses have the requisite knowledge and skills, self-reflection has often been overlooked as an evidence-based method of improving healthcare quality and safety. The challenge for NPD will be to develop innovative ways not only to foster appreciative inquiry and reflective practice, but also to provide recognition and award credit within existing continuing-education systems. Issues needing to be addressed include developing outcomes that are measureable, reliable, and valid, as well as demonstrating improvement in patient-centered outcomes that result from engaging in self-reflection.

Conclusions

Florence Nightingale began promoting nursing professional development over 150 years ago. Today, the evolution continues; from discipline-centric, provider-directed educational activities to new models that include more patient-focused, team-based education delivered via multi-modal formats with increased emphasis on self-reflection, and the future of the nursing profession is promising. Integrative nursing is at the heart of this evolution, helping nurses focus on competently caring in a meaning-based practice arena that promotes the wellbeing of both nurses and patients.

SELECTED REFERENCES

American Nurses Association and National Nursing Staff Development Organization. (2010). *Nursing Professional Development: Scope and Standards of Practice*. Silver Spring, MD: Nursesbooks.org.

Greiner, A. C., & Knebel, E., Eds. (2003). *Health Professions Education: A Bridge to Quality*. Washington, DC: The National Academies Press.

Institute of Medicine of the National Academies. (2009). *Redesigning Continuing Education in the Health Professions*. Washington, DC: Committee on Planning a Continuing Healthcare Professional Education Institute.

Institute of Medicine of the National Academies. (2010). *The Future of Nursing*. Washington, DC: Committee on the Robert Wood Johnson Foundation Initiative on the Future of Nursing, at the Institute of Medicine.

Interprofessional Education Collaborative Expert Panel. (2011). *Core Competencies for Interprofessional Collaborative Practice: Report of an Expert Panel*. Washington, D.C.: Interprofessional Education Collaborative.

Miller, G.E. (1990). The assessment of clinical skills/competence/performance. *Academic Medicine, 65*(9), S63–S67.

Moore, D. E., Green, J. S., & Gallis, H. A. (2009). Achieving desired results and improved outcomes: integrating planning and assessment throughout learning activities. *Journal of Continuing Education in the Health Professions*, 29(1), 1–15.

National Council of State Boards of Nursing. *Guiding Principles*. Retrieved from https://www.ncsbn.org/1325.htm

U.S. Department of Education (2013). Accreditation and Quality Assurance. Available at: http://www.ed.gov/ (last accessed April 18, 2013).

34

Integrative Nursing and Health Literacy

BONNIE L. WESTRA, ELIZABETH FINE WEINFURTER, AND CONNIE W. DELANEY

Health literacy is "the degree to which an individual has the capacity to obtain, communicate, process, and understand basic health information and services to make appropriate health decisions" (Centers for Disease Control and Prevention, 2011). The Institute of Medicine (IOM) found that engagement of consumers in their health management is essential and requires health literacy skills to understand and manage health information (Agarwal & Khuntia, 2009; Bipartisan Policy Center, 2012; Institute of Medicine, 2004; Institute of Medicine, 2009; Institute of Medicine, 2011). Health literacy skills are essential in order to find, understand, and choose appropriate treatments and practitioners whether they are conventional or within the realm of integrative health and medicine. According to Pew's *Mobile Health 2012* report, about 45% of U.S. adults use smartphones, and 19% of these smartphone users have applications to help them monitor or manage their health (Dolan, 2012). Respondents used smartphones to track their exercise, heart rate, diet or food, and their weight. Smartphones were used to look up health information and manage both medical crises and chronic conditions (Fox, 2010). The increasing use of the Internet and related technologies require multiple types of health literacy skills, including digital literacy.

According to the IOM 2004 report on health literacy, half of all American adults—approximately 90 million—are challenged by reading and understanding complex health information, such as insurance forms or medication labels. Persons 60 and older have a higher prevalence of low health literacy (Zamora & Clingerman, 2011), and nearly nine out of ten adults with health disparities may have low health literacy rates (Agency for Healthcare Research and Quality, 2008). Low health literacy may be due to lack of education, learning disabilities, cognitive declines, limited computer/Internet access, or having English as a second language (National Network of Libraries of Medicine, 2011).

Consequence of Low Health Literacy

Low health literacy is associated with poorer health outcomes and higher costs of care (Berkman et al., 2011; Evangelista et al., 2010). Consumers need an adequate level of health literacy to make informed healthcare decisions, such as whether to try acupuncture to treat pain associated with migraine headaches. Limited health literacy affects people's ability to find and use health information, adhere to treatments, take medications safely, receive preventive services, modify their behaviors towards health, or act on public health alerts (Ancker, Kern, Abramson, & Kaushal, 2012). Approximated costs related to low health literacy range from $106 billion to $238 billion annually, representing 7%–17% of all personal healthcare expenditures (Wolf & Bailey, 2009). These costs are associated with delayed diagnosis and treatment for illnesses, increased utilization of health services, and difficulties with adherence to remedies for managing health problems (Weiss et al., 2005). Costs also could be related to poor decisions related to integrative therapy.

Health Literacy Competencies

Health literacy is a complex multidimensional issue and involves more than reading skills. Health literacy also requires the ability to interpret medical and health language and apply it to one's own specific health status. There are variations in the dimensions identified for health literacy competencies. Common dimensions of health literacy include:

- Oral literacy (speaking and listening)
- Print/visual literacy (writing and reading, understanding graphical and visual information)
- Information literacy (obtaining and applying relevant information)
- Numeracy (the ability to calculate or reason with numbers)
- Computer/digital literacy (operating a computer or information device)

(Per the National Network of Libraries of Medicine, 2011; U.S. Department of Health and Human Services, 2012.) The last three are less-known areas; therefore, information literacy, numeracy, and computer/digital literacy are addressed in this chapter.

Information literacy is defined as the set of skills needed to find, retrieve, analyze, and use information (Association of College and Research Libraries, 2012). An example is a consumer with insomnia. The search results for "CAM and sleep" on the National Center for Complementary and Alternative Medicine's (NCCAM) website provide many alternatives for the treatment of sleep. But what are the skills required for consumers to effectively evaluate integrative therapies and choose the ones that are best for them (Long, 2009)? There is emerging interest in finding out how information literacy, and more specifically critical health literacy, relates to integrative health and medicine. A qualitative study was conducted to create a framework exemplifying critical health literacy for CAM (Long, 2009). The critical health literacy framework for CAM emerged from CAM clients and practitioners in three European countries. Long found that for CAM to be effective for self-management, advice-giving needed to occur within a supportive environment and relationship, and clients needed to be open to change and committed to maintaining their health. The philosophy of CAM is congruent with critical health literacy.

Health numeracy is the use of quantitative information for making health decisions, managing health, and adhering to treatments and procedures (Golbeck, Ahlers-Schmidt, Paschal, & Dismuke, 2005; Schapira et al., 2008). Numeracy ranges from basic mathematical skills, such as counting or calculating, to application and interpretation of numerical data for health situations. For example, the most basic numerical skill may be counting pills from a medication bottle or correctly using information such as dates, time, phone numbers, and addresses for scheduling appointments. More complex numeracy skills are involved when patients evaluate the effectiveness and costs of treatments, such as comparing conventional medical care with integrative therapies for neurological conditions (Wells, Phillips, Schachter, & McCarthy, 2010). Comparing survival curves of different treatments—such as chemotherapy, Chinese medicine, or nutritional treatments for cancer—has been found to be more challenging for people with low numeracy skills (Rakow, Wright, Bull, & Spiegelhalter, 2012).

Computer/digital literacy related to health is defined as the ability to find and apply health information from a variety of electronic sources. The availability of health information through electronic media and the Web has grown exponentially. Particularly important is the ability to apply criteria to determine if a website is credible or access personal health information electronically. Consequently, health literacy is impacted by the level of computer literacy of patients, clients, and the general population.

Assessing Health Literacy

Several tools exist that assess various dimensions of health literacy (Mancuso, 2009). Clinicians are especially interested in assessment tools that can be administered quickly. Several useful options for assessing health literacy are shown in Table 34.1.

To evaluate information literacy, providers may choose to observe for clinical "red flags" that may suggest a patient has limited literacy (American Medical Association, 2007; Ancker & Kaufman, 2007; Osborne, 2013). These red flags include the following behaviors:

- Identifying medications by looking at the pills, rather than reading the labels.
- When given written information, making an excuse such as "I forgot my glasses, can you read this to me?" or "I have a headache, I'll read this when I get home."

Table 34.1: Information Literacy Assessment Tools

METER (Medical Term Recognition Test) (Rawson et al., 2010)	This self-administered test presents patients with a list comprising both real and made-up medical terms. The patient is asked to mark the terms that are real medical terms. The test takes about two minutes to complete. The instrument measures information literacy and is available in the appendix at http://www.ncbi.nlm.nih.gov/pmc/articles/PMC2811598/.
Rapid Estimate of Adult Literacy in Medicine— Short Form (REALM-SF) (Arozullah et al., 2007)	This tool is a seven-item word recognition test based on the 66-item Rapid Estimate of Adult Literacy in Medicine (REALM) that measures patients' recognition of common medical words. Clinicians score and assess a patient's health literacy level in 1–2 minutes. Patients are asked to read seven words out loud, and clinicians score the number correctly pronounced. A drawback to this test is that it must be administered and scored with the clinician present, and low-literacy patients may be embarrassed at having difficulty pronouncing words (Osborne, 2013). This instrument is available at http://www.nchealthliteracy.org/instruments.html.
Short Assessment of Health Literacy for Spanish Adults (SAHLSA-50) (Lee, Stucky, Lee, Rozier, & Bender, 2010)	The Short Assessment of Health Literacy for Spanish Adults (SAHLSA-50) is a validated health literacy assessment tool containing 50 items designed to assess a Spanish-speaking adult's ability to read and understand common medical terms. The SAHLSA was based on the Rapid Estimates of Adult Literacy in Medicine (REALM). This instrument is available at: http://www.ahrq.gov/populations/sahlsatool.htm
Newest Vital Sign (NVS) (Weiss et al., 2005)	This tool is a bilingual (English and Spanish) screening tool that can be administered in approximately three minutes. The patient is given a label from an ice cream container and is asked six questions about how they would interpret and make decisions based on the information presented. The test assesses basic numeric and literacy skills related to health information, and is available at http://www.pfizerhealthliteracy.com/physicians-providers/NewestVitalSign.aspx.
University of Minnesota Computer Literacy	This website includes an assessment of an individual's general technology skills, including the ability to operate a computer, use e-mail and Internet, use word processing software, and create and manipulate spreadsheets, databases, and graphic files. It is available at: http://www.d.umn.edu/kmc/student/loon/acad/ComputLit.html.
Nursing Informatics Self-Test	Nursing Informatics Self-Test on technical competencies provides an overview of critical computer technology skills for nurses, but they also can apply to consumers as well. This instrument is available at: http://nursing-informatics.com/niassess/tests.html.

- Incompletely or incorrectly filled out forms.
- Asking family members to read written material aloud.
- Not knowing names of medications or what they are for.

These behaviors do not necessarily indicate that a patient has low literacy, but they are useful signs for clinicians to notice.

Improving Health Literacy

Much health information is presented as text, whether on the Internet or in printed form. For individuals with limited literacy, dyslexia, or simply a different learning style, it is essential for clinicians to use educational materials that are not text-based. Investigators have shown that visual aids, combined with written or spoken words, improve patients' understanding and recall of health information (Houts, Doak, Doak, & Loscalzo, 2006; Katz, Kripalani, & Weiss, 2006). Many of the patient health sites listed in Table 34.2 contain illustrations, videos, and more to give patients a different way to learn about health information. Medline Plus (online) offers a section called "Videos and Cool Tools" that contains interactive tutorials of diseases and conditions, tests and diagnostic procedures, surgery and treatment procedures, and prevention and wellness. The section also offers animated anatomy videos, surgery videos, and games to help patients learn and assess their knowledge.

INFORMATION LITERACY

There are two major categories of interventions providers can use to improve health literacy. The first is referring patients to reliable sources of information and educating them about the need to think critically about the source of information. The second category is creating and providing information at an appropriate level for patients.

Reliable Sources of Information

The Internet is an excellent source of health information, but it also has many unreliable sources and websites. For example, a Google search for "Alzheimer's treatment" lists over 6.6 million results, and even though much of that information may be credible, it is overwhelming to know where to start. To help patients find reliable information quickly without getting overwhelmed or attracted to websites requiring money, refer them to a few of the best general patient-health sources listed in Table 34.2.

There are thousands of reliable, patient-friendly, topic- or audience-specific websites on the Internet. To make it easier to find the best sources, many libraries and other health organizations maintain portals of links to consumer health information based on specific topics. One example is the University of Minnesota Health Sciences Libraries' Resources for Personal Health site (http://hsl.lib.umn.edu/personalhealth). The site is maintained by a librarian with a specialization in Consumer Health Information from the Medical Library Association (Medical Library Association, 2012).

In addition to providing health information, there are many tools to help consumers evaluate health information on the Internet (Table 34.3). The MedlinePlus Guide to Healthy Surfing (http://www.nlm.nih.gov/medlineplus/healthywebsurfing.html) organizes this essential information-literacy skill into specific steps to evaluate websites;

Table 34.2: Reliable Patient Health Internet Resources

Statistics on CAM National Health Interview Survey	The Centers for Disease Control, National Health Interview Survey includes a section on CAM. Available at: http://nccam.nih.gov/news/camstats/NHIS.htm.
Taking Charge of Your Health	University of Minnesota's Center for Spirituality and Healing and the Life Science Foundation have created a website that provides reliable information about alternative and integrative health practices. Available at: www.takingcharge.csh.umn.edu.
Cancer.gov	Hosted by the National Cancer Institute, the site provides information on different types of cancers, treatments, clinical trials, and more. One section includes integrative therapies. The site is for patients and their families, as well as healthcare providers. Available at: http://cancer.gov/.
MedlinePlus	Commercial-free, reliable, free health information from the National Library of Medicine including health topics, drug information, health news, medical encyclopedia and dictionary, interactive tutorials, and more. Available at: http://www.nlm.nih.gov/medlineplus/.
Kidshealth	The Nemours Foundation's Center for Children's Health provides sites for parents, children, and teens containing current information (in English and Spanish) about child development, nutrition and fitness, preventive health care, and diseases and conditions. Available at: http://kidshealth.org/.
NIH Senior Health	From the National Institutes of Health, this site provides information on many topics from cancer to mental health and is specifically designed for older adults, with features such as enlarged text and audio. Available at: http://nihseniorhealth.gov/.
Ethnomed	A joint program of the University of Washington Health Sciences Libraries and Harborview Medical Center, this site includes patient education materials on topics ranging from immunizations to asthma to smoking and more. It provides information in several languages, including Hmong and Somali. Available at: http://ethnomed.org/.
Healthy Roads Media	This site was created by Healthy Roads Media with support from the National Library of Medicine and others, and provides education materials in a number of languages and a variety of formats (including videos, handouts, and audio). Available at: http://healthyroadsmedia.org/.

specific teaching points for each skill are also given on the website. If there are concerns about particular websites, consumers should consult with their health provider.

Patient Education Material

Because there is so much excellent material already available through both Internet sources and institutional sources, providers rarely need to "reinvent the wheel." An example can be found at "Taking Charge of Your Health" (http://www.takingcharge.csh.umn.edu). However, if development is needed, there are many books and Internet resources that can help providers develop appropriate patient education materials. The basic principles of these resources align with good verbal techniques for

Table 34.3: Criteria for Evaluating Health Information on the Internet

Criteria	Evaluation Questions/ Issues
Consider the source	Use recognized authorities. Know who is responsible for the content.
Focus on quality	All websites are not created equal. Does the site have an editorial board? Is the information reviewed before it is posted?
Be a cyberskeptic	Quackery abounds on the Internet. Does the site make health claims that seem too good to be true? Does the information use deliberately obscure, "scientific" sounding language? Does it promise quick, dramatic, miraculous results? Is this the only site making these claims?
Look for the evidence	Rely on medical research, not opinion. Does the site identify the author? Does it rely on testimonials?
Check for currency	Look for the latest information. Is the information current?
Beware of bias	What is the purpose? Who is providing the funding? Who pays for the site?
Protect your privacy	Health information should be confidential. Does the site have a privacy policy and tell you what information they collect?

communicating with patients, and are shown in Table 34.4 (U.S. National Library of Medicine, 2011).

NUMERACY

The design of numerical information can influence comprehension and decision-making. One recommendation to increase understanding of numerical data is attending to consistent use of numbers and their meaning. Higher numbers should indicate higher quality of care, rather than lower numbers (Peters, Dieckmann, Dixon, Hibbard, & Mertz, 2007). A good example of using higher numbers to represent higher quality for integrative health modalities is shown in Table 34.5. Each column represents a different agency, and higher percentages represent better quality care.

In addition to having higher numbers represent better quality, displaying only essential data in tables improves comprehension, particularly for those with low numerical literacy (Greene, Peters, Mertz, & Hibbard, 2008; Peters et al., 2007). An example of a site that displays only essential information is Medicare's comparison of health savings plans (http://www.medicare.gov/Publications/Pubs/pdf/11206.pdf). Only the four most important questions are displayed in the table, followed by text explanations, shown in Table 34.6.

In addition to tables, pictographs are used to improve comprehension (Tait, Zikmund-Fisher, Fagerlin, & Voepel-Lewis, 2010). An example of a pictograph is shown in Figure 34.1, which represents the proportions of food by food groups recommended for a healthy diet.

Table 34.4: Basic Principles for Educational Material

Principle	Explanation
Know your target audience.	Consider reading level, cultural background and attitudes, age group, and English language proficiency (ELP).
Determine objectives and outcomes.	What do you want your target audience to learn? For example, if your objective is to show the proper use of asthma inhalers, emphasize the outcome of their proper use. A sample sentence might be: "Following the directions for your asthma inhaler may help you breathe easier."
Keep it simple.	Keep within a range of about a fourth- to sixth- grade reading level. Find alternatives for complex words, medical jargon, abbreviations, and acronyms. When no alternatives are available, spell complex terms and abbreviations phonetically and give clear definitions. Keep most sentences short. Use varied sentence length to make them interesting, but keep sentences simple.
Focus on key concepts.	Use bolded subheadings to separate and highlight document sections.
Be clear.	Use a clear topic sentence at the beginning of each paragraph. Follow the topic sentence with details and examples. For example, "Proper use of asthma inhalers helps you breathe better. Here are reasons why." Then give reasons. Examples and stories may help engage readers.
Personalize messages.	Use the "you" attitude. Personalization helps the reader understand what he or she is supposed to do.
Emphasize benefits.	Emphasize benefits of adopting the desired behavior. For example, "Following these directions will help you get enough medicine from the inhaler."
Check assumptions.	Do not make assumptions about people who read at a low level. Maintain an adult perspective. Many who are challenged by English are extremely fluent in a different first language.
Be consistent.	Be consistent with terms. For example, don't use "drugs" and "medications" interchangeably in the same document.
Maintain a positive message.	When possible, say things positively, not negatively. For example, use "Eat less red meat" instead of "Don't eat lots of red meat."
Use visual displays.	Use pictures and photos with close, concise captions Avoid graphs and charts unless they actually help understanding. Balance the use of text, graphics, and white space.
Consider formatting.	Use upper and lower case letters rather than all capital letters. When possible, use graphics or spell out fractions and percentages.
Keep a consistent writing style.	Use the active voice and vivid verbs. Structure the material logically. Some users prefer step-by-step instructions. Others may find concepts arranged from the general to the specific easier to understand.

Table 34.5: Sample Presentation of Quality Information for Integrative Health Consumers

Agency A	Agency B	Agency C	Minnesota Average	National Average
Does the provider listen to your needs and concerns?				
94%	96%	97%	95%	97%
For patients with back pain, how effective was the treatment received?				
85%	83%	69%	80%	80%
How satisfied are you with the length of time it takes to get an appointment?				
85%	83%	69%	80%	80%
For patients with heart disease, the provider gave options that were consistent with my preferences and lifestyle to lower my cholesterol.				
78%	98%	68%	80%	80%

Table 34.6: Display of Table Information Comparing Four Most Important Questions

	Plan A	Plan B
Yearly Deposit	$2,500	$1,500
Yearly Deductible	$4,000	$3,000
What You Pay after the Deductible	0%	0%
Out of Pocket Maximum	$4,000 same as deductible	$3,000 same as deductible

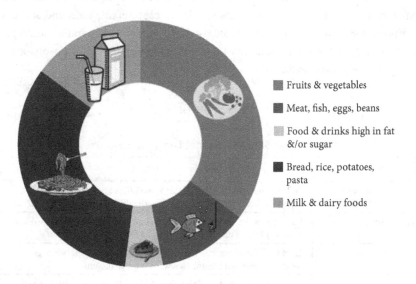

Fruits & vegetables

Meat, fish, eggs, beans

Food & drinks high in fat &/or sugar

Bread, rice, potatoes, pasta

Milk & dairy foods

FIGURE 34.1 Example of pictograph

Table 34.7: Computer Literacy Online Training Resources

Resource	URL
University of Minnesota—Twin Cities	Computer living and problem-solving: http://www.cehd.umn.edu/PsTL/DougRobertson/ODL/PsTL1571v8StudyGuidePart1.pdf
University of Minnesota—Duluth	Computer literacy: http://www.d.umn.edu/kmc/student/loon/acad/ComputLit.html
University Laboratory High School Library	Online computer literacy course that addresses "netiquette," copyright, online catalog and database exercises, search tools, website evaluation, and survey of Internet use: http://www.uni.illinois.edu/library/computerlit/index.php
Microsoft Office Training	Online modules for Microsoft Office products: http://office.microsoft.com/en-us/training-FX101782702.aspx

COMPUTER LITERACY

There are many resources that provide training in computer literacy, including community education, community colleges and university classes, books, and online resources. Examples of online classes, modules, or tutorials are shown in Table 34.7.

Providers and consumers alike are increasingly seeking information from websites and using smartphone applications ("apps") to manage their health. The Internet offers new opportunities for learning, as shown in Table 34.8.

The increasing use of the Internet and smartphone apps requires information and digital literacy skills, as well as numeracy skills, to capture, integrate, and accurately interpret information to optimize the value of the information. Integrative health practitioners may want to think about how they can take advantage of these evolving tools to improve health and wellbeing.

Table 34.8: Sample Internet Learning Resources

Resource	URL
Podcasts on Health Literacy Out Loud	Podcasts on Health Literacy Out Loud offers audio interviews with experts in health literacy. http://www.healthliteracyoutloud.com/
Body+Soul	Practitioners of yoga, tai chi, or meditation can find smartphone apps to support these practices. http://www.bodyandsoul.com.au/
MyFitnessPal	Tracks food and exercise and helps the user develop personal goals for weight management. http://www.myfitnesspal.com/
FitBit	Tracks exercise, diet, and sleeping. FitBit can connect with a smart scale and a computer or mobile device and graphically display information for managing health. http://www.fitbit.com/

Summary

In conclusion, health literacy is a major problem in the United States, with dire consequences for health. Health literacy is multidimensional concept with standard and valid assessment tools available. Often information literacy and numeracy are assessed with the same tool, while computer literacy is separately assessed. Resources are available, including significant research and interventions for consumers with and without problems in health literacy. Wise assessment and use of these resources are essential.

SELECTED REFERENCES

Agarwal, R., & Khuntia, J. (2009). *Personal Health Information and the Design of Consumer Health Information Technology: Background Report.* (Prepared by Insight Policy Research under Contract No. HHSA290200710072T). (No. AHRQ Publication No.09-0075-EF). Rockville, MN: Agency for Healthcare Research and Quality.

Ancker, J. S., Kern, L. M., Abramson, E., & Kaushal, R. (2012). The Triangle Model for evaluating the effect of health information technology on healthcare quality and safety. *Journal of the American Medical Informatics Association, 19*(1), 61–65.

Association of College and Research Libraries. (2012). Introduction to Information Literacy. Retrieved April 20, 2012, from http://www.ala.org/acrl/issues/infolit/overview/intro.

Berkman, N. D., Sheridan, S. L., Donahue, K. E., Halpern, D. J., Viera, A., Crotty, K., et al. (2011). *Health Literacy Interventions and Outcomes: An Updated Systematic Review.* (Evidence Report/Technology Assessment No. 199.) Rockville, MD: Agency for Healthcare Research and Quality.

Institute of Medicine. (2004). *Health Literacy: A Prescription to End Confusion.* Washington, DC: National Academies Press.

Institute of Medicine. (2009). *Measures of Health Literacy: Workshop Summary.* Washington, DC: The National Academies Press.

Institute of Medicine. (2011). *Improving Health Literacy Within a State: Workshop Summary.* Washington, DC: The National Academies Press.

Mancuso, J. M. (2009). Assessment and measurement of health literacy: An integrative review of the literature. *Nursing & Health Sciences, 11*(1), 77–89. doi:10.1111/j.1442-2018.2008.00408.x

Osborne, H. (2013). Assessing health literacy. In *Health Literacy from A to Z* (pp. 9–14). Burlington, MA: Jones & Bartlett Learning.

Zamora, H., & Clingerman, E. M. (2011). Health literacy among older adults: A systematic literature review. *Journal of Gerontological Nursing, 37*(10), 41–51. doi:http://dx.doi.org/10.3928/00989134-20110503-02

VI

Integrative Nursing: Global Perspectives—State of the Practice

35

Integrative Nursing in Germany

RANIER AMMENDE AND RENATE TEWES

Overview of Nursing and Healthcare

The history of nursing in Germany is long, and punctuated by persistent struggles to gain political influence, autonomy, and control of its destiny as profession. Prior to the sixteenth century, the profession was dominated by Roman Catholic and subsequently, by Lutheran religious orders. Secularization began in the nineteenth century with the rise of modern hospital systems and the Red Cross. With this fundamental shift from a religious to a modern scientific paradigm, the struggle for autonomy, definition of roles, and creation of a distinct knowledge accelerated. At the beginning of the twentieth century, the first German Nursing Association was founded and participated in the International Council of Nursing (ICN). In 1907, the first Act of Parliament regulating nursing in Germany was passed. World War I, the rise and fall of the Third Reich, World War II, and the division of Germany from 1945 to 1989 disrupted the development of nursing in Germany. Hilde Steppe (2011) described in her work on the history of German nursing the crippling impact of the wars and the influence of the ruling ideologies during these times.

The founding of the European Community and the European Union's Directive regulating healthcare professions in its member states supported the development of nursing and training in Germany. The Acts of Parliament regulating nursing education in 1985 and in 2003 were major steps that forced Germany to catch up with international developments of nursing in the EU. In the 1960s, East Germany introduced academic programs to prepare nurses, nurse educators, and nurse management. After the reunification, academic programs to educate nurses were implemented in many universities of applied sciences and some universities (www.pflegestudium.de). Nursing science develops and underpins the professionalization of nursing in Germany, yet funding for nursing research projects is very difficult to obtain. Established scientific communities of other professions have been most successful in garnering funds to support their research efforts.

Nursing has continued to proceed in developing its own domain and body of knowledge. The first translations of nursing theories from Great Britain and the United

States led to a dialogue about the redefinition and domain of nursing in Germany, from Virginia Henderson's definition of nursing in the 1950s, to the nursing model of Roper, Logan, and Tierney in 1988. In the 1980s, publishing houses in Germany and Switzerland started translating books on nursing from English into German at a large scale, and the number of nursing journals increased. In psychiatric nursing, the nursing theory of Hildegard Peplau was introduced and is still widely used.

There are multiple pathways to enter the nursing profession in Germany. Nurse aides complete one year of basic vocational training at a school of nursing following their ninth year of basic education. After ten years of basic education, students can pursue vocational training focusing in pediatrics, adult nursing, or geriatrics. (The pediatric and geriatric training is not fully EU recognized.) The entry requirement for the bachelor of nursing science degree is twelve years of schooling. Completion of the program takes four and a half years as it includes both a full academic program along with vocational nurse training. Academic programs to prepare teachers and managers are at the bachelor's and master's level. Master's programs focusing on advanced nursing practice are just being established.

As there is no registration of nurses in Germany yet, statistics are not very reliable. However, estimates show there were approximately 1.2 million nurses employed (all levels of preparation) in 2011. In 2011, there were approximately 60,000 nursing students in basic vocational training for adult nursing, 6,500 nursing students in basic vocational training for pediatric care, 52,000 nursing students in basic vocational training for geriatric care, and 6,500 students at universities of applied sciences earning a bachelor of nursing science degree to qualify for bedside nursing (*Bund-Län der-Arbeitsgruppe-Eckpunkte-Papier*, 2012).

In October 2011, the Gemeinsamer Bundesausschuss (G-BA) published a list of responsibilities in patient care that will be transferred from physicians to nurses, under the approval of the German Ministry of Health. Nurses will now be able to determine the length and need for home care and prescribe nursing items and materials needed for wound dressings. They will have extended competencies in the care of people suffering from chronic diseases as dementia, high blood pressure, and diabetes mellitus. Educational programs are needed to accommodate this shift of responsibility.

At present, the government also plans a reform of nursing education, introducing training for the "nurse responsible for general care," replacing the three basic nurse trainings used presently. This reform will be another step to catch up with EU standards. Yet politicians of all parties oppose the modernization of the EU Directive regarding new entry requirements for nursing education.

Since 1883 the healthcare system in Germany has been based on a compulsory insurance system. The federal government sets out the regulating framework for the health system. Approximately 91% of the population is insured with the compulsory insurance system; about 9% of the population take out private insurance or pay out of their own pocket (these options depend on a certain level of private income). Because of a decreasing working population, in 2010, Germany passed legislation to add state revenue to cover the cost of the healthcare system. The introduction of the German Diagnostic Related Groups (DRGs), demographic changes, and technical and medical innovations led to a more competitive system. There are currently 2,064 hospitals with 502,749 beds and an average length of stay of 7.9 days. It is understood that costs need to be drastically reduced, beds closed, and the average length of stay shortened. The aging population of Germany needs more efficient home care and nursing homes, as well as rehabilitative and health-promoting concepts. In 2010, Germany spent approximately 290 billion Euros in the healthcare system. Legislation setting a debt limit to cut federals spending will increase the pressure to reform the system.

In 2010, Germany developed an agenda of national health goals. These are

- Reducing diabetes mellitus type 2
- Reducing the mortality rate of women with breast cancer
- Reducing smoking
- Growing up healthy
- Increasing health competency of the population, empowerment of patients
- Decreasing depression
- Healthy aging

(Source: Bundesministerium für Gesundheit 2013)

These goals indicate less dominance by the medical model, and a tendency to re-empower the population, so that the people will regain more control over their own health issues. This will also save resources. Consumer protection and patient rights gain importance. This development is a challenge to the nursing profession in Germany, which did not actively participate in defining these goals, but now has the chance to create relevant nursing services for the population.

Integrative Nursing in Germany

HILDEGARD OF BINGEN

A variety of holistic and integrative healing methods are practiced throughout Germany. The famous saint and nun Hildegard von Bingen (1089–1179) experimented in medieval times with herbs and developed many recipes and special diets for different illnesses. Her work anticipated many of the concepts and principles of integrative nursing, including the idea that human beings are complex adaptive systems who are inseparable from their environment and that nature has healing and restorative properties. The idea of offering herbs and nutrition is consistent with the modern-day principle of integrative nursing that focuses on beginning with the least-intensive therapeutic modalities (von Bingen, 1151).

Interest in the mystic Hildegard von Bingen and her rich knowledge about holistic nursing care is now experiencing a renaissance. For example, the Hospital of Natural Healing in Munich (Krankenhaus für Naturheilweisen) uses some herbs (like Galgant) and methods (like bloodletting) that were described by von Bingen (www.focus.de). Nurses in this hospital participate in holistic treatments of patients and continue to use the same type of herbal packs as were first used in the Middle Ages.

ROSEN BODYWORK

Marion Rosen was born in Nuremberg in 1914 and developed a relaxation method in the 1940s that included bodywork, breathing, and movement. As she was a Jew, she fled to Berkeley, California, during the time of the Nazi regime, which is why today there are Rosen Centers in both Berkeley and Germany. It takes five years to train to be a certified Rosen Practitioner (www.rosenmethod.com). Nurses are using this method, but not in hospital settings.

AROMATHERAPY

The German nurse Maria Hoch (born 1957) developed a concept of aromatherapy and implemented it in the hospital in Munich where she worked as the chief nurse executive. She also offers educational programs for nurses (www.aroma-forum-international. de). Aromatherapy is very well received in German nursing. Many hospitals and caring homes use essential oils for room ventilation, massage, bed baths, applications, and herbal packs. Aromatherapy's uses are diverse and include beneficial relaxation or stimulation for body and soul; antipyretic and antiseptic treatment; and prophylaxis of thrombosis, pneumonia, pressure sores, ulcer, thrush, and parotitis (Price, 2012). Aromatherapy is also used with fungus infections, to promote pain relief, in wound management, and for different types of insomnia (Zimmermann, 1998). Nurses very often use essential oils in palliative and end-of-life care (www.hospiz-und-palliativmedizin.de). The German law allows the treatment of physical and psychological diseases with essential oils only by physicians and naturopaths (*Heilpraktiker*). Nevertheless, everyone is authorized to use aromatherapy for relaxation, wellness, and preventive healthcare. Education on aromatherapy is most often offered as training on the job and can last from two to six months. This method is less invasive, is aligned with the view that nature is a healer, and aromatherapy reaches not only the body, but also the spirit and mind.

SPAS AND THERMAL BATHS

Nowadays Bad Wörishofen (the *Bad* means "spa") is still popular for its spas and rehabilitation clinics. Nurses play an important role in offering water treatments to patients.

Furthermore, the concepts of the Bavarian priest and hydrotherapist Sebastian Kneipp are becoming popular in kindergarten, like the "Kneipp-Kita" in Dresden (www. kita.de). Children in these kindergartens are less often ill compared to children of other nurseries (www.kneipbund.de). A particular Kneipp concept that is often used is "walking barefoot in the morning dew on the grass," which is said to balance the immune system. In German nursing, the Kneipp concept is mainly used in rehabilitation as a less invasive therapy. The focus is on nature's ability to offer healing and restorative properties.

BASAL STIMULATION

Andreas Fröhlich and Christel Bienstein developed the method of "basal stimulation" for nursing (Fröhlich & Bienstein, 2003), which activates perception, stimulates body and movement experiences, and is a way of communicating with patients who are severely ill. This includes patients with craniocerebral trauma, hemiplegia, coma patients, or people with apallic syndrome.

Basal stimulation can stimulate all senses by touch (tactile, haptic), with colored light (visual), music (auditory), tasty meals (gustatory), using fragrances (olfactory), or a waterbed with loud speakers to experiencing the rhythms of music (vibration). The goals of this intervention vary and include relaxation reduction of anxiety, the establishment of a new body image, coordination of movement, enhancing the individual's experience of his or her own body, and fostering security and trust. This method has also been successfully implemented in intensive care units as a way to foster weaning (Nydahl & Bartoszek, 2003).

Basal stimulation is very well known in German nursing and part of basic vocational training. Research by Heimerl et al. (2010) showed that basal stimulation not only changes the nurse–patient communication but also influences the attitude of the organizational culture, process, and structure. Furthermore, Isfort et al. (2008) emphasized the positive impact of basal stimulation on premature babies if used by their parents. This less-invasive intervention is based on the person-centered relationship between the nurse and the patient. It activates the individual's innate capacity for health and wellbeing and emphasizes the idea that humans are inseparable from the environment.

NEURO-DEVELOPMENT TREATMENT

In 1943, physiotherapist Berta Bobath and her husband, neurologist and pediatrician Karel Bobath, developed the "Bobath concept." In English, this concept is called "neuro-developmental-treatment" (NDT). The NDT approach is used in the management and treatment of patients (children and adults) with central nervous system pathophysiologies. The basic assumption of NDT is that the damaged brain can be compensated by developing new synapses achieved by passive movement of paralyzed extremities.

NDT is not a set of methods to be used in the same way for all patients with brain impairments, but is a person-centered learning approach of position, handling, moving, and self-help (Dammshäuser, 2005). It is important to integrate the treatment into daily activities. NDT is most effective when the treatment is integrated into daily activities and used across all departments in a healthcare organization. For example, a patient who suffered a stroke is admitted to hospital and transferred to an ICU or stroke unit before moving on to a normal ward and then into a rehabilitation unit. If NDT is used continuously by all members of the healthcare team, the learning chances for the patient's brain increase (Lay, 2007). There is an international community of NDT members (www.ndty.org), but more evidence is needed to understand the efficacy of this approach on patient outcomes (Kollen et al., 2009). In Germany many hospitals offer trainings on NDT, and many nurses use this concept in their daily practice. This approach sees the human being as inseparable from the environment and having the innate capacity for health and wellbeing.

ANTHROPOSOPHIC NURSING

The term *anthroposophy* is from the Greek, meaning "the wisdom of the nature of man." This philosophy was founded by Rudolf Steiner (1861–1925). The central idea is the inner development of perceptive imagination, inspiration, and intuition to experience an objective spiritual world. The concept of free will is important and can be experienced by creative activity and independent thought (McDermott, 2007). Anthroposophical ideas have been applied in many areas including education, nursing, medicine, agriculture, architecture, and the arts (Heiner, 2010). Anthroposophical Societies have been established in fifty countries and about 10,000 institutions around the world (Grote, 2007).

In his *Theosophy* Steiner combines Christian ideas with Eastern tradition. Steiner speaks of reincarnation of the human spirit. He described some conditions that determine the interdependence of a person's life and his karma (Steiner, 1997). In nursing and medicine, his concepts of the human body play an important role. Beside the physical body and the ego, which anchor the faculty of self-awareness, he mentioned two more instances: the "life body," called the "etheric body," which nurtures, breathes, and grows the physical body; and the bearer of consciousness, called the "astral body" (Steiner, 2012).

These four bodies are all interconnected. In nursing it is important to focus on them all. In nursing assessment, the physical body is comprehensively described. Assessing the etheric body means describing the function of the seven life processes: nutrition, breathing, warming, circulation, maintenance, growth and maturation, and reproduction. The astral body is observed by watching prevailing mood, sympathies and antipathies, and behavior. Assessing the ego means focusing on biographical data, cultural and religious information, and state of consciousness (van der Star, 2010).

Besides the five senses of taste, smell, touch, sight, and hearing, anthroposophy offers seven more methods of perception: life, balance, self-movement, temperature/warmth, language, concept, and ego. The feeling of warmth is very important for identity (ego development) and does not just mean temperature, but also a warm and welcoming atmosphere. Anthroposophical nurses are trained to avoid hectic daily routines, to touch the patient gently, and to offer another blanket for those who tend to harden or stiffen, like people with cancer, diabetes, arteriosclerosis, or rheumatism. Some body parts loose warmth faster, like shoulders, the back, knees, kidneys, and feet. External applications in form of infusions, oils, and lotions are very helpful, as well as rhythmical body oiling (van der Star, 2010). Giving warmth and feeding the spirit can happen by showing motivation, idealism, enthusiasm, or by just being present. When the person feels sufficiently warm, the ego is able to open up for the outer world.

Based on the philosophies of Rudolf Steiner (1861–1925), anthroposophical nurse training covers the healing qualities of plants (e.g., teas and compresses), the theory and practice of holistic care, helping patients be responsible for their wellbeing, and exploring the individual meaning of illness with patients.

An example of an anthroposophical treatment is ginger, a medicinal plant used with patients with osteoarthritis. In a study by Black et al. (2010), it was shown that ginger is effective as a pain reliever for patients with osteoarthritis, though randomized controlled trials suggest that its effectiveness decreases after six weeks (Zahmatkash & Vafaeenasab, 2011).

Tessa Therkleson's phenomenological research on ginger-compress therapy for patients with osteoarthritis led to interesting results. Over a period of nine months, ten osteoarthritic patients received a hot ginger compress in kidney area for 30 minutes, which was followed by 20 minutes of rest. They recorded their pain by journaling and coloring human diagrams with red (warmth), blue (cold), and yellow (sensations).

The findings of this study identified seven responses to the ginger treatment: (1) meditative-like stillness and relaxation of thoughts, (2) constant penetrating warmth throughout the body, (3) positive change in thoughts, (4) increased energy and interest in the world, (5) deeply relaxed state that progressed to a gradual shift in pain and increased interest in others, (6) increased suppleness within the body, and (7) more comfortable, flexible joint mobility (Therkleson, 2010).

Central to the practice of anthroposophical nursing are the twelve "nursing gestures": creating space, relieving, nourishing, cleansing, protecting, confirming, enveloping, challenging, stimulating, awakening, balancing, and standing up/encouraging. Individual caregiving is based on common values anthroposophical nurses share. This goes along with respect for the dignity, the intact human core of patients despite their physical impairments, and ensuring privacy (Bopp & Heine, 2009).

Rhythmical body oiling is a well-established method in anthroposophical nursing. This technique of massaging in circles needs hands that touch without pushing, always keeping skin contact. Being present and staying connected with the patient is not just meant physically, but also psychologically and spiritually (Bertram, 2005). In his phenomenological research, Bertram (2005) found three patterns of reactions of patients after rhythmical oiling: solving, regaining the feeling of oneness, and gaining the ability to do something new.

One day after a breast removal, 44-year-old Mrs. Dierkes still felt too exhausted to meet her family members. In a conversation with the nurse, she was able to articulate her need for protection. Being a mother of two children (six and eight years), she used to be the caregiver of the family. The nurse decided to use the gesture of enveloping to bring Mrs. Dierkes a sense of safety and peace. First she used warming oil and gave her patient a foot massage. Research on reflexology shows a positive impact on fatigue (Lee et al., 2011). After the massage, the nurse helped Mrs. Dierkes dress herself and put a warm colored scarf around her shoulders. After brushing her hair, Mrs. Dierkes felt much better and was able to meet her family.

Herdecke Community Hospital in Germany has offered anthroposophical medicine and nursing since 1969. The hospital chose a non-hierarchical form of administration, which requires all members of the hospital to share the responsibility for making decisions (Schily, 2009). The entire work force is divided into self-organizing professional groups and a system of boards. This type of organization has proven flexible and encourages cooperation.

Challenges and Barriers to Integrative Nursing

Introducing integrative nursing in Germany is a slow process. To be able to offer integrative nursing, the profession needs to gain more autonomy in defining nursing and using complementary methods. The healthcare system in Germany focuses far more on physicians, their therapies, and prescriptions. The nursing profession needs more research to legitimize bringing integrative approaches into German nursing practice. Academically prepared nurses will be better positioned to conduct and disseminate research. The advancement of integrative nursing also requires that laws and regulations be changed so that integrative practices and complementary therapies are viewed as being sanctioned within the legally defined scope of practice.

Present healthcare legislation focuses on reducing costs and improving "efficiency." The lobbyists of the medical-industrial complex are very actively opposing cuts in their realms. The nursing profession needs to establish stronger political influence to have legislation and budgeting rules changed so that nursing has the time and personnel needed to offer integrative nursing. The compulsory health insurance system in Germany defines the treatments offered to the public, as well as their costs. Presently, additional treatments offered by physicians must be paid for privately by patients.

Over the centuries, a segment of the population in Germany preserved healing traditions that have not been embraced by the modern medical system. A great number of *Heilpraktiker* (naturopaths) offer complementary therapies to patients. A 1938 Act of Parliament regulates the therapies these providers can offer and defines which diseases can only be treated by physicians. After training in private schools, *Heilpraktikers* take exams with a board of physicians to obtain a license. Approximately 40%–50% of patients using the healthcare system in Germany also consult a *Heilpraktiker*, although they often pay for these services privately and do not tell their physicians about this additional treatment.

Other professions noted for offering complementary therapies are physiotherapy and midwifery. Most physiotherapists and midwives are working in their own practice and offer regular treatments prescribed by physicians and paid for by insurance companies, in addition to complementary therapies, if a customer is willing to pay for it.

Vision of Integrative Nursing in Germany

Heinrich Schipperges notes in his book *Der Garten der Gesundheit* ("The Garden of Health," 1994) that in the past, besides the "*res naturales*" (physiology), the "*res contra naturam*" (pathology), and "surgery and the *materia medica*" (pharmacy), the "*res non naturales*" (hygiene, the art of living and diet) played an important role in classical healing models. With the advent of modern science and modern medicine, the *res non naturales* was almost forgotten. The ancient holistic view of healthcare was kept alive, though, in models of care of the sick in monasteries, concentrating on activities of daily living. The best example of this is the life and work of Hildegard of Bingen, and in modern times, of the inspiring Liliane Juchli, a Swiss nun, teacher, and author of one of the most important textbooks on nursing in German language in the twentieth century.

The modern nursing profession in Germany will be able to merge a rich legacy of caring and healing traditions of the past and modern nursing science, and unfold a powerful caring-healing model for the benefit of the population. It will help reform the anachronistic system we are working in now.

It is a fact that with an aging population, a great increase of chronically ill people, decreasing tax revenue, and rising costs in health services, cuts of services will not solve the problems we face. Germany is changing into a multicultural society and is integrating large numbers of people with different conceptions of health and illness. Within the European Union, rules and regulations are being harmonized. Cross-border cooperations in healthcare systems are commonplace now, and insurance coverage is given within the EU. Health education in working environments and private lives is one central issue to be dealt with. Our highly developed medical-technical system will have to be used when necessary, and not used if not necessary. Integrative nursing will gain ground in Germany because the dominating medical-technical industry cannot solve the problems on its own. It loses control as people travel for treatments, use the Internet as a source of information, and explore different healing practices.

The increasing number of nursing students in bachelor's, master's, and doctoral programs will lead to more research and will bring new nursing knowledge into the system and improve and change services. Well educated nursing staff now participate in decision making and policy development. The transfer of more responsibility to treat and care for patients, as stated above, is the first step enabling nurses to offer their practice within the system or a joint practice with physicians and other health professions.

2013 in 4 Länder of Germany nurses voted for the establishment of Nursing Chambers, which will regulate the nursing profession, set professional standards, and create quality standards for further education in nursing. The governments of the Länder will transfer nursing issues to the Chambers, as they are self-regulating bodies. That will strengthen the power of influence of nurses regarding legislation and policy.

The Robert Bosch Foundation has financed a great many projects to improve the nursing profession in Germany over the past twenty years. One important project was the publication of papers on the importance of nursing research for the improvement of patient care in Germany. In 2011, the foundation also supported an interdisciplinary dialogue with the federal government on funding research grants for nursing scientists. Recent steps by the Ministry of Education and Science indicate that more funds for research will be relocated to schools of nursing at universities.

Integrative nursing is a paradigm change. It focuses on the patients as "unitary human beings" (Rogers, 1994). We are convinced that necessary changes in the highly complex healthcare system will be strongly influenced by the new generation of empowered and well-educated nurses. They will not use as much of their energy to survive in the healthcare system and please physicians and managers. They will concentrate more on the human beings in need of integrative nursing care.

SELECTED REFERENCES

Hafsteinsdottir, T. B., & Grypdonck, M. H. (2004). NDT competence of nurses caring for patients with stroke. *The Journal of Neuroscience Nursing: Journal of the American Association of Neuroscience Nurses, 26*(5), 289–294.

Kollen, B. J., Lennon, S., Lyons, B., et al. (2009). The effectiveness of the Bobath concept in stroke rehabilitation: What is the evidence? *Stroke: a Journal of Cerebral Circulation, 40*(4), 89–97.

Lee, J., Han, M., Chung, Y., Kim, J., & Choi, J. (2011). Effects of foot reflexology on fatigue, sleep and pain: A systematic review and meta-analysis. *Journal of Korean Academy of Nursing, 41*(6), 821–833.

McDermott, R. (2007). *The Essential Steiner* (pp. 3–11, 392–395). Aurora, CO: Lindisfarne Books.

Price, S. (2012). *Aromatherapy for Health Professionals*, 4th ed. London: Churchill Livingstone.

Rogers, M. E. (1994). The science of unitary human beings: Current perspectives. *Nursing Science Quarterly, 7*(33), 33–35.

Rosen Method. Retrieved April 11, 2013, from http://www.rosenmethod.com.

Steiner, R. (1997). *An Outline of Esoteric Science.* Hudson, NY: Anthroposophic Press.

Steiner, R. (2012). *Theosophie.* Basel: Rudolf Steiner Verlag.

Therkleson, T. (2010). Ginger compress therapy for adults with osteoarthritis. *Journal of Advanced Nursing, 66*(10), 2225–2233.

36

Integrative Nursing in Turkey

SEBAHAT GÖZÜM AND NURGÜN PLATIN

Overview of Nursing and Healthcare in Turkey

Turkey, often called Anatolia, is a transcontinental Eurasian country located between Southeastern Europe and Western Asia. The country's population in 2010 was 73.7 million. The age group 15–64 years old constitutes 67% of the population, with 26% aged 0–14 years, and senior citizens 65 years and older make up the 7% of the total population. Life expectancy is 71.1 years for men and 75.3 years for women, with an overall average of 73.2 years for the population as a whole (Turkish Statistical Institute, 2010).

Turkey's healthcare system went through radical changes when the Health Transformation Program started in 2003 (Akdağ, 2011). The program has three components. The first is provision of primary healthcare services staffed by family physicians and family health personnel, generally female nurses or midwives, who are responsible for the infant and female population. An average case load for the healthcare unit is 4,000 people. Their responsibilities include the follow-up of the growth and development of the newborn, health screening and immunization services, health education on family planning for women of reproductive age, and follow-up during the pregnancy and postpartum period. The family health personnel are also responsible for taking laboratory specimens for the outpatient population that the family physician is caring for. Services offered are free of charge.

The second component of the new system is the restructuring of health insurance. A general social insurance system is structured on the solvency ratio of the client to pay for services. Secondary and tertiary services are delivered at the inpatient government or private healthcare facilities. The expenses of these services are covered by the insurance system; however, people pay a contribution rate along with the insurance rate payment. The expenses of the people with insolvency are covered through public resources.

The third component of the new system was put into practice in November 2011, when the Government Hospitals Association Act converted the government in-service health organizations into autonomous businesses. The Health Transformation Program started with the philosophy of easy accessibility, equity, and service quality. However, the system has been criticized for its privatizing of the healthcare system, converting hospitals into businesses, increasing payments, and risking healthcare personnel's job security.

In many respects, the developments within the nursing profession occurred independently from the developments of the healthcare system. The first nursing training began in 1912 with three care-giving courses initiated by the Ottoman Red Crescent Association for male nurses in the military. The first Turkish nursing school with a diploma program was created in 1925, following the establishment of the Turkish Republic in 1923. However, Florence Nightingale's work in Turkey during the Crimean War in 1854 is often cited as the beginning of modern nursing.

The first university nursing baccalaureate degree program started in 1955 (Bahçecik & Alpar, 2009). In 1997, all nursing diploma and associate degree programs were changed into baccalaureate programs as well. Unfortunately, nursing diploma programs reopened in 2007 to meet the nursing shortage. Currently, there are 95 nursing schools offering baccalaureate degrees. Nursing students, male and female, are admitted through a highly competitive General University Entrance Examination, which is organized by the Turkish Higher Education Council (Thobaben et al., 2005; Görgülü & Dinç, 2007). Nearly all of the programs use the classical educational system. Only a few programs have an integrative curriculum or use the problem-based learning approach.

The first Master of Science program in nursing started in 1968, and the Ph.D. programs in 1972 (Bahçecik & Alpar, 2009). These graduate programs specialize in medical-surgical, pediatrics, psychiatry, obstetrics and gynecology, public health nursing, nursing administration, and fundamentals of nursing. Currently, there are 783 nurse academic teaching staff, of whom 65 are professors. However, this number is far below the number that is needed to meet the present demands for nursing education. Despite the struggles within nursing education in Turkey, the country is positioned favorably relative to international educational standards for nursing (Thobaben et al., 2005; Görgülü & Dinç, 2007; Dal & Kitiş, 2008; Can, 2010). Nursing education programs are being revised with the Bologna process and the norms of EU to optimize nursing education.

The exact number of nurses is not known, because there is no registration office for nurses. However, according to Ministry of Health's statements, there are 120,422 nurses in Turkey. It is estimated at least another 100,000 are needed. An insufficient number of nurses and the unequal distribution of nurses throughout the country are important barriers to providing quality nursing care in the country (Kocaman et al., 2008).

Integrative Nursing in Turkey

Anatolia has been the homeland for such civilizations as the Hittites, Sumerians, Urartians, Phrygians, Assyrians, Lydians, Romans, Ancient Greeks, Ionians, Byzantines, Seljuk Turks, Mongols, and the Ottoman Empire. Because of Turkey's culturally rich history, there are many culturally based beliefs and practices in disease prevention and treatment.

Turkey has also a rich philosophical and medical heritage from Rumi and Avicenna. Even traits from the shamanic beliefs and or practices remain in the society today, such as wearing a blue "evil eye" amulet for protection from the evil spirits, making wishes by tying colorful strings of cloth on the trees, or reading the Kur'an in a musical rhythms after a person's death. On the other hand, praying in the Islamic religion five times a day from sunrise to sunset is considered a good example of both daily exercise and meditation. Nurses encounter many of these practices in patient care and in public health practices.

As far back as 1206 in the City of Kayseri, and in 1484 in Edirne, there were psychiatric hospitals where the main treatment elements were music, water sounds from fountains, and special aromas in rooms with excellent acoustics. Currently the classical Turkish music tonalities and pentatonic melodies of Central Asian Turkish music are being used to regulate some mind and body functions and emotions. These music therapies are offered through commercial personal development programs and have become quite popular.

There are some traditional practices that are recommended or practiced by some physicians. These are the thermal baths and leech therapy. Thermal spring baths are commonly known for their use with the treatment of the rheumatoid disorders. The Turkish bath (*hamam*), including a deep rubbing of the skin with a silk cloth to provide stimulation for circulation, peeling, and general relaxation, has a traditional place in Turkish culture. Even some nurses working in some of these thermal spring baths take an active role with the treatments. Ancient thermal pools with special (toothless) fish living in 37° C spring water help with the healing of skin lesions such as psoriasis. This is a highly recommended therapy by dermatologists.

Medical leeches (*hirudo medicinalis*) have been used for thousands of years for the management of venous diseases of the lower extremities, migraines, and headaches. Current medical use includes adjunctive treatment with plastic-reconstructive surgery post-operatively to assist with the collateral circulation formation, relieve venous congestion around the surgical area, and help with the flap healing in venous insufficiencies (Köse et al., 2008; Thearle, 1998). Leeches are placed on the congested areas and encouraged to feed. While leeches feed, they also secrete a bioactive, heparin-like substance in their saliva called *hirudin*, which acts as a natural thrombin inhibitor (Zaidi et al., 2011; Gödekmerdan et al., 2011). There is also reported use of self-applied leeches in the case of severe pain related to advanced-stage cancer. In one case report, a patient reported outpatient self-treatment with seven leeches to the lumbar region that resulted in complete healing of pain (Kalender et al., 2010).

There are other practices, such as *hacamat* or cupping, which are being used widely. *Hacamat*, an old Islamic treatment method, is a traditional style of bloodletting therapy. It has been one of the most widely used traditional medicinal treatment modalities in

Turkey. The mechanism of its effectiveness is to drain and restore the affected area. Currently, the practice is used for hypertension, neck pain, and headaches (http://www.islamihacamat.com/). Cupping (application of glass suction cups on the skin) has been used since antiquity in the treatment of pain and respiratory congestion. Mechanically, it would be equivalent to postural drainage done with tapotement (tap done with cupped hands). Cupping is a medicinal practice that is very widespread in Asian countries. The practice is still being used especially by the elder population in rural areas of Turkey.

While the practices mentioned above have a long history of use within various regions of Turkey, testing these therapies for effectiveness is a relatively new phenomenon. Since 1997, numerous studies in Turkey describe the use of complementary and alternative medicine (CAM) in different regions of the country. Studies dealing with the impact of cultural health practices in Turkey have also gained momentum in the 2000s. Initial studies done by nursing teaching staff were mostly epidemiological studies focusing on the frequency and need for the use of CAM by healthy and/or sick individuals in Turkey (Gözüm et al., 2003; Tan & Uzun, 2004; Gözüm & Unsal, 2004; Algier et al., 2005; Unsal & Gözüm, 2010; Avci et al., 2012).

The prevalence of CAM usage was found to be between 32% and 60%, with herbal medicines being the most commonly used form. Herbal products are consumed in cooking, applied topically, or within tea (green-leaved plants, nettle, thyme and oleander, etc.) (Samur et al., 2001; Algıer et al., 2005; Işıkhan et al., 2005; Taş et al., 2005; Aslan et al., 2006; İnanç et al., 2006; Mazıcıoğlu et al., 2006; Avci et al., 2012). Herbs and plants have been used in the culture for centuries and are a vital part of folkloric/traditional Turkish medicine. Remedies such as medical leeches, cupping, thermal spring baths, plant and food therapies, praying, and spiritual practices have all been found to be effective, practical, easy to access, cost-effective, and supported by conventional medicine.

Herbal therapies such as linden, mint, chamomile, rosehip, ginger, wild thyme, cinnamon, and stinging nettle (*urtica dioica*) are the most commonly used herb teas for disorders as snuffle, flu, upper respiratory system infections, and digestive problems. They are also recommended for daily use as an alternative for the black tea by most health professionals. Herbal therapies are also often used by chronically ill patients with cancer, hypertension, diabetes, arthritis, COPD, asthma, kidney problems, and allergies. Stinging nettle, found in most areas of the country, is the most frequently used complementary therapy by cancer patients. Patients' rationale for using complementary and integrative therapies is to strengthen the immune system, to improve the quality of life, and to reduce the side effects of the treatment.

Eventually nurses', nursing students', and physicians' interest in CAM use was recognized (Uzun et al., 2004; Öztekin et al., 2007; Yildirim et al., 2010). In one study (Set et al., 2012), it was reported that health professionals working in primary healthcare settings had limited knowledge but positive attitudes towards the use of CAM and were ready to improve their knowledge. Eventually, public and medical interest led to a movement by the Ministry of Health to integrate some CAM therapies within the conventional healthcare system. The ministry issued a decree in November of 2011 that regulated the related tasks of offering CAM, creating the opportunity for nurses to use CAM practices with their professional practice.

Because of the keen interest in CAM's effect on cancer patients, the National Medical Oncology Association (UTOD) and the Ministry recommended that health professionals use the terms complementary and *integrative* rather than complementary and *alternative* practices. Along with the recommendation, they established a Web page to relate their position on the subject (http://www.kanser.org/toplum/?action=sayfa&id=2), which cites the Society for Integrative Oncology Association's (SIO) integrative medical guidelines. The website provides a list of the most commonly used herbal medicines, along with their risks when used concurrently with conventional medical treatment. Also listed are complementary therapies whose safe usage has been determined. Some medical staff do not recommend the use of these therapies until after conventional treatments are over. However, the general trend is to accept such techniques as massage, exercise, acupuncture, relaxation, music therapy, and other body–mind practices as supporters of the medical treatment that enhance the quality of life of the patient.

Studies of complementary therapies carried out by nurses have demonstrated promising outcomes. Examples include the effect of acupressure on nausea, vomiting, and anxiety in women with breast cancer (Genç, 2010), and the effect of aromatherapy on symptoms and quality of life of women with breast cancer receiving chemotherapy (Ovayolu, 2011). Other experimental studies report positive results on various patient groups and include using foot massage on physiological edema (Çoban & Şirin, 2010); back massage on the sleep quality of the elderly (Çınar & Eşer, 2012); massage on pain, itching, and anxiety levels of adolescents with burn wounds as complementary to medical therapy (Parlak Gürol, 2010); aromatherapy massage on dysmenorrhea with university students (Apay et al., 2012); and music therapy on post-operative pain and the physiological parameters of patients following open heart surgery (Özer et al., 2010). The effectiveness of organic honey verses ethoxy-diaminoacidrine plus nitrofurazone dressings on bed sores was reported in one nursing study (Güneş & Eşer, 2007). Another studies have reported the effects of various interventions such as the administration of massage, sucrose solution, herbal tea, and hydrolysed formula for the treatment of colic (Arikan et al., 2008), and breast milk and sucrose for pain reduction during examination for retinopathy of prematurity (Taplak and Erdem, 2012). Presently there are experimental studies in process to test the effectiveness of such traditional methods as honey, black mulberry, and walnut jam with chemotherapy-induced mucositis and post-partum nipple sores.

In a recent study (Koç et al., 2012), 129 midwives reported their results with complementary and integrative medicine for pregnant women. In the study, 58.9% of the midwives had suggested CAM to the women. Among the suggested treatments, CAM herbal treatment, diets, and exercises were used most (32.6%, 27.9%, and 28.7%, respectively), and acupuncture, relaxation techniques, and fast walking were used the least (1.6%, 6.2%, and 7.0%, respectively). Herbal therapy was most often recommended for such conditions as nausea/vomiting, anemia, gastric complaints, constipation, sore throat, insomnia, hypertension, sinusitis, cough, common cold, stress, hemorrhoids, and asthenia/fatigue.

It is anticipated that descriptive and experimental research will have an important impact on the development and use of integrative nursing in Turkey. The topic of cultural health practices is being discussed in the intercultural/transcultural Nursing Congress meeting held every two years. "*Intercultural Nursing* is a book that focuses on cultural health practices for chronic disease, child care, mental health and psychiatric nursing, reproductive health (infertility, prenatal and postnatal care), and pain with clear explanations to help nurses see the patient as a whole" (Seviğ & Tanrıverdi, 2012).

In addition to the practices mentioned above, nurses in Turkey often recommend the usage of natural foods and plants. For example, many nurses treat sore nipples by applying olive oil, onion juice, tea dressings, or the mother's own milk. Other practices worth mentioning are the application of egg yolk oil or organic olive oil for skin burns.

Integrative Nursing Models and Exemplars in Turkey

Turkey has culturally rich history of complementary and integrative practices. Nursing, however, has been slower in adopting these practices. Only a few nurses are practicing with an integrative nursing understanding at the bedside, and it is not common for nurses to have private practices where these therapies are offered. In general, these practices are mostly being used in private healthcare facilities \or as part of personal improvement programs.

Acupuncture is the most widely used complementary therapy for obesity, smoking cessation, and pain management, by both the public and physicians. In a few private hospitals, acupuncture is being used successfully for relieving chemotherapy-induced nausea and vomiting (Tek et al., 2012). In another private hospital, patients are taught basic yoga principles after gastric-bypass surgery to help with the control of their blood pressure and heart rate. In a few hospitals, women are offered a water birth if they choose (Memorial Hospital). Although it is not common, some private hospitals use some complementary therapies alone or with conventional medical treatment. A private oncology hospital (Medical Park Cancer Hospital) offers information on its website about the safe use of acupuncture, biofeedback, neurofeedback, and guided imagery (http://www.kanserhastanesi.com.tr/kanser-tedavisi/).

Oncology patients' use of CAM has triggered the interest of oncology nurses and the related professional nursing association. The Oncology Nursing Association's annual scientific meeting includes topics such as patients' psychological and spiritual care needs, and methods to reduce stress. The Turkish Oncology Nursing Association collaborated on a European study of CAM use in breast, colorectal, lung, head and neck, gynecological, and hematological cancers in 2004. Papers were published in various nursing and medical journals (Molassiotis et al., 2005; Molassiotis et al., 2005).

Currently, nurses interested in advancing the use of CAM therapies and cultural practices are focusing on generating scientific evidence that will be key to securing support for the integration of these practices with conventional treatments. While interest in integrative nursing is strong, it is still early in the movement and somewhat rare to see integrative nursing care being offered within clinical care settings.

Challenges and Barriers to Integrative Nursing Practice

As shown above, many non-pharmacological nursing care practices and interventions are supportive to medical treatment and care. These interventions are also well known as independent functions of nursing. For example, massage is a very basic nursing intervention that is also considered a complementary treatment method. Therefore, forming the bridge between independent nursing functions and non-invasive complementary practices such as music, relaxation exercises, spiritual care, aromatherapy, acupressure, and lymphatic drainage should theoretically be easy.

The challenge is that nursing tends to be very focused on medical tasks and is often limited to physical care, a situation that is exacerbated by a shortage of nurses. Therefore, success with integrative nursing practice among nursing colleagues will depend on other factors in Turkey, such as the nurses' active support, interest, and leadership on the topic. In addition, sharing the presently available experimental research results with both teaching staff and clinical nurses and emphasizing how integrative nursing fits with the non-pharmacological nursing interventions and with the independent nursing role are also important strategies, as are expanding publications and offering conferences and seminars on integrative nursing practices. These approaches are also believed to be helpful in keeping the cultural practices alive within the globalization of the world.

Vision of Integrative Nursing

We perceive integrative nursing as a strengthening factor for nursing in many ways, such as providing comprehensive self-care during wellness and illness, considering the full "bodymindspirit" in the healing process, and helping the patient or client find meaning. Professional integrative nursing expects nurses to guide and act as an advocate for the society with evidence-based integrative practices; expands and clearly redefines "holistic nursing" with a chance to integrate cultural practices; redefines the vogue complementary relations between empirical knowledge and the art of nursing; elaborately supports the development of personal knowledge, especially the tacit knowledge of the nurse; and defines a way to integrate the four ways of knowing of nursing into the practice.

However, nursing is still being dominated by the medical model and must urge a shift in its paradigm, which means redefining nursing, redefining its status quo, and readapting nursing into the complex healthcare system. The practice of integrative nursing would be a unique chance to approach human beings within the challenges, opportunities, and risks of the twenty-first century and the healthcare system, as well as a chance to actualize the concept of nursing as the nursing theorists have tried to define it since the time of Nightingale.

Initially, transforming nursing education and adapting it to nursing practice is expected to be a long process. Its comprehensive and abstract content needs to be handled delicately, perhaps with new teaching strategies. This, we believe, will eventually lead us to new nursing practice theories.

SELECTED REFERENCES

Aslan, O., Vural, H., Komurcu, S., & Ozet, A. (2006). Use of complementary and alternative medicine by cancer patients in Turkey: A survey. *Journal of Alternative and Complementary Medicine, 1*, 355–356.

Avci, A. I., Koç, Z., & Sağlam, Z. (2012). Use of complementary and alternative medicine by patients with cancer in northern Turkey: Analysis of cost and satisfaction. *Journal of Clinical Nursing, 21*(5-6), 677–688.

Bahcecik, N., & Alpar, S. (2009). Nursing education in Turkey: From past to present. *Nurse Education Today, 29*(7), 698–703.

Dal, U., & Kitis, Y. (2008). The historical development and current status of nursing in Turkey. *Online Journal of Issues in Nursing, 13*(2), 1–9.

Gözüm, S., Tezel, A., & Koc, M. (2003). Complementary alternative treatments used by patients with cancer in eastern Turkey. *Cancer Nursing, 26*(3), 230–6.

Isikhan, V., Komurcu, S., Ozet, A., Arpaci, F., Ozturk, B., Balbay, O. & Guner, P. (2005). The status of alternative treatment in cancer patients in Turkey. *Cancer Nursing, 28*, 355–362.

Koç, Z., Topatan, S., & Sağlam, Z. (2012). Use of and attitudes toward complementary and alternative medicine among midwives in Turkey. *European Journal of Obstetrics & Gynecology & Reproductive Biology, 160*(2), 131–136.

Tas, F., Ustuner, Z., Can, G., Eralp, Y., Camlica, H., Basaran, M., et al. (2005). The prevalence and determinants of the use of complementary and alternative medicine in adult Turkish cancer patients. *Acta Oncologica, 44*, 161–167.

Tek, I., Akgedik, K., Öztürk, S., Turhan, F., Kursak, N., Gürsoy, I. D., et al. (2012). The effect of acupuncture on the prevention of post-chemotherapeutic nausea-vomiting. *European Journal of Oncology Nursing, 16*(1) Supplement, 23–24.

Yildirim, Y., Parlar, S., Eyigor, S., Sertoz, O. O., Eyigor, C., Fadiloglu, C., et al. (2010). An analysis of nursing and medical students' attitudes towards and knowledge of complementary and alternative medicine (CAM). *Journal of Clinical Nursing, 19*(7-8), 1157–1166.

37

Integrative Nursing in the United Kingdom

SUSAN SMITH, JANINA SWEETENHAM, AND ANGELA BRADSHAW

Overview of Nursing in the United Kingdom

Since its inception in 1948, the United Kingdom's National Health Service (NHS) has provided most services cost-free at the point of care. The NHS is funded centrally by the government from public taxation, but it faces a challenging climate in the worldwide economic downturn and the continually increasing demand for a wider range of services. The NHS is currently addressing how to deliver services while maintaining and improving quality within a fixed financial envelope. As the largest group of staff, and a crucial part of the healthcare team, nurses have a pivotal role in this evolutionary process, and it is vital that they are fully prepared to fulfill that role.

Other than within the NHS, nurses are employed in the armed forces, independent schools, pharmaceutical companies, industry, charitable facilities, and the independent sector, which provides acute services for private patients. Private hospitals also support the Department of Health imperative in the reduction of waiting times, mainly through the provision of routine surgery.

ENTRY INTO NURSING

In September 2008, the Nursing and Midwifery Council (NMC, www.nmc-uk.org), which regulates the professions in England, Wales, Scotland, and Northern Ireland, ratified a crucial change in registration requirements, designed to lead to the creation of a workforce "fit" for the twenty-first century. As of early 2013, the academic award for registration as a nurse will be a degree in nursing, as diploma courses are being phased out. New entrants to the profession will have to study first-degree level (www.nhs.careers.nhs.uk).

The pre-registration degree comprises 50% theory and 50% practice, with time being split between the university and practical placements in a variety of healthcare settings. All student nurses engage with the basic principles of nursing during the

Common Foundation Programme, after which, they specialize in one of the following areas: adult, mental health, learning disabilities, and care of children.

SPECIALTY EDUCATION IN NURSING

There are two entry routes into midwifery. One route is direct, whereby the student undertakes a pre-registration three-year midwifery degree comprising 50% supervised midwifery practice in both community and hospital settings and 50% integrated study of theory. The second route to midwifery involves a 78-week full-time program for qualified nurses registered on the Adult Nursing branch of the Nursing and Midwifery Council register. Again, the student undertakes supervised midwifery practice integrated with theoretical study. Completion of either route leads to both an academic and a professional qualification.

The initial entry requirement to train for a Specialist Community, Public Health, or District Nursing role is to hold a registered nursing qualification. Such roles include: Health Visiting, Occupational Health, School Nursing, Sexual Health, Health Protection, and Family Health Nursing (in Scotland). Further study in each of these fields of practice is at master's degree level.

NURSING AND MIDWIFERY REGULATION

The Nursing and Midwifery Council requires all nurses, midwives, and specialist public health nurses to register if they wish to practice in the United Kingdom. A survey in 2008 estimated that there were 676,547 nurses and midwives on the register in the United Kingdom (35,305 of this total were registered midwives). More than 65% of those were over forty years of age, and 31% were over fifty. For the year ending April 2011, the total number of nurses and midwives was 655,132. Demography shows the United Kingdom not only has an aging nursing workforce to provide nursing services to an aging population, but there are fewer of them to do this.

Integrative Nursing in the United Kingdom

The term "integrative nursing" is not commonly found in the U.K. health literature; "holistic nursing," "person-centered care," and "therapeutic relationships" are major areas of emphasis that are aligned with the integrative nursing construct. "Integrative healthcare" is a more familiar phrase, as is "integrative medicine," which seeks to integrate traditional and complementary approaches in the treatment of a wide range of conditions and interconnect the work of multiple disciplines in striving for the best possible quality of patient care. These terms tend towards a potentially restrictive view of healthcare: integrative medicine, for example, relates to "treatment" rather than healing, "curing" rather than caring. Whilst nurses are part of, and integral to, such initiatives in the United Kingdom, they focus more on the expansive definition of "heal," which is of course "to make whole" (Chambers, 2003).

The Royal College of Nursing believes "holistic care" incorporates "the psychological, environmental and spiritual needs of a patient, as well as the physical, so that people are treated as whole human beings and the impact of the illness on their quality of life is evaluated too." Holistic nursing reflects significant elements of integrative care, and there are many fine examples of how British nurses relate holistically to their patients, intermingling complementary approaches with traditional practices and creating a unique care approach. One of the best demonstrations of this occurs when individuals receive palliative care in a hospice situation. Hospice care not only takes care of people's physical needs, but also addresses their emotional, spiritual, and social needs. Dame Cicely Saunders is credited with founding the first "modern" hospice in the United Kingdom, a facility that was significantly different from earlier "homes for the dying." She combined three key principles: excellent clinical care, education, and research. She always saw patients as at the centre of all activity:

> You matter because you are you, and you matter to the end of your life. We will do all we can not only to help you to die peacefully, but also, to live until you die. (Dunphy, 2011)

The Health Foundation, an independent charity that works to enhance the quality of healthcare in the United Kingdom (http://www.health.org.uk), sees patients as equal partners in planning, developing, and assessing care to make sure it is most appropriate for their needs. It involves putting patients and their families at the heart of all decisions. This, they say, is "person-centered care."

PERSON-CENTERED CARE

In England, Wales, Northern Ireland, and Scotland, person-centeredness and compassion are expectations of the National Health Service. Nurses, who spend so much time creating effective relationships with their clients, are the obvious people to advance such care in the rapidly evolving healthcare arena. Person-centered care for patients relates to a relationship with their nurse that helps them feel safe, understood, and valued as a unique human being. The focus is on the actual needs and wants of the patients themselves and relieving patients' anxiety through their inclusion in decisions about care and treatment. Person-centered nurses offer patients reassurance, security, and a sense of wellbeing, which not only improves the patient experience, but has been shown to positively impact health outcomes (e.g., reductions in length of stay and lower incidence of acquired infections). Person-centeredness for staff is about feeling valued, empowered, and supported in an environment where they are happy with the quality of care given and received. Organizations valuing person-centeredness identify this as a priority and monitor its achievement across the different levels of staff.

THERAPEUTIC RELATIONSHIPS

Holistic nursing draws on nursing knowledge, theories, expertise, and intuition to guide nurses in becoming therapeutic partners with patients or clients. Generally, the literature identifies the need for trust, respect, professional intimacy, empathy, and power as the basis of a therapeutic relationship.

In addition to these, Neal (2003) highlights the following crucial characteristics of effective partnerships:

- Independent professional practice
- Self-knowledge for both nurse and client
- Professional boundaries which must not be crossed

Jones (2009) describes therapeutic communication as a complex skill that only develops where the nurse has empathy or insight. Mitchell and McCormack (1998, p. 50) add:

Patients themselves value therapeutic relationships which offer respect, trust and care...such relationships may in themselves prove to be healing in the broadest sense.

Finally, Dame Christine Beasley, the (then) Chief Nursing Officer for England and Wales said in 2010:

Regardless of setting, nursing today requires an intricate interplay between fundamental care and high level technical competence, biomedical knowledge, decision making skills and the ability to develop therapeutic relationships based on compassionate and intelligent care.

Integrative Nursing

There are some common themes identifiable from the three approaches of holistic nursing, person-centered care, and therapeutic relationships. These are:

- The knowledge of the nurse, based upon sound evidence and her capacity to make/facilitate decisions about appropriate interventions in the mutually agreed best interests of the patient.

- The nature of the individuals involved and their preparedness to accept responsibility for themselves and their roles within the healing/caring process. This incorporates the self-knowledge and emotional intelligence (Goleman, 1995) of both nurse and patient.
- The creation of a unique relationship that is focused upon the needs and wishes of the patient. With the patient at the centre of all activity, such a relationship *must* be therapeutic in nature, and it must take account of the patient's potential vulnerability and the importance of professional boundaries that must be observed.

At the heart of these themes lies the nurse's way of "being-knowing-doing." Between them, the themes address the caring and healing relationship and the informed choice about traditional and emerging interventions. Together, these elements comprise the definition of integrative nursing that forms the backbone of this book.

We argue that nurses are often the central focus of the person's journey through healthcare; they relate to, and communicate with, many different professional groups and function within many different environments and contexts. They help their patients maintain their "selfhood" as they navigate through confusing and little-understood jungles of professional fiefdoms, egos, and bureaucracy. They facilitate a whole-systems approach (Bertalanffy, 1962). In all of healthcare, which other professional is so uniquely qualified to engage in truly integrative practice?

We therefore posit the working model below—the "Whole Systems Caring Model." Whilst we acknowledge there are gaps, we will use this model as the ontological basis for an exploration of selected initiatives within the NHS that enhance, support, and sometimes block an integrative nursing approach and the opportunities available for supporting an integrative nursing culture.

Several key concepts of the model are addressed in certain advanced roles held by nurses in the United Kingdom:

- Independent professional practice and expanding professional boundaries are integral to nurse prescribers. These nurses, under the vicarious liability of their employers and their own professional accountability, are able to independently prescribe a raft of drugs to their patients.
- Self-care and responsibility for self underpin the role of preceptor for newly qualified nurses and midwives.
- The role of the nurse consultant not only exemplifies independent professional practice and stretches professional boundaries, but also requires self-knowledge, personal responsibility, and self-care. As a result of this advanced role, there is a shift in the power balance between nurse and physician within specialist areas of practice.

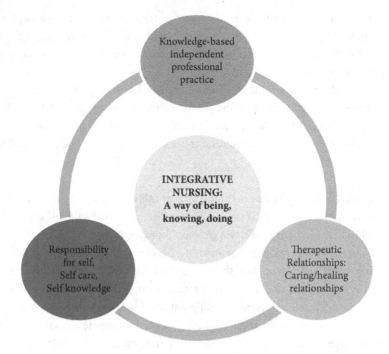

FIGURE 37.1 The Whole-System Caring Model

Integrative Nursing Exemplars in the United Kingdom

One exemplar illuminates the essence of integrative nursing practice in the United Kingdom: the Caring Behaviours Assurance System (CBAS).

THE CARING BEHAVIOURS ASSURANCE SYSTEM (CBAS)

"The Caring Behaviours Assurance System: Caring for Patients, Caring for Staff" is an evidence-based system for enabling and assuring the delivery of person-centered care. It addresses caring for patients and caring for staff in equal measures; it engages with individuals, teams, executive boards, and the national agenda in assuring the quality of the care experience for patients, their families, and staff. The values, process, and outcomes of CBAS are driven by an integrative nursing systems approach, which promotes whole-systems caring and healing, builds caring and healing relationships, and provides a platform for traditional and emerging interventions, selected to meet the unique needs of the individual patient.

CBAS was introduced into NHS Scotland in 2011 and continues to be implemented across the country, led by the Chief Nurse for Scotland, Ros Moore, and the creators of the system, Dr. Susan Smith and Janina Sweetenham (www.choice-dynamic-int.com).

The key elements of CBAS have been adapted to fit the categories of quality identified in the Quality Strategy for Scotland (The Scottish Government, 2010). The CBAS process is relevant to all staff who work within health and social care, although here we are clearly focusing on the *nurse's* involvement and leadership of the program. It can be argued that nurses are at the vanguard of improving the patient's and staff's experience of healthcare and are directly influencing the way in which all other healthcare professionals perceive, manage, and enhance the quality of care.

The essence of CBAS lies in the creation of effective relationships between the nurse and her patient, the nurse and her colleagues, and the nurse and herself. At the heart of integrative nursing lies the caring and healing relationship. The creation of such a therapeutic partnership inevitably requires the exploration of independent professional practice and professional boundaries, self-knowledge, self-care, responsibility, and an awareness of the balance of power between patient and nurse. Our working model helps us make sense of the interrelated elements underpinning the integrative nursing philosophy embedded within CBAS. Where true therapeutic relationships exist, they support whole-system/whole-person healing and facilitate the integration of different approaches, therapies, and interventions, depending on the unique needs of the patient. At the heart of the CBAS model is a "Person-centered Care Quality Instrument" (PCQI) used to guide debate about assuring quality, care, and compassion. The PCQI is tailored to each ward or unit by the staff. It is a number of evidence-based statements, drawn from the full array of national and international literature around quality, grouped together to reflect six categories reflected in "the 7 C's" of the Healthcare Quality Strategy (2010): Caring and compassionate staff and services; clear Communication and explanation about conditions and treatment; effective Collaboration between clinicians, patients, and others; Clean and safe care environment; Continuity of care; and Clinical excellence.

CBAS reminds the nurse of her original motivation to enter the profession; it gives her a chance to stand back and re-engage with her values, thus revisiting and extending her own self-knowledge. The education program for the implementation of CBAS comprises four days, during which three identified Quality Champions for each team come together to explore the principles, processes, and practice of CBAS. The program begins with a self-care workshop that incorporates some aspects of the HeartMath® (HM) System of tools and techniques, drawing on the book *Transforming Stress* by Childre and Rozman. (www.heartmath.com). We believe that it is not possible to address the quality of the patient experience unless we also explore the quality of the staff experience. So giving the Quality Champions the skills to engage in deeper and more effective self-care is crucial and underpins the whole of CBAS.

It is well documented that stress compromises the quality of care. HM offers techniques for managing stress in the moment. Instead of waiting for a day off, a massage, a walk in the country, or a holiday at some future point, HM techniques enable the

HeartMath is a registered trademark of the Institute of HeartMath.

practiced person to become physiologically coherent "in a heartbeat." "Physiological coherence" is achieved when all the bodily systems work together optimally, so that thinking is clearer, decision-making more incisive, and intuition honed. In such a state, the body and mind become like a fine-tuned motor, purring along the often challenging avenues of healthcare.

Integrative nursing focuses on the health and wellbeing of caregivers as well as those they care for. The HM programme offers a powerful way for the nurse to help herself and ultimately create an effective therapeutic partnership with her patient.

In addition to managing the stress reaction, HM tools help participants:

1. Understand that care is not just the "doing," it's also about the feeling the care and the experience that goes along with what is done/said. Patients may never remember exactly what the nurse said or did, but they will always recall how they felt when that nurse was near. "Doing without feeling" is not good for the patient or the nurse.
2. Create and nurture authentic relationships in which the nurse "gets in tune" with her patient and not only acts as a better transmitter and receiver of information but can actually pick up on what is *not* being said.
3. Reset a healthier baseline of resilience in the body when it has become used to living with high levels of stress.

Our working model is further endorsed as we see that HeartMath helps the nurse enhance her own self-knowledge. It also helps her look after herself and step up to the responsibility for maintaining her own health and wellbeing, which directly affects the patient's experience. HM tools help the nurse develop greater insight and empathy about her patient, which are requirements for the development of therapeutic communication (Jones, 2009).

HM tools include a simple technique with the potential for lifelong impact. In engaging with the CBAS program, the Quality Champions address their own independent professional practice, their professional boundaries, self-knowledge, self-care, and the nature of the power relationship between themselves and the patient. CBAS is shifting the balance of power from a mechanistic medical model to one that integrates all healthcare professionals into a unified decision-making group focused on care and compassion.

The following quote is just one of many similar comments made by CBAS participants: "I've always been taught to care for people in the way I would want to be cared for, but this is wrong—what I want may not be what my patient wants. We MUST ask them." The Quality Champions took the view that the enhanced communication between staff and patients and their families enabled the staff to bring in a wider range of therapeutic interventions and therapies, because they were more receptive and alert to the needs, sometimes unexpressed, of their patients.

Case Study

Six months after the implementation of CBAS into the Golden Jubilee Hospital in Glasgow, Scotland, a review was held by the executive nurse, senior managers, and the Quality Champions from the following wards and units: coronary care, orthopedics, general surgery, cardiothoracic, and thoracic. The Golden Jubilee Hospital has a national remit for specialist surgery and a high national reputation for quality of care. Even so, the group identified the following improvements, prompted by the CBAS program:

• More patient interviews are carried out.
• Improved communication with patients. More emphasis on "How are you feeling?" and always asking the question: "What we can do for you today?"
• Improvement in communication with relatives using a purpose-designed communication sheet.
• The unique team "Person-centered Care Quality Instrument" (PCQI) laminated on the wall for all to see and refer to.
• An "issue of the week"—one of the PCQI statements to focus on during the designated time.
• Improvement noted in patient experience questionnaires.
• Open visiting now established (following consultation with patients, relatives, and staff).

The nurse's being-knowing-doing, aimed at advancing the health and wellbeing of herself and her patient, is clearly developed through the CBAS process, as is the enhancement of the caring and healing relationship.

By placing the patient and relative firmly at the centre of activity, nurses are reviewing all interaction from that perspective. In terms of the impact of this approach on professional teams, not only do they get greater satisfaction from their engagement with happier, more contented clients, but their workload can be readdressed and even reduced. As one participant stated, "If we only listened to what the patient *really* wants—and did it—we wouldn't be nearly so busy." Such focused, authentic, coherent listening to patients moves nurses closer to an integrative model of practice.

Vision of Integrative Nursing in the United Kingdom

Many years ago, a very high-profile consultant physician addressed nurses at their graduation. He told them never to forget that they are the central cog in the wheel of care. He and his fellow doctors only ever "visit" to diagnose, carry out a treatment, or prescribe a drug. Important work, he told them; but the nurse who is with the patient every minute, who sees them in the context of their lives and their families—she is the person who really knows and understands. One of the authors of this chapter graduated that day, and she learned half the message that carried her through the subsequent forty years of her career. It took a few more years before the other half of the message got through: the person who *really* knows and understands is the patient. Together they are a formidable combination. Nurses have to move away from historical power plays and recognize their right to be out there, leading care and integrating traditional and emerging practices that the patient, his family, and the nurse deem to be of value. Integrative nursing begins with the nurse recognizing her unique and powerful role in ensuring that the patient is kept at the centre of a caring, healing, therapeutic relationship that brings together appropriate interventions to enhance health and wellbeing.

The major "Aha!" experience that the CBAS Quality Champions get when working through the Implementation Programme lends power to this view. If suitably challenged and supported in the raised awareness that results from this strategy, they should have no doubt about the increasing development of integrative nursing approaches.

Leadership in healthcare generally, and nursing in particular, needs to step up to the plate. Francis's 2013 report into the failings at Mid Staffordshire NHS Foundation Trust highlights how patients were failed by the system, which put the organization's interests before the safety of patients and their families.

The Vision for Nursing (DH 2012) sets out how the profession needs to be the leader of care and compassion. One of the most challenging aspects of the vision for nursing in the United Kingdom is developing nurses to lead with a broader sociopolitical leadership model and position themselves ready to influence health policy. Antrobus and Kitson (1999) noted the leadership discourse in the United Kingdom had to date been concerned with professional issues, and as a result it had focused upon developing nurses and nursing. However, the findings of the study question the political success of the internally focused nature of leadership in the previous century. They argued for nursing to interpret and translate between macro issues of policy and the micro issues of practice. Almost a decade later, we see the emergence of politically savvy leaders working closely with ministers not only to influence but to shape the policy. Some would argue that nursing is now seen to influence health policy at government levels, while others suggest there are still gaps, particularly in the leadership of education. Setting the patient at the centre of all activity needs to be addressed both operationally and strategically.

Nursing leaders in England, Northern Ireland, Scotland, and Wales are working in different cultures and policy timeframes. Nursing must work closely with the designers of the system, civil servants, ministers, and managers. National policy changes in 2013 in each of the countries will see a shift in power balance—for example, in England, the policy is driven by competition, contestability, and choice, while in Scotland by integration and collaboration. This tension in the system calls for education and practice to synergize their ideas and creatively seek new solutions. As the policy shift aims to both meet a holistic agenda where care is transferred to the home and encourage patients to self-manage and self-care, so, too, the education curriculum must change to a more holistic, integrative mode.

The further development of integrative nursing approaches requires a change in attitude and expectations. The nurse may engage in the creation of ways to effectively measure qualitative interventions, or she may need to accept that some things are immeasurable and let go of professional self-doubt while seizing personal courage. High-quality care requires compassion, kindness, effective communication between client and professional(s), collaborative decision-making based upon the expressed desires of the client, the creation of a psychologically safe environment in which concerns can be expressed and addressed, and, of course, clinically excellent interventions. Nurses are good at all of these.

In looking at the definition of integrative nursing, we were reminded of the work of Csikszentmihalyi (1993, p. 241) on wisdom. He says there are three components to wisdom:

- It is a way of knowing—a cognitive skill grasping at the universal truths underlying specific events or issues.
- It is a way of acting based upon a set of values which relate to personal and interpersonal harmony.
- It is personally desirable—inner wisdom leads to serenity, and this feel-good factor acts as both cause and effect in enabling people to let go of narrow, introverted goals for broader, universal harmony. Serenity also makes the individual less vulnerable to the cares and woes of "non-wise" beings.

The similarities between wisdom and integrative nursing are impressive. If nurses in the United Kingdom can truly use their whole selves in creating a space for clients and their relatives at the centre of all activity, accepting that people are the real experts on themselves and that we only have to discover how to gather that information, they would be in a position to protect them (serenely) from the attention of the non-wise beings who assume "patients must be done to."

> *There are moments when heart, mind, body and spirit combine to join the flow of caring*
> *so that healing happens. As nurses we are part of this healing stream.*
> *—Wright, 2006*

Let's create caring and healing relationships that truly support whole person and whole systems healing.

We believe nurses are wise.

Carpe Diem.

SELECTED REFERENCES

Department of Health. (2001). *The Expert Patient: A New Approach to Chronic Disease Management*. London: The Stationery Office.

Department of Health. (2012). *Compassion in Practice. Nursing Midwifery and Care Staff: Our Vision and Strategy*. London: DH.

Francis, R. (2010) *Interim Report on the Independent Inquiry into Care provided by Mid Staffordshire NHS Foundation Trust. January 2005—March 2009*. London: The Stationery Office.

Francis, R. (2013). *Report of the Mid Staffordshire NHS Foundation Trust Public Inquiry*. London: The Stationery Office.

Mitchell, A., & Cormack, M. (1998). *The Therapeutic Relationship in Complementary Health Care*. London: Churchill Livingstone.

Neal, K. (2003). Nurse-patient relationships. Cited in Hinchliff, S., Norman, S., & Schober, J. (Eds.), *Nursing Practice and Health Care*. 4th ed. London: Arnold.

Nursing and Midwifery Council. (2008). Statistical Analysis of the Register 1st April 2007 to 31st March 2008. London: NMC.

The Royal College of Nursing.http://nursingstandard.rcnpublishing.co.uk/students/clinical-placements/patientcentred-care/holistic-care.

The Scottish Government. (2010). The Health Care Quality strategy for Edinburgh, Scotland. Retrieved April 19, 2013, from www.scotland.gov.uk/Resource/Doc/311667/0098354.pdf.

Wright, S. (2006). The heart of nursing. *Nursing Standard, 20*(47), 20–23.

38

Integrative Nursing in Ireland

MICHAEL SHANNON AND MARTIN McNAMARA

Overview of Nursing in Ireland

A SUMMATION OF IRISH HEALTHCARE SERVICES

Significant health and nursing policy developments have had an impact on the nursing profession and practices over the last decade in Ireland. It is evident that nursing must demonstrate its value to those who have the power to affect or determine policy decisions and the allocation of resources. The nursing profession is evolving within the broader context of healthcare, healthcare policy, and society at large. Nurses working in Ireland presently face considerable challenges in providing increasingly specialized care to patients with ever more complex needs. There has been a public-sector employment control framework in operation, including a moratorium on staff recruitment and mandated reductions in admissions to nursing programs in recent years. These constraints place greater demands on practicing nurses to do more, and better, with fewer staff.

In the Irish context, as well as the economic downturn affecting health spending, two related sets of developments over the last decade are particularly relevant and are shaping the debate about the nursing profession. First, the Irish healthcare system has been through significant and far-reaching restructuring, including the creation of the centralized Health Service Executive (HSE), since 2005. Driving this restructuring, there has been an explicit policy goal to shift resources and services from acute care into primary care and for greater service coordination and integration of services. Secondly, changes have taken place in the profession of nursing, particularly in specialist and advanced clinical roles and responsibilities and in education and management roles, following the hugely influential *Report of the Commission on Nursing* (Government of Ireland, 1998).

EVOLUTION OF NURSING IN IRELAND

In the first part of the nineteenth century, following the loosening and subsequent re-
peal of the Penal Code, the Irish Catholic Church became active in establishing education, health, nursing, and poor-relief services, and in providing care for the elderly, the
insane, and the "fallen" (Inglis, 1998; Luddy, 1995; Magray, 1998; McKenna, 2006). By
the 1960s, periodicals in Ireland had begun to discuss the actual and potential contribution of nurses to the health services. *The Catholic Nurse* (1922) and *The Irish Nurses'
Journal* (1936) carried reports of research into nursing, including job analyses and time
and motion studies, and discussed previously unrecognized aspects of the nurse's role,
such as health educator (Fealy, 2004).

A major review of the role of nurses in the Irish health services and health service management commenced in 1975, when the Minister for Health established the
Working Party on General Nursing (Department of Health, 1975). It made 66 recommendations, among which was recognition of the role and function of nursing and the
provision of support staff to undertake non-nursing duties (Department of Health,
1980, para. 4.20.10). McGowan (1980) described the work of the nurse in Ireland as
complex, involving the application of a range of skills for an ever more complex clinical role that included care planning, administrative duties, problem solving, teaching,
and patient safety.

While the "good Irish nurse" ideal persisted in the public consciousness, by the
1990s, many Irish nurses considered the "good nurse" ideal to be a myth (Simons et al.,
1998). Nurses were now viewed as being well educated, having up-to-date skills and
knowledge, and they were perceived as open-minded, competent, confident, and ethical (Simons et al., 1998).

Numerous reports published between 1998 and 2011 have had a huge impact on
the nursing profession in Ireland. The most influential force for public and professional policy in relation to nursing has been the implementation of the *Report of the
Commission on Nursing: A Blueprint for the Future* (Government of Ireland, 1998),
which was a result of extensive consultation with nurses, midwives, and other interested parties.

In an extensive review of the changes in the professional role of nurses during
the seventeen years between 1980 and 1997, Condell (1998) concluded that the Irish
nursing profession needed to clearly state the parameters of nursing care so that role
boundaries could be established and defined. In her examination of the changes in
the professional role of the nurse outside Ireland, Savage (1998) identified a number
of problems associated with the role of the nurse, including role strain, role conflict,
and role ambiguity, which centered on issues such as definitive agreement on levels of
practice, legislation for advanced practice, criteria for entry to specialist and advanced
practice, and the scope of professional practice. In her review of management in the
health services, Flynn (1998) highlighted the diversity of roles undertaken by nurses

in the management of health services internationally and how the wider health system and hospital organizational structures determined nursing structures. The National Council for the Professional Development of Nursing and Midwifery (2001–2011) oversaw the development of clinical career pathways for nurses and midwives, including clinical nurse/midwife and advanced nurse/midwife practitioner roles.

Since the Commission on Nursing report in 1998, nursing and midwifery have undergone rapid change, and a number of publications have identified both the potential and under-utilization of nurses and midwives. These include *The Scope of Nursing and Midwifery Practice* (An Bord Altranais, 2000), which outlined a framework to support and empower nurses and midwives to determine and make decisions about the expansion of their scope of practice. The *scope of practice* is defined as the "range of roles, functions, responsibility and activities which a registered nurse is educated, competent and has the authority to perform" (An Bord Altranais, 2000, p. 3). The *Strategic Framework for Role Expansion of Nurses and Midwives* (Department of Health and Children, 2011) provides the current policy direction for the enhancement of nursing and midwifery roles. This framework explicitly requires a skill-mix assessment when examining role-expansion opportunities.

EDUCATIONAL SYSTEM

Up until the last decade of the twentieth century, the system of nurse training in Ireland was based on the Nightingale apprenticeship model, introduced as part of a process of nursing reform in the late nineteenth century. The Nightingale apprenticeship model began as a vocational extension of secondary education and was strongly insulated from the mainstream of higher education (Fealy, 2006). It was only at the start of the twenty-first century that nursing in Ireland gained entry to the academy and joined the other graduate professions in healthcare. A significant milestone in the reform of nursing education in Ireland was the *Working Party Report on General Nursing* (Department of Health, 1980), which called into question the apprenticeship model of training as a suitable method for meeting the education and training needs of nurses. In 1994, *The Future of Nurse Education and Training in Ireland* (An Bord Altranais, 1994) led to the establishment of links with higher education for the purpose of academic accreditation at diploma level. Finally, recommendations of the Commission on Nursing (Government of Ireland, 1998) resulted in the introduction in 2002 of a four-year bachelor of nursing degree as the sole route of entry to nursing practice in general (adult), psychiatric, and intellectual disability nursing. Until this time, degrees in nursing were offered by only a few centers to experienced registered nurses, mainly on a part-time basis. In 2006, a direct-entry midwifery degree was established, as well as a four-and-a-half-year integrated children's and adult nursing program.

The achievement of undergraduate student status for nursing students, all-graduate status for registered nurses, and full academic status for former nurse tutors was hailed as a major success for Irish nursing (Begley, 2001; Cowman, 2001). However, the extent to which the curriculum was based on a coherent and distinctive vision of the discipline of nursing and its epistemic basis, as opposed to perfectly legitimate social, economic, and political considerations related to improved pay, conditions, and parity of esteem with other healthcare occupations, has been an enduring issue in Irish nursing education (McNamara, 2008)

In late 2011, the Irish Minister for Health commissioned a National Strategic Review of Undergraduate Nursing and Midwifery Degree Programmes (Department of Health, 2012) to evaluate their alignment with the health service reform program, the future workforce needs of the public health system, and the need to achieve value for money. The content, structure, and delivery of degree programs was examined, as well as the number of student places required to meet projected workforce needs, given the anticipated patterns of service delivery in the health system of the future.

NURSING WORKFORCE

Nursing as both a profession and an occupational group has been through significant changes in the last decade and has faced challenges in recent years arising from funding cuts and restrictions on recruitment. At the end of September 2010, the largest employer in Ireland, the Health Service Executive (HSE), employed 108,801 whole-time equivalent (WTE) healthcare staff across all HSE-funded organizations (Health Service Personnel Census, 2010). Nurses and midwives comprise 34% of the HSE workforce and are collectively the largest group of employees within the public health sector. The number of nurses had fallen to 35,800 by September 2011 due to public-sector employment controls (Health Service Personnel Census, 2011); by December 2012, the number had fallen further to 34,900 (Health Service Personnel Census, 2012), though nursing remains by far the largest health professional group.

Irish nurses have also faced challenges in recent years in relation to the clarity of the various roles and grades of nurses working in the health system. The Commission on Nursing recommended that an examination of the nursing and midwifery resource be undertaken by a steering group under the auspices of the Department of Health and Children. The findings in the *Interim Report* (Department of Health and Children, 1997, p. 15) suggested: "In the tightening labor market there is likely to be a re-assessment and re-evaluation of professional roles and consideration to the concept of 'substitution' and 'redistribution of tasks' of nurses." This view was challenged by Shannon (2001) in the *Effective Utilization of Professional Skills of Nurses and Midwives Irish Report*, which recommended that a grade of healthcare assistant/maternity healthcare assistant be introduced as a member of the healthcare team to assist and support the nursing and midwifery function in Ireland. This report recommended that the nursing/midwifery function remain the preserve of nurses and midwives to ensure the profession is effectively regulated, educated, and developed. This view was further supported in an *Irish Department of Health and Children Report* that stated: "There is no substitution for the skilled expertise of the qualified nurse who must remain central to the assessment, planning, implementation and evaluation of patient care and to the supervision and delegation of all activities [in] relation to patient care" (Shannon & Murray, 2001, p. 11).

The Nursing and Midwifery Resource Steering Group Report, *Towards Workforce Planning* (Department of Health and Children, 2002), recognized that the profession of nursing can exert considerable influence on health service redesign. The report recommended the adoption of an integrated strategic approach to workforce planning with the nursing and midwifery professions as key participants in the creation of the skilled, competent, and qualified workforce required to meet the changing demands of the health system; however, the recommendations of this report were implemented only in 2009.

The Commission on Nursing also recommended that middle nursing managers should have a defined functional role in managing units of care, with clear responsibilities and explicit delegation of authority from directors of nursing. This would allow them to engage in professional and clinical leadership, staffing and staff development, resource management, and effective communications. Furthermore, the Commission recommended that the Department of Health and Children, health services providers, nursing management, and nursing organizations develop appropriate systems to determine staffing levels and examine opportunities for the increased use of care assistants and other non-nursing personnel in the performance of non-nursing tasks.

Integrative Nursing in Ireland

The Report of the National Strategic Review of Undergraduate Nursing and Midwifery Degree Programmes, published in December 2012 (Department of Health, 2012) highlighted some of the curricular and pedagogical issues that many nurse educators, nursing academics, and commentators had long believed militated against the transmission and enactment of a philosophy of nursing congruent with the principles of approaches such as integrative nursing (McNamara, 2010; McNamara et al., 2011). Although widely welcomed as a positive and progressive step in nursing education, the form and content of undergraduate nursing degree programs had for some time given rise to concerns about their tendency over time to become content-saturated and to institutionalize a rupture between theoretical and clinical learning. An investigation of the underlying principles structuring nursing curricula in Ireland suggested that they tended to lack an integrating, underpinning framework that was grounded in a distinct nursing standpoint and perspective. This gave rise to eclectic, fragmented, and at times incoherent curricula lacking the cohesion and direction required to undergird the formation of the strong professional and disciplinary nursing identities necessary not only for the enactment of a distinct nursing role, but also for meaningful and legitimate participation in multidisciplinary and interprofessional teams (McNamara, 2009).

It is reassuring to note, therefore, that the report stresses the importance of a philosophy of nursing and a unique disciplinary knowledge base to underpin curricula and support the professional identity of nursing. This should enable nurses to articulate their professional and disciplinary boundaries and to better represent their distinctive contribution to patient, family, community, and health system outcomes. Boundaries matter because they provide the basis for genuine interprofessional working; they should be neither rigid nor impermeable, but rather must be flexible, porous, and continually negotiated (McNamara et al., 2011). The concepts of the expert patient, self-care, and a recovery approach are highlighted in the report, as is effective communication within genuinely therapeutic relationships. Equality, patient involvement, and inclusiveness emerge as key principles, and better integration of theoretical and clinical learning is recommended. The dominance of a hospital and acute-illness model is challenged, and a rebalancing of the curriculum to foreground a community and health-promotion focus is advocated. Featured terms such as "emancipatory and person-centered care," the "management of key transitions," "clinical judgment and decision making," "quality and patient safety," and "respect for dignity and diversity" are encouraging. However, the challenge will be to embed these concepts and principles in a curriculum that is infused with a distinct nursing disciplinary perspective and that is experienced as coherent and cohesive by students across all the settings in which they learn. The overarching, comprehensive, and inclusive concept of integrative nursing may well offer a way to address this challenge.

Integrative Nursing Models and Exemplars in Ireland

In Ireland, the concept of integrative nursing has not been explicitly named or referenced. However, its meta-theoretical perspective and underlying tenets will by no means be unfamiliar to Irish nursing scholars or clinicians. Drawing on documentary sources from the nineteenth century, Meehan (2012) proposes the "Careful Nursing" philosophy and practice model based on the work and writings of pioneers of modern, professional nursing in Ireland, such as Catherine McAuley, Mary Aikenhead, and their contemporaries, as well as the work of Thomas Aquinas. The model is currently in use in Ireland and in New Jersey, Illinois, and Indiana in the United States (Meehan, 2012).

The philosophical assumptions underlying nursing practice in the Careful Nursing professional practice model are the human person, an infinite transcendent reality, and health. The human person is a unitary being in whom bio-physical and psycho-spiritual realities can be distinguished. Attention is paid to both the outward life of the body and senses and to the inward life of the mind, spirit, and communion with an infinite transcendent reality. After Aquinas, an infinite transcendent reality is the "abundantly loving source of all creation, unitary wholeness and healing in the universe" (Meehan, 2012, p. 2908). Health is human flourishing, described as the person's integrated experience of relative autonomy, harmony, personal dignity, contentment, and a sense of purpose. The ultimate source of flourishing lies in nature and in an infinite transcendent reality; it can be fostered by restorative psycho-spiritual, bio-physical, and social influences in individuals and in their environment.

These three basic tenets give rise to four elements of a nursing professional practice model: therapeutic milieu, practice competence and excellence, management of practice and influence in health systems, and professional authority. Each of these has a number of dimensions wherein the congruence with integrative nursing is evident. First, the therapeutic milieu dimensions are *caritas*, contagious calmness, nurses' care for themselves and each other, intellectual engagement, and a safe and restorative physical environment. Second, practice competence and excellence transcend the narrow biomedical model perspective on health and illness, emphasizing the range of evidence-based modalities that nurses, in "supportive participation" with families, friends, and the community, might draw upon in "fostering safety and comfort" using their clinical reasoning and decision-making capacities. Next, a whole-systems approach is discernible in the third element, which is concerned with the support of nursing practice at all organizational levels through trustworthy collaboration with other healthcare professionals, administrators, leaders, and policy makers based on "perceptiveness, prudent judgement and fortitude" (Meehan, 2012, p. 2912). Finally, "professional authority" encompasses both professional self-confidence and visibility. Both of these are crucial if nursing is to exercise influence at the systems level. Meehan recognizes the professional affirmation that arises from a deep commitment to a set of professional values that underpin the delivery of a skilled, informed, and valuable public service. Equally, influence and recognition require nurses to articulate their distinct yet complementary contribution to health and healing and to engage in public and professional debate on health issues.

McCarthy and Landers (2010) explore Celtic beliefs, meanings, and ideas for nursing practice, and drawing, *inter alia*, on the poetry and philosophy of John O'Donohue, attempt to recover for Irish nursing a view of the human person and the nurse–patient relationship that integrates insights from the humanities and sacred literature (Baumann, 2010). These insights lead McCarthy and Landers (2010) to propose a model of personhood based on seven assumptions that recognize:

(1) nursing's concern for the whole person;
(2) that the person is an existential being;

(3) that nursing is a caring force entailing a therapeutic relationship that includes caring, love, and hope;

(4) that nursing is a sensing process comprising presencing, hearing, touching, and seeing;

(5) that the nurse is the *Anam Cara* or "soul friend" to each patient;

(6) the influence of the internal and external environment on the individual's health and illness; and, finally,

(7) that the nurse takes responsibility for the restoration of a healing environment.

Having outlined distinctively Irish models of nursing and their views of persons, health, illness, and practice, it is possible to analyze policies and strategies to examine the extent to which the underpinning tenets are implicit but discernible. We now discuss recent developments in nursing education, nurse specialization, end-of-life care in acute hospitals, mental health, and the use of complementary and alternative medicine (CAM).

The Requirements and Standards for Nurse Registration Education Programmes (An Bord Altranais, 2005) have been criticized for being content-driven and over-prescriptive and for no longer reflecting the system changes that have impacted the nature of clinical placement opportunities for nursing students. However, the Nursing and Midwifery Board of Ireland has a statutory obligation to ensure the undergraduate nursing programs comply with all relevant Irish and European Union legislation and directives. The problem may rather lie, then, with the lack of exposure to, familiarity with, and in-depth knowledge of an explicit, integrating theoretical framework within which the various requirements and standards may be addressed in a coherent and integrative manner. A recent review of the representation of nursing programs on the website of Irish nursing schools (McNamara et al., 2012) compared the majority of them unfavorably with exemplar sites of schools in Canada, Norway, and Australia in terms of the extent to which an explicit, integrating nursing discourse was present. Nevertheless, one Irish school did succeed in articulating a distinct nursing perspective, demonstrating that it is possible to comply with the necessary statutory requirements while representing the discipline of nursing in a coherent and credible way. The same argument applies to graduate nursing education programs, including those for clinical specialist and advanced practice roles.

A pilot project underway at a major Dublin academic teaching hospital aims to identify a core set of nursing key performance indicators (KPIs) that are person-centered in focus and clearly relate to the patient experience. Initial work has identified eight KPIs: consistent delivery of care against identified need, patient confidence in the skills of the nurse, patients' sense of safety whilst under the care of the nurse, patients' involvement in decisions made about their care, time spent with patients, respect for patients' choices and preferences, nurses' support for self-care, and nurses' understanding of what is important to patients. These KPIs suggest nursing-sensitive and specific outcome measures that are consistent with some of the core principles of integrative nursing and could be integrated with other measures to demonstrate the impact of graduate registered nurses, clinical specialists, and advanced practitioners.

Until recently, nursing and midwifery education and practice in end-of-life care had largely been based on experiential learning wherein custom and practice generally dictated how care was planned and implemented in the final stages of dying and after death. Specialist Palliative Care teams have had a considerable influence on end-of-life care, particularly symptom management, education, leadership, and research. Yet, outside the remit of Specialist Palliative Care teams, practices can fall short of what is required to ensure optimal care.

In response to an identified need for improvements in end-of-life care, a national program of work has been underway since 2007 through the Irish Hospice Foundation's Hospice Friendly Hospitals Program. The program is based on core principles that support hospitals to develop effective end-of-life care systems and practices consistent with international best practice. One core principle targets the cultures and contexts in which end-of-life care occurs in acute and residential settings. The focus of this strategy is on creating the necessary infrastructure to support person-centered care and initiate and embed change in a range of practice settings. Nursing teams in major acute hospitals work together in practice development groups to critically review their current practices and to plan and implement change; the emphasis is on fundamental culture change, critical creativity, and teamwork, rather than technical skills.

Emancipatory practice development (Manley et al., 2008) starts with a critical exploration of attitudes and beliefs about end-of-life care. Through a process of facilitated inquiry, nurses are beginning to interrogate hitherto-unquestioned care practices and transform the clinical area so that it provides a more conducive environment for patients and their families. Early objectives include reductions in the level of staff-generated noise to create a more therapeutic atmosphere, better use of shared space for private conversations between staff and patients and between staff and relatives, and a greater emphasis on privacy and dignity. Learning to challenge and be challenged is initially daunting for many; nevertheless, participants are discovering that supportive challenge is a necessary process when making changes to their practice.

The Report of the Expert Group on Mental Health Policy, *A Vision for Change* (Government of Ireland, 2006), outlined a framework for fostering positive mental health based on an integrated and holistic view of mental illness and a multidisciplinary approach to dealing with the biological, psychological, and social factors contributing to mental health problems. The principles underpinning the framework are consistent with those of integrative nursing, emphasizing person-centered treatments, formulated in consultation with service users and their carers, the involvement of service users and their significant others, and harnessing the resources of service users and their social networks to achieve meaningful integration and participation in the life of the community. A focus on promoting mental health through enhancing protective factors, a recovery orientation, and an emphasis on the social determinants of mental illness reflects a holistic and integrative approach to care, consistent with the philosophy of integrative nursing and a template for policies for a range of other conditions.

In Ireland, individuals have a right to avail themselves of complementary and alternative medicine if they so wish, unless there are contraindications to its use. This is particularly important in the use of aromatherapy, herbal preparations, homeopathic preparations, and reflexology. Fox et al. (2010) found that the use of CAMs is increasing in the general Irish population, with the prevalence rate for visits to CAM practitioners increasing from 20% in 1998 to 27% in 2002. CAM practitioners most frequently visited were acupuncturists, reflexologists, homeopaths, chiropractics, and osteopaths. Pain, anxiety, and depression were found to be significant predictors of CAM use. Overall, Fox et al. (2010) conclude that the pattern of CAM use in Ireland is broadly in line with international trends; its use continues to grow, and it now represents a significant sector within Irish health care, mainly because of an increase in patient demand and in the number and diversity of providers that now exist.

The Nursing and Midwifery Board of Ireland has provided guidance to nurses and midwives in relation to the use of complementary therapies in two of its publications— *Guidelines for Midwives* (An Bord Altranais, 2001, Section 17) and *Guidance to Nurses and Midwives on Medication Management* (An Bord Altranais, 2003, Section 2.8). Nurses and midwives who wish to use CAM in the course of their practice must adhere to the following standards:

- Complete an educational program that develops the knowledge and skills required to use CAM therapies in a competent manner. Where this program is confined to a particular form of complementary therapy, practice must be confined to that therapy only. Where possible, training should be accredited by a body established for that purpose.
- Be fully aware of any contraindications or restrictions to the use of a particular therapy for an individual patient or client, taking full account of the client's medical history and current treatments. Therapies should complement and not replace conventional medical therapy.
- The individual patient or client must consent to the use of complementary therapies. Detailed and clear written information should be provided, a verbal explanation given and the client's understanding of both determined.
- Obtain the written agreement of their employer to use CAM in their practice.
- Exercise their accountability for the administration of CAM through accurate recording of the therapy and the patient's response to its use.
- Ensure ethical, evidence-based practice; the development by healthcare institutions of clinical guidelines for the utilisation of complimentary therapies is strongly recommended.

Nurses and midwives are also advised to enquire into and document a patient's or client's own use of complementary therapies when taking a history as part of the assessment.

There are many centers in Ireland that offer complementary therapies in addition to conventional medical therapy. For example, at St. Luke's Hospital in Dublin, aromatherapy and therapeutic massage are available to patients with cancer. Patients who may benefit from any of these therapies are referred for treatment by nursing staff, radiographers, or doctors. Additionally, Our Lady's Hospice in Harold's Cross has a department of Complementary and Supportive Therapies, which also conducts research on complementary therapies. In recognition of the interest exhibited by the public in complementary therapies, the Department of Health has funded three full-time clinical research nurses to carry out research. These nurses are currently based in Our Lady's Hospice.

Challenges and Barriers to Integrative Nursing

McNamara (2008, 2009) has identified the lack of preparation and lack of interest of many nurse educators and nursing academics as one of the key barriers to the enactment of philosophies and models such as integrative nursing in Ireland. This is primarily a systemic rather than an individual failing, as historically the education programs through which nurse educators were prepared and formed did not place much emphasis on the distinctive ways of being a nurse and of knowing and doing nursing. This was then reflected in the curricula that they developed and delivered. Without targeted interventions to interrupt this state of affairs, there is a danger of maintaining an undesirable status quo by which the education system reproduces nurses with only a tenuous grasp of the distinct and fundamental principles underpinning the professional and disciplinary practice of nursing. Recent critical scholarship (e.g., McNamara, 2010) and the recommendations of the National Strategic Review (Department of Health, 2012) provide some grounds for optimism that there is a growing awareness of the long-term consequences for the profession of being unable to articulate a distinct disciplinary perspective.

One such consequence emerged in a comprehensive national review of the clinical leadership development needs of nurses and midwives (Fealy et al., 2011; Casey et al., 2011; McNamara et al., 2011). Casey et al. (2011) found that the need to engage in the collective development of the profession was highest for all grades of nurse. Fealy et al. (2011) found that nurses, particularly those at staff and middle-manager levels, experienced a lack of influence in interdisciplinary care planning and policy, as well as a lack of recognition of the nursing contribution to care. McNamara et al. (2011) concluded that clinical leadership development should emphasize the development of all nurses as clinical leaders in the context of the delineation, clarification, and articulation of their distinctive contribution in multidisciplinary care settings. Nurses' recognition and influence in and beyond the immediate context of care depends greatly on their ability to articulate the distinct nursing contribution to patient care. This ability provides an essential resource to resist the ongoing blurring, effacement, and dilution of nurses' roles.

Vision of Integrative Nursing in Ireland

Ireland is currently facing economic challenges that are unprecedented in the history of the State. These affect the provision of all public services, particularly health and social care, which account for a significant proportion of the national budget. Concomitant with these financial constraints is the requirement to assure patient safety and to enhance the quality of services provided, in parallel with a service reconfiguration aimed at achieving greater effectiveness and efficiency. These challenges mirror those facing countries across the world.

In light of the scale of these challenges, it is imperative that all stakeholders, including nurses and midwives, work together to provide a safe, high-quality healthcare service that is responsive, timely, and accessible. This is a hugely challenging agenda, particularly in light of the planned introduction of a Universal Health Care funding model, the development of clinical risk and governance agendas, and the implementation of clinical care programs across acute, primary, and continuing care. Nurses and midwives in Ireland have the capacity, insight, dedication, and resilience to support and drive the necessary operational change agenda not only at the frontline, but also at managerial, corporate, strategic, and policy development levels. With the necessary educational infrastructure, informed by a distinctive nursing disciplinary perspective and the necessary organizational support, nurses and midwives have an unprecedented opportunity to play a central role in reengineering existing and developing new healthcare services in Ireland. Fundamental to nursing leadership and health service reform is the critical application of integrative nursing.

SELECTED REFERENCES

Baumann, S. L. (2010). Exploring Celtic beliefs, meaning, and ideas for nursing practice. *Nursing Science Quarterly, 23*(4), 341–342.

Fealy, G. M. (2006). *A History of Apprenticeship Nurse Training in Ireland.* London: Routledge.

Fealy, G. M., McNamara, M., Casey, M., Geraghty, R., Butler, M., Halligan, P., et al. (2011). Barriers to clinical leadership development: Findings from a national survey. *Journal of Clinical Nursing, 20*(13–14), 2023–2032.

Fox, P., Coughlan, B., Butler, M., & Kelleher, C. (2010). Complementary alternative medicine use in Ireland: A secondary data analysis of the SLAN studies. *Complementary Therapies in Medicine, 18,* 95–109.

McCarthy, G. M., Landers, M. G. (2010). A conceptual model of nursing: A model of personhood for Irish nursing. *Nursing Science Quarterly, 23*(4), 343–347.

McNamara, M., Fealy, G., Casey, M., Geraghty, R., Butler, M., Halligan, P., et al. (2011). Boundary matters: Clinical leadership and the distinctive disciplinary contribution of nursing to multi-disciplinary care. *Journal of Clinical Nursing, 20*(23–24), 3502–3512.

McNamara, M. S. (2009). Nursing academics' languages of legitimation: A discourse analysis. *International Journal of Nursing Studies, 46*(12), 1566–1579.

McNamara, M. S., Fealy, G. M., Geraghty, R. (2012). The visibility of the discipline on the websites of academic nursing schools. *Nursing Outlook, 60*(1), 29–36.

McNamara, M. S. (2010). Where is nursing in academic nursing? Disciplinary discourse, identities and clinical practice: A critical perspective from Ireland. *Journal of Clinical Nursing, 19*, 766–774.

Meehan, T. C. (2012). The careful nursing philosophy and professional practice model. *Journal of Clinical Nursing, 21*(19–20), 2905–16.

39

Integrative Nursing in Iceland

GISLI KRISTOFERSSON AND THORA JENNY GUNNARSDOTTIR

Overview of Nursing and Healthcare in Iceland

From the time Iceland was settled, around A.D. 870, until the late seventeenth century, Scandinavian- and European-influenced traditional folk healing was the only form of healthcare delivery available to Icelanders. Most widespread were the use of herbs, and later homeopathy, before formal medical training became more common. Official midwifery training was established in 1761. Today, Iceland has universal healthcare, like the rest of the Nordic countries. Healthcare expenditures in Iceland currently represent 9.7% of the gross domestic product (GDP), which is comparable to other that of Western nations with a similar healthcare model, and significantly lower than the United States, which has 17.4% of its GDP devoted to healthcare costs, according to latest Organization of economic cooperation and development (OECD) data. The United States cannot claim nearly the success Iceland can in areas such as infant mortality rate and general life expectancy (OECD, 2012). This being said, it should come as no surprise that 82% of nurses in Iceland work in the public sector, and 50% of all working nurses are employed by the nation's largest hospital, the National University Hospital of Iceland (NUHI). Private not-for-profit agencies deliver vital healthcare services in Iceland, but the majority of care is publically funded. Many nursing homes for the elderly operate according to this private-pay model. There is much debate about whether private for-profit organizations can play a more vital role in the Icelandic healthcare system. At this point, these organizations are few and play only an insignificant role in the delivery of healthcare to Icelanders. Public and political opinion is greatly divided on this issue, and there are no immediate plans to increase their role for now.

According to the Icelandic Nurse's Association (INA), there are approximately 600 registered nurses per 100,000 inhabitants in Iceland (INA, 2012). This is well below the EU average of almost 800 nurses per 100,000 inhabitants, and drastically below that of other Nordic countries like Denmark (more than 1,400 nurses per 100,000 inhabitants) and Finland (more than 1,500 nurses per 100,000 inhabitants)

(European Hospital and Healthcare Federation, 2012). Nurses in Iceland are regulated by numerous laws and regulations and are responsible for the care they provide according to those laws.

Since 1973, a nursing program at the university level has been offered at the University of Iceland. The only other university-level nursing program in Iceland is at the University of Akureyri in the northern part of the country. Both programs are four years in length, with two semesters each year consisting of sixty ESTS (European Credit Transfer System) credits. Students must complete a total of 240 credits within six years to graduate with the degree of bachelor of science in nursing. Iceland is one of the few countries in the world where a bachelor's degree is required for entry into the nursing profession. In addition students must complete a matriculation exam after attending four years of upper secondary education in a gymnasium to be admitted to college, making the process of nursing education in Iceland one of the most extensive in the world.

Both university programs offer a short introduction to complementary and alternative medicine (CAM), including massage, relaxation therapy, music therapy, and aromatherapy, emphasizing the use of these practices as supported by evidence-based knowledge. The students do hands-on exercises in relaxation and massage therapies. In 2008, the first course at the graduate level was offered to nurses through the University of Iceland and became quite popular. In its 2011 manifesto, the Icelandic Nurses' Association emphasized the role of complementary therapies by stating that: "health service users should be given the opportunity of complementary therapy grounded on evidence-based knowledge and provided by nurses who have specialized in the area in question" (INA, 2011, p. 6).

In 2010, nurses interested in complementary therapies set up the Chapter of Complementary Therapies for Nurses through the INA. The aims and goals of the chapter include plans to increase the use of evidence-based integrative therapies within the healthcare system and increase nurses' knowledge about these therapies.

Icelandic healthcare facilitates each have their own independent regulatory systems, but only a few have set up specific organization-wide regulations about the use of CAM in their facilities. There is language in Icelandic healthcare laws that patients should have access to the best care available at each time, which would include integrative therapies, but it remains unclear how organizations should enforce these laws. So the use of these therapies within a particular healthcare system is often limited, based on the knowledge and education of individual healthcare professionals. Furthermore, in 2012, there was a proposal set forth at the Althingi (the Icelandic parliament) to examine how the healthcare system could reimburse certain complementary therapies if they were shown to be beneficial to patients. However, mainly due to cost-related issues, the bill did not garner majority support, but it did stimulate an interesting discussion on the use of integrative therapies in the Icelandic healthcare system and possible reimbursement by the state.

Integrative Nursing in Iceland

In 2000, eight major societies of complementary therapies in Iceland merged to form a single organization called the Association of Complementary and Alternative Medicine in Iceland (ACAMI). About 600 practitioners are a part of this organization, whose major goals are to make continued progress on healers' work environments and to establish recognition and provide education on issues related to the work of healers in the community (ACAMI, 2012).

The legal environment for these practices is slowly improving, and a few important milestones have been reached. In 2005, the Ministry of Health in Iceland decided to commission a report on the regulatory status and future direction of integrative medicine in Iceland, which highlights the many challenges faced by nurses wanting to practice CAM in Iceland (Althingi, 2005). The authors of the report conducted many in-depth interviews with various stakeholders and parties of interest and made concrete recommendations based on their findings. Although most of these recommendations have only been followed in part at this point in time, it is of interest to review the highlights briefly, as they are pertinent to the growth of integrative nursing in Iceland:

- Educational facilities should be responsible for the education of healthcare professionals to increase their focus on integrating CAM successfully into the traditional healthcare system.
- An academic center will be established where healers and representatives from the social sciences, life sciences, and healthcare sciences unite in interdisciplinary research on the efficacy and utility of various CAM modalities.
- The Health and Rehabilitation Clinic in Hveragerdi (HRC) will be given the official role to introduce healers in the community and work for the integration of these areas in collaboration with the Association of Complementary and Alternative Medicine in Iceland.
- Healthcare authorities will encourage healthcare facilities to promote to their patients the utilization of the services of healers and encourage healthcare facilities to form a specific policy when it comes to CAM in their facility.

As a part of a larger study on the use of healthcare services in Iceland, the scope of the utilization of healers was assessed and the likely explanatory factors of their use explored (Helgadottir, Vilhjalmsson, & Gunnarsdottir, 2010). A sample of 1,532 Icelandic adults between the ages of 18 and 75 responded to a survey yielding a 60% response rate. Almost 32% of the respondents had visited a healer in the past twelve months, an estimated increase of 5% since 1998. Women and high-income individuals were more likely to use a healer than men and lower-income individuals. Individuals having negative or positive attitudes toward physicians' services were more likely to use a healer than those expressing a neutral attitude. Finally, repeated physician visits were related to an increased likelihood of CAM use. These results reveal that Icelanders use healers to a considerable degree, and it appears that the general healthcare system insufficiently meets the needs of the public in this regard. Finally, most CAM users appear to use CAM treatments as a supplement to the care provided in the general healthcare system, indicating that the utilization of both of these approaches is by no means mutually exclusive.

Studies have been done to assess the use of CAM in oncology patients at the NUHI. A final-thesis project of nursing students revealed that, among 120 patients receiving cancer treatment, all but one of these patients had used CAM in addition to medical intervention (97.5%) (Gretarsdottir, Thordardottir, & Gudmundsdottir, 2002). The most common forms of CAM used were natural products (70%), then spiritual coping mechanisms (69%), followed by various forms of physical exercise (69%). Very similar findings can be seen in the results of a thesis project from a pharmacy student in 2002 (Konradsdottir, 2002). The results of a European study ($n = 956$) of patients in cancer treatment reported that Icelandic patients' ($n = 43$) use of CAM was 30.2%, compared to 35.9% of the total group (Molassiotis et al., 2005).

In 2002, a survey within the NUHI (Baldursdottir et al., 2002) found that 26 of 54 nursing units responding used CAM in the care of their patients. The most common forms of CAM used were relaxation and massage to reduce anxiety and increase the quality of sleep. Whether CAM was offered was often decided by an individual nurse or a small group of nurses, and CAM was not integrated into the care model of the units or the application of appropriate outcome measurements.

INTEGRATIVE NURSING MODELS AND EXEMPLARS IN ICELAND

Nurses in Iceland have been practicing integrative nursing by using interventions that support the person as whole. This has been practiced within the hospital settings as well as in rehabilitation or in health clinics situated out in the countryside, where the intense Icelandic nature plays a big role in healing and wellness. Some therapies are provided to patients within the hospital setting, but institutions have not been up to date in enhancing guidelines regarding the matter, as previously discussed. However, nurses have often been at the forefront of proposing guiding principles in the use of CAM in their respective institutions and/or agencies in Iceland.

Nursing is perfectly situated at this time to lead the way in integrative healthcare delivery in Iceland. Nurses in Iceland appear to be open and positive towards increasing the role of CAM modalities in their practice. It can be assumed that CAM is being implemented all over the country, as the authors continue to receive news of individual nurses or isolated groups of nurses applying the principles of integrative nursing in to their practice. However, these are individual efforts, often lacking formal institutional oversight or appropriate quality control and outcome evaluations. The interest

The Health and Rehabilitation Clinic (HRC)

The relatively unspoiled nature of Iceland, with its hot springs and an abundance of clean water, offers many opportunities to improve health through integrative therapies. One such place is the HRC Spa and Medical Clinic, owned by the Nature and Health Association of Iceland (www.hnlfi.is). The natural surroundings are geothermally active and rich with hot springs. The grounds include multiple walking and hiking paths, swimming pools, and indoor exercise facilities. A key philosophy of the HRC is the belief that the body has its own power to heal and rejuvenate. Different CAM modalities are individually tailored to suit the healthcare needs of each guest. The clinic offers treatments to promote health, based on the philosophy of natural medicine, placing special emphasis on healthy nutrition, hydrotherapy, outdoor exercise, relaxing herbal and mud baths, meditation, physiotherapy, acupuncture, massage, and health education. Nurses play an important role and are responsible for many of the mind–body therapies that take place at the HRC, such as meditation and relaxation sessions.

Reykjalundur Rehabilitation Center

Reykjalundur is a rehabilitation clinic located just outside Reykjavik that specializes in the holistic rehabilitation of persons recovering from both physical and mental health problems. Nurses at Reykjalundur have long been known for their innovative strategies to aid in their clients' long road to recovery. They use CAM modalities such as progressive relaxation and relaxation massage, along with mindfulness-based interventions (www.reykjalundur.is).

Midwifery

Integrative therapies have been used by midwives in Iceland for some time. The use of acupuncture has increased in Western medical practice, and several midwives in Iceland are now using acupuncture as a therapeutic tool (Vernhardsdottir et al., 2009). Since 2002, midwives in Iceland have had the opportunity to take courses in acupuncture that are specifically tailored to benefit women who are pregnant. The courses have been certificated by the Icelandic Directorate of Health (the equivalent of the U.S. Surgeon General). In 2008, around 160 midwifes had earned the certificate to integrate acupuncture into their practice. Two studies in Iceland have evaluated the effects of acupuncture in this setting. One looked at the efficiency of acupuncture in actuating cervical ripening and spontaneous labor after 41 weeks of normal pregnancy (Vernhardsdottir, 2008). The findings showed that the intervention may have a positive effect on cervix ripening; however, a larger sample size is required to adequately examine the effectiveness of this intervention. Another study was designed to assess the effects of acupuncture on pelvic pain during pregnancy (Vernhardsdottir et al., 2009). Twenty women were given acupuncture treatments twice a week for four weeks by a pair of midwives. The women evaluated their pain on a visual analog scale (VAS) scale and answered three questionnaires over the research period. The results show that there was a significant reduction of pain, and approximately 75% of the women felt that the acupuncture treatment reduced their pelvic pain slightly or noticeably. The intervention also appeared to improve mobility, sleep, and the ability to perform daily activities. Icelandic midwives have also been using aromatherapy with good results to treat pain and nausea during delivery, although official outcome measures have not been implemented yet.

Nursing Homes

Pet therapy, aromatherapy, massage, and relaxation are among the therapies that appear to be used most frequently in long-term care settings in Iceland. Most of the therapies are provided by nurses or nursing assistants who have gained specific training in the area of the CAM being implemented. Outcomes of these programs have not been published.

Oncology Nursing

It is well documented that cancer patients are frequent users of CAM (Deng et al., 2007). It is also known that some CAM modalities have been shown to be effective and help patients cope better with symptoms and increase their wellbeing (Deng et al., 2007). However, not much is known about the effectiveness of many of the therapies or how some of the CAM modalities interact with other therapies that patients receive within the hospital. Therefore, the cancer unit at the NUHI has worked to apply guidelines for patients and healthcare professionals who use CAM and provide information on their use, developing a policy on the use of such therapies for cancer patients. The goal of this work was to make suggestions about how these services should be provided within the hospital setting and how outcomes could be evaluated most efficiently.

In 2006, a group consisting of three nurses and one physician was formed to examine how the integration of CAM could be achieved safely in the care of cancer patients at the NUHI. The group developed guidelines for the cancer units, which were introduced and accepted by physicians in these units in 2008. They are greatly inspired by guidelines from the Society for Integrative Oncology (SIO), which is supported by evidence-based practice in integrated medicine (www.integrativeonc.org). According to the Icelandic guidelines, only specific complementary therapies are to be used within the hospital. They are: massage, physical exercise, relaxation, and acupuncture. Furthermore, the guidelines discuss the importance of providing information on the potential usefulness and possible risks of the therapies for the patients and increasing research on their efficacy in this clinical setting.

A good example of the use of CAM within the NUHI is relaxation therapy. Relaxation therapy has been offered at the oncology and hematology outpatient clinic for more than a decade, as well as on various psychiatric units. Many patients have expressed great satisfaction with the therapy, but little is known about other outcomes. A study was conducted to assess changes in nine common symptoms among cancer patients who received relaxation therapy (Gunnarsdottir, Jonasdottir, & Fridriksdottir, 2011). Since 2007, patients who receive relaxation therapy at NUHI have completed the Edmonton Symptom Assessment Scale (ESAS) before and after each therapy session. ESAS includes nine symptoms, with severity scored on a 0–10 numeric rating scale, with higher scores indicating more severity. A retrospective chart review was completed on 251 patients who received relaxation therapy from January 2007 until August 2008. The results showed a significant decrease in symptom prevalence, mean number of symptoms, and symptom severity. The prevalence of worst wellbeing to best wellbeing decreased from 92% to 59%, tiredness from 87% to 65%, anxiety from 78% to 54%, and shortness of breath from 60% to 40%. The greatest difference in means was on the variables of wellbeing and tiredness. These results indicate that this individualized relaxation therapy is effective, at least in the short term, to reduce both symptom prevalence and severity of symptoms common in cancer patients. There are plans to conduct further studies on the role of CAMs within the NUHI.

Psychiatric Nursing

Psychiatric nurses have been quite engaged with CAM, but usually as individuals. Relaxation groups have been a common form of intervention, and hypnotherapy has also been offered by nurses within the specialty. And although not always implemented by nurses exclusively, massage, mindfulness, and yoga have also been available for specific populations of psychiatric patients at the NUHI for some time. In recent years, a nurse has been offering reflexology treatment to psychiatric patients at the NUHI. This therapy has become quite popular with the patients in the psychiatric units of the NUHI.

is clearly there; the next steps are to increase quality, efficacy, and patient safety in the delivery of integrative nursing approaches in Iceland. Integrative nursing, as it is discussed in this book, gives structure to this effort and offers valuable tools to continue on the right path.

Challenges and Barriers to Integrative Nursing

The challenges and barriers that can impede nurses from providing integrative nursing care are the same in Iceland as in other Westernized countries. Laws and regulations on the delivery of CAM in many institutions are virtually nonexistent or unclear. This creates a culture of providing CAM therapies in isolation and without proper quality assurance and outcome measurements. Also, it is less likely that the safety and efficacy of the modalities is ensured before they are implemented. This especially applies to large institutions meant to serve the entire population, like the NUHI. Apart from this, further improvement is needed in regulatory and credentialing practices for CAM, independent from institutional regulations. This would clarify the expectation and standards of practice for nurses wanting to practice or complement their nursing care with CAM and increase patient safety and provider integrity and quality.

Another challenge for nurses in applying and implementing CAM in their respective practices is the relative obscurity of advanced practice nursing in Iceland. Although one could argue that the role of the RN is relatively strong in Iceland, the same cannot be said about advanced practice nurses, who are relatively few and not very visible in society. Because of the weak position and tradition of advanced practice nurses in Iceland, the expertise needed to implement and develop new interventions outside of the mainstream medical knowledge is not present. But advanced practice nurses are in a unique position, due to their distinctive fund of research knowledge and clinical expertise, to implement budding or lesser-known interventions (Bjornsdottir, 2005).

Iceland also shares with the rest of the Westernized world the challenge that CAM remains on the periphery of academia but mainstream with the public. This divide needs to be bridged somehow. A common explanation is that CAM does not lend itself well to the traditional Western research paradigm of double-blind, placebo-controlled studies (Verhoef et al., 2005). In some cases qualitative methods might be a better fit, but these are often not high on the academic totem pole, especially when it comes to funding. This makes CAM research an underfunded and underdeveloped field, despite intense interest of patients, possible cost effectiveness, and paucity of side effects compared to those of many interventions based on traditional Western medicine.

In this book integrative nursing is seen as focused on integrating traditional Western nursing science with emerging therapies centering on a whole-person approach with a bodymindspirit emphasis. This includes a focus on communities, families, environment, and the physical, psychological, and spiritual dimensions of our clients. For the biologically focused medical paradigm that currently dominates the Icelandic healthcare system to change, much needs to happen. So much so, that nurses could not and should not think to bring about such changes by themselves. Nurses must reach out to other professions to achieve a paradigm shift in the Icelandic healthcare system. This means that nurses need to work with other healthcare professions, lawmakers, and the public to have their services be more person-centered, holistic in nature, and focused on an integrative approach. The barriers between professions are often necessary but sometimes impeding, especially when large-scale changes are needed. This is why an interprofessional dialogue needs to take place about acknowledging the possibilities of a whole-person, whole-system approach to patient care delivery using an integrative healthcare model.

Vision of Integrative Nursing in Iceland

Integrative nursing is the future of nursing, as well as its past. Many Westerners have lost faith in the way we view illness and health. The current paradigm of thinking about illness and health has brought us great advances and many wonders, but now is the time to pause and reflect and perhaps start making changes. Nurses need to start empowering their clients. Arguably the biggest health improvements of the last centuries were not due to the invention of medications or surgical techniques, although these have certainly played their part. The biggest improvements we have seen have been due to simple but effective public health measures such as improved sanitation and nutrition, proper handling of food, and use of disinfectants.

We are now faced with lifestyle illnesses as the main cause of health problems. The solution does not require inventing new medications to lower blood pressure or a new surgical technique to remove the fat from our bellies, although these can and will certainly play a part. A real solution must prevent these kinds of interventions from being necessary. The principles of integrative nursing help shape the nurse's role in the future because they are by their very nature preventative. Exercise, meditation, energy medicine to reduce stress, functional medicine, and dietary supplements can and should play a vital part in the healthcare system of the future.

Iceland's culture and clean environment offer endless possibilities as a center for many modalities in integrative nursing. As stated previously, there is some movement towards this goal, but more work is needed. Geographically, Iceland is situated between North America and Europe, the two continents where lifestyle illnesses are most rampant and therefore CAM is the most pertinent and needed. The unspoilt nature and plethora of geothermal pools, in addition to an extremely well-educated healthcare work force, especially when it comes to nurses, all make Iceland an ideal healthcare oasis that emphasizes the use of integrative nursing.

We encourage the founding of an interdisciplinary center on CAM as suggested in the 2005 healer report and feel this might create an academic way of thinking about CAM instead of academia writing it off as "hippie nonsense." But this might not be a realistic short-term goal, especially since the educational and healthcare systems have suffered greatly following recent budget cuts and the economic collapse of 2008. A more realistic short-term goal is to increase the role of complementary therapies in both nursing programs, including the development of a specific course in the undergraduate programs focusing on CAM, and a track in the University of Iceland's School of Nursing's master's program, where nurses would be able to specialize in the implementation of specific CAM modalities. This would lay a foundation of further development and implication of nurses as leaders in the CAM revolution we all know is coming.

Icelanders could greatly benefit from outside support and encouragement when it comes to integrating complementary therapies into the healthcare setting. There is no need to reinvent the wheel, and there are institutions all over the world that are successfully integrating CAM in to their paradigm of care. This is especially true for Scandinavia and the United States (e.g., the Integrative Care Science Center in Sweden and the Center for Spirituality and Healing at the University of Minnesota in Minneapolis). Some degree of cooperation is already underway in the implementation and training of nurses and nursing students in integrative approaches between Iceland and the other Nordic countries, and we hope this will only increase over time. It is our hope that collaborations be established between Iceland and these, and more, institutions to further develop the integration of CAM modalities into mainstream healthcare in Iceland.

Summary

The extent to which the principles of integrative nursing are aligned with nursing practice in Iceland remains somewhat unclear. In this chapter, the highlights of integrative nursing in Iceland have been reviewed to shed some light on this issue. This chapter cannot be seen as a comprehensive overview of the use of integrative therapies by nurses in Iceland, as such a vast undertaking lies outside the scope of this chapter. What remains clear, though, is that nurses are interested in providing integrative nursing care for their patients, and many are taking the first steps to do so. There is a unique opportunity for further rapid growth due to the excellent educational background of nurses in Iceland and the cultural acceptance of integrative modalities, to which the Icelandic healthcare system has thus far been extremely slow in responding. Nurses need to speed up. A revolution in the application of integrative therapies in the healthcare setting is coming, and those who miss the boat are doomed to watch from ashore as the future of healthcare unfolds.

SELECTED REFERENCES

ACAMI. (2012). The Association of Complementary and Alternative Medicine in Iceland. Retrieved on March 20, 2012, from http://big.is/page29/page29.html.

Deng, G. E., Cassileth, B. R., Cohen, L., Gubili, J., Johnstone, P. A. S., Kumar, N., et al. (2007). Integrative oncology practice guidelines. *Journal of the Society for Integrative Oncology,* 5(2), 65–84.

European Hospital and Healthcare Federation. Retrieved on March 5, 2012, from http://www.hope.be/03activities/quality_eu-hospitals/eu_country_profiles/00-hospitals_in_europe-synthesis_vs2011-06.pdf.

Helgadottir, B., Vilhjalmsson, R., & Gunnarsdottir, T. J. (2010). Notkun ohefdbundinnar heilbrigdisthjonustu a Islandi. [Use of complementary and alternative therapies in Iceland]. *The Icelandic Medical Journal, 96,* 269–275.

Icelandic Nurses' Association. (2011, May). Nursing knowledge for your benefit. Policy of the Icelandic Nurses' Association on Nursing and Healthcare, 2011–2020. Retrieved on March 21, 2012, from http://hjukrun.is/library/Skrar/Fagsvid/NursingPolicy2011%20loka.pdf.

Minister of Health. (2005, Jan.). *Report from the Minister of Health on Alternative Practitioners.* Retrieved on April 4, 2006, from www.althingi.is/altext/131/s/0731.html.

Molassiotis, A., Fernandez-Ortega, P., Pud, D., Ozden, G., Scott, J. A., Panteli, V., et. al. (2005). Use of complementary and alternative medicine in cancer patients: A European survey. *Annals of Oncology 16*(4), 655–663.

Organization for Economic Co-operation and Development. Retrieved on March 5, 2012, from http://www.oecd.org/document/16/0,3746,en_2649_33929_2085200_1_1_1_1,00.html

The Icelandic Nurse's Association. Retrieved on March 5, 2012, from http://www.hjukrun.is/english-information/nursing-in-iceland/.

Verhoef, M. J., Lewith, G., Ritenbough, C., Boon, H., Fleishman, S., & Leis, A. (2005). Complementary and alternative medicine whole systems research: Beyond identification of inadequacies of the RCT. *Complementary Therapies in Medicine, 13,* 206–212.

40

Integrative Nursing in Sweden

MATS JONG, MIEK C. JONG, AND TORKEL FALKENBERG

Overview of Nursing and Healthcare in Sweden

In Sweden, as in most European countries, formalized nursing emerged around 1400, when Catholic convents such as Vadstena kloster (http://www.birgittask-loster.se) were established in the southern parts of the country. The convent hospitals, and later on, the state hospitals, were from the beginning mostly dedicated to care for victims of major diseases of the time, such as the plague (*Pestis yersinia*), leprosy, and later on tuberculosis. Before the work of the nuns and monks of the convents, traditional healers called "old and wise men and women" (*Kloka gubbar och gummor*) were present in most villages during the farming society period. Among the nomadic people of Scandinavia, the Sami people, shamans called *Noaidi*, were numerous. These traditional healers played an important role in Scandinavia all the way into the twentieth century. Parts of the conceptual heritage of a "wise woman" are still evident today in the healthcare profession of midwifery, where midwives are sometimes referred to as *jordemor/jordgumma* (English, "earth mother"). During the witch hunt from 1666 to 1676, more than 300 women were killed, most likely wise old women with knowledge about birth and birth control. Beginning around 1680, the role of the midwife in Stockholm was regulated, and they were required to undergo training and examination by the chief physician of the town. Since 1951, it has been compulsory to first become a licensed nurse before undergoing midwife training.

Modern forms of nursing education made entrance in Sweden in the late nineteenth century, when one of Florence Nightingale's students, Emmy Rappe, founded the Red Cross Nursing School in Stockholm in 1867 (http://www.rkh.se/index.php?lang=eng). Licensed nurses have been educated on a university level since 1977 (two years of training) and since 1993 have undergone three years of theoretical and practical training.

Today, there are nursing schools at 25 different universities in Sweden, where approximately 4,000 nurses graduate each year. There are approximately 1,400 actively working licensed nurses per 100,000 inhabitants of Sweden (Socialstyrelsen, 2012). This is higher than the EU average of 800 nurses per 100,000 inhabitants (European Hospital and Healthcare Federation, 2011).

HIGHER EDUCATION IN SWEDEN

In 2006, the Swedish government ratified changes to comply with the Bologna Process (Joint Declaration of the European Ministers of Education, 1999), which aimed to make academic degree and quality assurance standards more comparable and compatible throughout Europe (Riksdagen, 1993, 1994, 2006). Put into action during 2007, this resulted in several changes to the system of higher education, which is now offered on three cycles (levels): Cycle 1 consists of three years of studies at the basic level (bachelor's degree), Cycle 2 involves one or two more years at an advanced level (master's degree), and Cycle 3 consists of four years of studies at the research level (doctorate).

NURSING EDUCATION

Basic Nursing Education—Cycle 1

In Sweden, the basic university level of nursing training contains three years of study and results in a bachelor's degree as well as a professional degree as a Licensed Nurse. The bachelor's degree is issued in the subjects of nursing, nursing science, or caring science.

In order to make Swedish nursing education more homogeneous, the Board of Health and Welfare issued a document describing the knowledge and competencies that are required for a Licensed Nurse (Socialstyrelsen, 2005) and aligned with the learning goals of the Higher Education Ordinance (Riksdagen, 1993). The document focuses on a model (Table 40.1) containing the three major areas of competence in the nursing profession, pinpointing the presence of a holistic view and ethical attitude (Socialstyrelsen, 2005).

Specialization in Nursing (Postgraduate Diploma in Specialist Nursing, 1 Year) and Master's Degree (2 years)—Cycle 2

After becoming a licensed nurse, there are a number of different specializations on the postgraduate level, leading to a Postgraduate Diploma in Specialist Nursing and a master's degree. These specializations include anesthesiology nurse, acute care nurse, intensive care nurse, operating room nurse, district nurse, and approximately ten others. The advanced level comprising two years of study represents more of an academic progression than a professional one.

Degree of Doctor in Nursing (PhD)—Cycle 3

The doctoral training consists of four years of full-time study, during which time students usually write three or four articles (published in international peer-reviewed journals), which then become chapters in their published PhD dissertation.

Table 40.1: Areas of Competence in the Swedish Nursing Profession

Major areas of competence	The theory and clinical practice of nursing	Research, development, and education	Leadership
A crosscutting presence of ethical and holistic values	*The nursing profession shall:* • *be founded on ethical values and a humanistic view of humans* • *show consideration, care, and respect for the patient autonomy, integrity, and dignity* • *value and respect the experiences and knowledge of the patient and his/her family* • *show openness and respect for different values and religious/spiritual beliefs* • *from the wishes or the needs of the patient or his/her family, speak in their cause* • *use existing research—ethical principles and conventions* • *make use of the knowledge and experiences of the working team and others in order to contribute to a holistic view of the patient*		

NURSES' ROLE IN HEALTHCARE AND SOCIETY

For decades, nurses in Sweden—in particular those who specialized in the areas of district nurse, child- youth healthcare, and school nursing—have had a unique and very important role in promoting health in the population. An example is the free antenatal and child healthcare, which provides services to promote child health and development and strengthen parents' ability to care for their newborn baby (Swedish Association of Midwives, 2007). Nurses also participate and work in the national vaccination programs and combine Physical Activity on Prescription (PAP) with Motivational Interviewing (MI) to help people develop their own inherent capacity to change.

THE SWEDISH NATIONAL SOCIAL AND HEALTH INSURANCE SYSTEM

Sweden has a national social and health insurance system that covers everyone who lives or works in Sweden. It provides financial protection for families and children, for persons with a disability, and in connection with work injury, illness, and old age. The system is financed primarily through taxes (70%), with additional funding from state support and patient fees. The economical risks and costs are shared by all people when a person or a family suffers from poor health and requires professional help (Försäkringskassan, 2013).

Healthcare is provided in accordance with the Health Care Act (Riksdagen, 1982) under the responsibility of the regional county councils or regional federations. Each healthcare provider receives funding based on an elaborate system of approximating the yearly healthcare cost per person living within its geographical borders (http://english.skl.se/). The individual pays a small subsidized fee for each visit to a care provider or care facility (approximately $0–$60US), with a maximum of $130–$150US per year for healthcare and a max of $1,300US for prescribed medications. For children, healthcare is free of charge (Försäkringskassan, 2013).

Integrative Nursing and Care in Sweden

Since the 1920s, intense lobbying of anti-quack movements in Sweden has led to national legislation that severely limits the possibilities of healthcare professionals to use complementary and alternative medicine (CAM) in their practice (Riksdagen, 1998). Until recently, licensed healthcare providers were only allowed to give CAM therapies to severely ill patients if no other treatment options were available, the interventions were not likely to cause harm, and the initiative came from the patient. As will be discussed later, the legal situation has recently changed, as the present law focuses more on patient safety (Riksdagen, 2010). Integration of CAM into conventional medicine relies and will continue to rely on its evidence (in accordance with Integrative Nursing Principle 5, see Chapter 1 of this book). Eklöf & Kullberg (2004) divide the practice of CAM and integrative care methods in Sweden into four categories:

I.   Patient-initiated treatments outside conventional medicine where treatment is paid by the individual patient "out of pocket" to the practicing CAM therapist. (CAM therapies are not included in the national health insurance or in most private insurances.)

II. Formal cooperation between conventional healthcare and CAM providers through referral of patients, stated by contracts, predominantly to licensed healthcare personnel (e.g., licensed naprapaths and chiropractors) or care facilities.

III. Licensed healthcare personnel practicing CAM within conventional care (e.g., massage, acupuncture, tai chi, yoga, mindfulness)

IV. Close cooperation under the "same roof" between licensed healthcare personnel and non-licensed CAM therapists

There exist only a few, relatively outdated population studies with respect to CAM use among the general population in Sweden. Studies conducted in 1999 and 2000 indicated that CAM usage is relatively high, with approximately 30% reporting use of natural remedies, nutritional supplements, and vitamins (Nilsson, Trehn, & Asplund, 2001). In a wider definition of CAM, 39% report to have used any CAM method in their life, and 20% in the last year, with massage, and the manual manipulative methods of naprapathy, and chiropractic care being the most common (Hanssen et al., 2005). Even though naprapathy and chiropractic therapy are licensed, evidence-based professions in Sweden, their services are not integrated in conventional healthcare.

A CAM treatment that has been integrated by nurses in a variety of care settings is tactile massage (TM). TM is a form of touch massage developed in Sweden during the 1970s by the pediatric nurse Siv Ardeby. It aims to stimulate attention, close contact, and communication through touch, and to reduce worry, stress, and pain, thereby promoting wellbeing (Ardeby, 2003; Airosa et al., 2011; Andersson, Tornkvist, & Wandell, 2009). TM is fully in line with the definition of integrative nursing as outlined in Chapter 1: it is an evidence-informed practice based on a caring and healing relationship that supports whole-person/whole-system healing (Lindgren, 2012). Acupuncture and TENS (transcutaneous electrical nerve stimulation) are other examples of CAM treatments that have become more or less accepted and integrated into conventional medicine.

NURSING PRACTICE OF COMPLEMENTARY AND ALTERNATIVE MEDICINE (CAM) IN SWEDEN

Little has been published on nurses' attitudes toward, use of, and practice of CAM in Sweden. A survey that investigated the practice of CAM among licensed nurses in Sweden (Jong, Jong, & Lundqvist, 2013) found that 15% of nurses who responded practiced some form of CAM. The majority, 69%, practiced CAM among family and friends, 25% within a private business, and 37% within public healthcare. The different CAM methods practiced are listed in Table 40.2. A total of 47% wish to practice CAM in the future.

INTEGRATIVE/HOLISTIC NURSING'S TRADITIONAL ROLE AND PLACE IN SWEDISH NURSING CURRICULA

Terms such as *integrative nursing* and *integrative medicine* are unfamiliar within the nursing profession in Sweden (Bjersa, Stener Victorin, & Fagevik Olsen, 2012). However, the concepts of holistic care and healing have been taught for a long time and are well integrated in curricula. There also continues to be a major focus on promoting health and preventing illness as well as the concept of salutogenesis (focusing on what keeps humans healthy as opposite to pathogenesis which focuses on what makes us sick).

During the late 1980s and early 1990s, Antonovsky's book *Unraveling the Mystery of Health* (1987) became popular among nursing educators in Sweden. The book elaborates on what makes people stay healthy and defines a sense of coherence in the terms of *comprehensibility, manageability,* and *meaningfulness.* Frankl's ideas (1997) about finding and maintaining meaning in suffering also influenced nursing education in

Table 40.2: Methods Practiced Today, and Those the Respondents Wish to Practice in the Future

| | a | | b | |
| | Practicing method today (n = 140) | | Wish to practice method in the future (n = 448) | |
	frequency	%*	frequency	%*
Massage	79	56.4	291	65.0
Dietary supplements/probiotics/ herbal remedies	54	38.6	147	32.8
Mind–Body Therapies	50	35.7	199	44.4
Spiritual treatments/therapies	33	23.6	60	13.4
Other**	27	19.3	40	8.9
Acupuncture	16	11.4	193	43.1
Anthroposophy	14	10.0	53	11.8
Creative therapies	13	9.3	95	21.2
Homeopathy	8	5.7	45	10.0
Ayurveda	7	5.0	60	13.4
Traditional Chinese medicine	3	2.1	53	11.8
Naprapathy	3	2.1	43	9.6
Chiropractic	2	1.4	47	10.5

*Percentages may exceed 100% due to the fact that respondents had the option of choosing multiple areas of practice.

**Among the other methods that are practiced today, different "home remedies" stand out. Other methods are mentioned, but there are no obvious categories; acupressure is the only method mentioned more than once. When it comes to what methods the respondents wish to practice in the future, the pattern is similar to that we saw in the CAM methods that are practiced today, the exception being that more people have mentioned tactile massage, aroma therapy, osteopathy, zone therapy, and the Rosen method.

Sweden. Both Antonovsky and Frankl support the notion of a holistic view of humans, a view that is expressed to some extent in the Swedish Healthcare Act but made more explicit by the Board of Health and Welfare in the "Description of Competence" that is required for a Licensed Nurse (Socialstyrelsen, 2005). Practically, the holistic view is present as a natural part of nursing curricula in all minor and major subjects of training, theoretical as well as clinical practice.

Some universities in Sweden (Karolinska Institutet, Gothenburg University/ Sahlgrenska Akademin, Karlstad University, Mid Sweden University, and Linköping University) offer possibilities for nursing and medical students to choose elective overview courses on integrative care and CAM. This includes experiential components in soft massage, breathing techniques, and mindfulness, as well as more specific courses in herbal medicine and acupuncture. Mid Sweden University has planned to start a full master's program in Integrative Health and Medicine.

INTEGRATIVE CARE/NURSING AND CAM—BELIEFS, KNOWLEDGE, AND ATTITUDES

Internationally, studies have reported that nursing students and faculty are open to including elements of CAM in the curricula (Avino, 2011; Kreitzer, Mitten, Harris, & Shandeling, 2002) and that the competency with CAM becomes greater after its inclusion (Booth-Laforce et al., 2010). A majority of oncology nurses believe that CAM can give added value to their patients (Damkier, Elverdam, Glasdam, Jensen, & Rose, 1998) and that nurses provide CAM in a high degree but express a lack knowledge (Shorofi & Arbon, 2010).

Then, what about Swedish nurses? A survey among licensed nurses (Jong et al., 2013) found that fewer than 12% ask patients about CAM use. The most common reason for not asking is that the nurses do not consider themselves knowledgeable about CAM. These findings are in line with the results of Shorofi and Arbon (2010) from Australia, and Bjersa et al. (2012) from Sweden. However, a high proportion (66%) of the nurses agrees that healthcare personnel should inform clients about CAM treatments when asked. This further supports our idea that there is a need for a higher degree of presence of integrative care and CAM in Swedish nursing education.

Exemplars of Integrative Care

HOSPICE/PALLIATIVE CARE

There are many facilities in Sweden dedicated to providing high-quality care for people who are close to dying. The care philosophies of these facilities, as well as their practical work, are based on holistic and integrative ambitions. Some are organized by the regional county councils, but most of them are run as nonprofit organizations (care foundations), often in collaboration with local municipalities and regional county councils, and also supported by gifts from individuals, companies, and churches. One pioneering example is Axlagården in Umeå (www.axlagarden.se), which has continuously provided humanistic-based care and holistic care at end-stage life. They provide qualified medical treatment integrated with generous nursing, which includes tactile massage, Jacuzzi, art therapy, and other activities to stimulate and increase the wellbeing of their guests.

ANTHROPOSOPHIC CARE—THE VIDAR CLINIC

The Vidar Clinic is the only fully integrative hospital and health central in Sweden, providing care based on conventional medicine as well as anthroposophic care. All licensed staff, physicians, and nurses are trained in both conventional and anthroposophic medicine. Anthroposophic medicine aims to stimulate patients' self-healing capacities by restoring the balance of bodily functions and strengthening the immune system, rather than primarily relieving the symptoms of disease. A broad variety of anthroposophic medicinal products originate from minerals, animals, and different parts of plants. In addition, non-medication therapies such as art therapy, rhythmic massage, eurhythmic movement therapy, and counseling are applied by nurses and specialized practitioners (Kienle, Kiene, & Albonico, 2006).

Challenges to Integrative and Holistic Nursing

LEGISLATION AND THE HEALTHCARE SYSTEM

Before 2012, healthcare staff were not allowed to offer CAM treatments, with the exception of terminally ill patients with no treatment options left. If they were practicing CAM, or any method not proven by scientific evidence, they would risk losing their license. In 2012, a case against a general physician who had been prescribing homeopathic remedies was brought to court. The prosecutor demanded de-legitimization of the physician based on the writing of the law. However, the Supreme Administrative Court (2011) ruled on interpretation of the Patient Safety Act (Riksdagen, 2010), declaring that the safety of the patient had not been at risk during the homeopathic treatment. On the basis of this verdict, licensed healthcare staff can now provide safe CAM treatments to fully informed and willing patients as long as they do not withhold from them any proven active treatment.

Although recent legal developments have created better opportunities for integrative care in Sweden, radical lobbyists and anti-quack movements will probably still remain a challenge for people working in the areas of CAM and integrative nursing. The increasing interest worldwide in individual patient-centered care, freedom of choice, and self-management may support CAM healthcare professionals in dealing with these challenges.

NURSING EDUCATION

Experience and research shows a high level of interest in promoting the whole-person view and including elements of integrative nursing within the nursing profession as well as in nursing schools (Jong et al., 2013). However, arguments often fall flat when discussions about teaching hours are made, where the hours for "hard, medical, physiological subjects" often win over the soft values of ethics and relational aspects of nursing. A similar view is shared by nursing students who are most interested in learning the technical aspects of nursing. Future employers more often ask for the technical skills and medical knowledge than the students' communication abilities and openness for integrative care. Herein is a true challenge for those active within the field: to put forth the evidence-based practices of integrative nursing and to demonstrate how they can add value to the direct care of patients, as well as in the training of future nursing staff.

A LACK OF NATIONAL SOURCES OF RELIABLE INFORMATION

In Sweden it is hard for patients, consumers, healthcare staff, and other stakeholders to find reliable information about CAM methods and integrative care. Internationally, there are some good examples of information providers, such as the National Center for Complementary and Alternative Medicine (NCCAM) in the United States (http://nccam.nih.gov/) and the National Research Center in Complementary and Alternative Medicine (NAFKAM) in Norway (www.nafkam.no). In Sweden, an initiative has been taken by the Integrative Care Science Center (IC) to provide online information to decision makers, press, and the general population on integrative care and CAM (http://www.integrativecare.se/en/). The IC initiative is presently in small scale, but hopes to develop more with support from stakeholders, to become a national competence center.

THE PUBLICLY FUNDED HEALTHCARE SYSTEM OF SWEDEN

The healthcare system of Sweden poses the greatest challenge for integrative nursing. Decisions regarding funding and prioritization of healthcare are made by politicians on a national, regional, and local level. This makes it hard for "new" interventions and treatments with roots in CAM to gain ground to be accepted, prioritized, and reimbursed by public caregivers. Decision makers in Sweden rely on advice and recommendations given by special advisory organizations such as the Swedish Council on Health Technology Assessment (www.sbu.se), which represents a view of evidence that is primarily based on quantitative biomedical data. In their systematic reviews of research, studies with qualitative methodology or complex interventions are seldom or never classified as having a high degree of evidence. The conclusion is often that more, larger randomized studies are necessary before such treatment options can be taken up in the public system.

Vision of Integrative Nursing in Sweden

The holistic, whole-person/whole-system point of view in healthcare has good support in the Swedish legislation (Riksdagen, 2010) and in the descriptions of competencies for registered nurses in Sweden (Socialstyrelsen, 2005), though it remains a question whether this will provide an opportunity for integrative nursing. Newspapers in Sweden are almost daily writing articles about patients who have experienced maltreatment, mostly caused by poor judgment and communication by medical staff who fail to create a relationship with the patient and thereby also hamper the possibility for patient-centered care and shared decision-making. These incidents stress the importance of reclaiming the integrative basis of caring and nursing, in which nurses are an integral part of the healing process (Integrative Nursing Principles 4-5, Chapter 1 and Chapter 3). Elements of this are taught at nursing schools and legislated, but not fully put to practice. In order to promote changes in the healthcare system at macro as well as micro levels, several actions are necessary to account for the principles of integrative nursing. The actions need to work from both top-down as well as bottom-up perspectives.

HOW TO INITIATE CHANGES AT DECISION-MAKING LEVELS

If decision makers will show interest and take actions to support whole-person care, it will generate positive effects throughout the healthcare system. Therefore, it is necessary to revisit the conventional, quantitative, biomedical view of evidence to take account of evidence generated in complex interventions from a whole-systems approach, in line with the circular model—taking account of evidence generated in multimethod research, where each method complements the other, (Walach, Falkenberg, Fonnebo, Lewith, & Jonas, 2006) as well as the complex system science (CSS) approach described in Chapter 1 of this book. The meta-theoretical perspective of CSS "provides a plausible explanation for the age-old adage that interventions must be considered within the context of the whole of the situation; what works in one case is not guaranteed success in another" (Chapter 1). Both the circular model and the CSS adhere to the first principle of integrative nursing: "Human beings are inseparable from their environments" (Chapter 1).

NURSING EDUCATORS, PRESENT AND FUTURE

A need exists for experiential courses for nurse educators, nursing students, and present staff to broaden their view on patient care, as well as to support their own wellbeing in line with integrative nursing Principle 6: "Integrative nursing focuses on the health and wellbeing of caregivers as well as those they serve" (Chapter 1; see also Chapter 3 about tending to the healer's vulnerability). This can be achieved by bringing in different elements of evidence-informed practices such as aromatherapy, massage, and mindfulness into nursing training. Since the spring of 2012, the Mid Sweden University has run an experiential Mind–Body program for staff and groups of nursing students, adapted from the program of Georgetown University in Washington, D.C. (Karpowicz, Harazduk, & Haramati, 2009; Saunders et al., 2007). By introducing a number of mind–body techniques (mindfulness, guided imagery, art, music, movement, writing, and more), the program aims to reduce stress and promote self-awareness, empathy, and openness. So far, preliminary results demonstrate that students embody a different attitude towards stressful events and to the biomedical paradigm, in line with the study by Karpowicz et al. (2009). As described by Janet Quinn in Chapter 2 of this book, "Self-awareness and self-knowledge are the beginning points of developing the multiple intelligences and skills necessary for integrative, person-centered, relationship-based caring and healing nursing practice."

These types of programs will certainly create awareness among university staff, students, and future healthcare professionals of the qualities of integrative practices, especially the importance of relaxation and meditation to promote and maintain health. This may facilitate integration of these techniques into clinical practice of healthcare.

SELECTED REFERENCES

Bjersa, K., Stener Victorin, E., & Fagevik Olsen, M. (2012). Knowledge about complementary, alternative and integrative medicine (CAM) among registered health care providers in Swedish surgical care: A national survey among university hospitals. *BMC Complementary & Alternative Medicine*, 12, 42. doi: 10.1186/1472-6882-12-42.

Damkier, A., Elverdam, B., Glasdam, S., Jensen, A. B., & Rose, C. (1998). Nurses' attitudes to the use of alternative medicine in cancer patients. *Scandinavian Journal of Caring Science*, 12(2), 119–126.

Försäkringskassan. (2013). The Swedish Social Insurance Agency (Försäkringskassan). Retrieved February 28, 2013, from http://www.forsakringskassan.se/sprak/eng/.

Hanssen, B., Grimsgaard, S., Launso, L., Fonnebo, V., Falkenberg, T., & Rasmussen, N. K. (2005). Use of complementary and alternative medicine in the Scandinavian countries. *Scandinavian Journal of Primary Health Care*, 23(1), 57–62.

Jong, M., Jong, M. C., & Lundqvist, V. (2013). A cross-sectional study on Swedish licensed nurses' use, practice, attitudes and knowledge about Complementary and Alternative Medicine (CAM). *Submitted for publication*.

Nilsson, M., Trehn, G., & Asplund, K. (2001). Use of complementary and alternative medicine remedies in Sweden. A population-based longitudinal study within the northern Sweden MONICA Project. Multinational monitoring of trends and determinants of cardiovascular disease. *Journal of Internal Medicine*, 250(3), 225–233.

Saunders, P. A., Tractenberg, R. E., Chaterji, R., Amri, H., Harazduk, N., Gordon, J. S., et al. (2007). Promoting self-awareness and reflection through an experiential mind-body skills course for first year medical students. *Medical Teacher*, 29(8), 778–784. doi: 10.1080/01421590701509647

Shorofi, S. A., & Arbon, P. (2010). Nurses' knowledge, attitudes, and professional use of complementary and alternative medicine (CAM): A survey at five metropolitan hospitals in Adelaide. *Complementary Therapies in Clinical Practice*, 16(4), 229–234. doi: 10.1016/j.ctcp.2010.05.008

Socialstyrelsen. (2005). Description of required competencies for Licensed Nurses [In Swedish: Kompetensbeskrivning för Legitimerad Sjuksköterska], artikel, nr 2005-105-1. The National Board of Health and Welfare (Socialstyrelsen). Sweden (p. 17). Stockholm: Socialstyrelsen.

White, A., & Editorial Board of Acupuncture in Medicine. (2009). Western medical acupuncture: A definition. *Acupuncture in Medicine*, 27(1), 33–35. doi: 10.1136/aim.2008.000372

41

Global Activism, Advocacy, and Transformation: Florence Nightingale's Legacy for the Twenty-first Century

DEVA-MARIE BECK, BARBARA M. DOSSEY, AND CYNDA H. RUSHTON

Integrative Nursing and Global Health

Global nursing practice is a large-scale contribution to human health. The missing link in the global goals discussion is often the missing voice of nurses who are striving to actually achieve these goals at grassroots levels with their extensive knowledge and experience. Large-scale global dialogue may seem to be beyond nursing's grassroots scope of practice. But if we can widen our nursing practice worldviews—to contribute our much-needed grassroots knowledge and experience to global dialogues—we can actually provide that essential missing voice. Today, nurses have unprecedented global networking and communications tools that do allow us to enter and contribute to the global arena in innovative ways. This can become the world's much-needed grassroots-to-global advocacy. (Dossey, Beck & Rushton, 2011). In Part VI, we will learn about the Caritas Path of Peace and integrative nurses' global endeavors to address universal needs for healing, health and wellbeing at grassroots levels in Germany, Turkey, England, Ireland, Iceland, and Sweden.

Integrative nursing recognizes health as an ever-changing pattern of creative, adaptive relationships—across all dimensions of human experience. Our integrative nursing lens acknowledges the fundamental unity within and between all beings and their environments. Thus, the health and wellbeing of people everywhere can be seen as having common ground—a worldview to secure a sustainable, prosperous future for everyone. Integrative nursing also focuses on the health and wellbeing of caregivers, as well as those they serve. Even as we see ourselves each as key contributors to global health, we also need to see our own essential self-care as a sustaining contribution to the overall health and wellbeing of all humanity.

Across this world, nurses actively serve on the front lines of healthcare—in rural communities, suburbs and cities, refugee camps, hospitals, war zones, and street clinics. Globally, more than 17 million nurses and midwives are involved in the being-knowing-doing required to advance the health and wellbeing of people, families, and communities (World Health Organization [WHO], 2006). Physically, mentally, emotionally, socially, and spiritually, nurses are prepared and educated to effectively accomplish traditional, integrative, and emerging interventions to support whole-person/whole-systems healing. Everywhere, our knowledge, expertise, wisdom, and dedication are required for humanity to be and remain healthy. Nurses have traditionally worked to achieve local goals. We understand grassroots needs and know how to be on-the-ground activists to meet these needs.

Severe health needs exist in almost every community and country. These are no longer isolated problems in far-off places. Across humankind, we all face common health concerns and global health imperatives. With globalization and global warming, no natural or political boundaries stop the spread of disease. In the developed world, healthcare is increasingly more complex and demanding. In the developing world, healthcare is marginalized and sometimes even nonexistent.

In almost every nation, the severe and chronic global nursing shortage continues to threaten the health of people across the world. This remains a major component of the continuing crises in global healthcare delivery and one of the key dynamics we, as nurses, continually address within our demanding workplaces (WHO, 2006). Struggling to achieve more than we can in any given day, wider global health needs directly impact our own professional and personal lives. In the next section, we review how Florence Nightingale's life remains vitally relevant to today—still helping us to respond to our twenty-first–century global health challenges—as we follow in her footsteps.

Nightingale: The Global Activist

Today, we recognize Florence Nightingale's (1820–1910) legacy as global nursing and global healthcare (Dossey, 2010a; Dossey, Selanders, Beck & Attewell, 2005). She envisioned what a healthy world might be and worked tirelessly to both articulate and realize this vision. Nightingale was a genius of both intellect and spirit, and her legacy resonates today as forcefully as during her lifetime. While most often remembered as the philosophical founder of modern nursing and the first recognized nurse theorist, she also ranks among the most brilliant sanitary, medical, and healthcare reformers in history.

After returning home from her famous achievements during the Crimean War (1854–1856), Nightingale continued—for nearly four decades—to work on the global challenges of her time. She analyzed data, wrote statistical reports, and informed politicians, crafting documents that resulted in legislation. She designed hospitals and sought to improve environments—in both rural and urban areas—by developing collaborative partnerships with others who agreed with her proposed reforms. She met with Queen Victoria, Prince Albert, and other royalty, dignitaries, viceroys, and military officers in India and from around the world, also serving as a consultant to both the North and South during the American Civil War. She changed political will by informing and interacting with government leaders across the British Empire and elsewhere.

Based on her own foundational experience with battlefield conditions, she actually drafted the British position papers presented to the first in a series of Geneva conventions that directly led to establishing the International Red Cross, then the League of Nations, and later, the United Nations. Anticipating the wider interconnected concerns we readily see today, she called for better conditions for women, children, the poor and hungry and for better education programs for marginalized people. She identified environmental health determinants (clean air, water, food, houses, and so on) and social health determinants (poverty, education, family relationships, employment)—local to global (Beck, 2010a).

With a worldwide network of colleagues and from a wide worldview of caring, Nightingale took her own courageous stand as a global advocate for the needs of others around the world. As a result, she gained new a ground of concern for the sick and impoverished people everywhere and sought to remedy the causes of this suffering. Although she faced many barriers, she stood on her own conviction to advocate changes that were necessary. In doing so, she became a catalyst for an emerging worldview that created nursing as we know it today (Beck, 2010b).

Nightingale also actively networked with a wide range of colleagues. As a result, 14,000 of her letters and her 200-plus official reports and books exist today in collections around the world. She also directly contributed to the print journalism of her time. For example, her *Notes on Hospitals* (Nightingale, 1859) clearly describes components of hospital design that we recognize today as factors of optimal healing environments. Her *Notes on Nursing* (Nightingale, 1860a) (79 pages) was written first for the general public and became an immediate bestseller upon first printing. Later, this text—published as a *Notes on Nursing, Revised* (Nightingale, 1860b)—was recognized as the first nursing textbook. While writing her own articles for newspapers and magazines, she also consciously cultivated her connections with the media professionals of her time, making sure they understood, communicated, and shared her messages.

She used these effective advocacy skills to shape public awareness, actively promoting health as a priority for people throughout the world. As a strong global advocate, she was a change agent who confronted apathy and indifference wherever she encountered them. Nightingale called all of these activities "health-nursing" and declared "health is not only to be well, but to use well every power we have" (Nightingale, 1893). In this way, she remains a model for nurses today, as we participate in achieving the UN Millennium Goals discussed next.

Global Activism and Achieving the United Nations Millennium Development Goals (MDGs)

During the year 2000, world leaders convened a United Nations Millennium Summit to establish eight Millennium Development Goals (MDGs) that must be achieved for the twenty-first century to progress toward a sustainable quality of life for all of humanity (United Nations Development Programme, n.d.). These interrelated goals, listed in Box 41.1, are an ambitious agenda for improving lives worldwide. Of these eight MDGs, three—#4: Reduce Child Mortality, #5: Improve Maternal Health, and #6: Combat HIV/AIDS, TB, malaria, and other diseases—are directly related to health and nursing.

World Health Organization Director General Margaret Chan has noted that efforts to achieve all the MDGs have clearly improved health across the world (WHO, 2013). This points directly back to the work Nightingale achieved in her time. Hence, all the UN goals have aims similar to those we as nurses work to achieve every day, at grassroots levels, everywhere. Nurses are engaged with various endeavors to address the global health included within the scope of the UN MDGs. Nurses are truly global activists who create new structures—widening health and healing worldviews with local dialogues and activities that shift behaviors and create new meaning-making towards health, including the process of health-making globally. We are continuing Nightingale's relevance and legacy for grassroots-to-global health with our authentic advocacy, as discussed next.

Authentic Advocacy

The word "advocacy" is derived from the Latin *advocatus*, "counselor," and *advocare*, "to summon or to aid." An advocate is a person who speaks or writes in support of something. Nursing organizations have codes of ethics recognizing advocacy as nursing's

---

Box 41.1 UN Millennium Development Goals (MDGs)

MDG 1: Eradicate extreme poverty and hunger.
MDG 3: Promote gender equality and empower women.
MDG 4: Reduce child mortality.
MDG 5: Improve maternal health.
MDG 6: Combat HIV/AIDS, malaria and other diseases.
MDG 7: Ensure environmental sustainability.
MDG 8: Develop a global partnership for development.

Source: United Nations Development Programme (UNDP), 2000. http://www.un.org/millenniumgoals/reports.shtml.

moral foundation—required for all those who take on the title and role of nurse. Examples include the International Council of Nurses (ICN) Code of Ethics for Nurses (International Council of Nurses, 2006) and the American Nurses Association (ANA) Code of Ethics with Interpretive Statements (American Nurses Association, 2008).

Coined by Rushton, "authentic advocacy" refers to actions taken on behalf of others that arise from a deep alignment of one's beliefs, values, and behaviors (Rushton, 2013). Rushton further develops authentic advocacy in her model of "compassion-based ethics"—the ability to be present for all levels of suffering, to acknowledge the suffering of others, to transform this suffering, and to engage in helping those who suffer (Rushton, 2007). This kind of authenticity in action is a fundamental element of integrity, as well as a foundation that allows for meaning, service, and fulfillment to arise. Similarly, in this context, *authenticity* also refers to alignment with the beliefs, values, and desired actions of those who are in need of advocacy. This connotes an "egoless" engagement with the other—or others—for the purpose of both benefitting them and serving from one's highest purpose.

When applied to nursing, authentic advocacy and compassion-based ethics form the intrinsic moral foundation of nursing where we are each morally required to demonstrate, in all our interactions, *respect* for the inherent human dignity of individuals—including the "self" of each nurse—as well as for patient safety and continuity of care. An authentic advocate (Rushton & Penticuff, 2007) understands the fundamental ethical principle of respect—the act of esteeming one another and attending to the whole person. For example, authentic advocacy involves patients and families in decision-making, provides family-centered care, and adopts broader perspectives marked by cultural humility. As authentic advocates, we demonstrate self-awareness with clearly defined values and the knowledge and skills of ethical discernment, analysis, and action.

Authentic advocates express opinions or preferences that stem from a deep sense of our own inner self, beliefs, and vision of what is possible. We inform and educate both others and ourselves about health and human rights. We understand and reflect our own beliefs as well as those learned from others and external sources. Instead of adopting a stance of "expert," we engage in discovering right actions through a process of inquiry, deep listening, and engagement to address the full spectrum of solutions stemming from individuals, systems, and underlying causes (Sharma, 2004).

Modeling a determined passion for what they care about, authentic advocates share their voice and soul's purposes and meaning, incorporating their very being and believing into the ability to facilitate change. They integrate co-advocacy through presence and deep listening to the stories of others in order to explore the suffering of others, as well as their own suffering. They seek language to express suffering and aim toward finding new expressions and insights, new meaning-making, and new identity around suffering and frustrations (Rushton, 2009).

Empowered, thus, to increase the health of the entire human family and the whole earth, authentic advocates connect with the larger goals of society. In all these ways, we can experience a sense of fulfillment, personal satisfaction, and accomplishment. As we become advocates for others, our lives are also impacted in profound ways.

The reflective questions of authentic advocacy include: (Rushton, 2009) How do you self-advocate, taking into account your own needs at home and work? How do you advocate strengthening relationships among your colleagues, patients, and others? How do you advocate by learning new behaviors and new communication skills for yourself? How do you advocate change in healthcare systems and structures and other grassroots-to-global conditions related to health?

Nightingale modeled authentic advocacy across her lifetime. She was an advocate for individuals, for soldiers, for families and communities, for the health of villages, cities, and nations, as well as for the health and wellbeing of her nursing students, urging them to integrate this mandate into their own work (Dossey, 2010a). Due to the prolonged illness she contracted in the 1850s during the Crimean War—recognized today as chronic brucellosis—Nightingale deeply understood what she needed to nurture herself and practice self-advocacy (Dossey, 2010b). Living until 1910, she worked on this for decades—practicing self-care at physical, emotional, mental, and spiritual levels. This component of her life continues to have deep relevance for the health and wellbeing of today's nurses, who regularly face rigorous working conditions and—in some parts of the world—severe hardships very similar to those Nightingale faced during the Crimean War. Her work gives us a deeper understanding of our role in global advocacy, discussed next.

Global Advocacy

The general public consistently rate nurses as the most trusted and well-respected profession in the world. But the roles we play in society are not well known, nor widely understood. The public sharing of our stories—related to both nursing and health—is not on nursing's traditional agenda. The strength of public advocacy for health has not yet fully evolved into nursing's capacity to voice our concerns through the wider public promotion of healthcare—to influence other groups and to dialogue and collaborate with other disciplines, particularly the media (Burish & Gordon, 2006).

We have always been good at communicating with each other—about our patients, our concerns, and our commitments to society. We know and tell each other how and why these issues matter. Like Nightingale, we have been excellent activists at the bedside of the suffering and for the promotion of health in local community settings. But we also need to discover—like Nightingale did—how to take our activism and evolve this work into global advocacy, providing nursing with new levels of global participation and impact.

At large-scale levels, the actions required to address global needs are related to global discussion and networking, to the telling of "news" stories to wider audiences, and to wider-scale communications to debate and share ideas. But when these global discussions carry on without being grounded in related grassroots knowledge and experience, this dialogue can become ineffective and even detrimental to achieving the global outcomes of health for all humanity.

An applicable approach to this global-to-grassroots gap is called Development Support Communications (DSC) (Food and Agriculture Organization of the United Nations [FAO], n.d.). It was first initiated by the United Nations Development Programme (UNDP) in the 1970s to empower people by mobilizing wider public opinion from grassroots "bottom-up" levels, rather than from the "top-down" global levels. From its beginnings, DSC was shaped as a community-level experiential process in which participants developed capacities to better articulate and widely communicate issues critical to their work and needs. Even in its early stages, this approach sought to empower individuals and small groups with networking and participatory communications—particularly through emerging media capacities—first in community-based print journalism, radio, and video broadcasts, and later through emerging Internet capacities.

DSC is also about people acquiring communication strategies as drivers of their own development. With communications skills at its core, DSC is a multifaceted process, encouraging people to use these emerging skills to identify problems, create solutions, and build wider consensus in doing so. Integrating the knowledge thus gained from these experiences, participants evolve new individual and interactive capacities to convey their knowledge beyond their own communities. To achieve these aims, DSC encourages the co-creation and sharing of grassroots knowledge globally—further calling for and contributing to sustainable change—particularly for the benefit of the most marginalized and impoverished people (FAO, n.d.).

DSC can be applied as a useful tool to extend nursing knowledge—the sharing of nursing's grassroots experience—for the wider promotion of twenty-first–century health. Using this approach, we can enhance and broaden our networking, advocacy, and media communications to the world beyond nursing' own circle to both strengthen nursing practice and widely promote the conditions required for the health of humanity. The DSC approach can provide global and virtual settings for nursing's voice and foster global networks to widely communicate the needs nurses see. This can more effectively articulate many aspects of our interactions with each other, including our continuing need for personal and interpersonal renewal, cross-cultural understanding, and effective communication outreach—going beyond our own nursing circles to include other disciplines. This approach can enhance our abilities to become global advocates for the wider issues that impact the health of every person we seek to help. It can directly promote solutions for healthier homes and workplaces. It can effectively articulate global concern to address the environmental and social determinants that directly impact the health and wellbeing of everyone. The use of DSC approaches can empower nurses to become stronger grassroots-to-global authentic advocates, facilitate the promotion of health, and enhance the connections of health to all development aims worldwide (Beck, Dossey, & Rushton, 2013)

An example of nurses' global advocacy is the "Nightingale Declaration for a Healthy World," crafted by the Nightingale Initiative for Global Health (NIGH) as seen in Box 41.2. One member of the founding NIGH team has indeed worked within United Nations networks since the 1970s and, within this work, has been involved in the application of Development Support Communications to meet the needs of people worldwide. Because of this direct connection, this declaration's opening phrase—"We, the nurses and concerned citizens of the global community"—was intentionally modeled after the Preamble to the Charter of the United Nations (1945), which begins with the words, "We, the peoples of the United Nations, [are] determined" and the subsequent Universal Declaration for Human Rights (1948). Recalling Nightingale's own exemplary work to communicate her concerns worldwide, this declaration was written to clarify and commit to communicating shared goals and purposes as we work together to build a better world for everyone. Its text challenges its signers—all nurses and all concerned citizens—to commit to our own emerging individual and collective global advocacy and to call for the achievement of a healthy world, together and each in our own way (Nightingale Initiative for Global Health [NIGH], 2007).

With communications tools unparalleled in human history, now is the time for us to find the courage and confidence to use these tools for the dynamic and innovative promotion of health at local, regional, national, and global levels. Now is the time to

Box 41.2 Nightingale Declaration for a Healthy World

An opportunity to participate in NIGH's outreach to individuals worldwide.

We, the nurses and concerned citizens of the global community, hereby dedicate ourselves to the accomplishment of a healthy world by the year 2020.

We declare our willingness to unite in a program of action, sharing information and solutions to resolve problems and improve conditions—locally, nationally and globally—in order to achieve health for all humanity.

We further resolve to adopt personal practices and to implement public policies in our communities and nations, making this goal for the year 2020 achievable and inevitable, beginning today in our own lives, in the life of our nations and in the world at large.

Source: Used with permission, Nightingale Initiative for Global Health (NIGH), 2007, www.nightingaledeclaration.net.

widen the scope of our nursing practice—to widely communicate the concerns we care about most with everyone else.

Like Nightingale in her time, nurses can effectively use media tools to demonstrate global advocacy. Our trusted voices can address many issues impacting health and nursing practice, including human conflict, poverty, lack of social justice, toxic environments, loss of family and community values, and even the forgetting to take personal care of one's own health and wellbeing. Nursing's voice can tell the stories of how we can and do contribute to solving these critical problems.

To achieve this, our challenge as global nurses and authentic advocates is to develop further collaborative pathways to positive interdisciplinary relationships with health-care colleagues, as well as with journalists, broadcasters, multimedia professionals, and other national and international networking groups. Our nursing practices can incorporate further the development of networking and communications capacities and media-related interviewing, writing and Internet skills, as well as health coaching (Hess et al., 2013). These contributions will further feed the flame of Nightingale's continuing global relevance—further building momentum toward the worldwide nursing activism and advocacy that will be needed in the months and years ahead for the global transformation discussed next.

Global Transformation

Our integrative nursing global challenges set the stage for newly articulated global desires to achieve health in every community throughout the world. As nurses continue their being-knowing-doing to advance the health and wellbeing of all, we can tap these global desires, which we also heartily desire for ourselves.

Researching how Nightingale achieved such deeply transformative work, Nightingale's biographers have noted that her life encompassed social action and sacred radical activism—a transforming force of compassion-in-action born of a fusion of deep spiritual knowledge, courage, love, passion and practice (Harvey, 2009). As well, she experienced and recorded her personal understanding of the awareness that something greater than she, the Divine, was present in all aspects of life (Dossey, 2009). Her deep inner work continually transformed her own life, allowing her to be a change agent and sustain her change agency for global transformation across her lifetime.

In today's specialized world, we may be tempted to compartmentalize our lives, placing our personal, professional, spiritual, political, and ethical concerns into different corners, without integrating these spaces. To Nightingale, this kind of fragmentation would have been unthinkable. As an icon of wholeness, an emblem of a united, integrated life, her shining example invites each of us to integrate our meaning and purpose across our own individual journey through life (Dossey, 2010d).

Monica Sharma, a physician who has worked through United Nations agencies to collaborate with people at the village level in Africa and India, has noted that "today, the most urgent and sustainable response to the world's problems is to expand solutions for problems—that are driven solely by technology—[to those solutions] generated from personally-aware leadership" (Sharma, 2004, 2007). This type of leadership, which Sharma calls "global architecture for personal to planetary transformation," can arise from applying ourselves to Nightingale's broader and deeper legacy. Sharma's philosophy can inspire and instill world-centric leadership values and capacities. It is also a transformative approach to develop nurses as global citizens—beyond the tasks of merely coping with today's local problems—so we may become agents of global transformation, creating new local-to-global solutions.

In the 1880s, Nightingale wrote letters indicating her belief that it would take 100 to 150 years before educated and experienced nurses would arrive to actually continue the global transformations she herself had begun. The nurses of the twenty-first century are literally the generations she foresaw and set her own hopes upon. We are twenty-first–century Nightingales who can carry forth her vision to achieve a healthier world together. Our own deep personal and professional integrative nursing mission can continually transform our own lives, thus allowing each of us to become effective catalysts for human health and to sustain our change agency for global transformation, across our lifetimes and to the generations who follow us.

Conclusion: Finding Our "Must"

Nightingale called her work her "must" (Dossey, 2010a). As we increase our awareness of the deepest needs of the world, this knowledge continues to help all of us—nurses and concerned citizens alike—identify our own "musts." This keeps us focused and empowered. Nightingale saw nineteenth-century problems and created twentieth-century solutions. We have seen twentieth-century problems and can continue to create twenty-first–century solutions by developing approaches that address global issues—such as the United Nations Millennium Goals (MDGs)—as well as the grassroots concerns we find in our own communities and healthcare settings. By increasing global public awareness about the priority of health and empowering nurses, nursing students, and concerned citizens to address the critical grassroots-to-global health issues of our time, these interrelated approaches will continue to keep Nightingale's deep and broad legacy alive across the twenty-first century and beyond.

Reflecting on Nightingale's global legacy of activism, advocacy, and transformation—and the possibilities for what we can achieve in our time—consider following these seven recommendations (Beck, 2010b):

- Make health—and activating positive health determinants—a top priority in human affairs.
- Value and sustain nurses in their caring to achieve health goals everywhere.

- Collaborate across disciplines and across cultures to promote health in community settings.
- Think globally; act to create and sustain local health literacy for everyone, across the lifespan.
- Make media a catalyst for nursing and for health.
- Keep health holistic, integrative, and transdisciplinary.
- Answer your own calling, your "must."

SELECTED REFERENCES

American Nurses Association. (2008). *Code of Ethics for Nurses with Interpretive Statements [Revised]*. Silver Spring, MD: American Nurses Association.

Beck, D. M. (2010a). Remembering Florence Nightingale's panorama: 21st century nursing at a critical crossroads. *Journal of Holistic Nursing Practice, 28*(4), 291–301.

Beck, D. M. (2010b). Expanding our horizons: Seven recommendations for 21st-century nursing practice. *Journal of Holistic Nursing Practice, 28*(4), 317–326.

Beck, D. M., Dossey, B. M., & Rushton, C. H. (2013). Building the Nightingale Initiative for Global Health—NIGH: Can we engage and empower the public voices of nurses worldwide? *Nursing Science Quarterly, 26*(10), 366–371.

Burish, B., & Gordon, S. (2006). *Silence to Voice: What Makes Nurses Know and Communication to the Public, Second Edition*. Cornell, NY: Cornell University Press.

Dossey, B. M. (2010a). *Florence Nightingale: Mystic, Visionary, Healer [Commemorative Edition]*. Philadelphia, PA: F.A. Davis Company.

Dossey, B. M. (2010b). Florence Nightingale and her chronic illness. *Journal of Holistic Nursing, 28*(1), 38–53.

Dossey, B. M. (2010c). Florence Nightingale: Her personality type. *Journal of Holistic Nursing, 28*(1), 57–67.

Dossey, B. M. (2010d). Florence Nightingale: A 19th-century mystic. *Journal of Holistic Nursing, 28*(1), 10–35.

Dossey, B. M. (2009). Nursing: Integral, integrative, and holistic—local to global. In Dossey, B. M., & Keegan, L. (Eds.). *Holistic Nursing: A Handbook for Practice* (6th ed.) (pp. 3–57). Burlington, MA: Jones & Bartlett Learning.

Dossey, B. M., Beck, D. M. & Rushton, C. H. (2011). Integral nursing and the Nightingale Initiative for Global Health: Florence Nightingale's legacy for the 21st century. *Journal of Integral Theory & Practice, 6*(4), 71–92.

Dossey, B. M., Selanders, L., Beck, D. M., & Attewell, A. (2005). *Florence Nightingale Today: Healing, Leadership, Global Action*. Silver Spring, MD: American Nurses Association NursesBooks.Org.

Food & Agriculture Organization [FAO] of the United Nations. (n.d.). *Development Support Communications (DSC)*. Retrieved from http://www.fao.org/DOCREP/005/Y4338E/y4338e07.htm.

Harvey, A. (2009). *The Hope: A Guide to Sacred Activism*. Carlsbad, CA: Hay House Inc.

Hess, D., Dossey, B., Southard, M. E., Luck, S., Schaub, B. G., & Bark, L. (2013). *The Art and Science of Nurse Coaching: The Provider's Guide to Coaching Scope and Competencies*. Silver Spring: MD: American Nurses Association.

International Council of Nurses. (2006). *The ICN Code of Ethics for Nurses*. Geneva, Switzerland: International Council of Nurses.

Nightingale, F. (1859). *Notes on Hospitals*. London, United Kingdom: Harrison.

Nightingale, F. (1860a). *Notes on Nursing*. London, United Kingdom: Harrison.

Nightingale, F. (1860b). *Notes on Nursing Revised*. London, United Kingdom: Harrison.

Nightingale, F. (2005). Sick-nursing & health-nursing (1893). In Dosssey, et al. (Eds). *Florence Nightingale Today: Healing, Leadership, Global Action (pp. 287-303)*. Silver Spring, MD: American Nurses Association NursesBooks.org.

Nightingale Initiative for Global Health—NIGH. (2013). *Why NIGH? Why now?* Retrieved from http://www.nightingaledeclaration.net/about-nigh.

Nightingale Initiative for Global Health—NIGH. (2007). *Nightingale Declaration for a Healthy World*. Retrieved from http://www.nightingaledeclaration.net/the-declaration.

Rushton, C. H. (in press). *One Heart: The Art of Compassion Based Ethics in Health Care*.

Rushton, C. H. (2009). Caregiver suffering: Finding meaning when integrity is threatened. In Haddad, A. & Pinch, W. J. (Eds.). *Nursing and Health Care Ethics: A Legacy and a Vision* (pp. 293-306).Washington, D.C.: American Nurses Publishing.

Rushton, C. H. (2007). Respect in critical care: A foundational ethical principle. *AACN Advanced Critical Care, 18*(2), 149–156.

Rushton, C. H., & Penticuff, J. C. (2007). A framework for analysis of ethical dilemmas in critical care nursing. *AACN Advanced Critical Care, 18*(3), 323–328.

Sharma, M. (2007). World wisdom in action: Personal to planetary transformation. *Kosmos*, Fall/Winter, 31–35.

Sharma, M. (2004). Conscious leadership at the crossroads of change. *Shift*, 12, 17–21.

United Nations Development Programme (UNDP). (2000). *The United Nations Millennium Development Goals Reports*. Retrieved from http://www.un.org/millenniumgoals/reports.shtml.

World Health Organization. (2013). *World Health Statistics*. Retrieved from http://who.int/gho/publications/world_health_statistics/2013/en/index.html.

World Health Organization. (2006). *World Health Report 2006: Working Together for Health*. Retrieved from http://www.who.int/whr/2006/en.

VII

Conclusion

42

Gazing with Soft Eyes

MARY KOITHAN

I f there is something that every sector of our global society can agree on, it is the need to transform our healthcare system. Stakeholders representing broad constituencies of consumers, educators, providers, policy-makers, executives, payers, and scientists have issued calls for sweeping change to address issues that include access, quality, safety, patient-centeredness, and affordability (IOM, 2001, 2010). Both consumers and providers long for relationship-centered care that is personalized and meaningful in a system where the administrative requirements actually support the delivery of care rather than detract from it. Recommendations abound and the points of agreement seem to recede into the swirl of political and ideological controversy.

As I watched the contents of this book unfold, the perennial wisdom of nurses captured my imagination. I have been particularly struck by the intricacies of expert nursing knowing—how we investigate, deliberate, decide, and ultimately recommend a particular course of action for a patient or family. The metaphor of "hard and soft eyes" (a term those of us who ride horses in an enclosed arena with other horses and riders understand) arose. It captures perfectly the insights that integrative nursing offers to the healthcare debate. Hard eyes are sharply focused, seeing very clearly but with limited range; almost oblivious to surroundings. Someone riding with hard eyes can almost run another rider over before realizing that they are there. Soft eyes see not only what is immediately in front of you, but also everything else in the environment. Riding with soft eyes helps prevent crashes, but it also provides all the data you need for deciding and correcting your course. Hard eyes see the individual limb on the individual tree. Soft eyes take in the whole tree and the surrounding forest.

Let's look for just a moment at the full meaning and consequences of integrative nursing—a way of being-knowing-doing that advances the bodymindspirit wellbeing of those entrusted to nurses through caring/healing relationships. Practicing nursing from a whole-person/whole-systems perspective begins with the recognition that the one we seek to help is a whole person who lives in a particular context (social, relational, temporal, geographical, cultural). It helps little to recommend therapies, whether biomedical, mind–body or manipulative, that a person cannot afford or access. Similarly, recommending interventions without considering downstream effects that could lead to a host of additional concerns is ineffective. Integrative nursing asks us to expand and soften our gaze to carefully consider the intervention within the context of the whole person and whole system, assuring that the interventions recommended are accessible, safe, and effective over both the short and long term.

When guided by the principle that people have innate healing capacity, the health-care system becomes supportive rather than directive; providers become partners rather than prescribers; and consumers become active rather than passive. Integrative nursing invites us to focus on building individual, family, or community resources (biopsychosocialspiritual) that restore and replenish; resources that support wellbeing and wholeness. Therefore, integrative nursing invites us to soften our gaze, recognizing that prevention and active partnership creates a more cost-effective, patient-centered system that decreases the incidence/prevalence of chronic diseases while improving the human and planetary condition.

Integrative nurses find meaning and purpose in relationship. Across each chapter of this book, what stands out is our commitment to provide opportunities for healing within a co-created relationship based on mutuality and participatory engagement. Some chapters emphasize the centrality of relationship in treatment decision-making, wherein the patient makes choices across a range of possible interventions that the nurse recommends; while others discuss the criticality of deep listening and presencing to wellbeing and health. Chapters on leadership and healthcare systems stress the central importance of collaborative interprofessional relationships built on trust and mutual respect. The soft, inclusive gaze of integrative nursing invites each of us to embrace the moral commitment of healthcare to be in right relationship with the earth, the people that we care for, our communities, and ourselves, creating a system that is responsive, compassionate, and caring.

Integrative nurses use a full complement of therapies to support and augment the healing process in a manner that first considers the least invasive and intensive therapy. Integrative nursing thus provides an individually nuanced and refined approach to symptom and illness management. I sit and marvel at the potential impact of this single principle. How many iatrogenic conditions could be prevented if we could teach children to treat pain by using heat or cold before reaching for medication? How much could we save if we tried manipulative, body-based therapies for recurrent headaches before we demanded an MRI and extensive neurological testing? What impact would we have on cost, quality of life, and productivity if we encouraged people to participate in stress-reduction activities rather than asking for the latest prescription advertised on television?

Integrative nursing invites us to turn soft eyes forward and envision the benefits of a system that returns us to our roots. By creating a system that is focused on "putting the patient in the best condition for nature to act," integrative nursing addresses accessibility, quality, safety, patient-centeredness, and affordability. With eyes that are softened and expansive, I stand in awe of the depth and breadth of the wisdom offered by this extraordinary group of nurses gazing forward, seeing so clearly the whole of the possibilities that integrative nursing has to offer our beleaguered healthcare system.

SELECTED REFERENCES

Institute of Medicine of the National Academies. (2001). *Crossing the Quality Chasm: A New Health System for the 21st Century.* Washington, DC: The National Academies Press.

Institute of Medicine of the National Academies. (2010). *The Future of Nursing.* Washington, DC: Committee on the Robert Wood Johnson Foundation Initiative on the Future of Nursing, at the Institute of Medicine.

Institute of Medicine of the National Academies. (2013). *Delivering Affordable Cancer Care in the 21st Century.* Washington DC: The National Academies Press.

INDEX